Management of Complications in Oral and Maxillofacial Surgery

Management of Complications in Oral and Maxillofacial Surgery

Editors

Michael Miloro, DMD, MD, FACS

Professor
Department Head
Program Director
Department of Oral and Maxillofacial Surgery
College of Dentistry
University of Illinois at Chicago
Chicago, Illinois

Antonia Kolokythas, DDS, MS

Assistant Professor
Associate Program Director
Director of Research
Department of Oral and Maxillofacial Surgery
Cancer Center University of Illinois at Chicago
College of Dentistry
University of Illinois at Chicago
Chicago, Illinois

WILEY-BLACKWELL

A John Wiley & Sons, Inc., Publication

Wiley-Blackwell is an imprint of John Wiley & Sons, formed by the merger of Wiley's global scientific, technical, and medical business with Blackwell Publishing.

Registered office: John Wiley & Sons Ltd, The Atrium, Southern Gate, Chichester, West Sussex, PO19 8SQ, UK

Editorial offices: 2121 State Avenue, Ames, IA 50014-8300, USA
The Atrium, Southern Gate, Chichester, West Sussex, PO19 8SQ, UK
9600 Garsington Road, Oxford, OX4 2DQ, UK

For details of our global editorial offices, for customer services, and for information about how to apply for permission to reuse the copyright material in this book, please see our website at www.wiley.com/wiley-blackwell.

Library of Congress Cataloging-in-Publication Data

Management of complications in oral and maxillofacial surgery / editors, Michael Miloro, Antonia Kolokythas.
    p. ; cm.
  Includes bibliographical references and index.
  ISBN 978-0-8138-2052-1 (hard cover : alk. paper)
  I. Miloro, Michael.   II. Kolokythas, Antonia.
  [DNLM: 1. Surgery, Oral.   2. Intraoperative Complications–prevention & control.
3. Oral Surgical Procedures–methods.   4. Reconstructive Surgical Procedures–methods.   WU 600]
  617.5′22–dc23
                                                                    2011036436

A catalogue record for this book is available from the British Library.

Wiley also publishes its books in a variety of electronic formats. Some content that appears in print may not be available in electronic books.

Set in 10.5/12.5pt Minion by Toppan Best-set Premedia Limited
Printed and bound in Singapore by Markono Print Media Pte Ltd

1   2012

To the students and residents who have managed, and learned from, complications with me over the years; and to the patients who have had to sustain these adverse outcomes, which are a critical part of the educational process for any surgeon.

To my wife, Beth, and our daughter, Macy, who make all of this possible and worthwhile.

MM

To my mentors who taught me that patients with less-than-ideal outcomes are the ones whom "you will always remember and the ones from whom you learn the most"; to the patients whose less-than-ideal outcomes became invaluable learning and teaching recourses for me, my students, and my residents.

To my husband, George, with much love and appreciation for his continuous support that makes it all possible.

AK

Contents

Contributors

Cole Anderson, DMD
Division of Oral and Maxillofacial Surgery
Carle Foundation Hospital
Urbana, Illinois

Jonathan S. Bailey, DMD, MD, FACS
Associate Clinical Professor and Program Director
Division of Oral and Maxillofacial Surgery
Division of Head and Neck Cancer
Carle Foundation Hospital
Urbana, Illinois

R. Bryan Bell, DDS, MD, FACS
Medical Director
Oral, Head and Neck Cancer Program
Providence Cancer Center
Attending Surgeon and Director of Resident Education
Trauma Service/Oral and Maxillofacial Surgery Service
Legacy Emanuel Medical Center
Affiliate Associate Professor
Oregon Health and Science University
Affiliate Assistant Professor
University of Washington
Head and Neck Surgical Associates
Portland, Oregon

Carl Bouchard, DMD, MSc, FRCD(C)
Massachusetts General Hospital
Boston, Massachusetts

Lauren Bourell, DDS
Resident in Oral and Maxillofacial Surgery
New York University Medical Center
New York, New York

Vernon P. Burke, DMD, MD
Department of Oral and Maxillofacial Surgery
School of Dentistry
Louisiana State University Health Sciences Center
New Orleans, Louisiana

John F. Caccamese, Jr., DMD, MD, FACS
Associate Professor and Program Director
Department of Oral and Maxillofacial Surgery
University of Maryland
Baltimore, Maryland

Eric R. Carlson, DMD, MD, FACS
Professor and Chairman
Department of Oral and Maxillofacial Surgery
University of Tennessee Graduate School of Medicine
Chief, Head and Neck Service
University of Tennessee Cancer Institute
Knoxville, Tennessee

Bernard J. Costello, DMD, MD, FACS
Professor and Program Director
Department of Oral and Maxillofacial Surgery
University of Pittsburgh School of Dental Medicine
Chief, Pediatric Oral and Maxillofacial Surgery
Children's Hospital of Pittsburgh
University of Pittsburgh Medical Center
Pittsburgh, Pennsylvania

Stephanie J. Drew, DMD
Private Practice
The New York Center for Orthognathic and Maxillofacial Surgery
West Islip/Lake Success/Manhattan, New York
Assistant Clinical Professor
Department of Oral and Maxillofacial Surgery
Stony Brook School of Dental Medicine
Stony Brook, New York
Assistant Clinical Professor
Hofstra North Shore–LIJ School of Medicine at Hofstra University
Hempstead, New York

Rui Fernandes, DMD, MD, FACS
Assistant Professor
Chief, Section of Head and Neck Surgery
Divisions of Oral and Maxillofacial Surgery and Surgical Oncology
Department of Surgery
University of Florida, College of Medicine–Jacksonville
Jacksonville, Florida

Savannah Gelesko, DDS
Resident
Department of Oral and Maxillofacial Surgery
Oregon Health and Science University
Portland, Oregon

Helen E. Giannakopoulos, DDS, MD
Assistant Clinical Professor
Department of Oral and Maxillofacial Surgery
University of Pennsylvania Hospital
Philadelphia, Pennsylvania

Robert Glickman, DMD
Professor and Chair
Department of Oral and Maxillofacial Surgery
New York University College of Dentistry
New York, New York

Kenneth C. Guffey, DMD, MD
Resident
Department of Oral and Maxillofacial Surgery
University of Alabama at Birmingham
Birmingham, Alabama

Pamela J. Hughes, DDS
Assistant Professor, Graduate Program Director
Division of Oral and Maxillofacial Surgery
Department of Developmental and Surgical Sciences
University of Minnesota
Minneapolis, Minnesota

Leonard B. Kaban, DMD, MD
Walter C. Guralnick Professor of Oral and Maxillofacial Surgery
Department Head
Harvard School of Dental Medicine
Harvard University
Chief of Oral and Maxillofacial Surgery
Massachusetts General Hospital
Department of Oral and Maxillofacial Surgery
Boston, Massachusetts

Vasiliki Karlis, DMD, MD, FACS
Associate Professor
Program Director
Department of Oral and Maxillofacial Surgery
College of Dentistry
New York University
New York, New York

Alexander Katsnelson, DMD, MS
Oral and Maxillofacial Surgeon
Private Practice
Chicago, Illinois

Dongsoo David Kim, DMD, MD, FACS
Associate Professor, Residency and Fellowship Program Director
Department of Oral and Maxillofacial/Head and Neck Surgery
Louisiana State University Health Sciences Center Shreveport
Shreveport, Louisiana

Antonia Kolokythas, DDS, MS
Assistant Professor
Associate Program Director
Director of Research
Department of Oral and Maxillofacial Surgery
Cancer Center University of Illinois at Chicago
College of Dentistry
University of Illinois at Chicago
Chicago, Illinois

Michael R. Markiewicz, DDS, MPH
Resident
Department of Oral and Maxillofacial Surgery
Oregon Health and Science University
Portland, Oregon

Michael Miloro, DMD, MD, FACS
Professor
Department Head
Program Director
Department of Oral and Maxillofacial Surgery
College of Dentistry
University of Illinois at Chicago
Chicago, Illinois

Daniel Oreadi, DMD
Assistant Professor of Oral and Maxillofacial Surgery
School of Dental Medicine
Tufts University Medical Center
Boston, Massachusetts

Bonnie L. Padwa, DMD, MD
Oral Surgeon-in-Chief
Section of Oral and Maxillofacial Surgery
Children's Hospital
Boston, Massachusetts

Jon D. Perenack, DDS, MD
Assistant Professor and Program Director
Department of Oral and Maxillofacial Surgery
School of Dentistry
Louisiana State University Health Sciences Center
New Orleans, Louisiana

Daniel Petrisor, DMD, MD
Sunset Oral and Maxillofacial Surgery
Portland, Oregon
Former Maxillofacial Oncology and Microvascular Reconstruction Fellow
Department of Oral and Maxillofacial Surgery, Louisiana State University Health Sciences Center
    Shreveport
Shreveport, Louisiana

Phillip Pirgousis, MD, DMD, FRCS, FRACDS (OMS)
Assistant Professor
Section of Head and Neck Surgery
Division of Oral and Maxillofacial Surgery
Department of Surgery
University of Florida, College of Medicine-Jacksonville
Jacksonville, Florida

Ramon L. Ruiz, DMD, MD
Director of Craniomaxillofacial Surgery and the Craniofacial Disorders Program
Arnold Palmer Children's Hospital
Orlando, Florida

Thomas Schlieve, DDS
Resident
Department of Oral and Maxillofacial Surgery
University of Illinois at Chicago
Chicago, Illinois

Miller Smith, DDS, MD
Fellow
Oral and Maxillofacial Surgery
Southern General Hospital
NHS Greater Glasgow & Clyde
Glasgow, United Kingdom

David C. Stanton, DMD, MD
Associate Professor
Program Director
Department of Oral and Maxillofacial Surgery
University of Pennsylvania
Philadelphia, Pennsylvania

Maria J. Troulis, DDS, MSc
Associate Professor
Massachusetts General Hospital
Department of Oral and Maxillofacial Surgery
Boston, Massachusetts

Peter D. Waite, MPH, DDS, MD
Diplomate, American Board of Oral and Maxillofacial Surgery
Diplomate, American Board of Cosmetic Surgery
Charles A. McCallum Endowed Chair, Professor
Department of Oral and Maxillofacial Surgery
School of Dentistry and Medicine
University of Alabama
Birmingham, Alabama

Brent B. Ward, DDS, MD, FACS
Assistant Professor and Program Director
Department of Oral and Maxillofacial Surgery/Oncology
University of Michigan Hospital
Ann Arbor, Michigan

Fayette Williams, DDS, MD
Clinical Faculty
Department of Oral and Maxillofacial Surgery
John Peter Smith Hospital
Fort Worth, Texas

Preface

"The years teach much which the days never know."

–Ralph Waldo Emerson

"We look for medicine to be an orderly field of knowledge and procedure. But it is not. It is an imperfect science, an enterprise of constantly changing knowledge, uncertain information, fallible individuals, and at the same time, lives on the line. There is science in what we do, yes, but also habit, intuition, and sometimes plain old guessing. The gap between what we know and what we aim for persists. And this gap complicates everything we do."
–Atul Gawande, *Complications: A Surgeon's Notes on an Imperfect Science*

Without a doubt, but unfortunately for the patient, we learn the most from our surgical complications; and it is our recognition, acceptance, and management of these complications that result in decreased patient morbidity and makes us better surgeons.

The specialty of oral and maxillofacial surgery is perhaps one of the most diverse in medicine and dentistry, with a continuously redefined scope of practice. Although several well-written comprehensive reference textbooks exist that cover the full scope of our specialty, this textbook, *Management of Surgical Complications in Oral and Maxillofacial Surgery,* is a comprehensive reference textbook that focuses primarily on the potential complications encountered in the routine practice of our specialty. The consideration of complications in reference textbooks is limited and sporadic and includes a textbook, *Complications in Oral and Maxillofacial Surgery,* which was published in 1997, and a volume in *Oral and Maxillofacial Surgery Clinics of North America* covering complications, which was published nearly two decades ago.

The clear purpose of this textbook is to provide a comprehensive, well-organized, up-to-date reference for the management of complications *for* oral and maxillofacial surgeons that results from procedures *performed by* and *is written by* oral and maxillofacial surgeons. *Management of Surgical Complications in Oral and Maxillofacial Surgery* provides a systematic approach to complication recognition and management for residents in training as well as clinicians practicing the full and expanded scope of oral and maxillofacial surgery. In addition to its function as a reference textbook, this book is an excellent resource for examination preparation purposes since a solid knowledge base in complication recognition and management is an essential component of clinical practice.

The outstanding contributors for each chapter were chosen based upon their unique training and practices in the specific topic of the specialty. These authors should be commended for their willingness to present their poor results and treatment failures in an honest and professional manner in the pages that follow. The authors attempt to use an evidence-based approach with a critical evaluation of the current literature, as well as their own clinical experience and expertise, in order to guide their management strategy recommendations. The clinical figures and radiographic patient information used by the authors of patients who have sustained complications serve to augment the manuscript portion of the textbook and provide an illustrative point of view for the clinician. The excellent contributions from each of the authors reflect their extensive experience and in-depth knowledge in their individual clinical areas of expertise. Each chapter highlights the potential complications encountered during the practice of oral and maxillofacial surgery, from those most commonly encountered to those occurring less often, and from the simple to the more-complex problems with which every competent oral and maxillofacial surgeon should be familiar. The authors attempt to focus on the prompt recognition of each complication, consider preventative measures, and describe precise management strategies considering the already-compromised clinical circumstances. The authors have done an impressive job of compiling this information in an organized fashion so that it could be presented to the reader in an easy-to-read format. We are indebted to the authors, as well as their patients, for providing the case presentations that are essential for this textbook, with the goal of providing an increased knowledge base of all oral and maxillofacial surgeons in training and in practice, thereby potentially reducing patient morbidity in the future.

Michael Miloro
Antonia Kolokythas

Management of Complications in Oral and Maxillofacial Surgery

1

Ambulatory Anesthesia

Vasiliki Karlis, DMD, MD, FACS
Lauren Bourell, DDS
Robert Glickman, DMD

INTRODUCTION

Ambulatory anesthesia is one of the more common adjunctive procedures performed by an oral maxillofacial surgeon (OMS) in private or academic practice. Anesthetic states ranging from mild sedation to general anesthesia are achieved, mainly through the use of intravenous agents but occasionally with inhalational agents as well. When indicated, the provision of anesthesia can greatly facilitate many dentoalveolar and other outpatient surgical procedures, and often enhances patient comfort and satisfaction as well as surgeon efficiency. Ambulatory anesthesia is frequently recommended to patients as an adjunct for particular procedures such as third molar removal, and many patients request anesthesia regardless of the planned surgical procedure. In the special case of pediatric patients, where patient cooperation can be unreliable and anxiety is frequently at a high level, the utility of ambulatory anesthesia can be even greater. In both children and adults, ambulatory anesthesia allows for more procedures to be performed in an outpatient setting that would otherwise require a trip to the operating room.

Given the many benefits of outpatient anesthesia, it is not surprising that a great number of anesthetics are performed each year by OMSs in outpatient settings. Adjunctive anesthesia is provided to thousands of patients per year, and the number of complications reported during the provision of ambulatory anesthesia remains quite low—less than 1% of anesthetic cases.[1] Of these reported complications, serious adverse events make up an even smaller number. Much conscientious effort has gone toward ensuring the safety of ambulatory anesthesia, particularly in the areas of surgeon training, prevention, patient monitoring, and emergency protocols. While OMSs can exhibit confidence in the use and safety of ambulatory anesthesia, we must also maintain a high level of vigilance in order to prevent anesthetic complications and appropriately manage them in the cases when they arise.

Many OMSs who provide anesthesia in an outpatient setting also perform surgery in a hospital operating room (OR), and there is frequently overlap in the types of surgical procedures that are performed in either setting. However, there are some notable differences in the anesthetic as it is conducted in the OR versus an outpatient facility. In the OR, the anesthesia is nearly always provided by someone other than the surgeon—an anesthesiologist or certified registered nurse anesthetist (CRNA). This allows the surgeon to focus single-mindedly on the surgery at hand. In contrast, in outpatient anesthesia, the OMS typically acts as surgeon-operator, or the "operator-anesthetist" model, providing both the anesthesia and performing the surgery simultaneously. Support for this dual role of the OMS can be gleaned from data demonstrating a very low incidence of anesthetic-related complications in outpatient settings where surgeon-operators administered the anesthesia.[1] The administration of outpatient anesthesia requires extra attention from the surgeon who must monitor both the anesthesia and the surgical procedure simultaneously. Maintaining

Management of Complications in Oral and Maxillofacial Surgery, First Edition. Edited by Michael Miloro, Antonia Kolokythas.
© 2012 John Wiley & Sons, Inc. Published 2012 by John Wiley & Sons, Inc.

this balance of attention can be challenging and may require a different set of skills than those utilized in the OR.

Other important differences between anesthesia administered in the OR and ambulatory anesthesia can contribute to the relative safety of outpatient anesthesia. Two important factors are the greater risk and complexity of surgical procedures performed in an OR setting, and the greater distribution of lower-risk patients (ASA I and II) in outpatient settings versus higher-risk patients (ASA III and above) who may be treated more frequently in the OR setting. These factors emphasize that careful patient and procedure selection contribute to the prevention of complications in outpatient anesthesia.

Lastly, emergency equipment and equipment available for patient monitoring is often more extensive in the OR than outpatient setting, though this difference is decreasing in large part due to the decreasing cost of equipment and technology. Certain invasive modes of patient monitoring, such as arterial or central venous lines, remain confined to the operating room; however, many of the same modalities of monitoring cardiac and respiratory function exist for both OR and outpatient use. In addition, the emergency equipment of the OR has been feasibly reproduced for efficient use in an outpatient setting. The OR, by virtue of being located within the hospital, will retain an advantage in terms of emergency preparedness, access to trained staff, blood and tissue products, and specialist consultation. However, anesthesia in the OR setting can have increased risk due to increased complexity of surgical procedures and/or higher-risk patient populations. These differences are important for the OMS who treats patients in both settings because they have important implications for the prevention and management of anesthetic complications.

PREVENTION OF COMPLICATIONS IN AMBULATORY ANESTHESIA

Patient Characteristics/Selection

The best and most effective management of anesthetic complications is to prevent their occurrence. There is well-documented evidence that certain perioperative patient characteristics contribute significantly to anesthetic and surgical risk. Some of these characteristics, such as patient age, are easy to quantify and have fairly predictable patterns of anesthetic risk. Other patient characteristics such as underlying medical conditions, medications, previous surgical history, allergies, cardiac and respiratory reserve, and body mass index can be more difficult to assign risk. A detailed history and physical examination with appropriate preoperative laboratory workup and communication with the primary care physician are paramount in identification of those patients who may safely undergo anesthesia in an outpatient setting.

Several algorithms and systems of classifying anesthetic risk based on patient characteristics are in common use, with the ASA (American Society of Anesthesiology) criteria being among the most widespread (see Table 1.1). The utility of the ASA classification has been shown in scientific literature that demonstrates a clear association between ASA status (I–V) and the risk of anesthetic complications.[2] The ASA classification is widely recognized and simple to use, and it is a valid starting point into which other patient risk determinants can be incorporated. The Duke Activity Index is another useful measure of a patient's physical status. It presents a functional assessment of physical capacity based on an individual's exercise tolerance and ability to perform various activities of daily living (see Table 1.2). The ability to engage in exercise or everyday physical activities is inversely correlated with risk of anesthetic complications and provides an additional parameter for patient screening.

An adjunctive measure of patient risk for ambulatory anesthesia includes specific classification of the airway. Mallampati's classification is a simple visual classification system, divided into four categories, which attempts to assess the posterior oropharyngeal airway patency based on the visibility of structures of the posterior oropharynx (uvula, fauces, soft and hard palates). The distance between the hyoid bone and the chin can be estimated as an additional, albeit crude, indicator of airway patency and ease of intubation with shorter mental-hyoid distances indicating greater airway risk. In addition, specific characteristics of patient body habitus such as obesity or the presence of a short, thick neck can be general predictors of risk of airway collapse during anesthesia.

Obesity, defined as a body mass index greater than 30, is a recognized risk factor for complications related to anesthesia. Obesity is associated with a decreased respiratory functional residual capacity (FRC) and can

Table 1.1. ASA Physical Status Classification

ASA I	No systemic disease
ASA II	Mild to moderate systemic disease, well-controlled disease states; e.g., well-controlled NIDDM, asthma or epilepsy; pregnancy
ASA III	Severe systemic disease that limits activity but is not incapacitating; e.g., IDDM; history of CVA, MI, or CHF >6 months ago; mild COPD
ASA IV	Severe systemic disease that limits activity and is a constant threat to life; e.g., history of unstable angina, CVA or MI within the past 6 months; severe CHF, severe COPD; uncontrolled DM, HTN, or epilepsy
ASA V	Patients not expected to survive 24 hours
ASA VI	Organ donors

NIDDM: non-insulin-dependent diabetes mellitus; IDDM: insulin-dependent diabetes mellitus; CVA: cerebrovascular accident; MI: myocardial infarction; CHF: congestive heart failure; COPD: chronic obstructive pulmonary disease; DM: diabetes mellitus; HTN: hypertension

Table 1.2. Duke Activity Scale Index

Functional Class	Metabolic Equivalents	Specific Activity Scale
I	>7	Patients can perform heavy housework such as moving furniture or scrubbing floors, and can participate in moderate recreational activities such as bowling, dancing, skiing, or doubles tennis.
II	>5	Patients can do light housework such as dusting or washing dishes, can climb one flight of stairs, can walk on level ground at 4 mph.
III	>2	Patients can dress themselves, shower, make the bed, walk indoors.
IV	<2	Patients cannot perform activities of daily living without assistance; may be bedbound.

lead to an increased incidence of respiratory complications, particularly airway collapse and desaturation. Obese patients have a fourfold increased risk of respiratory complications during ambulatory anesthesia procedures.[3] In the pediatric population as well, obesity has been recognized as a growing problem. A study by Setzer et al. found an increased incidence of respiratory complications and unexpected overnight hospital admission in a group of obese pediatric patients undergoing ambulatory anesthesia for dental surgery procedures (compared to their nonobese counterparts).[4] Patient positioning during surgery may play a role in preventing adverse respiratory complications in obese patients, as a recent study demonstrates an increase in time to desaturation in obese patients who were preoxygenated in an upright (90-degree sitting) position prior to induction of general anesthesia.[5] Maintaining obese OMS patients in an upright position during anesthesia may help to prevent respiratory complications by maximizing FRC and minimizing the effects of gravity on posterior oropharyngeal airway collapse.

Age is also an important determinant of anesthetic and surgical risk. Age is easily quantified and there is evidence that increased risk of complications occur at the extremes of very young and very old age. There is greatly increased risk associated with anesthesia and surgery in the first one month and one year of life.[6] In terms of increasing age and risk of complications, there remains a strong positive correlation though the association is more gradual and progressive. In the very young, much of the increased anesthetic risk can be attributed to the relative anatomical and physiological immaturity of infants and very young children. This makes the mechanics of anesthesia more difficult (airway management, fluid replacement, patient monitoring) while the decreased therapeutic index of anesthetic drugs in small children greatly increases their toxic potential. At the other end of the spectrum, advanced age leads to an increase in medical comorbidities and decreased physiological reserve from the normal aging process. This likewise decreases tolerance for physiologic insults and lowers the therapeutic index of many drugs and interventions.

Aside from patient characteristics, another factor that can help prevent complications in the postoperative period is to ensure that patients will have a responsible adult who can accompany them home and care for them after the anesthesia and surgical procedure.[7]

Procedure Characteristics/Selection

In addition to appropriately screening patients for in-office procedures, it is also important to bear in mind the surgical complexity and length of time needed for the planned procedure. Certain procedures, such as third molar removal, are nearly always performed in an outpatient setting. Other surgical procedures, such as minimally invasive temporomandibular joint procedures (TMJ arthroscopy) and extensive bone grafting or implant procedures, can be performed either in the OR or in an outpatient setting. This is largely dependent upon the preference of the surgeon and patient, the availability of appropriate instruments and equipment, as well as financial issues. The most important consideration in preventing complications is to ensure that the surgical procedure planned is not more complex or lengthy than can be accommodated in a particular outpatient setting. Patient risk factors and procedure risk factors should be balanced such that longer and more complex procedures are avoided in patients who already represent increased surgical risk. Complex or lengthy procedures may benefit from having an additional practitioner or trained person to assist with the anesthetic management of the patient. This will help to offset some of the increased attention required for the surgery itself. With proper planning, a majority of routine OMS surgical procedures can potentially be accomplished in an outpatient setting.

Patient Screening

The goal of patient selection for ambulatory anesthesia procedures is to determine a particular patient's risk factors for anesthesia and to identify those patients who may safely undergo the procedure in an outpatient setting. The first step is to perform a comprehensive history and targeted physical exam. Information to be elicited includes prior anesthetic experiences, prior hospitalizations, emergency room visits, prior surgeries, allergies or adverse reactions to any medications, and any and all medications taken (including over-the-counter medications and vitamins or herbal supplements). Herbal medications are surprisingly common (taken by almost 25% of patients) and garlic, ginkgo biloba, and ginseng (the "three Gs") may be particularly risky when taken perioperatively as they affect platelet function and may increase bleeding risk.[8]

A review of systems can ascertain whether a patient has any undiagnosed medical conditions that could impact the planned anesthetic procedure. In particular, questions designed to elicit underlying respiratory, neurologic, or cardiac disease are especially important. A history of snoring, allergic rhinitis, wheezing, shortness of breath (exertional or spontaneous), and recent upper or lower respiratory infections can provide important information about the possible risk of respiratory complications. Certain medical conditions and risk factors to look for include history of asthma, chronic obstructive pulmonary disease (COPD), and tobacco use. Chung et al. identified asthma with a fivefold increase in respiratory complications during ambulatory anesthesia, and smoking carries an increased fourfold risk.[3] Patients with COPD have twice the risk of respiratory complications during ambulatory anesthesia.[9] Ascertaining a patient's exercise tolerance can provide a great deal of information as well, including signs and symptoms of respiratory or cardiac disease, as well as musculoskeletal complaints or any limitations in range of motion. In patients who do not engage in regular exercise, one can substitute questions about activities of daily living such as walking several blocks, climbing more than one flight of stairs, grocery shopping, doing several loads of laundry, or performing vigorous housework.

It can be helpful to obtain a family history, particularly from patients who are young or present with few medical history findings, especially to ascertain whether anyone in the patient's immediate family has ever had an adverse event related to anesthesia, an unusual genetic illness, congenital heart defect, or premature or sudden unexpected death. Asking about a history of tobacco, alcohol, and illicit drug use is important. In a patient who drinks alcohol regularly, asking about usual intake and effects (e.g., drowsiness, tipsiness) can sometimes provide a crude indication of response to anesthesia. Vital signs should be recorded for every patient prior to the day of the planned procedure as they are helpful for establishing a particular patient's baseline. For example, this may help to differentiate a patient who, on the day of surgery, develops hypertension as a result of anxiety from a patient whose baseline blood pressure is usually elevated.

The history and physical exam forms the basis for deciding whether a patient will need further testing or evaluation prior to the anticipated anesthetic. Further evaluation can take many forms, including laboratory testing, ECG/chest radiography, or consultation with the patient's physician including referral to specialists as needed. Patients who give a complex medical history with multiple chronic conditions, recent surgeries or hospitalizations, multiple hospitalizations in the past year, clearly warrant further testing and consultation with the patient's physician. These types of patients are obviously at higher risk and may or may not represent suitable candidates for outpatient anesthetic procedures. Of more concern, however, may be those patients whose risk for outpatient anesthesia is unclear or unknown. In this case, the role of laboratory testing and other investigations is to clarify whether the patient may be safely sedated in an outpatient setting. Patients who give an unclear or ambiguous medical history obviously fall into this category, as do patients with several positive findings in the review of systems or patients with chronic medical conditions that appear to be poorly controlled. In addition, one should approach cautiously patients who report no medical problems and who have not had a routine medical exam within the past three years or longer, particularly if they are middle-aged or older, or have other obvious medical risk factors. Patients such as these may have undiagnosed medical conditions that could greatly impact the safety of the planned outpatient procedure.

A diversity of laboratory tests may be ordered for a patient, but for routine use, relatively few are necessary. A complete blood count (CBC) and basic metabolic panel represent two of the most common basic laboratory tests. The CBC can give information about the presence of infection or inflammation (elevated white blood cell count), the relative proportions of blood cells, the presence of anemia (hemoglobin and hematocrit) and type (red blood cell size and morphology), and verify an adequate number of platelets for hemostasis. The CBC does not provide information about platelet function or the clotting ability of blood for which a partial thromboplastin time (PTT) and prothrombin time (PT, commonly reported as an international normalized ratio, or INR) are needed. A bleeding time test will give information about platelet function, but it is infrequently used. The basic metabolic panel will provide information about electrolyte and acid/base balance as well as renal function [blood urea nitrogen (BUN) and creatinine levels], and may be substituted by a complete metabolic panel that also includes markers of liver function (typically, aspartate and alanine transaminase liver enzyme levels). Markers of renal and liver function should be considered for patients with diabetes, liver, or kidney disease as they can indicate the progression of disease as well as the potential need for modification of anesthetic drug dosages. In women of reproductive age, some practitioners will also order a beta-human chorionic gonadotropin test (B-HcG) to verify a patient's pregnancy status. A serum B-HcG is more sensitive, but urine B-HcG tests are less expensive and easy to administer. If a B-HcG will not be performed for a patient, it is important to ask about the possibility of pregnancy and document the conversation in the patient record. Laboratory tests performed within the preceding 30 days are generally considered recent enough and do not necessarily need to be repeated. Patients with more rapidly changing conditions, such as patients taking warfarin, will need more recent laboratory tests. B-HcG tests, if indicated, are ideally performed within 1 week of the scheduled anesthetic.

Special considerations exist for preoperative screening of patients with known or suspected cardiovascular disease. Cardiovascular disease is increasingly common and cardiovascular complications of anesthesia are among the most serious. Basic methods of screening for cardiovascular disease include the standard 12-lead ECG and chest radiography. More advanced diagnostic methods include echocardiography and cardiac stress testing. Depending on the institution and surgeon preference, some oral maxillofacial surgery practices routinely order ECGs and chest radiography for patients over a certain age. Sometimes this practice is restricted to patients who are scheduled for OR procedures and sometimes it extends to outpatient anesthetic procedures as well. For low-risk procedures in ASA I (and most ASA II) patients for whom a detailed history and physical exam have been performed, an ECG and chest radiograph are largely unnecessary. Cardiac testing may be considered for patients with clinical risk factors for cardiac complications, as assessed by the American College of Cardiology and American Heart Association in the 2007 *Revised Cardiac Risk Index*. These factors include a history of ischemic heart disease, compensated heart failure or prior heart failure, cerebrovascular disease, diabetes mellitus, or renal insufficiency.[10] Minor predictors of cardiac risk include being over 70 years of age, uncontrolled hypertension, abnormal ECG, and nonsinus rhythm, but these have not demonstrated utility as independent markers of cardiac risk during noncardiac surgery.[10] A patient's functional capacity as measured by "metabolic equivalents" is an important parameter assessed in the 2007 ACC/AHA guidelines on perioperative cardiovascular evaluation. Patients who have poor functional capacity represent a greater risk of cardiac complications than those with good functional reserve. The 2007 ACC/AHA guidelines recommend 12-lead ECG testing and noninvasive stress testing for asymptomatic patients with cardiac risk factors who will undergo intermediate-risk surgical procedures or vascular surgery, but are typically not recommended for low-risk surgeries such as ambulatory surgery. The guidelines were developed based on level of evidence from the professional literature indicating a clinical advantage to preoperative intervention in various patient groups prior to noncardiac surgery.

If additional testing is indicated, the patient's physician should be contacted prior to the planned anesthetic, as patients may have had an ECG or other cardiac test performed recently. Chest radiographs or ECGs that are abnormal are always an indication for further investigation, though further testing may not be needed. If previous ECGs or chest radiographs show an abnormality that has remained stable with time and if the patient's physician has indicated this, further testing is unlikely to change the clinical assessment. However, any abnormal finding that is new or has progressed from previous test results should result in follow-up with the patient's treating physician and additional testing as indicated.

Preoperative testing can help to identify abnormalities and quantify the level and type of disease a patient may have, but the clinician must ultimately gather this data and interpret it in a clinically useful manner. Several algorithms and classification schemes have been developed to aid in converting clinical data into a measure of anesthetic risk that can aid the surgeon in determining the relative risk of a particular patient for undergoing an outpatient anesthetic procedure. One of the most popular, the ASA classification, has already been mentioned. Several risk stratification schemes exist for cardiovascular risk factors in particular, including the most recent guidelines from the American College of Cardiology and the American Heart Association (described above).

Preoperative patient screening not only helps to identify those patients who represent a poor risk for outpatient anesthesia, but for low- and moderate-risk patients it can help to identify any patient-specific risks and aid in planning ahead.

Intraoperative Patient Monitoring

Technological advances have produced an increasing number of new and improved devices for the intraoperative monitoring of patient vital signs and sedation level. Patient monitors not only provide peace of mind that the patient is stable, but they can also provide an early warning when complications begin to occur. Ideally, effective intraoperative monitoring can allow for potentially serious situations to be recognized early and effectively managed. Basic measurements during outpatient anesthesia include pulse oximetry, a heart rate monitor, and intermittent blood pressure monitoring. Additional monitors can include capnography, BIS (bispectral monitoring), and a precordial (esophageal) stethoscope.

Pulse Oximetry

Pulse oximeters are designed to estimate blood oxygen saturation and work via measurements of infrared energy transmission. In smokers, pulse oximetry readings may be artificially increased due to the level of carboxyhemoglobin present in the circulation. This is especially true for those who have smoked tobacco within a few hours of the anesthetic procedure. The pulse oximeter cannot distinguish between carboxyhemoglobin and oxygen-carrying hemoglobin in the blood of smokers and thus provides an overestimate of the true blood oxygen saturation.

The reading provided by pulse oximetry is a good approximation of blood oxygen partial pressure, and 90% oxygen saturation is the standard cut-off value below which desaturation begins to have noticeable clinical effects. There is a time delay between a patient's true oxygen saturation and the pulse oximeter reading, and many oximetry machines will sound an alarm when a patient's oxygen saturation reading drops below 93% or 94% to allow for this. Most healthy adults will have an O_2 saturation of between 98%

and 100% on room air, but occasionally patients with underlying respiratory compromise will have a baseline O_2 saturation of 94–95%. It can be important to know this prior to beginning a procedure to avoid the erroneous assumption that a patient with a low baseline O_2 saturation is experiencing respiratory depression as a result of anesthesia.

Heart Rate and Rhythm Monitoring

A simple heart rate monitor will be sufficient in many circumstances; however, a 3-lead or 5-lead ECG monitor will provide a tracing of the cardiac rhythm, which can be indispensible if a complication arises that involves a cardiac arrhythmia, cardiac depression, or ischemia/infarction.

Blood Pressure

Blood pressure readings should be taken, at a minimum, both before and after an anesthetic procedure as well as prior to discharge. An automatic blood pressure cuff that can be set to take readings at different time intervals [noninvasive blood pressure (NIBP)] is an efficient choice. Routine interval blood pressure measurements are useful in all patients because even low-risk patients may experience anesthetic complications involving blood pressure changes. In higher-risk patients, blood pressure monitoring is especially important, particularly when there is concern about hypertension, hypotension, or changes in cardiac output.

Capnography

Capnography devices utilize a chemical probe that measures the level of expired carbon dioxide and can be used to monitor respirations. Capnography has been extensively utilized in the OR but much less frequently in outpatient settings. It can be extremely useful, however, as it provides a measure of tidal volume, respiratory rate, and respiratory depth. While it does not provide an estimate of blood oxygen saturation, it is more sensitive than pulse oximetry for detecting respiratory depression and apnea.

Precordial (Esophageal) Stethoscope

The precordial or esophageal stethoscope is a bell-type stethoscope that is placed on the pretracheal region of the patient's chest. By listening through one or two earpieces, or using a speaker system, a practitioner can auscultate a patient's respirations and will be immediately alerted to any change in respiratory rate, depth, or quality. While this method of intraoperative monitoring is sensitive, it does not appear to be particularly popular among OMSs. The study by D'Eramo reported only 36% of practitioners used a precordial stethoscope, compared to a 93% utilization rate for blood pressure and pulse oximetry monitoring.[1] The stethoscopes become less reliable in situations of increased ambient noise or excessive patient movement that can displace the bell of the stethoscope. Nevertheless, the esophageal stethoscope can provide additional clinical information regarding a patient's respiratory status. It may be most useful when treating small children (or others at increased risk of rapid respiratory compromise) and obese patients, in whom it can sometimes be difficult to observe chest rise and other signs of ventilatory effort.

Bispectral (BIS) Monitor

Of the available patient monitors, the BIS monitor is unique because it quantifies the level of anesthetic sedation at the level of central nervous system (CNS) activity. Consisting of an adhesive strip that is positioned on the forehead and a monitor that reads EEG activity, the BIS monitor is typically used in an OR setting. It can help to determine a patient's level of sedation and is useful for maintaining a desired level of anesthesia. It is also useful for accelerating emergence from anesthesia. There is some suggestion that the BIS monitor may increase patient safety by decreasing the amount of anesthesia given while also minimizing complications of anesthesia that is too light. However, most of the benefit of the BIS monitor may be outweighed by the cost of the system.

Personnel Preparedness

Specific guidelines, in addition to individual state law specifications, regarding the appropriate number of personnel and specifics of their training requirements when administering outpatient anesthesia exist and should be adhered to strictly. Familiarity with the equipment used for monitoring, as well as emergency

Table 1.3. Emergency Drugs and Equipment

Emergency Equipment:
Defibrillator
Suction (portable)
Oxygen tank with backup
Face mask (non-rebreathing with ambulance bag)
Laryngoscope with light source, blades, extra batteries
Endotracheal tubes, cuffed/uncuffed
Laryngeal mask airway
Oral airways
Nasal airways
MacGill forceps
Tracheostomy/cricothyroidotomy set

Emergency Drugs:

Epinephrine	Atropine
Vasopressin	Succinylcholine
Nitroglycerin	Glycopyrrolate
Adenosine	Lidocaine
Labetalol	Metoprolol
Esmolol	Diphenhydramine
Lorazepam or diazepam	Hydrocortisone
Glucagon	50% Dextrose
Naloxone	Flumazenil
Albuterol MDI	Aspirin

---

equipment and setup, medications, and dosages, are crucial for administration of safe outpatient anesthesia. In addition to emergency equipment setup and operation, the treating team should practice, at frequent intervals, emergency scenario response to ensure preparedness and to anticipate and prevent adverse events. In addition, frequent scheduled and unscheduled drug and equipment inventory examinations and testing for expiration dates and malfunctions should be implemented.

Equipment and Emergency Supplies

Some of the most common emergency drugs and equipment that may be needed in an outpatient anesthesia setting are listed in Table 1.3. Emergency drugs are available from the manufacturer in appropriate dilutions that are prepackaged into syringes designed for single-patient use. Though there is an increased cost when purchasing emergency drugs in this form, it allows a practitioner to select and administer an emergency drug as needed without the delays while potentially minimizing calculation errors.

Postoperative Monitoring

When the surgical and anesthetic procedure is completed, the patient is discharged to a postoperative area where patient recovery from anesthesia is typically overseen by someone other than the surgeon. Due to the short-acting nature of most anesthetic drugs currently in use, most patients begin to awaken by the end of the surgical procedure. Some patients may still be significantly sedated upon arriving to the recovery area, however, due to differences in patient response to anesthesia. Vital signs should continue to be monitored postoperatively. A trained staff member should be physically present in the immediate recovery area at all times and should observe the patient's condition including skin color, respiratory rate and effort (chest rise), response to verbal or physical stimulation, and any signs of agitation or inability to be roused. Once patients are reasonably awake, they may be joined by a family member or friend, if space permits in the recovery area.

INCIDENCE OF COMPLICATIONS IN AMBULATORY ANESTHESIA

Though little historical data are available, it appears that ambulatory anesthesia has increased in safety over the past several decades. A recent large study reported an incidence of outpatient anesthetic complications of 1.45%, compared to a 2.11% complication rate for inpatient anesthesia.[11] Improvements in equipment design for the provision of anesthesia and patient monitoring as well as improvements in engineering controls, safety practices, and practitioner training have contributed to the overall low rate of anesthetic complications. Some of the more common complications of anesthesia, such as nausea and vomiting, have relatively low morbidity although the institutional costs may be high. Other complications such as respiratory or cardiac arrest are so morbid that significant effort has been made to adequately prevent and manage them despite their very low incidence. A proportion of complications are due to underlying patient factors such as patient age and medical comorbidities over which the practitioner has little control, but evidence has also shown that many complications are the result of operator error, equipment malfunction, or systems failure. Preventable complications offer an opportunity for the individual clinician and the specialty as a whole to make improvements that increase patient safety and anesthetic success.

NEUROLOGICAL COMPLICATIONS

Syncope

Syncope, one of the most common anesthetic complications, typically occurs in the preoperative setting, but may be observed occasionally postoperatively as well. Syncope is defined as transient loss of consciousness with spontaneous return to consciousness. In a study by D'Eramo, syncope was the most frequently observed complication, occurring in 1 out of 240 parenteral sedation cases and 1 out of 521 general anesthetic cases.[1] It is usually related to patient's anxiety in the preoperative setting and is most frequently observed upon venipuncture for placement of an intravenous line.[12] Syncope responds well to placing the patient in the Trendelenberg position, as this places the patient's head lower than the thoracic cavity and speeds blood return to the brain. Supplemental oxygen is beneficial and should always be given; it is also useful in cases of near-syncope. Ammonia smelling salts may also be helpful and are usually applied in situations where Trendelenberg positioning and supplemental oxygen does not result in a rapid return to consciousness.

In the postoperative period, patients may experience syncope due to vasovagal response or transient orthostatic hypotension when rising too quickly from a seated or supine position. This complication may be prevented by assisting all patients when they stand or begin walking, since syncope under these circumstances carries the additional risk of injury from falling. Management consists of patient positioning, supplemental oxygen and ammonia salts if needed.

Any period of unexpected patient unconsciousness that lasts for several minutes is not considered true syncope. If a loss of consciousness episode lasts more than a few minutes, other causes should be investigated without delay, including the possibility of hypoglycemia, hypotension, dehydration, partial seizure, oversedation, or cerebrovascular accident.

Oversedation

Oversedation is a relatively common event observed during ambulatory anesthesia that can rapidly develop in a potential complication of variable severity. It initially manifests as lack of adequate patient response to appropriate stimuli. For example, a patient who previously responded to loud verbal or forceful physical stimuli may suddenly fail to respond. In cases of profound oversedation, a patient may fail to respond to increasingly painful stimuli, and when the plane of general anesthesia is reached, the patient will have lost protective airway responses. If allowed to progress without intervention, oversedation can rapidly advance to airway obstruction, hypopnea, or apnea leading to hypoxemia. In severe cases, respiratory depression can lead to respiratory arrest and depression of cardiac output will be observed.

Oversedation in ambulatory anesthesia takes two forms: unintended deep sedation or general anesthesia during the procedure, or prolonged or delayed awakening in the postoperative period. Intraoperatively, oversedation is produced by too high a dose of an anesthetic drug or a dose of anesthetic that is administered too quickly. Patient factors often figure prominently in cases of oversedation, as patients who are very sensitive to the effects of an anesthetic or who have greatly decreased elimination kinetics will have a narrowed therapeutic range compared to an "average" patient. It can be quite difficult to titrate anesthetic drugs in such a patient, with the result that oversedation is more likely to occur.

Age is an important factor in a patient's response to anesthesia. Sensitivity to anesthetic drugs and alterations in the dosages are required to achieve specified levels of sedation with extremes of age. While this may seem self-evident in the elderly, research shows that the reduction in required anesthetic dose begins as early as age 40 to 45.[13] For each decade past the age of 40, there is an observed 10% reduction in the dose of fentanyl required while for propofol, the dose reduction is about 8%.[13] The pediatric population in particular has a markedly idiopathic response to anesthetic drugs, and titration of sedation can be more challenging in this age group. Ironically, patients with very high anxiety levels may be prone to oversedation because they typically require a high initial dose of anesthetic to achieve sedation, but often markedly less medication to maintain a given level of anesthesia. Failure to reduce the dosage of anesthesia adequately after the initial induction bolus in these patients can result in oversedation.

Oversedation may be caused when boluses of a drug are given too quickly or too close together. This typically occurs during an anesthetic procedure when a patient begins to awaken or become agitated and additional medications are administered to rapidly deepen the anesthesia. Since all anesthetic drugs take some period of time to exert their effect, failure to wait for the drug to take effect can result in the observation that the dose was insufficient and the administration of an additional bolus. Subsequently, when the additional boluses have had time to take effect, the patient may be in a deeper plane of anesthesia than was intended. This can be partially prevented by the spacing of additional drug boluses and knowing the time to effective onset of the anesthetic drugs utilized. Not all pharmacologic agents demonstrate first order kinetics however, and rate of drug onset can be increased or decreased depending on the patient's plasma drug level.

Oversedation can sometimes result when the level of surgical stimulation is rapidly or dramatically decreased. Since surgical stimulation tends to counteract the sedative effects of anesthetic drugs, a higher dose of anesthesia is typically required for more stimulating surgical procedures. A patient who is at an appropriate level of anesthesia may quickly become over-sedated if stimulation is decreased or discontinued. In situations where changes in the level of surgical stimulation can be predicted, allowing time for the anesthetic drug to wear off or decreasing the rate of infusion can effectively prevent most oversedation in these cases.

Oversedation is a relatively common complication of ambulatory anesthesia which can rapidly develop in severity. It initially manifests as lack of adequate patient response to appropriate stimuli. For example, a patient who previously responded to loud verbal or forceful physical stimuli may suddenly fail to respond. In cases of profound oversedation, a patient may fail to respond to increasingly painful stimuli, and when the plane of general anesthesia is reached the patient will have lost protective airway responses. If allowed to progress without intervention, oversedation can rapidly progress to airway obstruction, hypopnea, or apnea leading to hypoxemia. In severe cases, respiratory depression can lead to respiratory arrest and depression of cardiac output will be observed.

Management of mild oversedation may consist of briefly interrupting the administration of anesthetic drugs and observing the patient for a return to the desired level of anesthesia. If any degree of respiratory obstruction or depression is noted, maneuvers aimed at opening the airway such as a chin lift or jaw thrust should be performed as well. Given the rapid redistribution and short duration of effects of many anesthetic drugs, mild oversedation is self-correcting with supportive measures within a matter of a few minutes.

Although not a mainstay of treatment, administration of reversal agents may be considered as an adjunctive therapy for oversedation. Few drugs used in ambulatory anesthesia have a reversal agent, but naloxone is able to reverse the effects of opioid agonist drugs and flumazenil is an effective antagonist of the benzodiazepine class of drugs. These reversal agents can be effective in reversing the effects of oversedation due to drug overdosage, but they reverse all actions of a drug including desirable effects such as analgesia, hypnosis, and anxiolysis. They may be considered for the treatment of oversedation and prolonged awakening in the postoperative period and are generally well tolerated. Research has not supported the routine use of reversal agents to speed recovery from ambulatory anesthesia procedures.

Seizures

Seizure activity, both partial type and tonic–clonic seizures, represents abnormal CNS excitation. Because anesthetic drugs act by causing depression of the CNS, seizure activity during an anesthetic procedure is unlikely to occur. In patients with seizure disorders, however, seizures may occur in the preoperative and postoperative periods. Management of seizures involves positioning the patient to avoid injury and loosening tight or restrictive clothing as much as possible. Most seizures will terminate after a few minutes and require no other treatment, though benzodiazepines such as midazolam, lorazepam, or diazepam may be given intravenously or intramuscularly to terminate seizure activity. Since patients will typically become hypoxic during the clonic phase of a tonic–clonic seizure, supplemental oxygen may be beneficial in the immediate postictal period.

CARDIOPULMONARY COMPLICATIONS

Respiratory Depression and Respiratory Arrest

The effects of anesthetic drugs are the most common cause of respiratory depression in ambulatory anesthesia. An overdose of anesthesia will produce respiratory depression in virtually all cases, and this may progress to full respiratory arrest if not promptly corrected. Even typical doses of anesthetic drugs will cause some degree of respiratory depression in a proportion of patients.

Primary respiratory depression, caused by the provision of anesthesia itself, refers to a deficit in ventilation or oxygenation or both. Respiratory depression may take the form of mechanical obstruction, caused by collapse of the oropharyngeal soft tissues or occlusion of the airway by the tongue or secretions. Central respiratory depression, characterized by hypopnea or apnea can also occur either separately or concurrently.

Typically, mechanical obstruction occurs more frequently and at lower anesthetic doses than central apnea does, and it occurs to some extent in susceptible persons. Obese patients, those with short thick necks, mandibular retrognathia, and patients with obstructive sleep apnea are among the most susceptible groups. In severe cases, this may render these patients unsuitable for ambulatory anesthetic procedures. In most other cases, patient positioning can play a role in airway obstruction. Respiratory obstruction due to mechanical airway obstruction can be managed by careful suctioning, repositioning of the tongue in a forward position, and either a chin lift or jaw thrust maneuver. If necessary, the level of anesthesia may be lessened, as increasing levels of sedation contribute to the degree of airway impediment. Rarely, an oral or nasal airway may be needed to overcome the obstruction in the posterior pharynx and stent the airway open. Supplemental oxygen can be helpful to decrease any oxygen desaturation associated with mild to moderate obstruction, although oxygen by itself does not alleviate the mechanics of obstruction.

Respiratory depression may also be "central," characterized by a decreased respiratory rate or periods of apnea. Narcotic drugs are most often implicated because of their effects on the medullary respiratory center of the brainstem that results in decrease respiratory drive and response to hypercapnia. At moderate levels of narcotic effect, the decreased respiratory rate is accompanied by a compensatory increase in tidal volume that prevents oxygen desaturation. At higher levels of narcotic sedation, respiratory depression can progress to apnea and respiratory arrest. A brief period of respiratory support in the form of supplemental oxygen via a face mask with cessation of anesthetic drug administration may be all that is necessary in terms of management—particularly with short-acting drugs in a patient with good respiratory reserve. Whenever there is desaturation in a setting of frank apnea, however, the patient's ventilation should be assisted by a positive pressure face mask until spontaneous respiration resumes.

Occasionally, mask ventilation with or without the placement of an oral or nasal airway will not be sufficient to overcome airway obstruction and provide oxygenation. In these cases, other means of establishing an airway and achieving effective ventilation should be employed. These include laryngeal mask airway (LMA) insertion or endotracheal intubation for administration of positive pressure ventilation with high oxygen flow. Because endotracheal intubation is a technically complex procedure and requires specialized equipment, it is subject to high rates of failure, especially in emergency situations. Intubation should only be considered in a patient who is hypoxemic and cannot be effectively mask ventilated. An LMA can be successfully used for the support of ventilation as an alternative to endotracheal intubation and has several advantages over the traditional endotracheal tube (ET). LMAs are quickly and easily inserted without the need for specialized equipment. Use of an LMA poses no risk of inadvertent intubation of the esophagus or mainstem bronchus or injury to the vocal cords. Airway stimulation is minimal and removal of the LMA can be easily accomplished once spontaneous respirations return. Regardless of the method used for airway establishment early recognition, preparedness, familiarity with the available equipment, and skill maintenance for their effective use are critical.

In addition to respiratory depression or arrest caused by anesthetic drugs, other causes of respiratory complications include stroke or myocardial infarction. The signs and symptoms of stroke or acute coronary syndrome can be significantly masked in a patient undergoing ambulatory anesthesia, and respiratory depression or arrest may initially be diagnosed as a case of oversedation. Any respiratory complication that does not respond to moderate interventions or progresses to a need for airway establishment and support of ventilation should be investigated for additional contributing factors or underlying conditions.

Laryngospasm, Bronchospasm, and Acute Asthma

A second group of respiratory complications that may arise in the course of outpatient anesthesia includes reactive airway conditions such as laryngospasm, bronchospasm, and acute asthma. One analysis of complications in ambulatory anesthesia identified laryngospasm, stridor, and obstruction as the most frequently observed adverse events, accounting for 40% of complications.[11] Acute asthma attacks are more frequent preoperatively and may be associated with patient anxiety. Laryngospasm and bronchospasm typically result from the combination of airway irritation and anesthetic sedation.

Acute asthma and bronchospasm are manifested clinically by audible wheezing (more prominent during expiration), tachypnea, shortness of breath, and are usually accompanied by decreasing oxygen saturation. They represent a hyperreactive process of the large airways that results in bronchoconstriction and obstruction to airflow. A number of factors may precipitate an asthma attack or bronchospasm, but in an oral surgical setting anything that causes airway irritation may be the predominant etiologic factor. Some examples include the production of aerosols during a procedure or decreased clearance of secretions that can irritate the airway and stimulate coughing. Laryngospasm, by contrast, is an acute upper airway obstruction that presents with stridor (incomplete laryngospasm) or failure of ventilation (complete laryngospasm with total closure of the glottis). Obstruction of the upper airway due to foreign body aspiration may also present with acute stridor and should be ruled out clinically. Laryngospasm results in reflexive closure of the glottis upon irritation and is a protective airway reflex. It does not occur in awake patients or in patients during general anesthesia, but can occur in a mild or moderate stage of sedation.[12]

Acute asthma attacks may be managed with inhaled beta-2-agonist bronchodilator medications such as albuterol. These drugs are typically administered via a metered-dose inhaler (MDI) either with or without an additional spacer device. Patients who are awake and alert may be allowed to self-administer the inhaled medication, while patients who are sedated may need assistance. In sedated patients, the use of a spacer may be particularly useful to assist delivery of the drug to the lungs and to prevent excess drug deposition in the oropharynx where it is has no therapeutic effect.

Inhaled bronchodilators are also the first choice treatment for bronchospasm and are administered similarly. In intubated patients these inhaled medications may be administered via ET tube or LMA, though the dosage must be greatly increased (up to 10 to 20 puffs) to account for the large amount of drug that coats the airway tube and does not reach the lungs. Both acute asthma and bronchospasm benefit from supplemental oxygen. In severe cases that do not respond to inhaled beta-agonists, intravenous or subcutaneous epinephrine may be considered as a rescue therapy. The adverse effects of epinephrine—particularly tachycardia and increased blood pressure—limit its use for reactive airway disease. It should be used with extreme caution, if at all, in patients with underlying cardiac disease.

The treatment of laryngospasm differs from that of asthma or bronchospasm. Because it occurs in patients who are at "lighter" levels of anesthesia, deepening the level of anesthesia will help to abolish the protective airway reflex and relax the vocal cords to allow the passage of air. Positive pressure ventilation, especially when instituted early in the course of the laryngospasm, is frequently successful at "breaking" the spasm. If it appears that secretions or bleeding in the oropharynx may be contributing factors, a brief period of suctioning with a tonsillar (Yankauer) suction may be helpful. Care should be taken that this does not delay positive pressure ventilation, however, and that the suction itself does not serve to further provoke the laryngospasm reflex. If neither deepening the anesthesia nor positive pressure ventilation proves successful, the treatment of choice for laryngospasm is the administration of the neuromuscular blocking agent succinylcholine. Succinylcholine for the treatment of laryngospasm is typically given at a dose of 20–40 mg initially, with an additional 20–30 mg given a minute or two later if the first dose proves insufficient.[14] This dose is less than the "standard intubating dose" of succinylcholine, but whenever a paralytic agent is given, it is safest to assume that complete paralysis may occur and the practitioner should be prepared to assist the patient's ventilation until the drug has adequately worn off and the patient is ventilating well without assistance.

Aspiration

Aspiration refers to the entry of substances such as blood, saliva, gastric contents, or foreign bodies into the lungs via inadvertent inhalation. Aspiration occurs due to decreased or absent protective airway reflexes and is exacerbated by decreased gastroesophageal tone. Patients with neuromuscular degeneration or history of stroke are at increased risk as are those undergoing sedation and general anesthesia. Additional risk factors include gastroesophageal pathology such as GERD (gastroesophageal reflux disease), hiatal hernia, or achalasia, as well as a history of esophageal surgery or gastric bypass.[15] The greatest risk from aspiration occurs with gastric contents that are due to complications from pneumonia (a chemical pneumonia causing damage to the lungs from the low pH of gastric fluids and the presence of peptic enzymes) or acute respiratory distress syndrome (ARDS). Either passive regurgitation of stomach contents or active vomiting during anesthesia can lead to aspiration. Any patient who begins to retch or vomit during an anesthetic procedure should be placed with their head lowered (Trendelenberg positioning) to prevent aspiration into the lungs, and any vomitus should be suctioned carefully from the mouth and oropharynx. Patients known or suspected to have aspirated vomitus should have their respiratory status carefully monitored as they may require elective intubation with lavage and suctioning of the bronchial tree. The role of steroids and antibiotic therapy in these patients has been questioned and they are not routinely administered. In the absence of signs indicating respiratory compromise, management of aspiration is expectant.

In the case of aspiration of a foreign body, the surgeon may make a careful attempt to visualize and retrieve the object if possible. A laryngoscope and MacGill forceps may be helpful in this situation. If the object cannot be visualized for removal, the patient's respiration should be monitored and supported as needed and the patient transferred to a hospital.

Preoperative Fasting Period (NPO Guidelines)

In order to decrease the risk of aspiration, a preoperative fasting period is typically required of patients undergoing an anesthetic procedure. The usual prohibition is nothing to eat or drink after midnight prior to the day of surgery, with the intent that a patient having surgery in the morning will have a completely empty stomach for the procedure. There has been some debate recently about the preoperative fasting guidelines both in recognizing the need to make them as patient-friendly as possible while also recognizing that due to individual differences in gastric emptying, there may be situations where patients will not have a completely empty stomach despite adhering to the fasting guidelines. Currently, the American Society of Anesthesiologists (ASA) recommends "light" solid food up to 6 hours before and clear liquids 2 to 3 hours prior to undergoing anesthesia. The goal is to minimize the risk of aspiration due to a full stomach while at the same time avoiding dehydration and hypoglycemia from prolonged fasting. Diabetic patients may require individualized fasting guidelines because they are especially susceptible to hypoglycemia and may also have delayed gastric emptying due to gastroparesis. Young children are another group for whom special consideration may be necessary when prescribing preoperative fasting guidelines.

Acute Vascular Events

Acute vascular events are among the most serious perioperative complications and include myocardial ischemia, myocardial infarction, and cerebrovascular accident (stroke). Due to the high prevalence of cardiovascular and atherosclerotic diseases in adults, complications of this nature should be anticipated in any office emergency plan.

Myocardial ischemia and myocardial infarction are most common in the postoperative period[12] and can be related to the surgical procedure, the anesthesia, or both. In a very anxious patient with a history of ischemic heart disease, the preoperative period presents a risk of acute angina. Risk factors for acute vascular events include history of heart disease or cerebrovascular disease, increasing length and invasiveness of surgery, and significant changes in heart rate, respiration, or blood pressure due to anesthetic drugs or surgical manipulation. Though profound fluctuations in heart rate, blood pressure, or respiration should be avoided in any patient, this is critical for individuals with underlying risk factors for acute coronary or cerebrovascular complications. In these patients, vital signs should be maintained close to baseline to avoid hemodynamic decompensation.

Acute angina is characterized by a sensation of pain, tightness, or crushing in the substernal region of the chest and may be accompanied by shortness of breath, anxiety, and diaphoresis. It can be difficult to differentiate acute angina from a panic attack or GERD/acute gastritis unless the patient has a history of angina episodes. Acute angina should be treated by discontinuing any stimulating procedure, administering a dose of sublingual nitroglycerin, applying supplemental oxygen via face mask or nasal cannula, and continuous monitoring of vital signs. If the pain does not subside completely within 10 minutes, a second dose of nitroglycerin may be given. Up to three doses of nitroglycerin have been recommended to alleviate symptoms of angina, but the surgeon should take into account the patient's medical history and level of distress in deciding when to call EMS (emergency medical services). It is recommended that EMS be notified immediately and that emergency medical drugs and supplies be readily available [advanced cardiac life support (ACLS) protocol] in cases of moderate to severe chest pain lasting 30 minutes or more, when the pain appears to be getting worse, if two to three doses of nitroglycerin are not sufficient to provide relief, and in any patient who is hemodynamically unstable.

In situations where a myocardial infarction (MI) is suspected, the patient should be given 325 mg of aspirin (chewed or crushed is preferable as it speeds absorption of the drug), sublingual nitroglycerin, and supplemental oxygen. If morphine is available, this should be given as well, both for pain relief and because it causes peripheral vasodilation, which enhances cardiac output. The patient's vital signs should be monitored continuously until EMS arrives, particularly the ECG (arrhythmias may accompany myocardial ischemia and can signal imminent cardiac arrest) and blood pressure. If the patient deteriorates to a situation of cardiac arrest, the ACLS protocol should commence without delay. (NB: Adequate and uninterrupted chest compressions are now recognized as a key to successful resuscitation efforts. If the patient is in a dental chair without a hard, flat back or which does not recline completely, it is preferable to place the patient on the floor so that adequately forceful chest compressions can be delivered against a firm supporting surface.)

The management of a patient where stroke/cerebrovascular accident is suspected includes notification of EMS and supportive measures. Supplemental oxygen should be given and the patient's vital signs monitored. A brief neurological examination may distinguish true cerebrovascular complications from confusion or disorientation that may result from anesthetic drugs. Aspirin should not be given to a patient suspected of suffering a stroke because intracerebral hemorrhage may be present. Patients who develop signs of neurocognitive deficit in the setting of severe hypertension (systolic >200, diastolic >110 mm Hg) should be treated with medication to decrease blood pressure. Of the intravenous agents, labetalol (a combination alpha- and beta-blocking agent) is frequently preferred for the management of acute severe hypertension (see the section on hypotension and hypertension).

Cardiac Arrhythmias

Cardiac arrhythmias may arise spontaneously or they may be associated with myocardial ischemia, respiratory depression, metabolic disorders, or other physiological derangements. Some anesthetic agents can cause or contribute to arrhythmias, particularly in susceptible individuals. Arrhythmias may be divided based on rate into tachyarrhythmias and bradyarrhythmias, or based on location of supraventricular ectopic rhythm generation versus ventricular arrhythmias. Some cardiac rhythm abnormalities such as premature ventricular contractions (PVC) and premature atrial contractions (PAC) occur spontaneously in an otherwise normal population and require no intervention. Likewise, certain instances of tachycardia (mild, associated with anxiety) and bradycardia (due to chronic treatment with beta-blockers, or in a competitive athlete) may be within acceptable limits. Any arrhythmia that is symptomatic, that carries a risk of conversion to a more dangerous cardiac rhythm, or that is accompanied by hemodynamic instability should be promptly addressed, however. If the arrhythmia is attributable to an underlying physiologic disturbance, efforts should be made to treat the underlying condition. Otherwise, the management strategies for cardiac arrhythmias include pharmacologic interventions or cardioversion/ defibrillation.

Tachycardia due to stress, anxiety, or pain usually responds to a deepening of anesthesia and additional analgesia. The administration of a beta-adrenergic blocking medication can be considered for refractory cases. Selective beta-1 medications are preferred so as to avoid undesirable bronchoconstriction. Esmolol is a beta blocker with a fast onset and short-acting duration. Metoprolol is another beta-1-selective medication with a longer acting-duration. Both are available for intravenous use and may be titrated to effect. In general, beta blockers are best avoided in patients with low cardiac output states such as acute MI or acute exacerbation of congestive heart failure due to negative inotropic effects. When tachycardia is secondary to hypotension, hypovolemia, or fever, it is preferable to treat the underlying physiological derangement.

For cases of paroxysmal supraventricular tachycardia, the drug adenosine is typically recommended. Supraventricular tachycardias that do not respond to drug therapy or wide-complex tachycardia (ventricular tachycardia) should be treated with synchronized/unsynchronized cardioversion (electric shock). Cardioversion is also preferred for tachycardia associated with hemodynamic instability. Cardiac rhythms associated with cardiac arrest, i.e., ventricular fibrillation or pulseless electrical activity, should be treated according to the ACLS protocols.

Bradycardia, defined as a heart rate <60 bpm, may occur in sinus rhythm (sinus bradycardia) or as a result of heart block (atrial–ventricular dissociation). Any new onset of heart block is cause for evaluation by a specialist (e.g., chronic heart block can be a stable condition in patients with cardiac pacemakers). Sinus bradycardia during ambulatory anesthesia can be a sign of myocardial depression and is cause for concern. It may be treated with atropine or glycopyrrolate (both vagolytics), or with sympathomimetic drugs such as ephedrine or epinephrine.

Hypertension and Hypotension

During the course of an anesthetic, both hypertension and hypotension may be encountered. Hypertension is typically associated with patient anxiety, painful stimulus, or anesthesia that is too light. Hypertension may also be seen in the hypertensive patient who neglects to take their regular antihypertensive medications the day of the surgical procedure. Hypertension may be treated by deepening the anesthesia or by judicious use of an antihypertensive medication. Labetalol, a combined alpha-adrenergic and beta-adrenergic blocker is often preferred, but selective beta-blocking agents such as metoprolol or vasodilating agents such as hydralazine may also be used. In patients whose baseline blood pressure is elevated (above 120/80), it is important not to decrease blood pressure too rapidly or profoundly so as to avoid inducing a decrease in cardiac output.

Hypotension may also be encountered in the course of an anesthetic. Several commonly used medications such as propofol can induce a transient decrease in blood pressure, particularly when given as a bolus. In a young patient without underlying cardiac disease, small to moderate decreases in blood pressure are usually well-tolerated. However, because hypotension may also be a sign of low volume status or of impending cardiovascular collapse, it should be closely monitored and treated aggressively when indicated. In pediatric patients particularly, hypotension typically precedes cardiac arrest and is an important warning sign.[16] Decreasing the anesthetic depth, increasing the rate of IV fluid infusion, or giving a bolus of IV fluids are all appropriate first steps in the management of hypotension. If these steps are not corrective, a vasopressor medication such as ephedrine or phenylephrine may be given while also investigating for any causative factors such as an underlying medical condition, anaphylaxis/allergic reaction, or increased vagal stimulation.

GASTROINTESTINAL COMPLICATIONS

Nausea and Vomiting

Postoperative nausea and vomiting (PONV) is frequently cited as the most common complication of anesthesia, and it is one that patients frequently complain about. Many drugs used in ambulatory anesthesia are potentially capable of causing nausea and vomiting, particularly the halogenated gases (isoflurane, halothane, sevoflurane) and anticholinesterases. Narcotic medications such as morphine and fentanyl may also cause nausea and vomiting, as do barbiturates. Benzodiazepine medications have not been cited as a cause of PONV, and propofol is known to have antiemetic properties.

In addition to the effects of the anesthetic drugs, there are several patient factors that are known to increase the risk of PONV. Female gender, obesity, gastroparesis, past history of PONV, and a history of motion sickness may all predispose toward nausea and vomiting post anesthesia. Dehydration may also be a factor.

Prevention is an important consideration given that PONV is a frequent cause of delayed discharge to home after ambulatory anesthesia procedures.[12] Treatment of nausea and vomiting once it occurs is more difficult and less successful than efforts at prophylaxis. Avoiding dehydration and hypoglycemia by maintaining a reasonable preoperative fasting period and giving IV fluids during surgery will benefit most patients. In addition, screening prospective patients to identify those at risk of PONV will allow the surgeon to consider pharmacological methods of nausea and vomiting prophylaxis. Several effective medications are available that can be given by mouth or intravenously prior to the procedure in order to prevent and treat nausea and vomiting (see Table 1.4).

ENDOCRINE COMPLICATIONS

Hypoglycemia

Hypoglycemia is a potential complication of ambulatory anesthesia anytime a preoperative fasting period has been observed. Diabetics, young thin females, and the elderly are particularly at risk but any patient may experience signs and symptoms of hypoglycemia. Minimizing the preoperative fasting period and giving IV fluids preoperatively (or having them available) may help to prevent hypoglycemia. In addition, recognizing patients who are at risk (such as diabetics) and monitoring their blood glucose via fingerstick is a very effective management strategy. Hypoglycemia may present with nonspecific signs and symptoms such as dizziness, tachycardia, hypotension, sweating, shaking, or nausea but can be easily diagnosed with a simple handheld glucometer. Hypoglycemia is easily treated with an oral or intravenous sugar source. In situations of severe symptomatic hypoglycemia, an injection of D50 (50% dextrose) or glucagon may be given.

Table 1.4. Common Antiemetic Medications

Dolasetron	5-HT3 receptor antagonist (PO, IV)
Ondansetron	5-HT3 receptor antagonist (PO, IV)
Metoclopramide	Pro-motility agent (PO, IV, IM)
Prochlorperazine	Phenothiazine derivative (PO, IV, IM, PR)
Trimethobenzamide	Acts on chemoreceptor trigger zone (IM, PR)
Scopolamine	Anticholinergic agent (transdermal patch)
Dexamethasone	Adjunct (PO, IV, IM)

PO: by mouth; IV: intravenous; IM: intramuscular; PR: rectal suppository

Adrenal Crisis

Adrenal crisis is a rare but serious complication of suppressed adrenal release of cortisol and can rapidly cause hemodynamic collapse if the cortisol deficiency is not promptly diagnosed and rectified. Risk factors for acute adrenal crisis include both patient and procedure factors. Surgical procedures that are invasive and cause high levels of physiologic stress carry the highest risk. Patients most at risk for adrenal crisis are typically those with a lengthy history of moderate- to high-dose exogenous corticosteroid supplementation, though adrenal crisis has been classically associated with Addison's disease (primary adrenocortical insufficiency). Since most procedures that will be performed in an outpatient setting will be minimally invasive and of short duration the risk of adrenal crisis is low. Patients should be screened for a history of Addison's disease or corticosteroid use, and preoperative adjunctive corticosteroid supplementation should be considered for any patient deemed to be at risk. Acutely, the management of adrenal crisis involves intravenous cortisol administration and supportive measures.

IMMUNOLOGIC COMPLICATIONS

Hypersensitivity Reactions

Hypersensitivity, or allergic, reactions are common in the general population and may be produced in the ambulatory anesthesia setting by a variety of common substances. Patients with a history of allergic asthma, atopy, or autoimmune disease may be most at risk. Mild reactions include urticaria, flushing, and pruritis, while more severe reactions can be characterized by angioedema, wheezing, nausea and vomiting, or anaphylaxis. The most common complication is a localized skin reaction, frequently to an adhesive tape used to secure an IV line, for example. Some of the medications used in ambulatory anesthesia (propofol or succinylcholine) have been implicated in allergic reactions, but this is generally rare.[16] Likewise, a true allergy to local anesthetic agents is very infrequent. Most hypersensitivity reactions will be mild and can be managed symptomatically. More serious reactions involving angioedema or a skin rash covering the full body require more aggressive management such as the use of an antihistamine drug (e.g., diphenhydramine) and possibly corticosteroids. Angioedema or other acute allergic facial swelling should be carefully monitored for the development of airway compromise—an unlikely but possible sequela. Anaphylactic reaction is a life-threatening emergency that is treated with epinephrine, corticosteroids, antihistamines, beta-2-adrenergic agonist inhalers, and cardiopulmonary resuscitation as needed.

PSYCHIATRIC AND EMOTIONAL COMPLICATIONS

Patient anxiety is the most commonly encountered emotional complication in ambulatory anesthesia, but patients may also experience euphoria, delirium, agitation, or hallucinations. Children and the elderly are most at risk, and certain anesthetic medications such as ketamine have been associated with a higher likelihood of emotional or cognitive disturbance. These types of complications may be distressing to the patient but are typically self-limiting and mild. Preventing patient injury due to agitation or delirium is the primary goal of management, and close supervision remains the best strategy.

Many anesthetic medications (particularly the benzodiazepines) produce some degree of amnesia. Amnesia is often an intended effect of anesthesia and therefore not a complication per se, but the practitioner should be aware that any instructions or information given to a patient may be affected by amnesia or cognitive distortion. Patients may not be able to distinguish between dreaming and events that actually occurred during anesthesia, leading to inappropriate associations with the anesthetic experience. It is not known how often this may occur as a complication of ambulatory anesthesia, but whenever medications are given that alter a patient's consciousness and perception there is a risk of cognitive and emotional distortion.

COMPLICATIONS RELATED TO PATIENT POSITIONING

In an outpatient surgical procedure of limited duration, the risk of injury to a patient from malpositioning is relatively small. In susceptible patients, or for longer procedures, special care in patient positioning is prudent to avoid musculoskeletal injury. The provision of anesthesia causes relaxation of the musculoskeletal system that can lead to hyperextension of the joints. Also, prolonged patient immobility can contribute to venous stasis, peripheral blood pooling, and the creation of pressure points. Elderly patients, patients with a history of musculoskeletal injury or arthritis, and obese patients are at increased risk for complications related to patient positioning. Patients with Marfan syndrome, Ehlers-Danlos, or other disorders of joint hypermobility may also be at risk. Down syndrome (trisomy 21) patients have increased range of motion of the cervical spine vertebrae and are at increased risk for vertebral dislocation if the head or neck becomes hyperextended. Of specific concern to oral maxillofacial surgeons is the potential for injury to the temporomandibular joint (TMJ) that can occur in sedated patients due to prolonged or exaggerated opening of the mouth during surgery. Key preventive measures are positioning patients in neutral body positions, minimizing length of surgery in susceptible individuals, and ensuring that dental chairs are cushioned and sized appropriately for the patient.

COMPLICATIONS RELATED TO IV LINE PLACEMENT

Complications related to placement of an intravenous line are some of the most common and troubling to patients. Pain, ecchymoses, and infiltration at the IV site are the most frequently encountered and can be managed symptomatically. More serious complications include phlebitis and thrombophlebitis at the injection site and are associated with certain irritating medications (such as intravenous diazepam), particularly when given in a small vein or at a high concentration. Phlebitis may take several weeks to resolve completely and may necessitate analgesia and anti-inflammatory medications. A rare but potentially serious complication involves the inadvertent intra-arterial injection of a medication, most commonly a barbiturate, with resultant extreme pain and vascular necrosis. With careful IV placement technique and the use of a full IV setup allowing proper dilution of medications, the incidence of complications can be minimized and have a measurable impact on patient satisfaction as well as safety.

ANESTHETIC COMPLICATIONS IN PEDIATRIC PATIENTS

Complications of ambulatory anesthesia in pediatric populations are similar in many ways to those that may be encountered in adults. As higher incidences of adverse events are reported for children with higher ASA classifications, and children less than 1 month old and less than 1 year old are particularly prone to anesthesia-related complications.[17] For pediatric and adult patients, much of the risk of complications from anesthesia can be attributed to underlying disease states and surgical risk factors. Nonetheless, there is an additional element of risk in the pediatric population due to decreased physiological reserve.

Children, far from being miniature adults, are different in fundamental anatomical and physiological ways. The immature cardiac, hepatic, renal, and respiratory systems in the child mean that large differences in drug effects, drug metabolism, and cardiac and respiratory compensations exist. Some of these differences are predictable whereas others are not. In general, the interpatient variability in the pediatric patient can be far greater than in an adult, necessitating more caution in the provision of anesthesia and complicating the titration of common anesthetic drugs.

Since children are smaller and weigh less than adults, the total doses of anesthetic drugs that may be safely given will be less in total. Due to the immaturity of the hepatic liver enzymes at birth, infants do not metabolize drugs as effectively as adults, and the clearance of many drugs can be prolonged significantly, with most individuals attaining full liver microsomal function at about 1 year of age.[12] Other physiologic systems take longer to reach maturity, particularly the cardiovascular and respiratory systems.

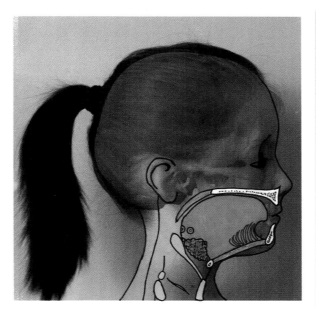 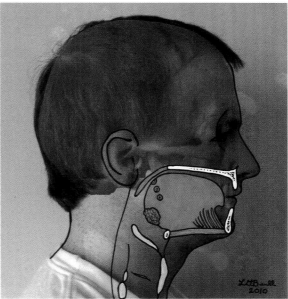

Fig. 1.1. Compared to an adult airway, the pediatric airway demonstrates more cephalad position of the vocal folds, a wider and angled epiglottis, a relatively larger tongue and lymphoid tissue (including lingual tonsil), and a narrower funnel-shaped cricoid cartilage.

The pediatric airway is characterized by a more cephalad position of the larynx, a thicker epiglottis, and angulation of the true vocal folds, which can make direct visualization more challenging (see Fig. 1.1).[16] In addition, the narrowest part of the pediatric airway occurs at the level of the cricoid cartilages just below the vocal folds; in contrast, the narrowest portion of the adult airway is typically the glottis itself. The chest wall and upper airway of the infant and young child are more compliant such that collapse of the airway occurs more easily and leads to airway obstruction.[16] Not only are children more prone to airway obstruction, but their increased oxygen and metabolic demand makes them more sensitive to hypoxia. Respiratory arrest can quickly lead to cardiac arrest if not promptly addressed.

The pediatric cardiovascular system is different from that of adults as well. In children, cardiac output is maintained primarily through heart rate rather than systemic vascular resistance. A sudden or sustained drop in heart rate can precipitate a severe drop in blood pressure and cardiac output in a child due to the relative lack of compensation via increase in peripheral vascular resistance. In practice, this means that most cardiac arrests in children are preceded by bradycardia.

Children also have an increased body surface area relative to their mass and are more susceptible than adults to hypothermia and insensible fluid losses. They may be more prone to hypoglycemia and dehydration and less able to tolerate prolonged preoperative fasting.

Children are frequently less able to communicate effectively, less cooperative, and more prone to anxiety and emotional outbursts. The increased emotional lability of some children can make these patients challenging to manage preoperatively and can complicate and prolong the postoperative recovery period. The age and anticipated level of cooperation of a given child patient often dictates the anesthetic plan, with pediatric patients sometimes requiring oral premedication prior to the planned procedure.

The range of complications that can occur in pediatric patients during ambulatory anesthesia is the same as for adults, though not all complications occur with similar frequency. In children, respiratory complications are among the most frequently reported serious adverse effects. The overall rate of adverse events is higher in children than in adults, ranging from 1.45% to as high as 6% in different studies.[11,18,19]

Pediatric Respiratory Complications

Respiratory complications in the pediatric population are the most frequently observed adverse event and are typically mild in nature, responding well to supplemental oxygen or head repositioning. The most common complication in children is respiratory depression and oxygen desaturation and ranges from less than 1% to 11% of subjects, depending on the study.[19] More frequent respiratory depression and desaturation are observed with combinations of intravenous medications, particularly combinations of narcotics and benzodiazepines or narcotics and propofol.[19] In a recently published report from the Pediatric Sedation Research Consortium on the use of propofol sedation/anesthesia for outpatient procedures, the number of respiratory complications outnumbered other complications significantly and included the following specific events in decreasing order of frequency: desaturation less than 90% for greater than 30 seconds; airway obstruction; cough; excessive secretions; apnea; and laryngospasm.[18] The authors of the study identified 1 in 65 anesthetics as being complicated by adverse respiratory events, and 1 in 70 anesthetics required airway interventions including placement of an oral or nasal airway, positive pressure ventilation, or endotracheal intubation.[18] A study by Kakavouli et al. reports an overall incidence rate of intraoperative respiratory complications of 1.9% with laryngospasm and bronchospasm identified as the most common adverse events.[17] Two separate studies on perioperative cardiac arrest in children list respiratory events[6] and airway-related causes[2] as the main causes of cardiac arrest attributable to anesthesia. Cravero reports two cases of cardiac arrest in children, one of which occurred secondary to laryngospasm and profound hypoxia, and the second that resulted after an apneic episode and bradycardia.[18] These cases underscore the fact that cardiac arrest in children is frequently preceded by respiratory arrest, whereas adults more frequently experience cardiac arrest secondary to MI or arrhythmia.

Pediatric Cardiovascular Complications

Children typically do not suffer from systemic hypertension, coronary artery disease, or congestive heart failure as in adult patients. Though there is always the possibility of undiagnosed congenital heart disease, most children who present for ambulatory anesthesia will be free of cardiac disease. Notwithstanding this, cardiac complications do occur in the pediatric population though at a much lower rate. In the study by Kakavouli et al., cardiac complications accounted for 8.6% of all observed complications.[17] Cravero et al. reported a rate of cardiac complications (defined as a change of more than 30% in heart rate, blood pressure, or respiratory rate) of 60.8 events per 10,000 anesthetic cases.[18] Cardiac arrest, though rare, does occur in children who undergo anesthesia and has a reported incidence rate of between 4.95 per 10,000 (Ref. 2) and 22.9 per 10,000.[6] While the majority of anesthesia-related causes of cardiac arrest are due to respiratory complications, the remainder may be attributed to bradycardia or anesthetic drug-induced cardiac depression (halogenated inhalation agents).

Other Pediatric Complications

In many other regards, the anesthetic complications that may occur in children are similar to those that occur in adults. The rate of aspiration (between 1 and 4 per 10,000 cases) is similar in adults and children as is the rate of postoperative nausea and vomiting, though children may experience more emesis with certain medications such as ketamine. Children may experience a paradoxical reaction and become stimulated or excited when given certain sedative-hypnotic drugs. In addition, children may be more prone to agitation, delirium, or hallucinations upon emerging from anesthesia. Research studies have estimated the incidence of post-procedure agitation, nightmares, and/or behavioral problems in children given ketamine to be between 4% and 17%.[19] Ketamine is also associated with higher rates of postoperative nausea and vomiting (6–12%).[19] The combination of midazolam and ketamine appears to reduce the incidence of emesis but not the incidence of postoperative agitation.[19]

PREVENTION AND MANAGEMENT OF PEDIATRIC ANESTHETIC COMPLICATIONS

Preoperative screening of the pediatric patient will be simpler as most will have an uncomplicated medical history. Laboratory testing is rarely indicated in these patients. Of special interest is a medical history of asthma or recent upper respiratory infection, as both these conditions may predispose toward respiratory complications during anesthesia. Upper respiratory tract infections are notoriously common in school-age and younger children, and adverse airway effects have been noted by some to persist for several weeks after the resolution of acute symptoms.[16] Parents should be asked about any cough, sore throat, or "runny nose," and the procedure should be rescheduled if there is any doubt about the child's condition.

Management of anesthetic complications in children is similar to that of adults with a few differences. The pediatric advanced life support protocol (PALS) mirrors the ACLS protocol for adults, except that PALS guidelines recommend beginning chest compressions for children with significant bradycardia (<60 bpm) and signs of hypoperfusion. Oxygen face masks (bag masks), endotracheal tubes, laryngoscopes, oral and nasal airways, and laryngeal mask airways of appropriate size should be available for use with pediatric patients. A frightened child may become increasingly uncooperative and inadvertently injure themselves at various stages during ambulatory anesthesia. Additional staff members may be required to be present during ambulatory anesthetic procedures to calm and distract the child at the start of the procedure and assist during recovery.

Postoperative monitoring of the pediatric patient is similar to that of adults. Children benefit from a prompt reunion with a parent or caregiver and effort should be made to have parents present in the postoperative recovery area as soon after the procedure as possible. Having a parent or family member present can help to calm an anxious child and may aid in the management of any postoperative drug-induced agitation.

In conclusion, anesthesia in outpatient settings for oral maxillofacial surgical procedures has an admirable track record of safety, and recent advances in the field have increased its safety and reliability. Complications, though infrequent, do occur during ambulatory anesthesia but with adequate knowledge and preparation many serious adverse events can be prevented or managed effectively.

SUGGESTED READINGS

1. D'Eramo EM. 1999. "Mortality and morbidity with outpatient anesthesia: The Massachusetts experience." *Journal of Oral and Maxillofacial Surgery* 57: 531–536.
2. Ahmed A, Ali M, and Khan M. 2009. "Perioperative cardiac arrests in children at a university teaching hospital of a developing country over 15 years." *Pediatric Anesthesia* 19: 581–586.
3. Chung F, Mezei G, and Tong D. 1999. "Preexisting medical conditions as predictors of adverse events in day-case surgery." *British Journal of Anaesth* 83: 262–270.
4. Setzer N, and Saade E. 2007. "Childhood obesity and anesthetic morbidity." *Pediatric Anesthesia* 17: 321–326.
5. Altermatt FR, Munoz HR, Delfino AE, et al. 2005. "Pre-oxygenation in the obese patient: Effects of position on tolerance to apnoea." *British Journal of Anaesthesia* 95: 706–709.
6. Gobbo Braz L, Braz JR, Módolo NS, do Nascimento P, Brushi BA, Raquel de Carvalho L. 2006. "Perioperative cardiac arrest and its mortality in children. A 9-year survey in a Brazilian tertiary teaching hospital." *Pediatric Anesthesia* 16: 860–866.
7. Borkowski RG. 2006. "Ambulatory anesthesia: Preventing perioperative and postoperative complications." *Cleveland Clinic Journal of Medicine* 73(Suppl 1): S57–S61.
8. Michota FA., Jr. 2006. "The preoperative evaluation and use of laboratory testing." *Cleveland Clinic Journal of Medicine* 73: S4–S7.
9. Arozullah AM, Khuri SF, Henderson WG, and Daley J. 2001. "Participants in the National Veterans Affairs Surgical Quality Improvement Program. Development and validation of a multi-factorial risk index for predicting postoperative pneumonia after major noncardiac surgery." *Annals of Internal Medicine* 135: 847–857.
10. Fleisher LA, Beckman JA, Brown KA, et al. 2008. "ACC/AHA 2007 guidelines on perioperative cardiovascular evaluation and care for noncardiac surgery: Executive summary." *Anesthesia & Analgesia* 106(3): 685–712.
11. Fecho K, Moore CG, Lunney AT, Rock P, Norfleet EA, Boysen PG. 2008. "Anesthesia-related perioperative adverse events during in-patient and out-patient procedures." *International Journal of Health Care Quality Assurance* 21(4): 396–412.
12. Dunn PF. 2007. *Clinical Anesthesia Procedures of the Massachusetts General Hospital*, 7th ed. Philadelphia: Lippincott Williams & Wilkins.
13. Martin G, Glass PS, Breslin DS, MacLeod DB, Sanderson IC, Lubarsky DA, Reves JG, Gan TJ. 2003. "A study of anesthetic drug utilization in different age groups." *Journal of Clinical Anesthesia* 15: 194–200.
14. American Association of Oral and Maxillofacial Surgeons. 2006. *Office Anesthesia Evaluation Manual*, 7th ed. Rosemont, IL: AAOMS.
15. Sakai T, Planinsic RM, Quinlan JJ, Handley LJ, Kim TY, Hilmi IA. 2006. "The incidence and outcome of perioperative pulmonary aspiration in a university hospital: A 4-year retrospective analysis." *Anesthesia & Analgesia* 103: 941–947.
16. Miller RD, Eriksson LI, Fleisher LA., et al. 2009. *Miller's Anesthesia*, 7th ed. Philadelphia, PA: Churchill Livingstone.
17. Kakavouli A, Li G, Carson MP, et al. 2009. "Intraoperative reported adverse events in children." *Pediatric Anesthesia* 19: 732–739.

18. Cravero JP, Beach ML, Blike GT, et al. 2009. "The incidence and nature of adverse events during pediatric sedation/anesthesia with propofol for procedures outside the operating room: A report from the Pediatric Sedation Research Consortium." *Anesthesia & Analgesia* 108(3): 795–804.

19. Mace SE, Barata IA, Cravero JP, et al. 2004. "Clinical policy: Evidence-based approach to pharmacologic agents used in pediatric sedation and analgesia in the emergency department." *Annals of Emergency Medicine* 44(4): 342–377.

2

Third Molar Surgery

Thomas Schlieve, DDS
Antonia Kolokythas, DDS, MS
Michael Miloro, DMD, MD, FACS

INTRODUCTION

Any tooth that fails to erupt into the dental arch within the expected time frame and is no longer expected to do so is, by definition, an impacted tooth. Failure of a tooth to erupt into the arch in a timely fashion can be due to several factors such as crowding from inadequate arch length (Bolton discrepancy), retarded maturation of the third molar, malpositioned adjacent teeth, associated pathology (odontogenic cysts and tumors), trauma, previous surgery, dense overlying bone (lateral positioning) or soft tissue and systemic conditions (syndromes). The mandibular and maxillary third molars are the most common impacted teeth, followed by the maxillary canines and mandibular premolars. It is of no surprise that extraction of third molars, usually impacted, is the procedure performed with the highest frequency on daily basis by oral and maxillofacial surgeons.

The indications and timing for removal of impacted teeth and specifically third molars are set forth by the American Association of Oral and Maxillofacial Surgeons (AAOMS) parameters of care and are not discussed further here. Complication rates from the removal of impacted third molars range from 4.6% to 30.9% with an average of approximately 10%.[1-6] The incidence of these complications varies with surgeon experience, patient age, and depth of impaction. Several factors are known to increase the risk of complications and these include increased age, female gender, presence of pericoronitis, poor oral hygiene, smoking, depth of impaction, and surgeon inexperience.[2,5,6] The aim of this chapter is to provide a comprehensive review of the common as well as rare peri- and postoperative complications associated with impacted third molar surgery and their management.

ALVEOLAR OSTEITIS

Alveolar osteitis (AO) or "dry socket" is a clinical diagnosis with an incidence of between 1% and 37%.[1,4-6,7] This wide range can best be explained by varied definitions of AO. Some studies define AO as pain that requires the patient to return to the surgeon's office, while others define it as simply based on a clinical diagnosis of AO. In addition, some studies report only those teeth that required surgical extraction or use varied surgical protocols.[5-8] The average incidence of AO in a private practice setting based on a survey of AAOMS members was 6.5%.[6] Contributing factors to the development of AO include the use of oral

Management of Complications in Oral and Maxillofacial Surgery, First Edition. Edited by Michael Miloro, Antonia Kolokythas.
© 2012 John Wiley & Sons, Inc. Published 2012 by John Wiley & Sons, Inc.

contraceptives, smoking, increasing age, female gender, presence of pericoronitis, surgical time, surgical trauma, and compromised medical status.[6,7,8]

AO is often described as the loss, lysis, or breakdown of a fully formed blood clot prior to its maturation into granulation tissue. Patients will present with a myriad of symptoms and signs for approximately 3 to 5 days following extraction. The most common complaints are pain, malodor, and foul taste that do not respond well to oral analgesics and often keep a patient up at night. Clinically, a gray-brown clot or the complete absence of an organized clot may be present in the extraction socket. Food debris may or may not be present and the surrounding tissue may be erythematous and edematous. The site is exquisitely tender and often patients will have referred pain to other areas of the head and neck including the ear, eye, or temporal and frontal regions.

The incidence of AO can effectively be decreased through a variety of interventions, all of which focus on decreasing bacterial counts at the surgical site. Chlorhexidine gluconate 0.12% presurgical irrigation either with or without postoperative rinses has shown to be beneficial in decreasing the incidence of AO.[7–9] Copious irrigation and lavage of the surgical site with normal saline has been reported to decrease AO. In one study, it was as effective as pre- and postoperative rinses with chlorhexidine, "Cepacol," and normal saline. Others have demonstrated no significant difference between pulse lavage and hand syringe irrigation. Intra-alveolar antibiotics, specifically tetracycline, lincomycin, or clindamycin may also decrease the incidence of AO.[8] Postoperative antibiotics have not consistently shown an ability to influence the development of AO and the evidence to support preoperative or intraoperative systemic antibiotics is controversial.[3,7,8] Most studies do not demonstrate a significant difference. Overall, good surgical technique with minimal trauma, copious irrigation, and the use of chlorhexidine rinses or topical antibiotics have shown promise in decreasing the incidence of AO.

The goal in treatment of AO is to relieve pain until adequate maturation of the healing socket has occurred. Most treatment regimens focus on gentle irrigation with or without mechanical debridement and placement of obtundant dressings. Interestingly, there is very little evidence to support the use of a certain dressing or medicament over another. Commonly, iodoform gauze and eugenol are used to "pack" the socket and this packing is changed QD or QOD.[4,8] Eugenol is a member of the phenylpropanoid class of chemical compounds and is beneficial due to its inhibition of neural transmission and neurotoxicity. Iodoform is an organoiodine compound that has antibacterial properties and has been used since the early 20th century as an antiseptic wound dressing. Most commercially available dry socket pastes or dressings include eugenol in combination with various other medicaments such as guaiacol, chlorobutanol, balsam peru, and butamben. The use of gelfoam as a carrier and obtundant dressing has also been reported. Patients should be seen regularly for follow up to ensure elimination of symptoms and if iodoform packing is used, to change or remove the packing. It is important to avoid the use of eugenol and other neurotoxic chemicals in the presence of an exposed inferior alveolar or lingual nerve. The use of systemic antibiotics is not recommended for treatment of AO.[8] Typically, patients will have resolution of symptoms within 3 to 5 days; however, in certain patients it may take up to 14 days for complete resolution.[4,8] In summary, AO is one of the more common complications of third molar surgery. Its incidence can be decreased though a combination approach of preoperative rinses, irrigation, and/or local antibiotic application, and its treatment is straightforward.

INFECTION

Surgical wound infection rates as a result of third molar extraction range from 0.8% to 4.2%, and almost exclusively involve the mandibular third molar sites.[1–6,10,11] According to most general surgery and infectious disease literature, any surgical procedure within the oropharynx is considered a clean-contaminated wound, a class II wound, and carries a less than 10% risk of surgical site infection (SSI). If inflammation without purulence is noted, such as that with pericoronitis, the wound is then classified as contaminated, class III, and carries an SSI rate of 20%. The presence of purulence or necrotic tissue at the time of surgery results in a 40% risk of SSI. Class I data are available to support the use of preoperative antibiotic prophylaxis for clean-contaminated wounds; however, there are no data to support continued antibiotic administration beyond the first 24 hours after surgery.[12,13,14] In relation to third molar surgery, 50% of infections are localized subperiosteal abscess-type infections occurring approximately 2–4 weeks after surgery.[10] This type of infection is attributed to debris left under the surgically created mucoperiosteal flap and would likely not be prevented with the use of antibiotic prophylaxis. The remainder of third molar SSI cases are rarely severe enough to necessitate further surgery or antibiotics. SSI within the first postoperative week occurs only 0.5–1.0% of the time.[10,11,15]

The risk of developing an SSI associated with the removal of third molars increases with degree of impaction, need for bone removal or sectioning of the tooth, the presence of gingivitis, periodontal disease and/or pericoronitis, surgeon experience, increasing age, and antibiotic use. The benefit of systemic antibiotic administration on the incidence of SSI in relation to third molar extractions is questionable and is not currently recommended since the incidence of complications from antibiotic administration is higher than the incidence of SSI: 11% and 0.8% to 4.2%, respectively.[10,11,15] It is also unlikely that perioperative systemic antibiotics are of any benefit in delayed, subperiosteal-type infections due to the nature of these infections as described previously.[10]

Signs of SSI can vary from localized swelling and erythema to fluctuance and trismus or systemic manifestations with fevers, dehydration, etc.[10] The treatment of SSI due to third molar surgery involves surgical incision and drainage in addition to the administration of systemic antibiotics. Penicillin is often used, as the vast majority of infections are caused by a mixed flora of micro-organisms with anaerobic and gram positive streptococci being the most common. Amoxicillin has a slightly wider spectrum of activity and metronidazole can be added to cover anaerobic organisms. For the penicillin-allergic patients, clindamycin is a good choice of antibiotic and can also be used when aerobic and anaerobic coverage is desired. Most often, patients will present with a vestibular, body of the mandible, or localized subperiosteal abscess. A rare occurrence is the spread of infection along fascial tissue planes and involvement of multiple potential spaces. This situation requires surgical drainage, IV antibiotics, and close follow-up as progression to parapharyngeal, submandibular, and retropharyngeal spaces can lead to airway embarrassment and even mediastinal abscess formation with potentially fatal result.[10,15]

BLEEDING/HEMORRHAGE

The incidence of clinically significant bleeding as a result of third molar surgery ranges from 0.2% to 5.8%.[4–6] According to the AAOMS Age-Related Third Molar Study, approximately 0.7% occur intraoperatively and 0.1% postoperatively.[1] Significant bleeding or hemorrhage is most often associated with mandibular third molar surgery (80%) when compared with maxillary third molar surgery (20%).[16] Specific risk factors include advanced age, distoangular impactions, and deep impactions.[6] Massive intraoperative bleeding is a rare occurrence and is often attributed to the presence of an arteriovenous malformation (AVM).[16] As such, examination of the surgical site for gingival discoloration, palpable thrill, or bruit is necessary. Imaging may demonstrate a multilocular radiolucency in the area of AVM in proximity to the third molar tooth (Fig. 2.1). In these patients, angiography is essential to confirm diagnosis and treatment with embolization is often necessary.

The most common inherited bleeding disorder, von Willebrand disease, affects an estimated 1% of individuals. Hemophilia A or B is present in 1 in 5,000 live births. Depending on patient age and sex, the first surgical procedure a patient undergoes may be third molar extraction as patients with mild to moderate forms of certain coagulopathies may be undiagnosed. Patients with an acquired or congenital coagulopathy will require further workup prior to surgery. Depending on the specific condition, recent laboratory values, factor replacement, hematology consultation, or inpatient surgery may be necessary.

Antithrombotic treatment with medications such as warfarin, thienopyridines, or aspirin is commonly encountered among patients requiring extractions. Warfarin and clopidogrel rank among the top 100 prescribed medications in the United States, an estimated 25% of individuals over age 75 currently take warfarin, and, according to the FDA, over 100 billion aspirins are taken each year. Most current literature does not recommend withholding these medications for tooth extraction. The risk of a thrombotic event outweighs any benefit of holding the medication. In patients taking warfarin, a preoperative INR (international normalized ratio) may be of value. According to Potoski, a value of 4.0 is acceptable for minor

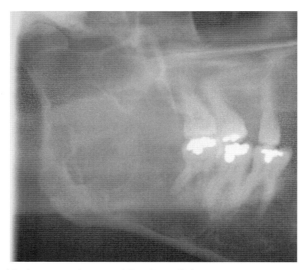

Fig. 2.1. Panoramic radiographic demonstrating a multilocular radiolucency arteriovenous malformation (AVM) associated with a third molar tooth.

surgical procedures, 3.0 if also taking clopidogrel, aspirin, or other antiplatelet medications, and 2.5 for more involved surgery.[16]

The treatment of bleeding or hemorrhage begins with local measurements, pressure with gauze, and packing. Intraoperative bleeding from soft tissues can usually be controlled with cautery, taking care to avoid any neurovascular structures. Bone bleeding or bleeding from extraction sockets can be controlled through a variety of measures. Intra-alveolar hemostatic agents such as gelfoam, surgicel, avitene, collaplug, collatape, thrombin, tiseel, or bone wax may be used alone or in various combinations. Over suturing and primary closure of the wound can also assist in hemostasis and containment of the various hemostatic agents. Oral rinsing with an antifibrinolytic such as Amicar® (epsilon-aminocaproic acid) or Cyclokapron® (tranexamic acid) can aid in maintenance of an organized clot.[16]

In the case of prolonged postoperative bleeding, the patient should be instructed to remove loose clots and bite firmly and continuously on a moist gauze pack for 30 minutes. If this is unsuccessful, exploration and debridement of the wound should be completed under local anesthesia without vasoconstrictor to allow for diagnosis of the cause of bleeding. Granulation tissue should be debrided, irregular sharp bony edges removed, and hemostatic agents used within the alveolus to assist in bleeding control. As with intra-operative bleeding, over suturing and primary wound closure can assist in hemostasis and maintenance of the various hemostatic agents.

MANDIBULAR FRACTURE

Mandibular fracture following third molar surgery is a rare occurrence and most often associated with deeply impacted third molars in patients over 40 years of age.[17] The reported incidence of mandibular fracture both intraoperative and postoperative ranges from 0.00490% to 0.00003% with a mean time to fracture ranging from 6.6 to 14 days following surgery according to studies by Iizuka and Krimmel respectively.[18,19] Fractures up to 28 days following surgery have been reported and no fractures reported beyond 6 weeks after surgery.[18,19] This time period correlates with increased masticatory forces due to decreased trismus, pain, and edema. Libersa, in his review of 37 fractures from 750,000 extractions, found that 8 of 10 late fractures occurred in men with 6 occurring during mastication.[17] Risk factors for fracture include age over 40, male, advanced atrophy, associated pathology such as cysts or tumors, osteoporosis, full dentition and bruxism.[17-19] The angle region of the mandible is of particular risk for fracture due to its relatively decreased cross-sectional area. The presence of a deeply impacted, fully developed third molar can occupy

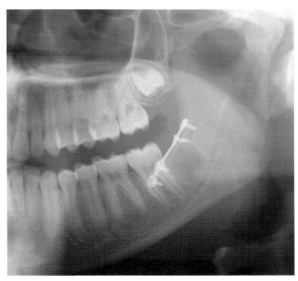

Fig. 2.2. Panoramic radiograph demonstrating open reduction and fixation of mandibular fracture after extraction of third molar.

a significant portion of this cross-sectional area leaving little support following surgical extraction.[18] Intra-operative mandibular fracture is almost exclusively due to the application of excessive force during third molar surgery. Often, it occurs during the use of dental elevators combined with the application of heavy pressure beyond that required to extract the tooth.[4] In patients over 40 years of age presenting with partial bone impactions (loss of external oblique ridge) and risk factors, even light force can cause fracture.[17]

Should a fracture occur during or after third molar surgery, it should be treated immediately. Open reduction and internal fixation can be easily accomplished in this region using the Champy technique with tension band plating (Fig. 2.2). Alternatively, closed reduction with intermaxillary fixation may be appropriate in certain cases. Regardless of the technique, the complication should be communicated to the patient and/or guardian and treatment initiated.

ORAL-ANTRAL COMMUNICATION

The extraction of maxillary molars can lead to a communication between the maxillary sinus and oral cavity. If this communication does not heal, or is treated inappropriately, it can lead to development of an oral-antral fistula (OAF). The incidence of oral-antral communication (OAC) from third molar extraction ranges from 0.08% to 0.25%; however, documented cases may under represent the actual number of cases due to the self-limiting nature of most communications and flap closure following impacted third molar removal.[1–6] It should be noted that OAC is more common at the first molar site followed by the second molar site and all patients should be alerted to the possibility of OAC and even OAF following removal of maxillary molars.[3,4]

When extracting maxillary molars in close approximation to the sinus, especially when sinus pneumatization and widely divergent roots are noted radiographically, excessive force should be avoided and consideration for sectioning of roots made. Predisposing factors include pneumatization around the tooth roots, periapical infection, acute/chronic sinusitis, adjacent edentulous spaces, and traumatic extraction (Fig. 2.3).[3,4,6] The assessment of an OAC should include the etiology, location, and size of the defect. Identification of an OAC can be assisted by having the patient perform the nose-blow test. The patient should pinch the nostrils together preventing air flow out of the nares. Next, have the patient attempt to blow gently though the nose while observing the extraction site. If an OAC exists, air will pass through it and bubbling of blood/fluid in the socket is observed. Another method also uses the nose-blow test but instead of observing the site directly, a mirror is placed near the site and is observed for fogging of the mirror. This

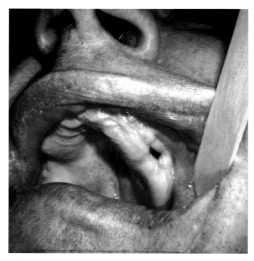

Fig. 2.3. Oral-antral communication after extraction.

test can be of particular use in third molar OAC due to the inability to visualize the depth of the socket in certain patients. Additionally, if upon inspection of the extracted tooth a segment of bone remains attached to the tooth toward the root apices, it is likely a communication exists. However, if no bone is present, this does not rule out the possibility of an OAC. The surgeon must avoid the temptation to probe or explore the extraction site as this can perforate an intact membrane and introduce foreign material, including bacteria, into the sinus cavity.

Once the surgeon has determined an OAC exists, the size of the defect should be appreciated. Defects less than 2 mm in diameter will close spontaneously. If desired, measures can be taken to ensure stability of a quality blood clot in the extraction site. A collagen plug, gelfoam, and/or sutures can be placed to assist in clot formation and maintenance. A moderately sized defect of 2–6 mm in diameter will require additional measures to aid closure of the OAC. A figure-of-eight stitch should be placed over the tooth socket to assist in clot maintenance, and gelfoam or a collagen plug can be placed within the socket to assist in formation of a stable clot. In addition, multiple medications should be prescribed to prevent congestion and development of maxillary sinusitis. Amoxicillin, cephalosporins, augmentin, or clindamycin can be prescribed. Nasal decongestants such as oxymetazoline and pseudoephedrine should be prescribed along with a nasal irrigant (saline nasal spray) to ensure patency of the ostium and normal sinus drainage. Oxymetazoline should only be used for a period of 3 days, as rhinitis medicamentosa can occur. Also, patients should be placed on sinus precautions to avoid increasing or decreasing pressure within the sinus. Specific instructions should be given to the patient to avoid sneezing though the nose, smoking, drinking with a straw, or blowing their nose. Smokers who cannot abstain should be informed of an increased risk of OAF development and smoke in small puffs to avoid changes in sinus pressure. A large defect, 7 mm or more in diameter, will require additional surgical procedures. Buccal or palatal flaps can be rotated to allow for primary closure. Gelfoam or collagen should be placed within the socket and the patient followed closely.

Patients with OAF may present weeks, months, or even years following extractions. Symptoms of unilateral sinus pain and pressure, nasal congestion, intraoral discharge/purulence, bad taste, or fluid communication between the mouth and nose may be noted. On exam, the area may be edematous and erythematous with granulation-like tissue bulging from the fistulous tract. Gentle probing of the area and X-ray examination with a radiopaque material within the tract can confirm the presence of an OAF. Treatment involves an initial period of antibiotic, nasal decongestant, nasal irrigant, and sinus precautions. Following resolution of acute infection and decreased sinus inflammation, surgical repair can be undertaken. Treatment should include excision of the sinus tract with inversion into the sinus to close the sinus side of the communication. The oral side can then be closed with a buccal advancement flap or palatal finger flap, buccal fat pad advancement flap, pedicle tongue flap, cheek mucosal flap, or temporalis myofascial flap. Excellent sources with detailed description of these techniques are available in the published literature.[4,20] An interpositional material such as bone graft, gold foil, or bioabsorbable material can be used as a third layer of closure. Recently, Watzak described a press fit, autogenous bone graft, technique for closure of OAF with subsequent conventional sinus lift and implant placement.[21] Following surgery the patient should be placed on sinus precautions for 3 weeks and continued on antibiotics, decongestants, and nasal irrigations.

INJURY TO ADJACENT TEETH/WRONG TOOTH EXTRACTION

The most common injury to an adjacent tooth is loosening or fracture of a large restoration.[3,4] Other injuries can include tooth loosening due to inappropriate use of elevators, crown fracture due to caries, and inadvertent extraction of an adjacent tooth.[3,4] The incidence of injury to an adjacent second molar when performing third molar surgery is between 0.3% and 0.4%.[1,2,5,6] Limited data exist regarding inadvertent extraction of an adjacent tooth specifically during third molar surgery; however, the overall incidence of wrong tooth extraction ranges from 0.026% to 0.047%.[3]

Adjacent teeth with large restorations, caries, or recurrent decay pose a risk for inadvertent injury. Evaluation of adjacent teeth both clinically and radiographically should be completed prior to beginning a procedure, and patients should be made aware of the possibility of injury. If an adjacent tooth poses a high risk for injury, attempts should be made to avoid luxation with elevators adjacent to the tooth or consideration should be given to not using an elevator at all. To avoid injury to the opposing dentition during extraction, excessive traction forces should be avoided. If a tooth suddenly releases, this can result in instrument damage to opposing cusps. Also, placing a finger or suction tip in between the forceps and opposing dentition can prevent contact with the instrument or absorb some of the blow. Wrong tooth removal should never occur if adequate attention is given to planning and appropriate time out. The tooth to be extracted should be marked on the radiograph and confirmed with both the patient and the assistant in terms the patient can understand (Fig. 2.4). Referrals should be contacted if confusion exists as to the correct procedure.[3]

If an injury occurs, it should be promptly treated and all parties involved notified. A fractured tooth or restoration can be temporized and the referring practitioner notified. Loosened or avulsed crowns can be recemented if no recurrent decay exists or temporarily cemented if caries are noted. If an adjacent tooth is loosened it should be repositioned and stabilized. Often, this requires only minimal repositioning, and the tooth can be left alone. If significant loosening has occurred, stabilization for 10–14 days with the least rigid method of stabilization should be used to avoid risk of ankylosis or root resorption. Extraction of the wrong tooth, if immediately noted, can be treated as an avulsion. The tooth should be implanted back into the extraction site and stabilized. If the tooth is being extracted for orthodontic reasons, the remaining teeth should not be extracted and a call should be placed to the referring orthodontist.[3] Occasionally, modification of the treatment plan can be done to utilize the tooth that should have been removed and

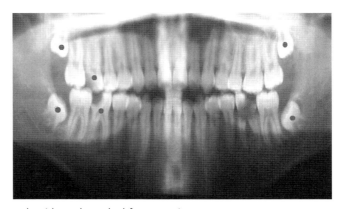

Fig. 2.4. Panoramic radiograph with teeth marked for extraction.

treatment can proceed with the new plan. If the original tooth planned for extraction needs to be removed, the health and stability of the accidentally extracted tooth should be confirmed prior to proceeding with further extractions. When the error goes unnoticed at the time of extraction, the tooth can obviously no longer be replanted. It is important to document thoroughly any case of wrong tooth extraction and inform all parties involved. According to data from the Oral and Maxillofacial Surgery National Insurance Company (OMSNIC), 46% of all wrong-site tooth extraction claims are settled with an indemnity payment. Thus, documentation and communication with both the patient and referring dentist are important to avoid litigation.

INJURY TO ADJACENT OSSEOUS STRUCTURES

During the process of third molar extraction, and more specifically maxillary third molar extraction, the surrounding bone is at risk for inadvertent fracture. The most likely places for bone to fracture during removal of maxillary third molars are the buccal cortical plate and maxillary tuberosity. The incidence of maxillary tuberosity fracture in association with third molar extraction is approximately 0.6% and is most often caused by excessive force with forceps or elevators. The combination of Type IV bone, no distal support, and often significant space involvement by maxillary sinus contribute to the potential for tuberosity fracture (Fig. 2.5).[3,22]

Maxillary tuberosity fracture or buccal cortical plate fracture can compromise future prosthetic rehabilitation as the maxillary tuberosity is an important anatomical retention point for complete dentures. Buccal plate fracture can lead to soft tissue tearing and irregular remaining alveolar bone. To avoid these complications the surgeon should ensure appropriate force application and remove bone in a controlled fashion when excessive force is necessary for extraction. In addition, placement of a periosteal elevator distal to the third molar to elevate the tooth and separate it from the periodontal ligament and tuberosity can assist the surgeon in avoiding a tuberosity fracture.

When a fracture of the buccal cortical plate occurs, the surgeon should asses the stability, size, and soft tissue attachment of the fractured segment. If the surgeon has been supporting the alveolus with finger pressure during extraction, early cortical plate fracture can be assessed. At this point, the cortical plate should be dissected free from the tooth with an elevator or other sharp instrument while the tooth is stabilized with forceps. Once the bone and soft tissue are dissected free, the tooth is extracted and the tissues approximated and secured with sutures. If a soft tissue flap is reflected from bone, the blood supply to the segment has been compromised, and that segment will become necrotic if not removed. Maxillary tuberosity fractures should be treated in a similar manner. Once recognized, the fractured segment should be dissected free from the tooth. Using a handpiece, the bone segment can be separated from the tooth and the roots sectioned to allow for atraumatic extraction. If adequate soft tissue attachment remains, the tuberosity is stabilized through good soft tissue closure with sutures. In the event that the tuberosity cannot be dissected free from the tooth, the reason for extraction should be revisited. If asymptomatic, the tooth

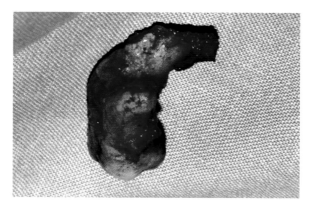

Fig. 2.5. Fractured tuberosity with extraction of maxillary third molar.

and attached tuberosity segment can be fixated for 6–8 weeks via an arch bar or orthodontic fixation followed by surgical extraction with controlled bone removal and tooth sectioning on a later date. If symptomatic, the tooth must be extracted and in doing so, the tuberosity will be removed. The remaining bone should be smoothened and soft tissues approximated with sutures. The overall goal of treatment in a tuberosity fracture is to maintain the bone in place unless its removal is absolutely necessary.[3,22]

PAIN AND SWELLING

Postoperative pain and swelling following third molar surgery is an expected and inevitable consequence of the inflammatory process of healing. The onset of swelling and pain is directly related to an increase in local levels of prostaglandins, leukotrienes, and thromboxane A2. Pain usually reaches its peak in 3–5 hours following surgery. On the other hand, swelling reaches its peak in 24–48 hours and then generally begins to decline on postoperative day 3 or 4. Contributing factors in the development of pain and swelling include operating time, difficulty in extraction, excessive retraction, and the degree of surgical trauma.[3,4]

"Treatment" of swelling and pain can begin prior to surgery. Preoperative IV steroids have been shown in multiple studies to decrease postoperative swelling, pain, and improve health-related quality of life.[23] During surgery, good surgical technique, copious irrigation, and the use of long-lasting anesthetics such as bupivicaine have been shown to decrease pain and swelling. Postoperative scheduled use of nonsteroidal anti-inflammatory (NSAID) drugs has been shown to be more effective in pain reduction than narcotic medications, and as such, narcotics can be better reserved for breakthrough pain.[3,4]

TMJ INJURY

The occurrence of temporomandibular joint (TMJ) injury as a result of third molar surgery is not supported in the literature. In a study by Threlfall, patients with diagnosed anterior disk displacement were no more likely than the control group to have had prior third molar surgery.[24] Also, only 9.5% of patients with anterior disk displacement reported third molar extractions within the past 5 years. Complaints of limited opening are most often due to trauma from injections, inflammation of the muscles of mastication, and/or the body's own protective mechanism to limit function and further trauma.[24]

Injury may occur if excessive force is used, a bite block is not in place when extracting lower third molars, or the patient's mouth is opened excessively.[4,24] This transient injury often resolves with soft diet, moist heat, jaw rest, and NSAID use. An acutely "stuck disc" can be treated effectively with arthrocentesis when observed.[24]

It is important to evaluate all patients undergoing third molar surgery for preoperative joint disease or myofacial pain and thoroughly document all such history. Clicks, pops, crepitus, opening and excursive movements, and any tenderness of the muscles of mastication should be noted. If prior TMJ dysfunction is present, contemplation for surgical extraction of teeth to avoid trauma to the joint should be made.

DISPLACEMENT OF TEETH

The iatrogenic displacement of maxillary and mandibular third molars into adjacent spaces is a rare complication with an unknown incidence.[25] Maxillary third molars can be displaced into the maxillary sinus, buccal vestibule, or posteriorly through periosteum and into the infratemporal fossa (Fig. 2.6).[3,4] Contributing factors for the displacement of maxillary third molars include superior-distal impaction, poor visualization and access, inadequate bone removal, lack of a distal stop, and careless elevation.[25] Displacement of mandibular third molars into the submandibular, sublingual, pterygomandibular, and even lateral pharyngeal spaces has been reported along with displacement of roots into the inferior alveolar canal.[3,4] The lingual cortex becomes progressively thinner in the more posterior regions of the mandible, and this often results in an extremely thin or even dehisced lingual plate. Any apically directed force may easily displace root segments or an entire tooth into the aforementioned spaces.[3]

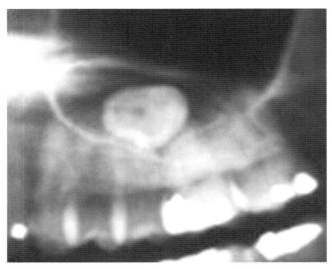

Fig. 2.6. Panoramic radiograph demonstrating third molar displaced into the maxillary sinus.

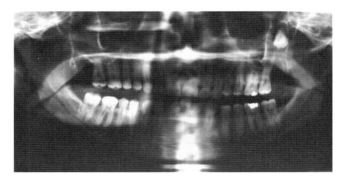

Fig. 2.7. Panoramic radiograph demonstrating tooth displaced into the infratemporal fossa.

The management of a displaced third molar tooth or root varies depending on the space involved. Maxillary third molars displaced into the maxillary sinus should be removed. Root tips less than 3 mm can be left to fibrose into the sinus mucosa if no previous infection of the tooth or sinus is present and initial attempts at retrieval are unsuccessful.[3] The morbidity of additional surgical procedures outweighs the benefits of removal in this case. An attempt to remove the tooth through the socket can be made by placing the suction near the opening into the sinus. Additionally, the sinus can be irrigated through the OAC and suction placed at the opening in an attempt to flush the tooth or root segment out. If the segment is visualized, the opening can be enlarged to allow retrieval. If this is unsuccessful the surgeon should abandon further attempts at removal through the socket and remove the tooth segment via a Caldwell-Luc approach into the maxillary sinus. This can be completed at the time of initial surgery or in a second procedure. If delayed retrieval is planned, the patient should be placed on antibiotics, decongestants, and the OAC closed as described previously.[3,4]

The retrieval of a maxillary third molar displaced into the infratemporal fossa can be complicated by bleeding from the pterygoid plexus, poor visualization, or inability to locate and stabilize the tooth.[25] In general, the tooth is located lateral to the lateral pterygoid plate and inferiorly to the lateral pterygoid muscle. Lateral and PA cephalometric films can assist in localizing the tooth (Fig. 2.7). The surgeon should extend the original incision distally to the tonsillar fauces and with blunt dissection, attempt to locate the tooth. If this attempt is unsuccessful, the tooth should be left in place and the patient placed on antibiotics. Never attempt to grab or probe for the tooth as injury to adjacent structures or further displacement of the tooth can occur. If asymptomatic, the tooth can be left in place and the patient followed closely. Pain, infection, limitation of opening, and patient desire are all indications for removal. This is completed in 4–6 weeks to allow for fibrosis to occur, the tooth to stabilize, and appropriate imaging [CT, cone beam CT (CBCT)] to be obtained. Multiple approaches have been described in the literature including CT-guided surgery, needle-guided fluoroscopic retrieval, transoral retrieval, and hemicoronal flaps.[3,4,25]

Displaced mandibular third molars are most often located in the submandibular space, inferior to the mylohyoid muscle. Attempts at removal should begin with digital pressure against the lingual surface of the mandible to try and force the root segment back into the mouth/extraction site. The opening into the floor of the mouth can be slightly enlarged to assist in retrieval; however, this should be completed cautiously to avoid injury to the lingual nerve. A lingual full thickness flap can be carefully reflected and the mylohyoid muscle incised to gain access to the submandibular space. Due to limited space, hemorrhage, and poor visibility, it may be very difficult to remove the tooth or root segment via this method. Allowing for fibrosis to occur and returning at a later date to remove the tooth or root is acceptable. Often, this is completed via an extraoral approach in the operating room and after CT scanning completed. Yeh has described an intraoral/extraoral approach where a 4-mm skin incision is made to allow for insertion of a hemostats and/or Kelly forceps and stabilization of the tooth while the tooth is located and removed via an intraoral lingual full thickness flap.[4]

Displacement of a root into the inferior alveolar canal should be approached with caution. Attempts at retrieval can further damage the nerve or further displace the root. If the root segment was not infected and the patient does not complain of neurologic findings, leaving the root segment is acceptable. If the root is infected or the patient has complaints of neurologic involvement, it must be removed with caution and consideration should be made for referral to a microneurosurgeon if neural repair becomes necessary.[4]

ASPIRATION/INGESTION

The incidence of foreign body aspiration or ingestion is likely underreported in the literature. Approximately 92.5% of objects are ingested while the remaining 7.5% are aspirated.[3,4] Patients who undergo the surgical removal of third molars are often sedated, which results in their gag and cough reflexes being obtunded. A pharyngeal curtain should be utilized in all patients to prevent aspiration or ingestion during surgery. If the patient is not coughing or in any respiratory distress, it is likely the tooth has been ingested and prompt referral to an emergency room for abdominal and chest radiographs to confirm the location of the object should be made. Coughing that continues or leads to respiratory distress should alert the surgeon to probable aspiration. An attempt to suction the object from the oral pharynx should be made and ACLS protocols activated. The Heimlich maneuver should be used to attempt to dislodge the object. If a patient becomes cyanotic or unconscious, an attempt at retrieval under direct laryngoscopy can be made. If this fails, cricothyrotomy may be necessary to secure the airway. An object that passes through the vocal chords will most likely end up in the right main stem bronchus or right lung, and the patient should be transported to the emergency room and arrangement for bronchoscopy and object retrieval should be made (Fig. 2.8).

NEUROLOGIC COMPLICATIONS

The incidence of neurologic complications as a result of third molar surgery ranges from 0.4% to 11%.[1,2,5,6,26] Injury to the inferior alveolar nerve (IAN) is associated with spontaneous recovery in 96% of cases and spontaneous recovery of lingual nerve injury is approximately 87%.[26] Sensory deficits that last longer than 1 year are likely to be permanent; recovery of sensation should begin within the first 8 weeks following surgery.[26] According to the AAOMS white paper on third molars, the incidence of IAN injury 1 to 7 days postoperatively is 1–5% and persistent alteration in sensation after 6 months ranges from 0.0% to 0.9%.[1] Lingual nerve injury 1 day after surgery was reported in 0.4–1.5% of patients, with persistent sensory alteration at 6 months in 0.0–0.5% of patients.[1] The use of lingual retraction increased the incidence of

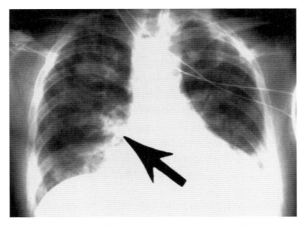

Fig. 2.8. Chest X-ray demonstrating aspirated tooth into right mainstem bronchus.

temporary paresthesia; however, the incidence of persistent findings remained the same. In a study by Tay et al., 192 inferior alveolar nerves in 170 patients were exposed during third molar surgery. Twenty percent reported paresthesia at the 1 week follow-up, and 6% had persistent paresthesia at 1 year.[27]

An increased risk of IAN injury is associated with increased age, complete bony impaction, horizontal angulation, sectioning of the tooth multiple times, bone removal, surgeon's experience, and duration of surgery.[26] Additionally, Rood et al. has described several radiographic predictors of potential nerve injury.[28] These include diversion of the IAN canal, darkening of the root, and interruption of the white line. One in three patients with canal diversion, and one in four patients with darkening of the root or interruption of the white line, exhibited impairment of sensation. These signs are highly sensitive but not highly specific for risk of injury, and the absence of all signs has a strong negative predictive value.[28] Therefore, patients without any significant indicators of injury are unlikely to have injury, patients with an injury are likely to have at least one of the predictors, and patients without injury commonly have predictors of injury radiographically. Other reported radiographic indicators such as deflected roots, narrowing of the root, dark bifid roots, and narrowing of the canal were statistically unrelated to nerve injury.[28]

Lingual nerve injury is associated with distoangular inclination, lingual orientation, and perforation of the lingual cortex.[29,30] Often, flap reflection, tooth sectioning with extension into the lingual plate, or lingual plate fracture are the cause of injury.[29,30] Due to the nerve's variable position, care must be taken when incisions are made and flaps reflected. Miloro et al. reported 10% of lingual nerves positioned superior to the lingual crest and 25% in direct contact with the bone.[31,32] The mean vertical distance from the crest is 2.75 mm and the mean horizontal distance from the lingual plate is 2.53 mm.[31]

Injury to the lingual or inferior alveolar nerve due to local anesthetic injection occurs in approximately 1 in 785,000 cases with 79% affecting the lingual nerve and 21% the IAN. The highest incidence is associated with prilocaine or articaine injection. The majority of cases (85%) resolve within 8 weeks and of the remaining 15%, one-third will eventually resolve.[33] Unfortunately, patients with persistent paresthesia are not candidates for microneurosurgical repair.

All patients who report paresthesia should be followed closely for resolution and appropriate objective testing should be performed. The clinical neurosensory test should be performed to determine the degree of impairment and whether microneurosurgical intervention is necessary. Mechanoceptive testing begins with Level A testing. It comprises brush stroke directional discrimination and two-point discrimination. It is important to test both normal and abnormal areas, map out the area of impaired sensation by marking directly on the patient's skin, and photograph the markings for future reference. Two-point discrimination can be tested using a Boley gauge or the noncotton end of a cotton tip. Testing should be completed in 2-mm increments until the patient can no longer discern two separate points. Normally, the IAN tests to 4 mm and the lingual nerve to 3 mm.[26] Level B testing involves contact detection and Level C pin-prick and thermal discrimination. The indications for repair are complete anesthesia beyond 1–2 months, profound hypoesthesia with no improvement after 3 months, early dysesthesia, and a clinically observed Sunderland

V transection.[26,34] Referral to a surgeon proficient in microneurosurgery should be made if any of the above criteria are met or if unfamiliar with nerve testing and possible treatment protocols.[26]

Bony sequestra and lingual plate exposure are potential complications of low significance but require thorough and prompt attention. Small bony sequestra will spontaneously extrude through the soft tissues and usually cause only temporary discomfort. Reassuring the patient or parent that there is no remaining tooth in the area, the usual concern at presentation, and removing the loose bone is all that is required. The injury to the soft tissues is resolved within few days, and the patient is instructed to avoid trauma from chewing in the area until this occurs. Exposure of the lingual plate or a portion of the mylohoid ridge is not uncommon since the overlying mucosa in this area is excitingly thin. The common complaints will be pain upon swallowing and sharp bone detected in the area. Application of topical anesthetic to allow for a bone file or fine rongeurs to gently smooth or remove any sharp bone is all that is required. The patient is instructed to avoid further injury to the area with certain foods such as popcorn or potato chips and is reassured that the area will spontaneously heal. Oral hygiene and rinses with chlorhexidine will facilitate coverage of the area.

OSTEOMYELITIS

The incidence of osteomyelitis as a result of third molar extraction is not reported in the literature however it is a known complication of infection, fracture, and/or extraction in medically compromised patients. Osteomyelitis is an inflammation of the bone marrow and is most common in the mandible due to its dependence on blood supply from the inferior alveolar artery and poorly vascularized thick cortical bone. Because the maxilla has a rich vascular supply from multiple vessels it is less likely to develop osteomyelitis. The presence of bacteria within the marrow space leads to inflammation and edema with subsequent compression of blood vessels and a decrease in blood supply. This decrease in blood flow results in ischemia, bone necrosis, and proliferation of bacteria. Purulence and bacteria can spread within the marrow via Haversian and Volkmann's canals and extend into cortical bone. Once the cortical bone and periosteum are involved, the blood supply is further compromised and perforation of soft tissues can occur resulting in fistula formation. Predisposing factors in the development of osteomyelitis involve suppression of host defenses in some form. Diabetes, alcoholism, autoimmune disease, radiation therapy, chemotherapy, steroid use, osteopetrosis, myeloproliferative diseases, and malnutrition can contribute to the development of osteomyelitis.[35]

The classification of osteomyelitis offered by Hudson is commonly cited in the literature and essentially breaks down into acute and chronic forms based on disease presence greater than 1 month (Table 2.1).[36]

Patients with osteomyelitis will often present with complaints of a dull and deep pain, swelling and erythema of overlying tissues, paresthesia of the inferior alveolar nerve, trismus, adenopathy, fistula, fever, and malaise.[35,37] In patients with chronic osteomyelitis, signs of acute infection such as fever are often not present; however, fistulas, both intra- and extraorally, are more common. Radiographs typically demonstrate a "moth-eaten" appearance of bony sequestrum. CT scanning can assist in the demarcation of lesion extent although it should be noted that 30–50% demineralization of bone is necessary before radiographic changes.[35] In chronic osteomyelitis there may be radiopacity due to an osteitis-type reaction and proliferation of bone. A laboratory workup will demonstrate leukocytosis in acute forms, elevated erythrocyte sedimentation rate (ESR) and C-reactive protein (CPR). Further laboratory evaluation of ESR and CRP levels

Table 2.1 Types of Osteomyelitis

Acute	Chronic
a. Contiguous focus	a. Recurrent multifocal
b. Progressive	b. Garre's
c. Hematogenous	c. Suppurative or nonsuppurative
	d. Sclerosing

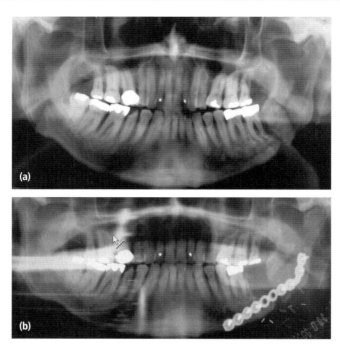

Fig. 2.9. (a) Panoramic radiograph demonstrating pathologic fracture due to osteomyelitis after third molar extraction. (b) Panoramic radiograph after open reduction and fixation of pathologic fracture due to ostemmyelitis after third molar extraction.

during treatment can assist in assessment of healing. Culture specimens will often reveal bacteria traditionally responsible for odontogenic infections such as *Bacteroides*, *Peptostreptococci*, *Fusobacterium*, and *Streptococci*. Occasionally, less common odontogenic bacteria are present. These include *Lactobacillus*, *Eubacterium*, *Klebsiella*, *Acinetobacter*,and *Pseudomonas aeruginosa*. Osteomyelitis of the jaws is different from osteomyelitis of other bones in that *Staphylococci* are not the predominant bacteria.[35]

The treatment of osteomyelitis is combination of surgical and medical management. Treatment of systemic diseases must be considered along with medical consultation when appropriate. Empiric antibiotics should be administered while awaiting final culture results. Penicillin/metronidazole or clindamycin are excellent first-line antibiotics. In chronic cases, sequestrectomy, decortication, and saucerization are necessary and extend to vital, bleeding bone. Removal of the cortex with placement of periosteum directly on the marrow space assists with blood flow. After aggressive debridement, that may lead to further weakening of the mandible, fixation may need to be employed to prevent fracture or for stabilization of a known fracture. External fixation, rigid internal fixation, or intermaxillary fixation may be used with the fixation type dependent on the surgeon's preference and degree of success of surgical debridement (Fig. 2.9).[35,37] Other methods of treatment have been proposed such as local antibiotic administration with both resorbable and nonresorbable carriers and hyperbaric oxygen. Polymethylmethacrylate beads impregnated with gentamycin have been discussed in the orthopedic literature; however, results can be disappointing due to inadequate local release and subinhibitory antibiotic levels.[38,39] Also, a second surgery is necessary to remove the beads. Hyperbaric oxygen (HBO) has not been demonstrated to have a significant effect on outcome based on the limited available literature.[40,41] Esterhai et al. studied the use of HBO on 28 patients with chronic refractory osteomyelitis and this controlled trial concluded that HBO had no effect on length of hospitalization, rate of wound repair, or recurrence of infection.[40]

SUGGESTED READINGS

1. Haug RH, Perrott DH, and Gonzalez ML. 2005. "The American Association of Oral and Maxillofacial Surgeons age-related third molar study." *J Oral Maxillofac Surg* 63: 1106.

2. Osborn TP, Frederickson G, Jr., and Small IA. 1985. "A prospective study of complications related to mandibular third molar surgery." *J Oral Maxillofac Surg* 43: 767.

3. Peterson LJ. 2003. *Prevention and Management of Surgical Complications. Contemporary Oral and Maxillofacial Surgery*, 4th ed. St Louis: CV Mosby.

4. Ness G. 2004. "Impacted teeth." *Peterson's Principles of Oral and Maxillofacial Surgery*, 2nd ed. London: BC Decker Inc.

5. Bouloux GF. 2007. "Complications of third molar surgery." *Oral Maxillofac Surg Clin North Am* 19(1): 117–28; vii.

6. Bui CH, Seldin EB, and Dodson TD. 2003. "Types, frequencies, and risk factors for complications after third molar extraction." *J Oral Maxillofac Surg* 61: 1379.

7. Larsen PE. 1992. "Alveolar osteitis after surgical removal of impacted mandibular third molars: Identification of the patient at risk." *Oral Surg Oral Med Oral Pathol* 73: 393.

8. Alling C. 1994. *Biology and Prevention of Alveolar Osteitis (Selected Readings in Oral and Maxillofacial Surgery)*, 1–19. University of Texas Southwestern Medical Center at Dallas.

9. Larsen PE. 1991. "The effect of chlorhexidine rinse on the incidence of alveolar osteitis following the surgical removal of impacted mandibular third molars. *J Oral Maxillofac Surg* 49: 932.

10. Figueiredo R, Valmaseda-Castellon E, and Berini-Aytes L. 2005. "Incidence and clinical features of delayed-onset infections after extraction of lower third molars." *Oral Surg Oral Med Oral Pathol Oral Radiol Endod* 99: 265.

11. Sweet JB, Butler DP, and Drager JL. 1976. "Effects of lavage techniques with third molar surgery." *Oral Surg* 42: 152–168.

12. Kirby JP. 2009. "Prevention of surgical site infection." *Surg Clin North Am* 89(2): 365–389, viii.

13. Mangram AJ, Horan TC, and Pearson ML. 1999. "Guideline for prevention of surgical site infection." *Infect Control Hosp Epidemiol* 20: 250–278.

14. Bratzler DW, and Hunt DR. 2006. "The surgical infection prevention and surgical care improvement projects: National initiatives to improve outcomes for patients having surgery." *Clin Infect Dis* 43: 322–330.

15. Goldberg MH, Nemarich AN, and Marco WP. 1985. "Complications after mandibular third molar surgery: A statistical analysis of 500 consecutive procedures in private practice." *J Am Dent Assoc* 111: 277–279.

16. Pototski M, and Amenábar JM. 2007. "Dental management of patients receiving anticoagulation or antiplatelet treatment." *J Oral Sci* 49(4): 253–258.

17. Libersa P, Roze D, and Cachart T. 2002. "Immediate and late mandibular fractures after third molar removal." *J Oral Maxillofac Surg* 60: 163.

18. Iizuka T, Tanner S, and Berthold H. 1997. "Mandibular fractures following third molar extraction: A retrospective clinical and radiological study." *Int J Oral Maxillofac Surg* 26: 338.

19. Krimmel M, and Reinert S. 2000. "Mandibular fracture after third molar removal." *J Oral Maxillofac Surg* 58: 1110.

20. Egyedi P. 1977. "Utilization of the buccal fat pad for closure of oro-antral and/or oro-nasal communications." *J Maxillofac Surg* 5: 241.

21. Watzak G. 2005. "Bony press-fit closure of oro-antral fistulas: A technique for pre-sinus lift repair and secondary closure." *J Oral Maxillofac Surg* 63(9): 1288–1294.

22. Ngeow WC. 1998. "Management of the fractured maxillary tuberosity." *Quintessence Int* 29: 189.

23. Beirne OH, and Hollander B. 1986. "The effect of methylprednisolone on pain, trismus, and swelling after removal of third molars." *Oral Surg* 61: 134–138.

24. Threlfall AG, Kanaa MD, and Davies SJ. 2005. "Possible link between extraction of wisdom teeth and temporomandibular disc displacement with reduction: Matched case control study." *Br J Oral Maxillofac Surg* 43: 13.

25. Oberman M, Horowitz I, and Ramon Y. 1986. "Accidental displacement of impacted maxillary third molars." *Int J Oral Maxillofac Surg* 15: 756–758.

26. Ziccardi V, and Zuniga J. 2007. "Nerve injuries after third molar removal." *Oral Maxillofac Surg Clin North Am* 19: 105–115.

27. Tay AB. 2004. "Effect of exposed inferior alveolar neurovascular bundle during surgical removal of impacted lower third molars." *J Oral Maxillofac Surg* 62(5): 592–600.

28. Rood JP, and Shehab BA. 1990. "The radiological prediction of inferior alveolar nerve injury during third molar surgery." *Br J Oral Maxillofac Surg* 28(1): 20–25.

29. Pichler JW, and Beirne OR. 2001. "Lingual flap retraction and prevention of lingual nerve damage associated with third molar surgery: A systematic review of the literature." *Oral Surg Oral Med Oral Pathol Oral Radiol Endod* 91: 395–401.

30. Queral-Godoy E. 2006. "Frequency and evolution of lingual nerve lesions following lower third molar extraction." *J Oral Maxillofac Surg* 64(3): 402–407.

31. Miloro M, Halkias LE, and Slone HW. 1997. "Assessment of the lingual nerve in the third molar region using magnetic resonance imaging." *J Oral Maxillofac Surg* 55: 134–137.

32. Seddon HJ. 1943. "Three types of nerve injury." *Brain* 66: 237–288.

33. Pogrel MA, and Thamby S. 2000. "Permanent nerve involvement resulting from inferior alveolar nerve blocks." *J Am Dent Assoc* 131(7): 901–907.

34. Sunderland S. 1951. "A classification of peripheral nerve injury producing loss of function." *Brain* 74: 491–516.

35. Marx RE. 1991. "Chronic osteomyelitis of the jaws." *Oral and Maxillofacial Surgery Clinics of North America* 24(2): 367–381.

36. Hudson JW. 2000. "Osteomyelitis and osteoradionecrosis." In: *Oral and Maxillofacial Surgery*, Vol. 5, Fonseca RJ, ed. Philadelphia: W.B. Saunders.

37. Coviello V. 2007. "Contemporary concepts in the treatment of chronic osteomyelitis." *Oral Maxillofac Surg Clin North Am* 19(4): 523–534, vi.

38. Alpert B, Colosi T, Von Fraunhofer JA, et al. 1989. "The in-vivo behavior of gentamicin PMMA beads in the maxillofacial region." *J Oral Maxillofac Surg* 47: 46.

39. Chisholm B, Lew D, and Sadasivan I. 1993. "The use of tobramycin impregnated polymethylmethracrylate beads in the treatment of osteomyelitis of the mandible." *J Oral Maxillofac Surg* 51: 444.

40. Esterhai JL, Pisarello J, Brighton CT, et al. 1987. "Adjunctive hyperbaric oxygen therapy in the treatment of chronic refractory osteomyelitis." *J Trauma* 27(7): 763–768.

41. Van Merkesteyn JP, Bakker DJ, and Van der Waal I. 1984. "Hyperbaric oxygen treatment of chronic osteomyelitis of the jaws." *Int J Oral Surg* 13(5): 386–395.

3

Implant Surgery

Pamela J. Hughes, DDS

INTRODUCTION

It is fair to say that the discovery and universal application of osseointegration has revolutionized the prosthodontic, surgical, and, increasingly, orthodontic rehabilitation of partially or fully edentulous patients, and in some cases, fully dentate patients. Although integration failure of implant devices occurs at very low rates, an implant that has not achieved osseointegration can certainly be considered a failure from a restorative or functional perspective. Fortunately, many complications that are associated with implant placement are considered reparable, even if it means removing the implant and starting over. However, failures sometimes can have devastating consequences on a patient's (or surgeon's) physical, psychosocial and financial well-being. This chapter will focus on the more commonly reported complications associated with dental implant surgery. Consideration will be given to (1) preoperative planning and the avoidance of complications during the treatment planning phase; (2) intraoperative contributions to integration failure and acute intraoperative complications; (3) early postoperative failures; and (4) late postoperative failures including peri-implantitis.

PREOPERATIVE PLANNING

Patient Assessment

There are many factors that are important to assess when evaluating a patient for implant reconstruction. Even before the actual *clinical* assessment is performed, the clinician should have a reasonable idea whether the patient is a good candidate for a successful outcome.

The patient's ability to cooperate with treatment and subsequent hygiene and maintenance should be a primary concern when evaluating the patient for implant reconstruction. The immediate surgical outcome, although a concern, does not mean much if the patient does not possess the skills or understanding important to the long-term success of implant rehabilitation. Additionally, the patient's expectations are key in determining whether or not the patient will consider his/her own treatment as a success.

There have been several systemic conditions cited in the literature that traditionally have been accepted as risk factors for integration failure. A number of articles cite specific conditions that are considered absolute or relative contraindications to implant placement. Typically these have included diabetes, osteoporosis, corticosteroid therapy, chemotherapy, and head and neck radiation.[1] Recently, several outcomes studies have alluded to the fact that each of these indeed may not be contraindications, and that other factors, not normally included on that list, may be bigger contributors to failure. A study by Klokkevold and Han[2] analyzed data from 35 articles that included failure rates in diabetic patients and smokers. The

Management of Complications in Oral and Maxillofacial Surgery, First Edition. Edited by Michael Miloro, Antonia Kolokythas.
© 2012 John Wiley & Sons, Inc. Published 2012 by John Wiley & Sons, Inc.

findings suggest that smoking significantly contributed to failure, but there was no difference for the diabetic patient. In a study reviewing 4,680 implants, Moy et al.,[1] however, found that there was a significant increase in implant failure for the diabetic patient and the smoker. Also, additional conditions related to increased risk for failure included patients age greater than 60 years of age, head and neck radiation, and postmenopausal estrogen therapy. Conversely, gender, hypertension, coronary heart disease, pulmonary disease, steroid therapy, chemotherapy, and not being on hormone replacement therapy (in postmenopausal women) were all *not* associated with increased incidence of implant failure.

Although the literature supports the fact that there may not be any absolute contraindications to implant placement, the clinician needs to understand how certain systemic conditions may affect the integration of implants. This will help direct proper judgment with respect to treatment planning in patients with systemic diseases or disorders. For example, in the diabetic patient, decreased vascularity and circulation of the recipient bed due to microvascular abnormalities such as thickening of capillary basement membranes contribute to impaired wound healing, and abnormalities in neutrophil chemotaxis and phagocytic activity may make the diabetic more susceptible to infections.[3] In the case of metabolic bone diseases (osteoporosis, hyperparathyroidism, Paget's disease, etc.), one must consider the potential for proper mineralization that is important to integration.

In most instances, the literature does not distinguish the difference between implant failure and medical complications associated with implant placement.[4] However, the clinician should differentiate the possible conditions that simply may cause implant failure versus conditions that may directly cause harm to the patient. For example, a patient who has had radiation to the jaws or has been treated with a potent bisphosphonate may be at risk for osteoradionecrosis or bisphosphonate-related osteonecrosis, respectfully, as well as implant failure. In these patients, "The option of implant therapy should be chosen restrictively, and the patient should be informed specifically, taking into account the current level of uncertainty with regard to the consequences."[4]

In general, if a patient has the proper physical and mental attributes to maintain implants after restoration, has reasonable expectations, and can safely undergo the surgical procedure without putting undue risk on their physical well-being, they are a candidate for implant reconstruction. The informed consent discussion should be tailored to each patient, taking care to identify issues that may cause increased risk of failure or medical/physical risk to the patient.

Clinical Assessment of the Patient

Thorough clinical examination prior to implant treatment planning is imperative to assess not only the recipient site itself, but also to evaluate the patient's current dentition and dental/gingival health, signs of parafunctional habits, malocclusion, or other factors that may be of importance with respect to implant failure. The clinician must keep in mind that the recipient site may be optimal for implant integration, but if the implant cannot be restored to proper function and aesthetics, then it may be deemed a failure.

The idea of placing implants in a patient with a history of periodontal disease has been a topic of controversy in the literature. Behind these studies, there exist several factors that make it difficult to compare outcomes. For example, each study may have different parameters with respect to the definition of periodontitis, the severity and treatment of periodontitis, the outcomes measures, the periodontal status at the time of placement, etc. Because of this variability, one cannot say for certain that a patient who experiences tooth loss due to periodontitis has a higher risk of developing peri-implantitis or integration complications.

Bruxism has been implicated in implant component fractures (implant platforms, abutment screws, implant bodies, etc.). Although no actual causal relationship exists, the general consensus in the literature recognizes an association between implant fracture and parafunctional habits. When developing an implant treatment plan for a patient with bruxism, the clinician should plan to minimize eccentric forces, eliminate cantilevers and potentially place additional implants to share the occlusal load (Fig. 3.1). When considering implant fracture, two other main causes have been implicated: manufacturing error and poor prosthetic fit.[5] Although these factors also may contribute to implant fracture, they are much less cited when compared with parafunction. Implant fractures are commonly preceded by multiple incidents of broken abutment screws and bone loss, and may give the clinician an indication that there is an underlying problem. Balshi et al.[5] performed an analysis of 4,045 implants placed in function for 5 years. He found eight fractured

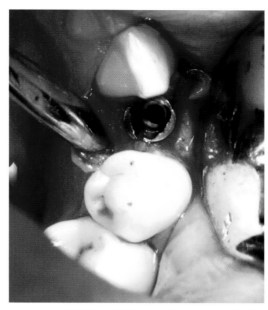

Fig. 3.1. Implant platform fracture caused by over-torquing the final abutment. This implant required removal and replacement.

implants (0.2%). Six were supporting posterior prostheses, and all patients were diagnosed with parafunctional habits. Most of these patients also had preceding problems with loosening or fractured prosthetic or abutment screws prior to fracture.

When examining the soft tissues surrounding the areas of interest, traditionally it was thought that there must be a proper amount of keratinized gingiva present for proper maintenance of implants. Recent studies, however, show that the amount of keratinized gingiva may only be a matter of cosmesis. There are no studies that show an increased loss of implants in areas of inadequate (<2 mm) keratinized mucosa. Kim et al.[6] suggest that there may be an increased risk of gingival recession and marginal bone loss in areas of deficient keratinized mucosa, but this does not necessarily cause adverse effects unless it is in the aesthetic zone and aesthetics are affected. Schrott et al.[7] reported similar findings as part of a prospective 5-year follow-up study of patients who underwent edentulous reconstruction with a fixed, mandibular implant prosthesis. They found that plaque accumulation and bleeding upon probing on the lingual surfaces were greater in patients with less than 2 mm of keratinized mucosa surrounding the implants. Buccal soft tissue recession was also reported to be greater over a 5-year period in patients with inadequate keratinized gingiva. These studies may suggest that patients with inadequate keratinized mucosa around implants may have greater challenges with hygiene leading to subsequent periodontal issues that may or may not impact the overall success of the reconstruction.

Bone quality has been implicated as one of the most important factors for initial implant osseointegration, but is unfortunately difficult to evaluate preoperatively and it is a factor that cannot be changed prior to surgery. It is widely accepted that Misch type 2 and 3 bone is the most favorable for initial osseointegration,[3] but many times, the surgeon may be faced with type 1 or 4 bone at the time of surgery, even if the patient has a fairly normal anatomic and radiographic examination. Sometimes it is not difficult to predict based on the patient's presentation. For instance, a patient with a severely atrophic mandible will most likely have nearly all cortical bone in the anterior mandible. Surgeons need to familiarize themselves with these presentations to make adjustments for bone quality. For instance, a tapered implant may be preferred, healing time may be extended, or a two- versus one-staged procedure may be indicated.

Prosthodontic and Surgical Treatment Planning

Implant reconstruction treatment planning is a team concept. The restorative dentist and surgeon must both provide input for a successful outcome. Failure to include the restorative dentist in the treatment

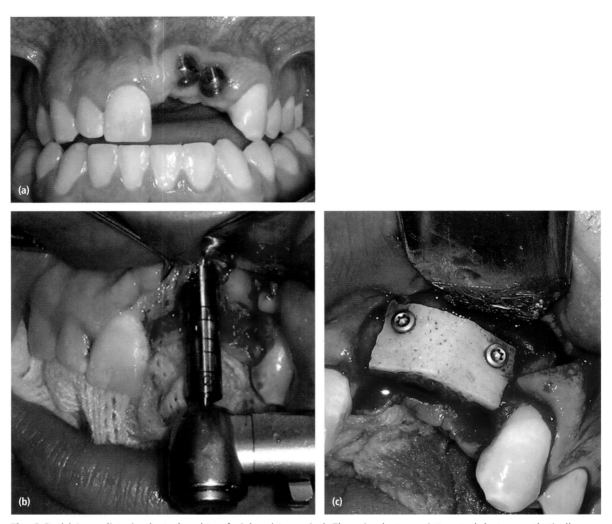

Fig. 3.2. (a) Immediate implant placed too facial and too apical. These implants are integrated, but are esthetically non-restorable. (b) Implant removal with a trephine. (c) An onlay/veneer graft was placed to facilitate proper placement of the implants. (Courtesy of James Q. Swift, DDS)

planning phase could lead to prosthodontic failures because of unrestorability of the implant due to location, angulation problems, or aesthetic failures. Both parties should communicate their preferences with respect to implant location. Many times it is helpful when the restorative dentist provides a surgical guide to assist with implant location and angulation [Figs. 3.2(a)–(c)]. Surgical guides are not always necessary depending on the location of the implants and the skill of the surgeon but can be very helpful for complex cases and aesthetic zone cases, especially those involving multiple implants. Recently, there has been great attention paid to computer-aided treatment planning, surgical guide fabrication, and computer-guided surgery. Currently, there exist no clinical trials indicating the superiority of such techniques. There may be some benefit of obtaining CT imaging when treatment planning sites that may have significant anatomic limitations, but in general, most of the information provided on the CT scan can be obtained by a good clinical examination, mounted models, and plane radiography.

Treatment planning not only addresses location of implants but also time between extraction and implant placement, time to implant loading, and time to final restoration. All of these factors may play a role in the initial integration and implant stability. The alveolar ridge undergoes hard and soft tissue dimensional change after tooth extraction. Several studies have looked at the amount of bone loss that occurs over time after extraction. These studies show a loss of horizontal width between 30 and 50% at 3 to 12 months after extraction.[8–11] Immediate and early implant placement has become an accepted technique to attempt to offset this anatomical change. However, Boticelli et al.,[12] placed 21 immediate implants in 18 patients, and upon re-entry at 4 months found resorption of the bone around the implants: approximately 50% on the buccal plate and 30% on the lingual. Covani[13] found similar outcomes and concluded that immediate implant placement cannot prevent resorption in the alveolar process. Although these studies suggest that bony resorption continues to take place regardless of when the implant is placed after extraction, there is no evidence to suggest that early or immediate placement techniques have a significantly lower rate (or higher rate) of integration success as those placed in a more delayed fashion. The author acknowledges, however, that more clinical studies need to be done in a randomized fashion with clearly defined long-term outcomes to help guide treatment strategies.

Timing to loading of implants is also well debated in the literature, and presumably has an effect on the overall success of implant integration. Jokestad and Carr[14] performed a systematic review of the literature examining timing to loading of implants. Only 22 papers were thought to be adequate for inclusion in the study. Due to the heterogeneity, variable clinical applications, variable outcomes, and lack of quality of evidence, the authors could not make a definitive conclusion. They stated that the average outcome was in favor of delayed loading, but there are no indications that immediate or early loading cannot be a safe procedure. With so many variables to consider (bone quality, type of implant, timing of implant placement relative to extraction, patient factors, prosthetic plan, stability of implant at time of insertion, etc.), one cannot, at this point, prove any superiority to any one loading plan.

Another factor to consider with respect to timing of implant placement and loading includes the augmented ridge or sinus. Aghaloo and Moy[15] performed a systematic review of the literature to determine which hard tissue augmentation procedures are the most successful in furnishing support for implant placement. The study included 90 articles that were acceptable for data extraction and analysis. Regarding sinus augmentation, the authors found that sinus augmentation with allogeneic/nonautogenous composite grafts had the best retention for implants (93%). Autogenous grafts were a close second at 92%, followed by alloplastic grafts at 82%. When looking at alveolar ridge augmentation, Aghaloo and Moy[15] reported the most success for implant survival in sites augmented with guided bone regeneration, onlay veneer grafting, and distraction osteogenesis. The authors, however, did acknowledge the limited number of acceptable studies and the variation in those studies that prevented the development of a definitive conclusion regarding the best hard tissue augmentation to support implant survival.

INTRAOPERATIVE COMPLICATIONS

Intraoperative complications during implant surgery can happen despite the most meticulous planning and preparation. For the most part, few are of large consequence and can be corrected with minor surgery or alteration in the prosthodontic plan. Few are life threatening or leave the patient with a permanent disability, but the chance of such complications is not zero. It is the responsibility of the clinician to include a discussion of risk during the informed consent process. The discussion should include risks of bleeding, pain, swelling, infection, damage to adjacent teeth, sensory disturbance, failure of integration, failure to obtain restorability, displacement of implants (for instance, in the maxillary sinus), and the possibility for the need for additional procedures.

Poor placement with respect to adjacent dentition can be a frustrating problem [Figs. 3.3(a)–(c)]. This can cause an aesthetic problem with the shape or emergence of the crown, and the periodontal health of the adjacent tooth can be affected as well (Fig. 3.4). Planning for implant surgery in locations of anatomic difficulty requires meticulous preoperative planning. Occasionally, complications happen regardless of preparation. In the posterior mandible for instance, care must be taken to plan for the positioning of the implant to avoid the inferior alveolar nerve. Most authors agree that placing the implant within 2 mm of the superior cortex of the inferior alveolar nerve (IAN) can cause a permanent sensory disturbance. Damage can be caused by the implant drill, or submerging the implant itself too apically. Goodacre et al.[16] reported an overall immediate (post stage 1) neurosensory disturbance of 6.1% upon reviewing 13 reports in the literature. The range in incidence was 0.6–39.0%. Most data indicate that the incidence decreases significantly over time.[16] In the case where it appears that there is not sufficient bone height superior to

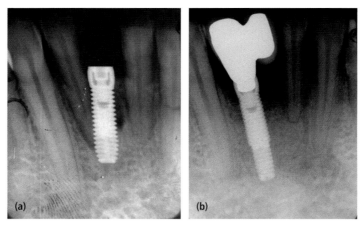

Fig. 3.3. (a) This implant is placed too close to the adjacent tooth and violates the periodontal ligament (PDL) space. (b) Subsequently, there is significant bone loss around the adjacent tooth that required removal of the tooth and the implant. One implant is used to restore both mandibular incisors due to limited space. (All images courtesy of James Q. Swift, DDS.)

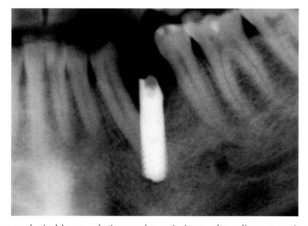

Fig. 3.4. Implant placed at an undesirable angulation and proximity to the adjacent canine. Note the bone loss distal to tooth number 22. The implant abutment is also fractured. This implant and tooth number 22 required removal with guided bone regeneration (GBR) prior to replacing the implants and restoration.

the IAN on plane radiography, alternate imaging techniques may be utilized to obtain a more precise measurement of the existing bone. Of course, if an inadequate height of bone exists, augmentation procedures or a nerve repositioning procedure may be undertaken; however, these procedures also carry risk with regard to sensory disturbance [Figs. 3.5(a), (b)]. Some surgeons would argue that obtaining contemporary forms of imaging (CT, cone beam imaging), and computer-assisted design/computer-assisted manufacturing (CAD/CAM) fabrication of surgical guides would negate this potential complication; however, there are no current published studies that directly compare these groups. Theisen et al.[17] suggested that displacement of implants in the posterior mandible can be attributed in part by the quality of the medullary spaces of bone in that anatomic region. They propose that the cancellous portion of bone in the posterior mandible is more abundant but less dense than in the anterior mandible, and this lack of bone density causes minimal resistance upon penetration of the cortex. In these cases, the drill tends to "drop" into spaces during the preparation, thus rendering the inferior alveolar nerve susceptible to damage if the drill is not properly controlled. When the implant is seated, there is also less resistance, and the implant

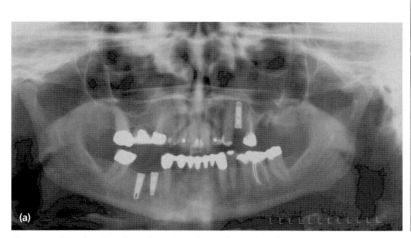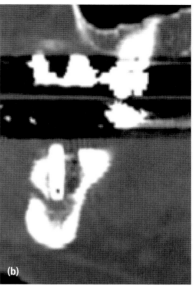

Fig. 3.5. (a) The distal implant (number 30) is placed too apically, encroaching on the IAN. (b) CT confirmation of the position of the implant into the nerve canal.

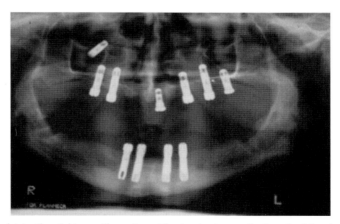

Fig. 3.6. Implant displaced into the right maxillary sinus. The implant was displaced while placing the healing collar.

may be seated deeper than the prepared osteotomy, particularly while tightening the healing abutment or cover screw. The true incidence of inferior alveolar nerve damage during implant placement is not truly known, but diligent preoperative planning and meticulous, controlled surgical technique will minimize this complication. Nonetheless, patients should be made aware of the potential for altered sensation as part of the informed consent process.

The displacement of dental implants is not just confined to the inferior alveolar canal, although that particular region probably poses the chance for the most serious long-term effects. The maxillary sinus has seen its share of displaced substances. Teeth and dental implants are probably the two most common objects that find their way into the maxillary sinus, and several reports in the literature discuss these incidents. Migration of implants into the maxillary sinus can be an acute or delayed event (Fig. 3.6). More commonly, an implant is displaced at the time of placement, although several reports describe implants that have migrated into the maxillary sinus several years after initial integration and restoration. Lida et al.[18] reported the migration of an implant into the sinus 10 years after initial placement. It is unclear what causes the migration of such implants, but the most accepted theory is a combination of osteopenia and excessive occlusal forces.[18] After such an incident, whether acute (at the time of initial surgery) or delayed, the implant should be retrieved via lateral antrostomy, and the surgeon may elect to augment the sinus at the same time if continued reconstruction is desired.

Several reports of severe sublingual hematoma formation have been reported in the literature.[19–22] Most articles reviewed involved patients undergoing two mandibular interforaminal implants to support an overdenture; however, one incident was related to an implant placed posterior to the mental foramen. Most patients experienced some degree of airway compromise necessitating intubation or a surgical airway. The reported etiology was lingual plate dehiscence with vascular injury. Three of four recent case reports reviewed noted significantly elevated systolic blood pressure at the time of hematoma formation.[19–21] Most were observed at the time of implant placement; one was delayed 3 hours after placement of the implants.[19] In most instances, treatment included hospital admission with airway management, steroids, and antibiotics. Surgical management was aimed at airway management and not necessarily drainage of the hematoma or ligation of the offending vessels. It has been suggested that in such instances, arterial ligation may be very technically difficult due to the engorgement of the tissues and the retraction of the offending vessel into the deeper tissues of the floor of the mouth and should only be performed in uncontrollable bleeding.[21] A secure airway and access to vessels via a neck incision require sterile conditions, and this is performed on the operating table. In all recently reported instances, the hematomas resolved after several days of close observation with a range in hospital stay from 3 to 11 days. Hofschneider[23] and Bevitz[24] have performed anatomic studies that suggest that branches of the submental or sublingual arteries are most at risk for injury in the floor of the mouth due to their potential intimate proximity to the lingual cortex of the mandible.

The rare, fatal complication of air embolism has been associated with implant placement.[25,26] In all cases, air was introduced into the cancellous marrow spaces in the mandible, forming an air embolism into the venous system. The air embolus then travels to the superior vena cava and subsequently into the right atrium resulting in cardiopulmonary collapse, leading to cardiac arrest. In all reported cases, implant drills with a combination of air and water internal irrigation were used. This complication can be prevented by using implant drills that are not air driven and do not have irrigation systems that are driven by air pressure. This complication is not limited to implant surgery, as several incidents have been reported in patients undergoing other dental procedures. Again, in these cases, air–water irrigation drills have been implicated as the source of the introduction of air into the venous system.

Early Postoperative Complications

Although the incidence of postoperative infections following implant surgery is low, the idea of antibiotic prophylaxis remains controversial. Several conflicting reports regarding the use of antibiotic coverage either preoperatively or postoperatively currently exist in the literature. Binahmed et al.[27] performed a two-center prospective study administering either a single preoperative dose of antibiotics before implant surgery or a 1-week postoperative regimen. It is unclear if the patients were randomized. In the study, 215 patients were enrolled and 747 implants were placed. There were slightly more patients and implants placed in the group that received a single preoperative dose (125 patients vs. 90 patients; 445 implants vs. 302 implants). There were no control patients who were not given antibiotics. The authors found no statistical difference between the groups, indicating that long-term postoperative antibiotics are of no advantage over a single preoperative dose. Kashani et al.[28] performed a similar study and concluded the same outcomes. Again this study evaluated a single preoperative dose compared to a 1-week postoperative regimen, and there were no controls receiving no antibiotic therapy. Mazzocchi et al.[29] performed a retrospective study including 437 consecutively treated patients undergoing implant placement. This population of patients did not receive antibiotic therapy but received anti-inflammatory therapy for 3 days following surgery. The authors found similar outcomes to success rates published in the literature and concluded that the use of antibiotics for routine implant placement may not be beneficial. In this study the published outcomes acted as a control, but there was no direct comparison between patients receiving antibiotics and those who were not. There are no large, randomized clinical trials to compare antibiotic prophylaxis with no antibiotic coverage at the time of implant surgery, but it appears from the published literature that a single preoperative antibiotic dose is similar in implant success outcomes to a 1-week postoperative course.

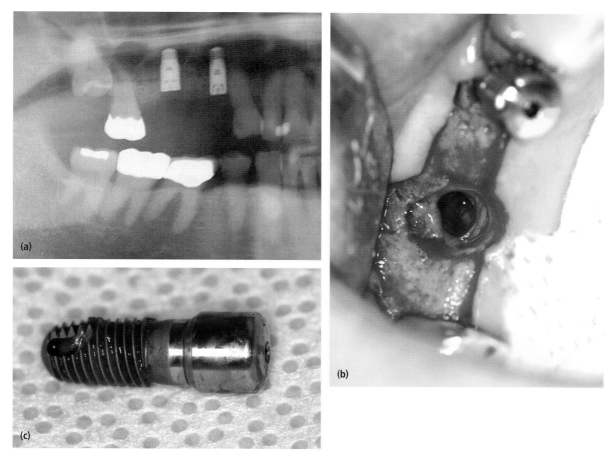

Fig. 3.7. (a) Panoramic radiograph showing implant at tooth number 3 site with peri-implant radiolucency and sinus contact with implant. (b) Site after implant removal; note the fibrous tissue lining the osteotomy site. (c) The implant was removed with finger pressure. (All images courtesy of Mark E. Engelstad, DDS, MD.)

Delayed Postoperative Complications

Fibrous Integration

Fibrous integration occurs when there is a lack of osseointegration [Figs. 3.7(a), (b)]. In such cases, many times the patient does not have any symptomatology, and the fibrous integration is discovered at the second stage surgery for implant uncovery or abutment placement. In these cases, the patient usually experiences pain upon manipulation or tightening of the healing or final abutment. Subsequently, the clinician finds that the implant is mobile and nonintegrated. The two most often assumed causes of fibrous integration are overheating of the bone during initial implant surgery or overpreparation of the osteotomy. In the latter instance, the implant typically will not torque to 20 newton cm at the time of placement. At least two articles[30,31] describe the threshold for bone necrosis at increased temperature. It has been shown that temperatures greater than 48°C cause necrosis of surrounding osteocytes.[32] A study by Senar[33] showed that *in vitro*, more heat is generated in the superficial portion of the osteotomy and concluded that external irrigation at room temperature can provide sufficient cooling during implant preparation.

Sinusitis

Most reports of chronic sinus disease or infection in the case of dental implants are usually related to sinus augmentation. It is a rare finding to see chronic sinus symptoms with successfully integrated maxillary implants near a nonaugmented sinus, even when the apices of the implants violate the floor of the maxillary sinus. Raghoebar et al.[34] reported a case of rhinosinusitis in 69-year-old woman who underwent reconstruction of a completely edentulous maxilla with six implants and an implant-supported overdenture. There were no sinus augmentation procedures performed to facilitate implant placement. The patient complained of rhinorrhea, nasal congestion, and paranasal headaches. Thorough examination via endoscopy revealed that two implants extended through the nasal floor, the nasal mucosa, and the ostium of the maxillary sinus was hyperemic. Instead of removing the implants, the surgeon amputated the apical portion of the implants that extruded through the nasal floor, and the patient's symptoms resolved.

Mandible Fracture

Mandible fracture is an uncommon complication due to implant reconstruction, and has been reported almost exclusively in the atrophic, edentulous mandible. Several factors need to be addressed when treatment planning for these cases. Imaging needs to clearly delineate not only the height of the mandible, but also the width. A minimum height of 7–10 mm and a minimum width of 6–8 mm of bone is required for implant placement.[35] In most reports, mandible fracture occurred after the restoration of the implants, and the prosthesis was in function for a period of months to years [Figs. 3.8(a)–(d)]. Mandible fractures secondary to implant reconstruction are rare and typically occur in atrophic edentulous mandibles. The treatment should follow basic trauma principles regarding atrophic mandible fractures. Immobilization and fixation with a large reconstruction plate is necessary for stability, and bone grafting may be necessary given the cortical, noncancellous nature of the bone that renders the healing capacity of the atrophic

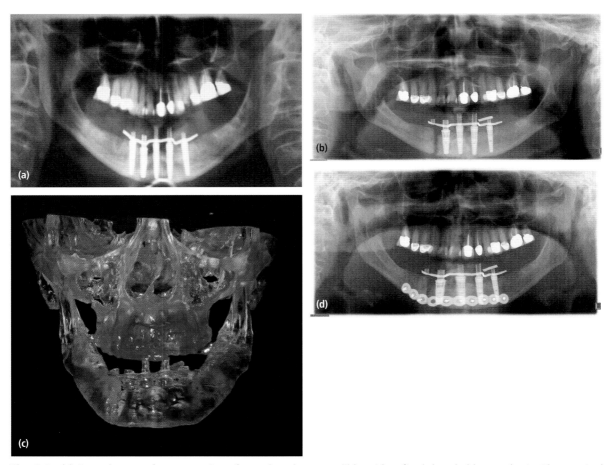

Fig. 3.8. (a) Several years after restoration of an edentulous mandible with a fixed-detachable prosthesis. The terminal implant on the right failed and was subsequently removed. (b) Mandible fracture through the site where the implant was removed. (c) Stereolithography (SLA) model used to create a jig to help position the reconstruction plate and screws while avoiding implant fixtures. (d) Postoperative panorex after reconstruction. (All images courtesy of David L. Basi, DMD, PhD.)

mandible. Additional bone grafting for augmentation may also be considered before implant placement in the atrophic, edentulous mandible. Several techniques have been described to facilitate the reconstruction. Also, the use of the transmandibular implant has been advocated in severely atrophic mandibles, but a recent study suggests that the long-term outcomes may not be superior to traditional techniques of implant placement as originally reported.[36]

Peri-implant Disease

Peri-implant disease is probably the most frustrating finding with respect to late implant complications. Heitz-Mayfield[37] suggested that peri-implant disease is the result of an imbalance between bacterial load and host defense. She further defines the disease as two entities, peri-implantitis, and peri-implant mucositis. What makes these entities so frustrating is the fact that there no clear clinical guidelines with respect to the cause of the problem, and there are no clear clinical guidelines to successfully treat these problems with any overwhelming success.

A recent review of the literature attempted to evaluate diagnosis and risk indicators of peri-implant disease.[37] The review identified 138 acceptable articles out of 1,113 published articles on this topic. In this meta-analysis the definition of the entities was as follows: Peri-implant mucositis is inflammation of the tissues surrounding the implant; peri-implantits implies the additional involvement of the supporting bone such as the case in marginal bone loss. Both have been related to the presence of bacterial invasion. Diagnosing peri-implant disease is not different from diagnosing periodontal diseases. Bleeding on probing (BOP) was shown to have a 100% positive predictive value for progression of peri-implant disease and therefore is considered a valuable parameter for diagnosis.[38] Furthermore, Luterbacher[38] found that the presence of specific bacteria along with BOP enhanced the prognosis of disease progression. The bacteria that were cultured were *Aggregatibacter actinomycetemcomitans*, *Prevotella intermedia*, *Porphyromonas gingivalis*, and *Treponema denticola*. Recent research has also been centered around salivary biomarkers, and although promising at present there is no correlation between biomarkers and disease severity or progression.[37] Because of the length of time that it takes for peri-implant diseases to develop, large, prospective, longitudinal studies are required to determine risk factors. Unfortunately, there are very few reported in the literature and most are retrospective, cross-sectional studies. The latter have been used in several literature reviews to determine risk factors. In one such study, the presence of periodontal disease, smoking history, diabetes, genetic traits, poor oral hygiene, alcohol consumption, and implant surface were examined as possible risk indicators.[37] The author found that there was substantial evidence that poor oral hygiene, history of periodontitis, and cigarette smoking are associated with peri-implant disease. There was limited evidence that diabetes and alcohol consumption are associated with peri-implant disease. There was conflicting and limited evidence for any conclusions regarding genetic traits and implant surface.

Once peri-implant disease is diagnosed, the clinician must decide how to treat the problem. Basically, surgical or nonsurgical therapy can be employed. Renvert et al.[39] reviewed the literature to evaluate nonsurgical treatment of peri-implant mucositis and peri-implantitis. First and foremost, they found that the literature was significantly lacking. Twenty-four studies were included in the review out of a possible 437 articles that were identified and included human and animal studies. The review evaluated mechanical therapy alone, mechanical therapy with adjunctive chlorhexidine rinse, and mechanical therapy with adjunctive systemic antimicrobials. They concluded that in the case of peri-implant mucositis, mechanical nonsurgical therapy can be effective, and the use of antimicrobial mouth rinses enhanced the mechanical therapy outcomes. In peri-implantitis cases, nonsurgical therapy was not found to be effective, and adjunctive antimicrobial (CHX) application had limited benefit. Adjunctive systemic antimicrobial therapy was shown to reduce BOP and probing depths.

Surgical therapy for peri-implant diseases has been reported in the literature, but the study designs are less than optimal. Also, there are tremendous variables involved in surgical treatment of peri-implantitis. Variables include surgical approach, implant surface decontamination procedures and substances, presence and type of bone grafting, presence and type of antimicrobials, and presence and type of membranes. Because of this large variability, one cannot equivocally advocate for a particular treatment. In addition, there have been no studies that include controls that have not received therapy to compare to the treatment groups.

SUMMARY

Implant complications can, for the most part, be avoided by diligent patient evaluation, multidisciplinary treatment planning, and a thorough understanding of and respect for the physiologic and clinical contributions of implant integration and wound healing. Nonetheless, complications do happen. If clinicians can anticipate or prepare for problems ahead of time, the more likely they will be able to manage complications most appropriately.

SUGGESTED READINGS

1. Moy P, Medina D, Shetty V, and Aghaloo T. 2005. "Dental implant failure rates and associated risk factors." *Journal of Oral and Maxillofacial Implants* 20(4): 569–577.
2. Klokkevold P, and Han T. 2007. "How do smoking, diabetes, and periodontitis affect outcomes of implant treatment?" *The International Journal of Oral and Maxillofacial Implants* 22(suppl): 173–206.
3. Martin R, Carter J, and Barber HD. 2000. "Surgical implant failures." In: *Oral and Maxillofacial Surgery*, Vol. 7, 1st ed. Fonseca R, Powers M, and Barber HD, eds. Philadelphia: W.B. Saunders Company.
4. Cochrane D, Schou S, Heitz-Mayfield LJA, Bornstein MM, Salvi GE, and Martin WC. 2009. "Consensus statements and recommended clinical procedures regarding risk factors in implant therapy." *The International Journal of Oral and Maxillofacial Implants* 24(suppl): 86–89.
5. Balshi T. 1997. "An analysis and management of fractured implants: A clinical report." *Journal of Oral and Maxillofacial Implants* 11(5): 660–666.
6. Kim BS, Kim YK, Yun PY, Yi YJ, Lee HJ, Kim SG, and Son JS. 2009. "Evaluation of peri-implant tissue response according to the presence of keratinized mucosa." *Oral Surgery, Oral Medicine, Oral Pathology, Oral Radiology, and Endodontology* 107(3): e24–e28.
7. Schrott AR, Jimenez M, Hwang JW, Fiorellini J, and Weber HP. 2009. "Five-year evaluation of the influence of keratinized mucosa on peri-implant soft-tissue health and stability around implants supporting full-arch mandibular fixed prostheses." *Clin Oral Implants Res* 20(10): 1170–7.
8. Schropp L, Kostopoulos L, and Wenzel A. 2003. "Bone healing following immediate versus delayed placement of titanium implants into extraction sockets: A prospective clinical study." *Int J Periodontics Restorative Dent* 23(4): 313–323.
9. Schropp L, Wenzel A, Kostopoulos L, and Karring T. 2003. "Bone healing and soft tissue contour changes following single-tooth extraction: A clinical and radiographic 12 month prospective study." *Int J Periodontics Restorative Dent* 23: 313–323.
10. Camargo PM, Lekovic V, Weinlaender M, et al. 2000. "Influence of bioactive glass on changes in alveolar process dimensions after exodontia." *Oral Surgery, Oral Medicine, Oral Pathology, Oral Radiology & Endodontics* 90: 581–586.
11. Lasella JM, Greenwell H, Miller RL, et al. 2003. "Ridge preservation with freeze-dried bone allograft and a collagen membrane compared to extraction alone for implant site development: A clinical and histologic study in humans." *J Periodontol* 74: 990–999.
12. Botticelli D, Berglundh T, and Lindhe J. 2004. "Hard-tissue alterations following immediate implant placement in extraction sites." *J Clin Periodontol* 31: 820–828.
13. Covani U, Bortolaia C, Barone A, and Sbordone L. 2004. "Bucco-lingual crestal bone changes after immediate and delayed implant placement." *J Periodontol* 75: 1605–1612.
14. Jokstad A, and Carr A. 2007. "What is the effect on outcomes of time-to-loading of a fixed or removable prosthesis placed on implant(s)?" *Int Journal of Oral and Maxillofacial Implants* 22(suppl): 19–48.
15. Aghaloo TL, and Moy PK. 2007. "Which hard tissue augmentation techniques are the most successful in furnishing bony support for implant placement?" *Int J Oral Maxillofac Implants* 22(suppl): 49–70.
16. Goodacre CJ, Kan JYK, and Rungcharassaeng K. 1999. "Clinical complications of osseointegrated implants." *Jounal of Prosthetic Dentistry* 81(5): 537–552.
17. Theisen F, Shulz R, and Elledge D. 1990. "Displacement of a root form implant into the mandibular canal." *Oral Surgery, Oral Medicine, Oral Pathology, Oral Radiology & Endodontics* 70(1): 24–28.
18. Lida L, Tanaka N, Kogo M, and Matsuya T. 2000. "Migration of a dental implant into the maxillary sinus: A case report." *Int J Oral Maxillofacial Surg* 29: 358–359.
19. Ferneini E, Gady J, and Lieblich S. 2009. "Floor of mouth hematoma after posterior mandibular implants placement." *J Oral Maxillofac Surg* 67: 1552–1554.
20. Pigadas N, Simoes P, and Tuffin JR. 2009. "Massive sublingual haematoma following osseo-integrated implant placement in the anterior mandible." *British Dental Journal* 206: 67–68.
21. Niamtu J. 2001. "Near-fatal airway obstruction after routine implant placement." *Oral Surgery, Oral Medicine, Oral Pathology, Oral Radiology & Endodontics* 92(6): 597–600.
22. Givol N, Chaushu G, Halamish-Shani T, and Taicher S. 2000. "Emergency tracheostomy following life-threatening hemorrhage in the floor of the mouth during immediate implant placement in the mandibular canine region." *J Periodontol* 71(12): 1893–1895.

23. Hofschneider U, Tepper G, Gahleitner A, and Ulm C. 1999. "Assessment of the blood supply to the mental region for reduction of bleeding complications during implant surgery in the interforaminal region." *Int J Oral Maxillofac Implants* 14: 379–383.

24. Bavitz JB, Harn SD, and Homze EJ. 1994. "Arterial supply to the floor of the mouth and lingual gingivae." *Oral Surgery, Oral Medicine, Oral Pathology, Oral Radiology & Endodontics* 77: 232–235.

25. Davies JM, and Campbell L. 1999. "Fatal air embolism during dental implant surgery: A report of three cases." *Can J Anaesth* 37(1): 112–121.

26. Girdler NM. 1994. "Fatal sequel to dental implant surgery." *Journal of Oral Rehabilitation* 21: 721–722.

27. Binahmed A, Stoykewych A, and Peterson L. 2005. "Single preoperative dose versus long-term prophylactic antibiotic regimens in dental implant surgery." *Int J Oral Maxillofac Implants* 20(1): 115–117.

28. Kashani H, Dahlin C, and Alse'n B. 2005. "Influence of different prophylactic antibiotic regimens on implant survival rate: A retrospective clinical study." *Clin Implant Dent Relat Res* 7: 32–35.

29. Mazzocchi A, Passi L, and Moretti R. 2007. "Retrospective analysis of 736 implants inserted without antibiotic therapy." *J Oral Maxillofac Surg* 65: 2321–2323.

30. Li S, Chien S, and Branemark PI. 1999. "Heat shock-induced necrosis and apoptosis in osteoblasts." *Journal of Orthopaedic Research* 17(6): 891–899.

31. Eriksson RA, and Alberksson T. 1983. "Temperature threshold levels for heat induced bone tissue injury: A vital microscopic study in rabbit." *Journal of Prosthetic Dentistry* 50: 101–107.

32. Yoshida K, Uoshima K, Oda K, and Maeda T. 2009. "Influence of heat stress to matrix on bone formation." *Clin Oral Impl Res* 20: 782–790.

33. Sener BC, Dergin G, Gursoy B, Kelesoglu E, and Slih I. 2009. "Effects of irrigation temperature on heat control in vitro at different drilling depths." *Clin Oral Impl Res* 20: 294–298.

34. Raghoebar GM, van Weissenbruch R, and Vissink A. 2004. "Rhino-sinusitis related to endosseous implants extending into the nasal cavity." *Int J Oral Maxillofac Surg* 33: 312–314.

35. Raghoebar GM, Stellingsma K, Batenburg RHK, and Vissink A. 2000. "Etiology and management of madibular fractures associated with endosteal implants in the atrophic mandible." *Oral Surgery, Oral Medicine, Oral Pathology, Oral Radiology & Endodontics* 89: 553–559.

36. Paton G, Fuss J, and Goss A. 2002. "The transmandibular implant: A 5- and 15-year single center study." *J Oral Maxillofac Surg* 60: 851–857.

37. Heitz-Mayfield L. 2008. "Peri-implant diseases: Diagnosis and risk indicators." *J Clin Periodontol* 35(suppl 8): 292–304.

38. Luterbacher S, Mayfield L, Bragger U, and Lang NP. 2000. "Diagnostic characteristics of clinical and microbiological tests for monitoring periodontal and peri-implant mucosal tissue conditions during supportive periodontal therapy." *Clinical Oral Implants Research* 11: 521–529.

39. Renvert S, Roos-Jansaker AM, and Claffey N. 2008. "Non-surgical treatment of peri-implant mucositis and peri-implantitis: A literature review." *J Clin Periodontol* 35(suppl 8): 305–315.

4

Maxillofacial Trauma

R. Bryan Bell, DDS, MD, FACS
Michael R. Markiewicz, DDS, MPH
Savannah Gelesko, DDS

INTRODUCTION

Complications in the treatment of cranio-maxillofacial injuries occur regularly and, even in the most experienced of hands, should be expected. Many, but not all, complications can be prevented by adherence to proper surgical technique and established treatment protocols, and by recognizing the potential for functional or aesthetic complications. While expected surgical complications such as infection and non-union of mandibular fractures are still associated with excellent outcomes if managed properly, those related to inaccurate reduction of midfacial and orbital fractures that result in facial widening and/or enophthalmos, respectfully, are exceedingly difficult to correct secondarily. The ultimate outcome for patients with cranio-maxillofacial trauma is thus less dependent upon the occurrence of complications and more upon the recognition of pitfalls during treatment and management of complications when they inevitably occur.

SOFT TISSUE INJURIES

Soft tissue injuries to the maxillofacial region may be complicated by infection or functional impairment of regional anatomy. Identification of risk factors for the development of complications is of paramount importance. Primary repair is both feasible and preferred for most facial wounds, and neurovascular and ductal injuries, even in the severely contaminated wound [Figs. 4.1(a)–(c)]. The rationale for this approach is that a significant number of patients will not develop infections and thus can benefit from the aesthetic and functional advantages of primary wound healing. Secondary reconstruction may be considered for highly contaminated wounds, or those with avulsive components. Administration of tetanus prophylaxis and appropriate antibiotics for contaminated wounds is the standard of care and should follow current guidelines; however, this topic is beyond the scope of this chapter.

Animal Bites

Dog and cat bites comprise an estimated 1% of emergency room visits per year in the United States.[1–2] An estimated 60% of animal bites are from dogs, and 10–20% are from cats, although the incidence of dog bite injuries is declining.[3] Death associated with dog bites is very rare, with only 300 dog-bite related deaths occurring from 1979–1996.[4] The incidence of fracture or laceration associated with dog bite injuries is between 4% and 7%.[5]

Infection is the most common complication associated with dog and cat bites, occurring in approximately 20% of cases.[6] The most common bacteria implicated in animal bite-related infections are

Management of Complications in Oral and Maxillofacial Surgery, First Edition. Edited by Michael Miloro, Antonia Kolokythas.
© 2012 John Wiley & Sons, Inc. Published 2012 by John Wiley & Sons, Inc.

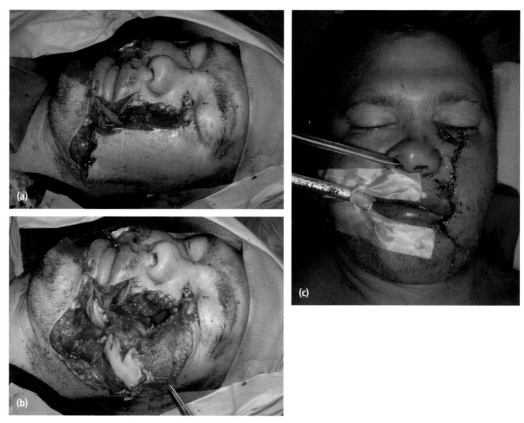

Fig. 4.1. Complex soft tissue injury. Primary repair is both feasible and preferred for most facial wounds, neurovascular, and ductal injuries, even in the severely contaminated wound. (a) Preoperative appearance. (b) Intraoperative view prior to anatomic layered closure. (c) Postoperative appearance.

Capnocytophaga, *Canimorsus*, and *Pasteurella species*. Infections from *C canimorsus* are aggressive in nature, and laboratory diagnosis is often difficult; therefore, antibiotic therapy should be started as early as possible when *C canimorsus* infection is suspected.

Canine Bites

Larger dog breeds such as Pit bull terriers, Rottweilers, and German shepherds, which lead the list of aggressive dog injuries, mostly cause high pressure crush injuries, while smaller breeds most often cause soft-tissue skin injuries.[6] While adults most often sustain bites to the hand, children are most commonly bitten in the face.[7,8,9] Bacteria specific to dog bite wounds include aerobes such as *Pasteurella*, *Streptococcus*, *Staphylococcus*, and *Neisseria*, and anaerobes such as *Fusobacterium*, *Bacteroides*, *Porphyromonas*, *Prevotella*, and *Capnocytophaga canimorsus*.[8]

Severe "mauling" type of dog bites can cause devestating neurovascular complicaitons, resulting in cranial neuropathy or exanguinating hemmorhage [Figs. 4.2(a) and (b)]. Injuries involving the neck or parotid region in particular should undergo thorough clinical and radiographic interrogation prior to definitive repair. Primary neurorraphy, duct repair, and/or vascular repair should be considered for major neurovascular injury or disruption of the nasolacrimal or parotid duct.

Feline Bites

Cat bite injuries are more likely than dog bites to cause injury to the face.[10] In addition, due to cats' narrow and sharp teeth, they are more likely to "inoculate" the victim by inflicting puncture wounds to the deeper soft tissue layers, which results in a higher complication rate than dog bites. The most common complications related to cat bites are localized wound infection, septic arthritis, and osteomyelitis.

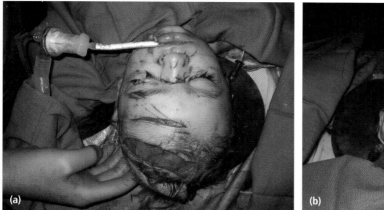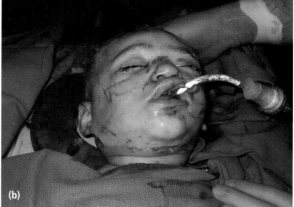

Fig. 4.2. Three-year-old child involved in "mauling" injury from dog. (a) Bird's-eye view. (b) Worm's-eye view.

Human Bites

Unlike animal wounds that become infected from the oral flora of the offending animal, infections from human bite wounds are usually secondary in origin and can occur in an estimated 10–20% of human bite wounds.[11,12] Primary closure is safe and advised after proper wound cleansing.[13,14]

Management of Bite Injuries

Animal bites presenting for treatment more than 8 hours after injury are at high risk for the development of suppurative complications, with cat bite wounds progressing at a faster rate than dog bite wounds.[8] Prophylactic antibiotics should be given in selected cases with coverage based on specific animal type. *Capnocytophaga canimorsus* and *Pasteurella species* are not susceptible to clindamycin, erythromycin, dicloxacillin, or cephalexin; therefore, these antibiotics should not be used. Amoxicillin–clavulanic acid provides excellent coverage against *Pasteurella multocida*, *Capnocytophaga canimorsus*, anaerobes, and susceptible *S aureus*, and should be considered first-line antibiotic therapy. Doxycycline combined with metronidazole should be considered in penicillin-allergic patients. If *Methicillin-resistant Staphylococcus aureus* (MRSA) is highly prevalent in the community, doxycycline can be considered as oral prophylaxis. For inpatient management, ampicillin–sulbactam, piperacillin–tazobactam, or ticarcillin–clavulanic acid should be considered first-line agents. Ceftriaxone, aztreonam, or a fluoroquinolone have good gram-negative coverage; combined with metronidazole, they are adequate alternatives. Monotherapy with a carbapenem such as ertapenem, meropenem, doripenem, or imipenem–cilastatin may also be considered. Indications for hospitalization include fever, sepsis, uncontrolled cellulitis, edema or fracture injury, loss of function, patients with immunocompromised status, or noncompliant patients.

Parotid Duct Injury

Injury to the parotid gland and duct should be suspected with any deep laceration to the cheek or neighboring structures. Van Sickels[15] divided the parotid gland and duct injuries into three different anatomic regions: region A, the area of the gland; region B, the site of the duct as it runs superficial to the masseter muscle; and region C, the region of the duct from the masseter muscle to where the duct meets the oral cavity exiting the buccal mucosa adjacent to the maxillary second molar. Initial assessment should include a full cranial nerve examination. Since the buccal branch of the facial nerve travels with the parotid duct after it crosses the superficial layer of the masseter muscle after exiting the parotid gland, facial motor function should also be assessed with any parotid duct injury—specifically motor function of the upper lip. Prior to primary closure, the wound should be explored to ascertain the integrity of the parotid duct and facial nerve.

Surgical options for parotid duct repair include: (1) primary repair; (2) ligation; and (3) fistulization of the duct into the oral cavity.[16] Stenting and primary repair of the duct becomes increasingly difficult with

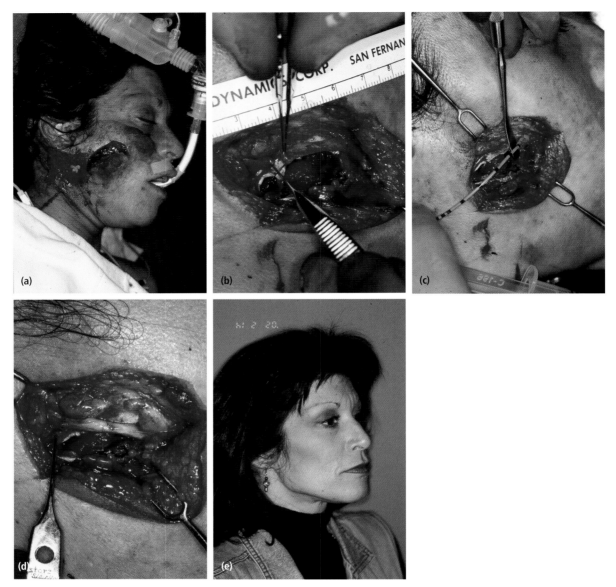

Fig. 4.3. Forty-three-year-old woman involved in a knife assault. (a) Preoperative appearance; (b) Identification of the proximal and distal stumps of Stenson's duct. (c) Stenting of Stenson's duct. (d) Primary anastomosis with 7-0 nylon suture. (e) Postoperative appearance.

surrounding soft tissue edema and maceration. Some authors suggest leaving stents in for several weeks following duct repair,[17,18] while others recommend stent removal following primary closure of the duct.[16,19] Detractors of long-term stent placement cite a higher occurrence of sialocele formation. Delayed parotid duct reconstruction has been successfully reported and may be more feasible from a technical standpoint. In a study by Lewis and Knottenbelt,[20] nineteen patients with parotid duct injuries underwent primary closure of the wound. Though ten patients had complications (seven with salivary fistula and four with sialoceles), all healed without surgical intervention. Primary repair whenever feasible is preferred [Figs. 4.3(a)–(e)]. If the proximal and distal ends of the parotid duct cannot be reapproximated, a pseudo-duct can be created by placing a drain with its origin at the parotid gland and terminal end in an orifice created into the buccal mucosa (fistulization).

Sialocele Formation

Sialoceles are common sequelae following parotid duct injury and repair. Sialoceles more proximal to the gland have been shown to respond to medical treatment, including the administration of antisialogogues and antibiotics. Surgical management include aspiration and pressure dressing placement, as well as fistulization as described above. The use of botulinum toxin injection into parotid glands with fistulas has also been shown to produce resolution of sialocele.[21,22] Long-lasting complications to the duct and gland that are unresponsive to previously described management may be definitely treated by parotidectomy, although the need for this is exceedingly rare.

Peripheral Facial Nerve Injury

Extracranial facial nerve injury may occur with any trauma to the region between the tragus of the ear and the commissure of the lip. The House-Brackmann classification of facial function is helpful in quantifying and documenting facial nerve function after an injury [Figs. 4.4(a)–(e)]. An accurate assessment of the

Grade	Definition
I	Normal symmetrical function in all areas.
II	Slight weakness noticeable only on close inspection. Complete eye closure with minimal effort. Slight asymmetry of smile with maximal effort. Synkinesis barely noticeable, contracture, or spasm absent.
III	Obvious weakness, but not disfiguring. May not be able to lift eyebrow. Complete eye closure and strong but asymmetrical mouth movement with maximal effort. Obvious, but not disfiguring synkinesis, mass movement or spasm.
IV	Obvious disfiguring weakness. Inability to lift brow. Incomplete eye closure and asymmetry of mouth with maximal effort. Severe synkinesis, mass movement, spasm.
V	Motion barely perceptible. Incomplete eye closure, slight movement corner mouth. Synkinesis, contracture, and spasm usually absent.
VI	No movement, loss of tone, no synkinesis, contracture, or spasm.

(a) House, J.W. and Brackmann, D.E. (1985) Facial nerve grading system. *Otolaryngol. Head Neck Surg.,* **93**, 146–147.

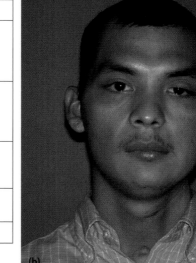
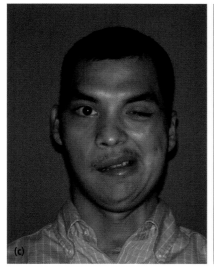
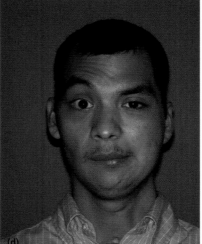
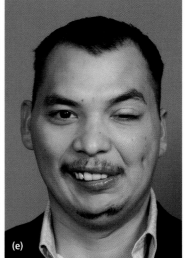

Fig. 4.4. House-Brackmann scale of facial function. (a) Outline. (b) Facial nerve injury, repose. (c) Facial nerve injury, animation. (d) Facial nerve injury; animation. (e) Facial nerve injury, 5 years after nerve grafting, note synkinesis.

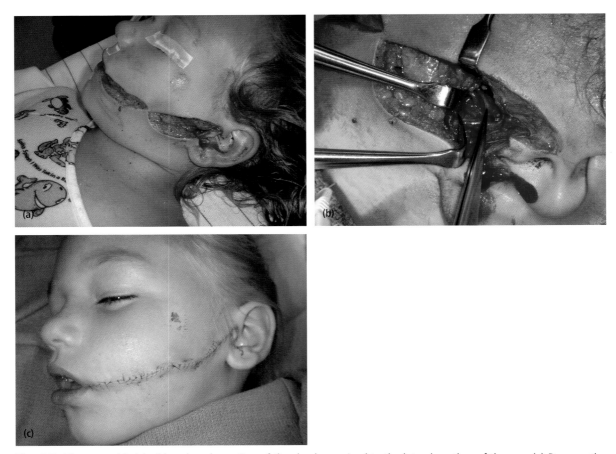

Fig. 4.5. Five-year-old girl with a deep laceration of the cheek, proximal to the lateral canthus of the eye. (a) Preoperative appearance. (b) Intraoperative exploration of facial nerve. (c) Wound closure.

involved anatomy and identification of the location of an injury following cranio-maxillofacial trauma is most important for determining the most ideal therapeutic intervention.

Following a complete neurological examination (if possible), the wound should be thoroughly evaluated prior to repair. Injury to the peripheral segment of the facial nerve proximal to a line drawn vertically from the lateral cantus of the eye is preferentially repaired by direct coaptation using microsurgical technique, without grafting if possible [Figs. 4.5(a)–(c)]. The goal in facial nerve repair should be restoration of facial tone, facial symmetry, and voluntary facial movement.[23] If tension-free coaptation is not possible, consideration can be given to the use of an interpositional nerve graft. The great auricular nerve is usually available and can be harvested without a second incision. Alternatively, a sural nerve graft may be harvested for this purpose. Another option is the hypoglossal-facial nerve (XII to VII) neurorrhaphy with or without grafting, although this technique may be preferred in the secondary setting due to the donor site morbidity.[24,25] Lagophthalmos should be managed with a gold weight relatively soon after injury and neurorrhaphy.

Nasolacrimal Injury

Injury to the nasolacrimal apparatus commonly occurs following injury to the eyelids and is associated with nasoethmoidal fractures approximately 20% of the time. The presenting sign is typically epiphora. Primary disruption of the nasolacrimal apparatus must be distinguished from eyelid malposition such as ectropion, in which the punctum is not opposed to the globe, both of which result in epiphora.

Additionally, facial nerve paresis may be associated with epiphora secondary to paralytic ectropion or weakness of the orbicularis muscle that is required for normal lacrimal pump function. Chronic inflammation and obstruction of the puncta may be complicated by dacryocystitis, which produces a red, swollen, and painful mass in the medial canthus, requiring prompt attendtion.[26]

The Schirmer secretion test can be used to assess and quantify tear production. After topical anesthetic is administered, white filter paper strips are placed at the junction of the middle and lateral thirds of the lower eyelids and held there with the patient's eyes closed for 5 minutes. The test is normal with greater than 10 mm but less than 30 mm of tear production. A fluorescein dye disappearance test may also be used and is performed by administering topical anesthetic and placing fluorescein dye at the inferior fornix of both eyes. Tear films are compared over a period of 5 to 10 minutes. The dye should drain rapidly through a patent outflow system. Dye in the tear film after 10 minutes indicates an abnormality of lacrimal outflow. Punctal dilation and canalicular probing, as well as lacrimal irrigation, Jones tests, dacryocystography, and dacryoscintigraphy are also used to evaluate lacrimal function.

In the primary setting, disruption of the nasolacrimal duct may be managed by cannulation anastomosis and intubation of the lacrimal duct [Figs. 4.6 (a)–(d)].[27] Chronic lacrimal duct obstruction is most successfully managed with dacryocystorhinostomy,[28] which today is performed endonasally, with an operating microscope to provide increased visualization.

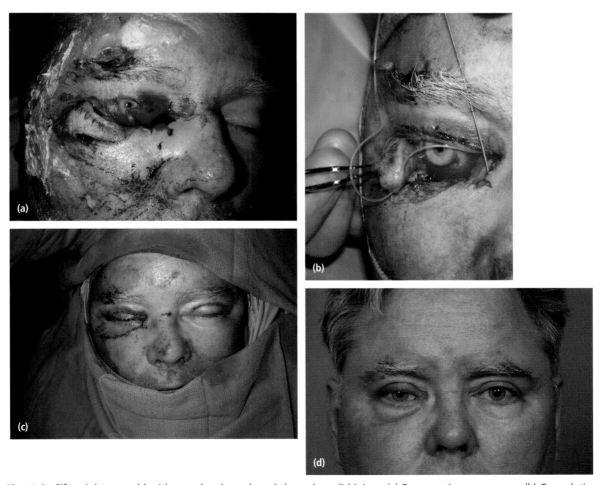

Fig. 4.6. Fifty-eight-year-old with complex through-and-through eyelid injury. (a) Preoperative appearance (b) Cannulation of the lacrimal duct. (c) Eyelid repair with canthopexy and upper eyelid skin graft. (d) Postoperative appearance.

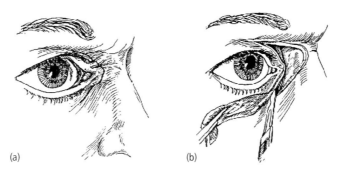

(a)   (b)

Fig. 4.7. Technique for medial ectropion repair. (a) "C-shaped" incision. (b) Tissue advancement with skin grafting the defect.

Ectropion

Several types of eyelid ectropion exist, including congenital, senile, cicatricial, and neurogenic. Cicatricial ectropion is most common in the post-traumatic setting. Scarring involving the midface may cause contracture of the lower eyelid and the resultant scleral show. Alternatively, the complication may be iatrogenic, resulting from improper lid position following lower lid approaches to the orbit. Ectropion may involve the upper lid, lower lid, or both, and result in epiphora and/or other ocular complications. The scar contracture may be medial or lateral, and it may include vertical shortening, horizontal shortening, or both.

Medial Ectropion

Medial ectropion may result from burns or tissue loss on the nasal dorsal skin, which causes scar contracture of the medial canthus in a medial and forward vector. This is often manifested as epicanthal folding, epiphora, and corneal exposure. The general principle of treatment is to restore the original size and location of distorted tissues, and to replace missing tissues with those of the similar structure. Scar release for medial ectropion involves a C-shaped incision over the upper eyelid, lateral nose, and lower eyelid (Fig. 4.7).[29] The resulting defect requires coverage with a full thickness skin graft to minimize secondary contraction. To optimize results and limit recurrence, the skin over the nose beyond the release incision is undermined to allow maximal release, and the periosteum over the frontal process of the maxilla is excised to allow adherence of the graft to the underlining periosteum. Adjunctive medial canthoplasty may be required and can be performed.[30]

Lateral Ectropion

Lateral ectropion is a relatively common iatrogenic complication related to lower eyelid approaches to the orbit (Fig. 4.8). While ectropion is inevitable in maxillofacial trauma surgery, avoiding the traditional "subciliary" approach, in favor of the transconjunctival and midlid incisions, can minimize its incidence.

The initial description of the Z-plasty by Denonvilliers was employed for treatment of lateral ectropion of the lower eyelid (Fig. 4.9).[31] The Z-plasty has the advantage of transposing the retracted lower eyelid tissue superiorly and posteriorly, achieving better adaptation of the lid margin to the globe. However, the additional scar that results from a Z-plasty in this area may be unsightly.[32]

Cicatricial ectropion of either eyelid with vertical shortening is approached with a subciliary release, or alternatively via a subconjuntival approach. The incision is made short of the medial and lateral canthi. Skin flaps are raised to allow approximation of the upper and lower eyelid margins. A bone-anchored lateral canthopexy is performed followed by skin graft if necessary. The eyelids can be separated either immediately, or in delayed fashion, if recurrence is of concern. If necessary, the C-shaped release can be combined with this approach, but should be completed first [Figs. 4.10(a)–(f)].[30] In addition to release and grafting, various local flaps have been described and can be employed for repair of lower eyelid cicatricial ectropion.[32,33]

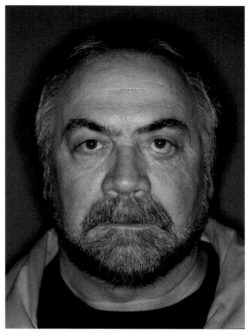

Fig. 4.8. Lower eyelid ectropion with increased scleral show.

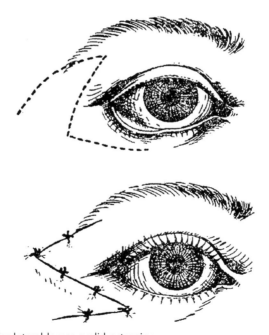

Fig. 4.9. Denonvilliers Z-plasty for lateral lower eyelid ectropion.

Entropion

Post-traumatic entropion is usually seen as complication of lower eyelid approaches which turn the eyelid and lashes inward toward the globe and is associated with increased scleral show and eye injury (Fig. 4.11).[34] Complications of entropion include ocular discomfort, trichiasis, corneal abrasion, microbial keratitis, corneal vascularization, and visual loss.[35] While senile entropion is caused by different pathological

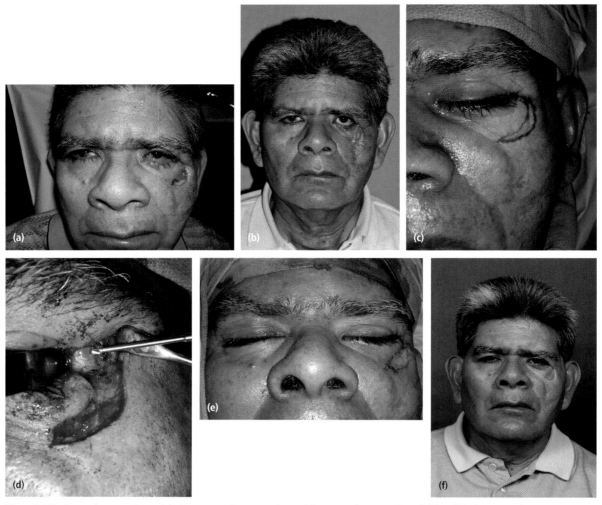

Fig. 4.10. Lateral ectropion. (a) Exposure keratopathy with secondary conjunctivitis. (b) Preoperative appearance demonstrating lateral ectropion secondary to scar contracture. (c) "C-shaped" incision outline. (d) Bone anchored lateral canthopexy. (e) Full thickness skin graft of the defect with lower lid repositioning and lateral canthopexy. (f) Postoperative appearance.

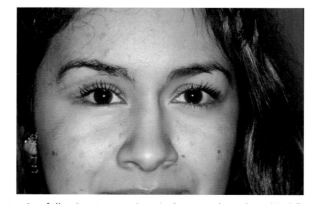

Fig. 4.11. Right lower lid entropion following transconjunctival approach to the orbital floor with lateral canthotomy.

mechanisms such as loss of lid laxity, loss of tension of lower lid retractors, and alterations to the musculus orbicularis, post-traumatic entropion is virtually always cicatricial in nature, and typically associated with transconjunctival approaches to the orbit. Cicatricial entropion can be treated by a keratinized tissue graft from the hard palate.[36] Management may also include anchoring the lateral tarsal tip to the orbital rim and using a single stitch lateral wedge technique. Description of these techniques is outside the scope of this chapter, but abundance of texts and articles are available for further reading.[37]

HARD TISSUE INJURIES

Mandibular Fractures (Symphysis, Body, Angle)

The primary goals of treating mandibular fractures are: (1) to restore form and function by returning the patient to the pre-injury occlusion and achieving anatomic reduction when possible and (2) to achieve osseous union predictably. The appropriate technique to achieve these goals varies based upon location of the fracture, the energy of the injury causing the fracture, and whether or not there is load sharing potential. The most common complications of mandibular fractures include infection, malunion, nonunion, tooth injury, and the need for hardware removal. Adherence to proper surgical techniques and the principles of reduction, stabilization and fixation with appropriate means will assist in minimizing these complications.

Principles of Fixation

A fixation system will provide either absolute (rigid) stability or functional stability. *Rigid stability* occurs when no movement whatsoever occurs across the fracture gap; *functional stability* occurs when movement is possible across the fracture gap but is balanced by external forces and remains within the limits that allow for the fracture to progress to union. While excessive mobility at a fracture site will lead to bone resorption and fibrous tissue ingrowth, absolute rigidity also will not achieve bony union. When excessive mobility is present, any fixation device will promote bone resorption and infection.

Functionally stable fixation is all that is necessary for successful healing of most fractures in the maxillofacial skeleton. Micromotion occurs in this paradigm that permits for secondary bone healing to occur. An example of nonrigid fixation is the use of a single miniplate at the angle of the mandible as described by Champy.[38] Thus, functionally stable fixation may also result in osseous healing and achieve predictable results.

Fixation requirements are considered by the ability of the host bone to share some of the functional loads. *Load-bearing fixation* is of sufficient strength to resist the functional masticatory forces during the healing phase, and the host bone fracture sites share none or little of the functional load. In contrast, *load-sharing fixation* refers to a scheme whereby the functional load is shared between the hardware and the bone along the fracture site. The indications for providing load-bearing fixation are those fractures with comminuted segments, atrophic mandibular fractures, and fractures with avulsed or missing segments. Load-sharing fixation is indicated in cases where no comminution or bone defects are present, and when intact bone cortices are opposed to one another after fracture reduction. The majority of mandibular fractures can be adequately treated with load-sharing fixation.

Teeth in the Line of Fracture

The management of teeth in the line of fracture has been a source of controversy in the literature for decades.[39] While it is clear that retaining grossly mobile or infected teeth in the line of fracture may invite wound healing complications, it is not clear how teeth in the line of fracture in all patients should be managed.

Various authors have attempted to use specific criteria such as tooth mobility, interference with fracture reduction, pulpal pathology, and location of the fracture to determine whether or not the tooth should be removed.[39–46] The preponderance of evidence suggests that teeth in the line of fracture (including third molars) may be retained providing that they do not interfere with favorable reduction, stabilization, and fixation of the fracture, and are not grossly mobile or infected. This approach has yielded a complication rate similar to other reported complication rates, regardless of the presence or absence of teeth in the line of fracture.[47]

Infections

Infection is the most common complication in patients undergoing treatment of mandibular fractures, occurring between 1% and 32% of the time.[48–58] Numerous risk factors have been associated with postoperative infection, including substance abuse or patient noncompliance with postoperative care regimens,[48] as well as significant delay in treatment.[59] Antibiotics have been shown to be effective in preventing infection when instituted before the repair of mandibular fractures.[60,61] However, the same effect for postoperative antibiotic administration has not been demonstrated.[62,63] While some investigators have concluded that the timing of treatment of mandible fractures following injury does not seem to have any prognostic value in success with infection rates relatively equal in early and late repairs,[64–67] others have shown that treatment within 3 to 5 days after trauma is optimal in terms of minimizing the rate of infection.[68,69] Other risk factors include high-velocity injuries and severe comminution or gross contamination.

Most infections related to mandibular fractures are polymicrobial, with both aerobes and anaerobes routinely cultured. The most common organisms are *Staphylococcus, alpha-hemolytic Streptococcus,* and *Bacteriodes,* as well as gram-negative organisms. Penicillin G, (with or without Flagyl, depending on the gram stain) or clindamycin are the drugs of choice.

Successful management of the infection requires adequate drainage, removal of the source, and appropriate antibiotic coverage. If the cause of the infection is related to mobile hardware and there is favorable bony union, removal of the loose hardware may be all that is necessary. Alternatively, if inadequate stability of the fractured segments is apparent, the previously placed fixation should be removed and replaced, usually with more rigid fixation. With careful patient selection, immediate bone grafting of infected mandibular fractures can be employed. This approach, in conjunction with appropriate fixation and intraoperative debridement, can result in bony union.

Malunion/Malocclusion

Malunion occurs when the fractured segments achieve osseous union in a position that results in either dysfunction or deformation. Complex or high velocity injuries increase the risk for malunion, as does patient noncompliance with postoperative instructions. Unfavorable functional or esthetic outcomes can also occur when the surgeon violates the basic principles of reduction, stabilization, and fixation.

Mandibular Symphysis, Parasymphysis, and Body Fractures

Malocclusion following treatment of mandibular fractures that involve the dentate portions of the mandible typically occurs when the fractured segments are not adequately reduced and stabilized, and appropriate fixation is not applied [Figs. 4.12(a)–(c)]. Evaluation of the occlusion for the presence of crossbite, accurate positioning of occlusal wear facets, as well as evaluation for mandibular angle flaring are important prior to fixation. Preexisting anterior open bite malocclusion can be challenging to assess, but careful examination for the lack of wear facets and the presence of mamelons on the incisor teeth should be of assistance.

Fig. 4.12. Principles of rigid internal fixation of the mandible. (a) Load-sharing fixation, with linear fracture of the right parasymphysis (left); stability is provided by a fixation system in conjunction with stabilizing forces provided by anatomic abutment of noncomminuted fracture segments (right). Fixation is applied to the inferior border (zone of compression) and superior border (zone of tension). (b) Load-bearing fixation, with comminuted fracture of the right mandibular body (left); functional stability is provided solely by the fixation system (right). Contemporary fixation systems involve 2.3- or 2.4-mm locking reconstruction plate at inferior border combined with secondary fixation of comminuted segments at the superior border. (c) Functional stabilization along Champy's ideal lines of osteosynthesis. Fractures located proximal to the first premolar may be safely stabilized with a single miniplate placed in the midbody position (2.0 mm). Fractures anterior to the first premolar should be stabilized with two plates (a tension band and compression band) separated by 4–5 mm and generally placed on either side of the mental nerve. (All images: Prein J, ed. 1997. *Manual of Internal Fixation in the Craniofacial Skeleton: Techniques Recommended by the AO/ASIF Maxillofacial Group.* Springer.)

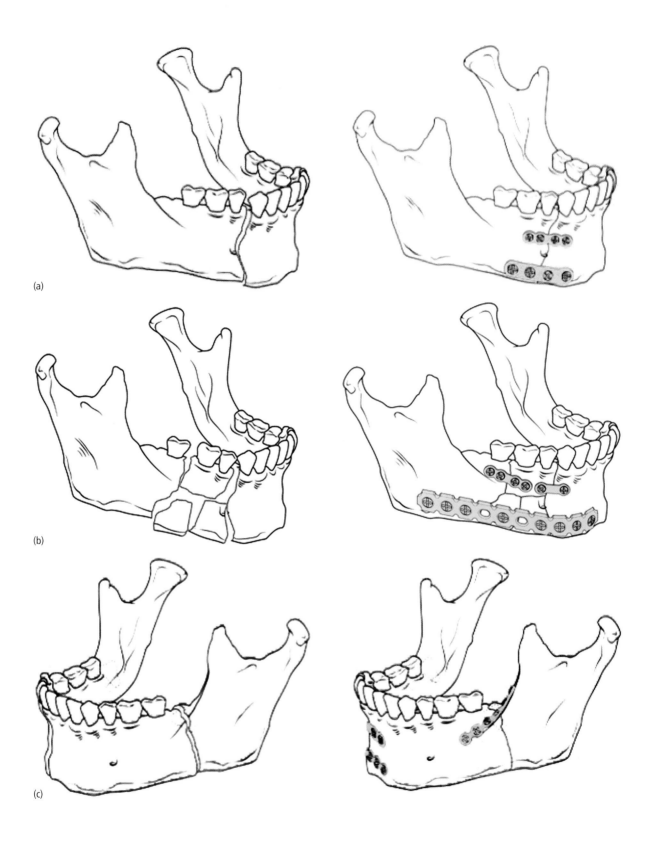

(a)

(b)

(c)

Following reduction, stabilization, and fixation of the fracture, the patient is assessed for the presence of a malocclusion. If one exists, then the fixation is removed and the procedures repeated. If malocclusion is recognized in the first or second postoperative week, it is advisable to take the patient back to the operating room for revision. If the malocclusion is recognized later than 2 to 3 weeks postoperatively, it is advisable to allow for bone union to occur and then consider secondary treatment if necessary.

Secondary correction of a mild occlusal discrepancies occurring from treatment of fractures of the dentate portions of the mandible should include consideration for comprehensive orthodontics to level and align the dentition. Orthodontic treatment alone in certain cases may be all that is necessary to correct spacing or step problems. If the occlusion cannot be corrected with orthodontic means alone, or if there is a significant aesthetic concern, then mandibular osteotomies are generally necessary.

Mandibular Angle Fractures

The ideal treatment of mandibular angle fractures has been controversial. Fractures of the mandibular angle, often complicated by the presence of a third molar, have been shown to have the highest rate of postoperative complications of all mandibular fractures.[45,70,71,72] Numerous techniques have been utilized to treat mandibular angle fractures.

Complication rates for the treatment of mandibular angle fractures of 0% to 32% have been described, depending upon the technique utilized.[49–58] Complication rates are often difficult to interpret, as the definition of a complication is variable. Bell and Wilson[47] described a complication rate of 32% in a series of 162 angle fracture patients. However, this number is misleading because virtually all patients had a favorable outcome with successful bony union and a return to premorbid occlusion. All but two patients had their complications managed on an outpatient basis, under local anesthesia or IV sedation, and almost always after bony union had been achieved. The majority of complications consisted of hardware removal, which is a limitation inherent to some fixation techniques employed for treatment.

Malocclusion resulting from angle fractures typically results in an ipsilateral posterior open bite in the case of unilateral fracture, or in an anterior open bite in the case of a bilateral angle fractures. In contrast to the malocclusions associated with the tooth-bearing segments of the mandible, which can often be treated with orthodontics alone, the open bite associated with angle fractures typically requires osteotomies for correction [Figs. 4.13(a)–(b)]. Typically, a unilateral or bilateral sagittal split osteotomy or combination

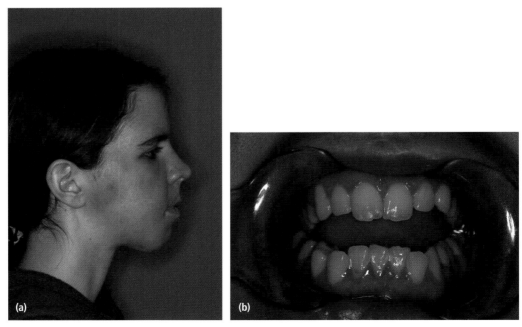

Fig. 4.13. Malunion of untreated bilateral mandibular angle fractures. (a) Lateral view (note facial elongation). (b) Occlusion (note anterior open bite).

with vertical ramus osteotomy are required for correction. Concurrent orthodontic treatment, although recommended, may not be essential for excellent treatment outcomes.

Nonunion

Nonunion of mandibular fractures is an uncommon sequela of treatment, but may occur even in the most experienced hands. High velocity injuries resulting in severe comminution, inadequate or improperly placed fixation, and poor patient compliance are common etiologies [Figs. 4.14(a)–(d)].

Comminuted fractures require load-bearing fixation because the surrounding bony fragments are incapable of sharing any of the functional loads transmitted during healing. Once the major proximal and distal segments are adequately stabilized, the remaining segments may be further secured. In cases of severe

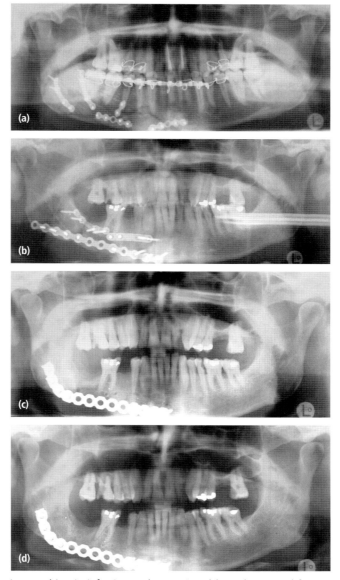

Fig. 4.14. Inadequate fixation resulting in infection and nonunion. (a) Nonbuttressed fractures, such as this comminuted fracture of the mandibular body are at high risk for healing complications. (b) Similarly unbuttressed fracture treated with inadequate (2.0 mm plates) and improper (DCP) fixation. (c) Postoperative panoramic radiograph of patient in (b) following repair with load-bearing 2.4-mm locking reconstruction plate. (d) Radiographic evidence of long-term union.

comminution, it is often helpful to stabilize the smaller fractures with miniplates first and then apply rigid fixation to the remaining construct in order to provide load-bearing support. Reoperation for debridement of necrotic soft tissue and nonviable bone and further stabilization potentially with grafting may be required in these cases.

Atrophic Edentulous Mandibular Fractures

Fractures of the atrophic edentulous mandible have traditionally been a major risk factor for nonunion. The attached muscular forces often cause significant displacement, patients are unable to wear dentures, and associated pain and masticatory dysfunction quickly renders these patients oral cripples. Furthermore, fracture-healing potential is impaired because there is little endosteal or periosteal blood supply and there is a severely diminished surface area that allows no load sharing capacity. Because of this, load-bearing fixation is necessary to achieve bony union. The use of miniplates is contraindicated due to high rates of nonunion [Figs. 4.15(a)–(c)].

Although controversy still exists with regard to the efficacy or necessity of simultaneous bone grafting in the primary setting,[73,74] there is little disagreement over the need for bone grafting in secondary reconstruction of nonunited mandibular fractures in general or in management of nonunion of a severely atrophic mandible fractures in particular. The theoretical advantage of primary bone grafting is that a corticocancellous bone graft would augment the osteogenic potential of the bone at the fracture gap and enhance healing.[75]

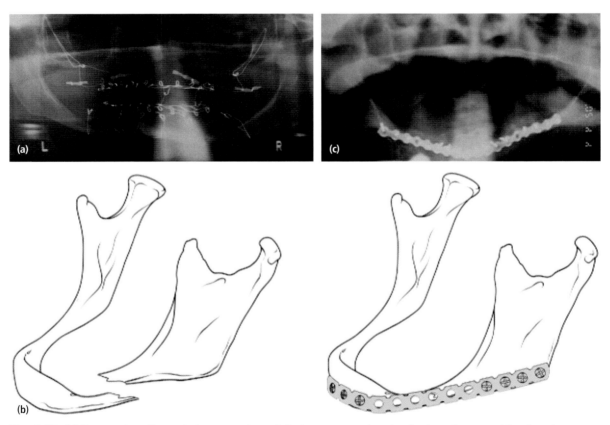

Fig. 4.15. (a) Panoramic radiograph demonstrating a failed attempt at closed reduction of an atrophic edentulous mandible fracture with Gunnings splints and skeletal fixation with circummandibular and circumzygomatic wiring techniques. (b) Diagram demonstrating the appropriate use of load-bearing fixation with a reconstruction plate to provide adequate stability in the case of an atrophic edentulous mandible fracture. (c) Panoramic radiograph showing adequate reduction and stabilization of an atrophic edentulous mandible fracture with a load-bearing reconstruction plate.

Mandibular Widening

Careful attention should be paid to cases of bilateral mandibular fractures involving the symphysis or parasymphysis. Lateral muscular forces will cause widening of the mandible by splaying the angles outward and creating a defect on the lingual aspect of the anterior-most fracture. Failure to adequately account for the lateral muscular forces will result in a gap along the lingual cortex and facial/mandibular widening [Figs. 4.16(a), (b)]. Treatment, if necessary, involves "re-osteotomizing" the symphysis fracture, over-reducing the fractures by pressing in at the mandibular angles, and applying load-bearing fixation to stabilize the symphysis.

Facial Asymmetry

Cillo and Ellis[76] recognized the importance of managing so-called "double unilateral" fractures of the mandible to prevent facial asymmetry [Figs. 4.17(a)–(d)]. In a review of 1,287 patients with mandibular fractures, they found that approximately 2.5% of the patients had more than one fracture on the same side, and in 25% of this subgroup, complications involving gonial flaring and cross bite occurred.

In order to prevent facial asymmetry, absolute anatomic reduction of all fractures must be achieved and adequate fixation should be applied.

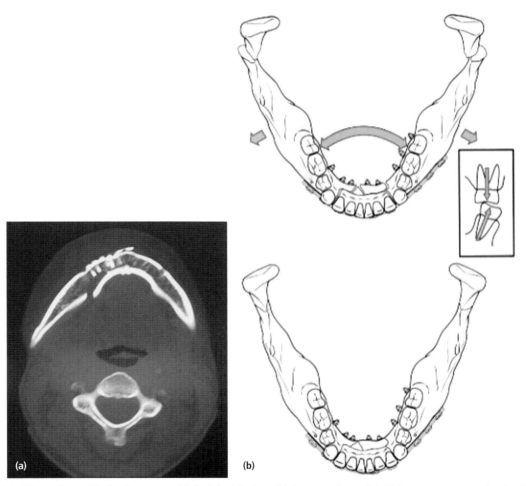

Fig. 4.16. Bilateral mandibular fractures with facial widening. (a) Preoperative axial CT image demonstrating inadequate reduction and fixation of the symphysis fracture (note diastasis at the lingual border of mandible). (b) Illustration of planned surgical treatment to include load-bearing fixation placed at the symphysis and open reduction with internal fixation (ORIF) of the mandibular condyles bilaterally (overbent plate). (All images: Prein J, ed. 1997. *Manual of Internal Fixation in the Craniofacial Skeleton: Techniques Recommended by the AO/ASIF Maxillofacial Group.* Springer).

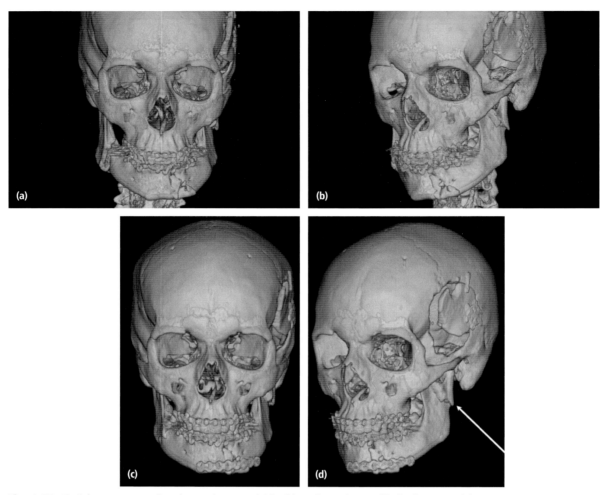

Fig. 4.17. Facial asymmetry related to undertreated "double unilateral" mandibular fractures. (a) Preoperative 3D CT image of patient with fractures of the right angle, left parasymphysis (comminuted), and left condyle. (b) Oblique view. (c) Post-operative CT image of patient following ORIF of the right angle fracture and left parasymphysis with closed treatment of the left subcondylar fracture (note: medial rotation and shortening of the left ramus with flaring of the left angle). (d) Oblique view (note: shortening of the left condyle ramus unit and medial displacement of the ramus/body segment. Ideally, double unilateral fractures should have both ipsilateral fractures reduced and stabilized.

Mandibular Condyle Fractures

Complications of trauma to the mandibular condyle can occur and include disturbance of occlusal function, facial asymmetry, ankylosis of the temporomandibular joint, limited mouth opening, and degenerative joint disease. The goals of treatment include prevention of functional limitations and establishment of a pain-free maximal incisal opening to preoperative levels; symmetrical pain-free movement of the jaw in all excursions; preinjury occlusion; and good facial symmetry. The methods used to achieve these goals are several and controversial. Currently these methods include the use of maxillomandibular fixation for a finite period of time followed by functional therapy; immediate functional therapy without the use of maxillomandibular fixation; and open reduction and internal fixation. The optimal treatment approach has not been universally agreed upon and indeed is probably one of the most controversial topics in the of maxillofacial surgery field.

Favorable results have been reported by a number of authors in large series of patients utilizing only closed treatment.[77–83] From these data it is clear that the goals of treatment for the great majority of patients with mandibular condyle fractures can be met utilizing closed methods. The question is "Which fractures, if treated closed, will most likely result in complications?"

The existing literature suggests that there are a number of potential predictors of complications following closed treatment. These include significant loss of ramus height, comminuted intracapsular fractures,[84] increased age,[85] bilateral subcondylar fractures, double unilateral mandibular fractures,[76] and condyle fractures associated with midface or panfacial fractures. In each of these instances, consideration is given to the risks, benefits and options of open treatment.

Malunion/Malocclusion

Malunion or malocclusion following closed or open treatment of mandibular condyle fractures is typically the result of loss of vertical dimension of the ramus/condyle unit [Figs. 4.18(a)–(g)]. Most of the time, the consequence of this loss in height is deviation of the mandible to the affected side, although occlusal prematurities and centric relation/centric occlusion discrepancies are also relatively common. In some cases of unilateral fracture, a malocclusion will manifest itself as an ipsilateral open bite. An anterior open bite may result in cases of bilateral condylar or subcondylar fractures.

Treatment of significant malocclusions ideally involves a combination of orthodontics and surgery to reposition the tooth-bearing segment by surgically rotating the mandible in a counterclockwise fashion. The choice of technique is dependent upon the level of the original fracture. For fractures located within the mandibular condyle, intraoral sagittal split osteotomy is the preferred method of mandibular repositioning. If the original fractures were in the subcondylar or ramus regions, then the "inverted L" osteotomy may be required, as it allows for greater lengthening of the pterygomasseteric sling.

Facial Asymmetry

Ellis and Throckmorton[86] in 2000 emphasized the differences in facial symmetry related to open and closed treatment of fractures of the mandibular condylar process. Patients with overriding fractures or significant angulation who were managed with closed treatment developed facial asymmetry by virtue of the shortening of the condyle ramus unit on the affected side.[87] While they did not provide objective guidelines for open reduction, a study by Kleinheinz and colleagues[87] found that displacements less than 37 degrees from the sagittal axis of the ascending ramus had negligible loss of vertical height when treated by conservative techniques [Figs. 4.19(a), (b)]. Therefore, to prevent complications associated with closed treatment, their recommendations for open repair of condyle fractures included displacement in excess of 37 degrees and significant decrease in vertical ramus height.[87]

Mandibular Hypomobility/Temporomandibular Joint Ankylosis

The etiology of post-traumatic mandibular hypomobility is unclear. One proposed mechanism is related to temporomandibular joint trauma, which causes hemarthrosis and initiation of a cascade of events that includes altered disc mechanics, cartilage degeneration, and the release of inflammatory mediators. These mediators of inflammation in turn cause effusion, internal derangement, fibrous adhesions, and hypomobility. Prevention of hypomobility following trauma to the mandibular condyle is of paramount importance.

The management of nonankylotic temporomandibular joint (TMJ) hypomobility, once it occurs, is beyond the scope of this chapter. In general, nonsurgical management, with nonsteroidal anti-inflammatory medications, soft diet, heat, and physical therapy with aggressive range of motion exercises is the best approach.

TMJ ankylosis is a severe complication that may arise following mandibular condyle fracture. The etiology of post-traumatic TMJ ankylosis is unclear but may be related to the fracture pattern. He et al. examined a series of patients with TMJ ankylosis secondary to condylar fractures and observed that a significant percentage of their patient population had sustained intracapsular fractures in addition to a second concomitant fracture. The authors postulated that the combination of sagittal intracapsular fractures, an associated fracture of the body or symphysis, and inadequate reduction of the fractures, led to a widening of the mandible and displacement of the lateral pole of the condyle or condylar stump laterally or

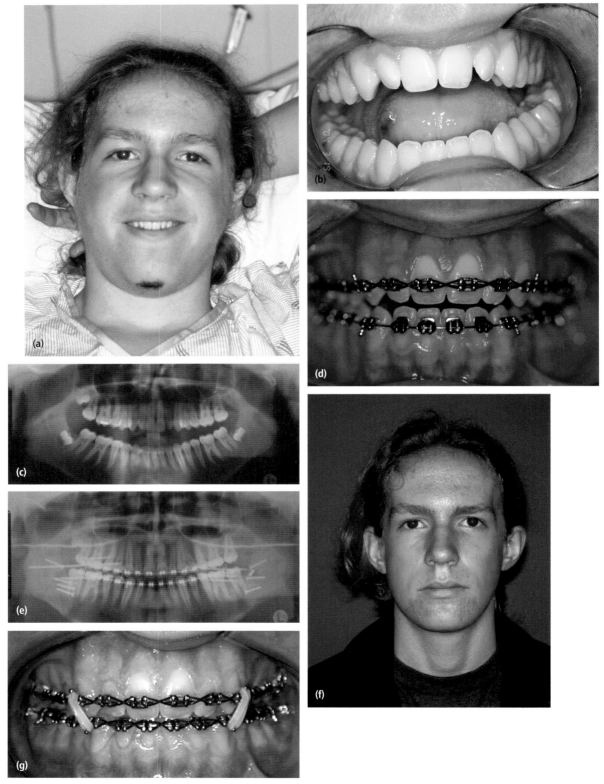

Fig. 4.18. Fifteen-year-old male with bilateral mandibular condyle fractures, treated closed, and complicated by anterior open bite. (a) Pretreatment appearance. (b) Pretreatment occlusion. (c) Post closed-treatment panoramic radiograph. (d) Post closed-treatment occlusion. (e) Panoramic radiograph 6 weeks following bilateral sagittal split osteotomies (BSSO) for correction of occlusion. (f) Facial appearance 6 weeks following BSSO. (g) Occlusion 6 weeks following BSSOs.

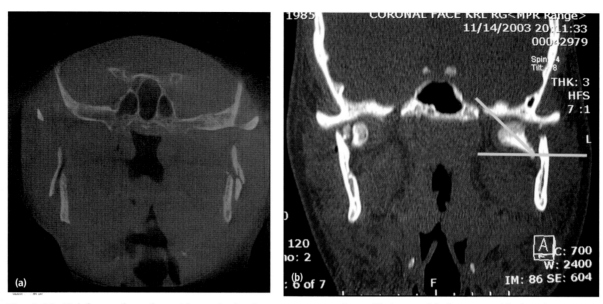

Fig. 4.19. Risk factors for unfavorable results for the management of mandibular condyle fractures with closed treatment. (a) Overlapping left mandibular condyle fracture with loss of vertical dimension. (b) Angulations of less than 37–45 degrees will result in negligible loss of vertical height when treated by closed techniques.

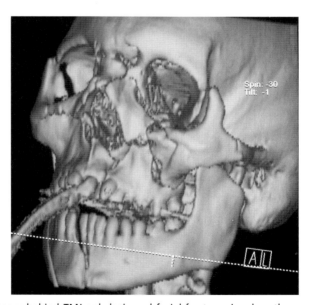

Fig. 4.20. The postulated theory behind TMJ ankylosis and facial fractures involves those with a combination of sagittal intracapsular fractures, an associated fracture of the body or symphysis, and inadequate reduction of the fractures, which leads to widening of the mandible and displacement of the lateral pole of the condyle or condylar stump laterally or superolaterally in relation to the zygomatic arch, where it fuses.

superolaterally in relation to the zygomatic arch, where it fuses (Fig. 4.20). The authors concluded that anatomic reduction of the fractures in this population of patients may minimize the incidence of post-traumatic TMJ ankylosis.

Bony ankylosis should be managed with gap arthroplasty and TMJ reconstruction. Numerous autogenous options are available for the purpose of reconstructing the mandibular condyle, and they have a long history of success. Custom alloplastic total joint prostheses for reconstruction of the condyle and temporal fossa following gap arthroplasty for bony ankylosis is an excellent, and perhaps preferred, alternative.

Facial Nerve Injury

The facial nerve may be encountered in open approaches to the condylar neck and head. The marginal mandibular branch that innervates the depressor anguli oris, depressor labii inferioris, and lower fibers of the orbicularis oris and mentalis may be encountered during standard submandibular or Risdon, low cervical, retromandibular, and preauricular approaches. In standard approaches, when posterior to the facial artery, the marginal mandibular branch of the facial nerve will be roughly 1 cm below the inferior border of the mandible, whereas when crossing the facial artery, the marginal mandibular branch is usually above the inferior border of the mandible.[88] However, some patients may show two, three, or even four branches of the marginal mandibular branch of the facial nerve between the angle of the mandible and the facial artery and vein. The facial vessels lie deep to the facial nerve; therefore, risk to the facial nerve is low once the plane of facial vessels is reached. It has been advocated to dissect to the level of the capsule of the submandibular gland to protect the marginal mandibular branch.[89] Using this approach, the capsule of the submandibular gland is included in the flap that is elevated toward the mandibular border and contains the marginal mandibular branch.

Alternatively, a transmasseteric approach can be performed where an incision is made though the masseter, 10–20 mm above the mandibular basilar edge.[90] In addition, endoscopically assisted fixation of condylar neck fractures, though time consuming, is associated with less morbidity to the facial nerve.[91]

Trigeminal Nerve Injuries

Injuries to the all three branches of the trigeminal nerve can occur following maxillofacial trauma.[92] The prevalence of inferior nerve injury following mandibular trauma approximates 58.5%. Causes of nerve injuries include soft tissue edema, secondary ischemia, transection and crush injuries of the nerve, and when the line of fracture occurs at a foramen and bony fragments impinge on the nerve.[92] The latter cause can lead to permanent anesthesia, parathesia, and dysesthesia if not addressed in a timely manner. Additionally, disruption of the inferior alveolar canal may cause bony proliferation and stenosis of the canal.[93]

Bagheri and colleagues described an algorithm for the approach to the patient with trauma-related trigeminal nerve injury.[92] In the preoperative period, in patients with neurosensory dysfunction, exploration and repair of the nerve should be carried out. However, if microsurgical repair is not possible, open reduction of the fracture should be performed and neurosensory testing should be conducted for 3 months. Patients with persistent neurosensory dysfunction after 3 months should be referred to a microneurosurgeon. Nerve exploration and repair should take place when there is no improvement after 3 months or if symptoms are not acceptable to the patient after fracture treatment.

FRONTAL SINUS FRACTURES

Frontal sinus injuries are relatively common occurrences, representing approximately 4–8% of all facial fractures.[94] Motor vehicle accidents are the most common etiology, and the fact that a high degree of force is required to fracture the frontal bone (800–2,200 pounds) means that many of these patients will have concomitant injuries that require a multidisciplinary approach. Immediate or delayed complications, some of which can be life threatening, occur in 10–20% of the patients with frontal sinus fractures.

The goals in the treatment of frontal sinus injuries are to provide an aesthetic outcome, restore function, and prevent complications. It has never been completely clear, however, whether the frontal sinus is the culprit in the development of postoperative complications, or a victim of improper or ill-advised surgery. In either case, complications occur both in patients treated surgically as well as in those who are observed. Chuang and Dodson[95] recently attempted to identify the frequency of serious complications of operated patients compared to patients who did not undergo surgery by applying the principles of evidence, based on the existing literature. A Medline search was conducted by identifying pertinent articles from 1980 to 2003 that were related to inflammatory complications associated with frontal sinus injuries. Excluding reviews and single case reports, serious inflammatory complications were reported in sufficient detail to estimate the frequency of such complications in only 25 studies.[96–119] Study design in these papers was generally considered poor (level 4 evidence), and the inclusion and exclusion criteria were variable or unidentifiable. Despite numerous limitations, it was estimated that the rate of serious complications is approximately 9% (range 0% to 50% with the 95% confidence interval from 0% to 21%). Additionally, in an effort to estimate the rate of complications from untreated frontal sinus fractures, an attempt was made to extrapolate data from the craniofacial surgery literature by reviewing outcomes of procedures that often involve disruption of normal frontal sinus anatomy. They identified nine studies from which comparable data were available and determined the incidence of complications following nonoperative management of iatrogenic frontal sinus injuries to be approximately 3% (range 0% to 12% with a 95% confidence interval ranging from 0% to 14%).[120–128] While a prospective study directly comparing nonsurgical treatment versus surgical treatment of frontal sinus fractures is neither feasible nor ethical, the current paper suggests that patients with less severe injuries can be safely observed with little risk of short-term complications and that more severely injured patients benefit from surgical repair with a relatively low risk of adverse short-term sequelae.

Principles of Frontal Sinus Management

There is no universal consensus as to how to best achieve the goals of treatment for frontal sinus injuries. Unfortunately, the questions that Stanley[117] proposed in 1989 still lack definitive answers more than 20 years later: (1) "Which fractures, if left untreated, will lead to an immediate or delayed complication?" and (2) What is the appropriate surgical procedure if treatment of the fracture is deemed necessary?"

The decision to operate should be based upon the question of whether or not the injury will result in adverse functional or cosmetic sequellae.[129–131] If the anterior table is depressed greater than its thickness, it is assumed that the injury will create a cosmetic deformity. If the nasofrontal duct (NFD) is obstructed or has the potential to be obstructed, then the patient may be at risk for suppurative complications. Once the decision is made to operate, the surgeon must first determine whether to preserve a functional sinus or to separate the sinus from the nasal cavity. Sinus function is maintained by simply repairing the anterior table by stabilizing the bony fragments with low-profile titanium plates and screws or biodegradable fixation. Patients with displaced anterior tables, evidence of NFD obstruction, and little or no posterior table involvement should have the frontal sinus obliterated. Patients who have severely displaced and comminuted frontal sinuses fractures with significant posterior table involvement, dural lacerations, persistent cerebrospinal fluid (CSF) leak and/or brain injury will often benefit from cranialization.

Bell et al.[94] reported the results of a series of 116 patients with frontal sinus fractures who were treated utilizing the above approach. Sixty-six patients presented with nondisplaced frontal sinus fractures that were managed nonoperatively. Fifty patients had frontal sinus injuries that required surgical repair with follow-up ranging between 0 and 90 weeks; there were no known complications in the group treated nonoperatively. Eighty-two percent of the patients maintained normal sinus function and anatomy, and the overall complication rate was 6.9%. Complications occurred in 16% of those patients treated surgically. Short-term complications (those occurring less than 1 month following operative intervention) occurred in five patients and included brain abscess (n = 1), frontal osteomyelitis (n = 1), hematoma (n = 2), CSF leak (n = 1), and meningitis (n = 1). Long-term complications occurred in four patients (between 1 month and 2 years postoperatively) including mucoceole (n = 2) and contour deformity (n = 2). At the time of revision surgery, both patients with mucoceles were noted to have incompletely removed sinus mucosa.

Infection/Sinusitis

Localized wound infection, hematoma, and/or seroma formation can occur in the immediate postoperative period. These complications can generally be prevented by utilizing suction drains for the first 2 to 3 postoperative days. If they do occur, surgical drainage and appropriate antibiotic therapy will usually resolve the problem without significant long term sequelae.

On the other hand, if a postoperative infection extends through a fracture of the posterior wall of the frontal sinus or through rents in the dura, the result may be acute epidural abscess or brain abscess (Fig. 4.21). Meningitis may also result, particularly in patients with severe injuries that involve the anterior and

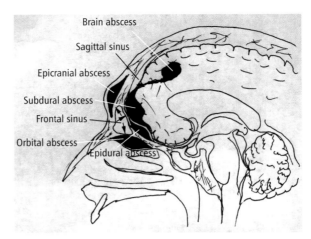

Fig. 4.21. Potential complications related to frontal sinus fractures. (Bell RB, Dierks EJ. 2007. "Paranasal sinuses: Function, dysfunction, and surgical complications." In: *Oral and Maxillofacial Surgery Knowledge Update*, Vol. 4, p. 74.)

posterior table and who undergo craniotomy. Prompt recognition and treatment with antibiotics and neurosurgical intervention are necessary for successful outcomes.

Complications of Sinusitis

Mucocele and Mucopyocele

Chronic sinusitis that causes inflammation and scarring of the sinus ostia can result in mucocele formation. Mucoceles are found most often in the frontal or maxillary sinuses and are a feared complication of frontal sinus fractures. The danger lies primarily in their propensity to become infected (mucopyocele), which can lead to potential intracranial infection or brain abscess. Frontal mucoceles (or mucopyoceles) should be managed by osteoplastic frontal sinus obliteration or, in rare cases, cranialization (discussed later).

Mucocele formation refers to an expansile mucous-filled lesion of the sinus that occurs due to obstruction of the nasofrontal recess. Continued secretion of mucous causes expansion and an increase in pressure, which leads to osteolysis and devascularization of bone. Osteomyelitis may occur from the compressive forces, or the lesion may extend intracranially or involve the orbits. When the lesion becomes infected, the term "mucopyocele" is used. Once a mucocele becomes infected, it may quickly spread to involve the epidural space or cause a brain abscess. It may also lead to frontal bone osteomyelitis or to orbital cellulitis/abscess.

Diagnosis of a mucocele may be difficult in the postoperative setting, as they may occur long after the initial trauma and repair (1 to 25 years). Symptoms are often nonspecific. If the mucocele is confined to the frontal sinus, frontal headache is the most common presenting symptom. If the orbit is involved, the patient may develop diplopia, proptosis, and limitation in ocular motility. Periorbital cellulitis, with or without ocular symptoms, is a common presentation in the post-traumatic setting. CT imaging is the diagnostic study of choice, which allows for accurate assessment of the size and location of the lesion.

Treatment of mucoceles is surgical [Figs. 4.22(a)–(d)]. Generally this will involve either obliteration of the frontal sinus with autogenous grafting (fat, bone, cement), or cranialization. Care must be taken to ensure that all mucosa is removed, including any remnants of the invaginated mucosa within the foramina of Breshet. As mentioned previously, the nasofrontal duct should be sealed with a robust pericranial flap. If the orbital roof has been destroyed, it must be reconstructed using either autogenous bone or alloplastic materials.

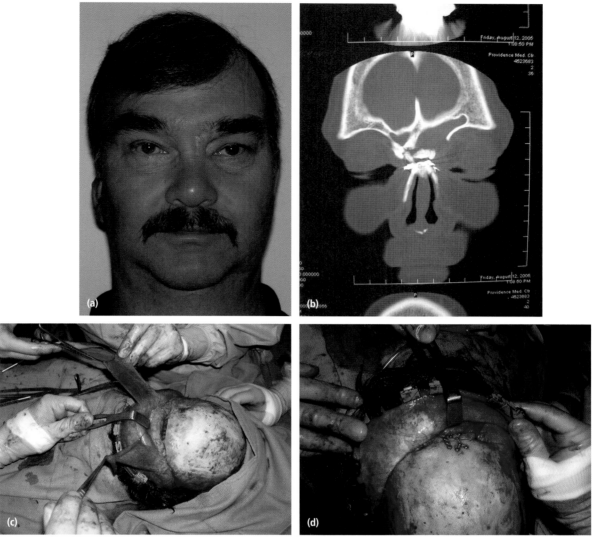

Fig. 4.22. Fifty-two-year-old male with chronic frontal sinusitis 12 years following repair of nasal orbital ethmoidal fractures associated with frontal sinus fractures. The patient failed multiple endoscopic attempts at restoration of nasofrontal drainage. (a) Preoperative appearance. (b) Coronal CT image demonstrating previous surgery and nasofrontal duct obstruction. (c) Intraoperative view of patient undergoing obliteration of the frontal sinus with autogenous fat and pericranial flap. (d) Intraoperative view, osteoplatic flap in place.

Orbital Complications

Complications can occur as a result of either sinusitis or sinus surgery. The major complications of sinusitis involve the orbit or the intracranial structures. Orbital complications are common and are due to the close proximity of the paranasal sinuses and the thin lamina papyracea separating the ethmoids from the orbit [Figs. 4.23(a), (b)]. An additional factor involved in spread of infection to the orbits is related to vascular anatomy. The superior and inferior ophthalmic veins are valveless and allow communication to and from the nose, ethmoids, face, orbit, and cavernous sinus.

Orbital infection has been classified into five categories:

- Group 1: Inflammatory edema, characterized by upper eyelid edema, normal extraocular movement, and normal vision

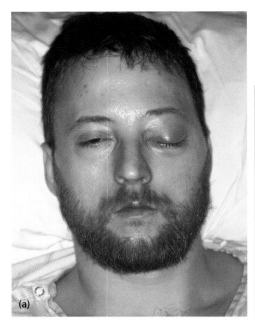
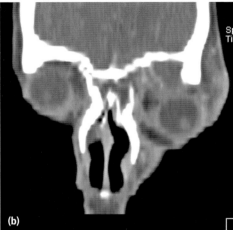

Fig. 4.23. Periorbital cellulitis secondary to pansinusitis. (a) Preoperative appearance. (b) preoperative axial CT image (note the intraobital stranding and globe displacement).

- Group 2: Orbital cellulitis characterized by severe, nonsuppurative periorbital edema, often resulting in proptosis, chemosis, impaired extraocular muscle function, or visual impairment
- Group 3: Subperiosteal abscess characterized by a collection of pus at the medial aspect of the orbit that causes downward globe displacement, impaired extraocular muscle function, and changes in visual acuity
- Group 4: Orbital abscess characterized by an abscess within the orbit, resulting in severe proptosis and complete ophthalmoplegia and visual impairment, often leading to blindness
- Group 5: Cavernous sinus thrombosis, which is infection of the cavernous sinus characterized by sepsis, orbital pain, chemosis, proptosis, and ophthalmoplegia

Treatment for Groups 1 and 2 consists of parenteral antibiotics. Suppurative infections, such as Groups 3, 4, and 5, require urgent surgical drainage, most often via an external approach.

Frontal Osteomyelitis

Osteomyelitis of the frontal bone is occasionally seen as a complication of frontal sinusitis, mucocele or mucopyocele formation. When characterized by subperiosteal abscess and swelling, it is referred to as Pott's Puffy tumor (Fig. 4.24). These entities can be associated with cortical vein thrombosis, epidural abscess, subdural empyema, and brain abscess. The cause of venous thrombosis is explained by venous drainage of the frontal sinus, which occurs through diploic veins, which communicate with the dural venous plexus. Septic thrombi can potentially evolve from within the frontal sinus and propagate through this venous system. Treatment therefore is by aggressive surgical debridement of the affected bone and soft tissue as well as appropriate antibiotic therapy.

Meningitis

Meningitis generally is regarded as the most common intracranial complication of sinusitis. Diagnosis is made after examination of CSF obtained via lumbar puncture. CSF cultures are used to guide antibiotic therapy that generally consists of high-dose parenteral antibiotics with good CSF penetration.

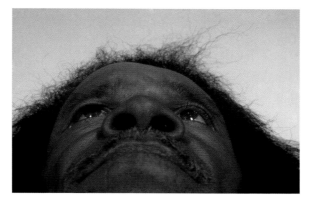

Fig. 4.24. Pott's Puffy tumor.

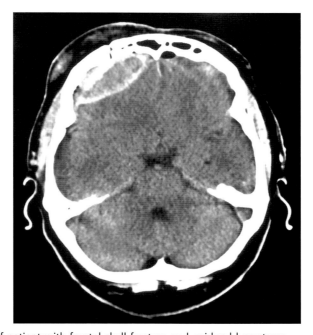

Fig. 4.25. Axial CT image of patient with frontal skull fracture and epidural hematoma.

Intracranial Abscess

Epidural, subdural, or brain abscess is the most feared complication of sinusitis, with mortality rates approaching 20% to 30% (Fig. 4.25).[3,14] Most abscesses occur in the frontal lobe and present with signs and symptoms such as headache, behavioral changes, fever, and sepsis. CT scan and laboratory tests are diagnostic. Treatment involves prompt neurosurgical consultation, craniotomy, and sinus drainage.

Cavernous Sinus Thrombosis

Cavernous sinus thrombosis results from retrograde spread of infection through the valveless veins of the face, sinuses, and orbit. The presentation is dramatic and is characterized by massive periorbital edema, ophthalmoplegia, proptosis, chemosis, and occasionally visual changes [Figs. 4.26(a)–(d)]. CT scan may be suggestive of the diagnosis, but angiography is diagnostic. Treatment consists of high-dose parenteral antibiotics, heparinization, and sinus drainage. Mortality is 30% if isolated to the cavernous sinus and 80% with progression to the sagittal sinus.[14]

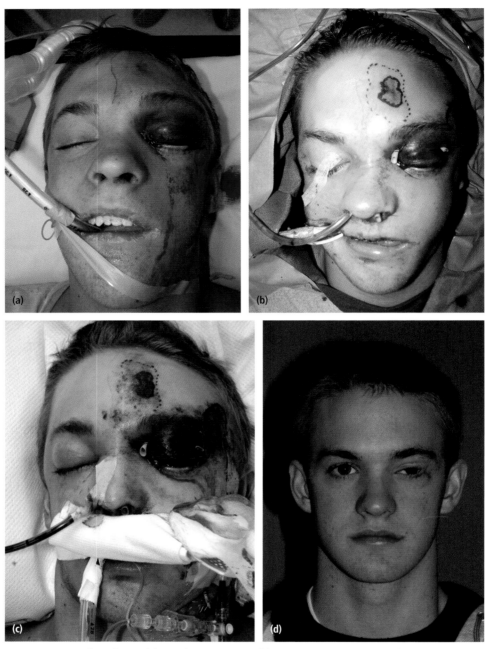

Fig. 4.26. Cavernous sinus thrombosis. (a) Initial presentation. (b) Progression at 48 hours after admission. (c) Progression 72 hours after admission. (d) 1 year following recovery.

Cerebrospinal Fluid Leak

Bell et al.[129] reported the outcome of a series of 735 patients with basilar skull fractures and noted an incidence of CSF leak of approximately 4.6%. Persistent CSF leaks (those lasting more than 7 days) occurring from anterior skull base fractures are unusual but can generally be prevented if the injury is properly managed in the primary setting. Many of these patients will have significant neurological injury as part of complex craniofacial fractures that requires neurosurgical intervention to inspect and repair dura tears, evacuate hematomas, and debride brain tissue. If the frontal sinus is involved and the NFD obstructed, it is prudent to cranialize the frontal sinus in the primary setting, to separate the neurocranium from the

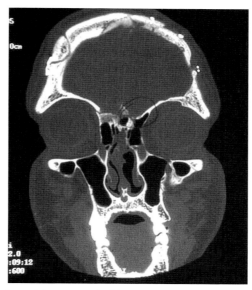

Fig. 4.27. Coronal CT image of patient with anterior skull base fractures complicated by cerebrospinal fluid leak. Cerebrospinal fluid leak should be suspected in patients with fractures of the anterior skull base and frontal sinus.

nasopharynx and prevent CSF rhinorrhea. A robust pericranial flap should be developed at the time of the coronal approach, which is used to line the skull base and seal the nasofrontal recess. Meticulous attention to removal of all sinus mucosa is critical, as is debridement of foreign material or devitalized tissue. If the brain injury is so severe as to warrant a decompressive craniectomy that involves the frontal sinus, the sinus membrane should be removed, a peripheral ostectomy performed, and the frontal bone reconstructed at a later date.

Recognition of CSF rhinorrhea in the immediate post-injury period can be difficult due to the associated nasal secretions, blood, and soft tissue edema. Various laboratory tests have been used to assist in the diagnosis of CSF rhinorrhea, including glucose, beta-2 transferrin, and beta trace protein (prostaglandin D synthase). Glucose assays lack sensitivity or specificity, and while beta-2 transferrin is highly specific, it is not always practical. Intrathecal injection of fluorescein, radioactive serum albumin, or indium may aid in detection both preoperatively and/or intraoperatively and when combined with high resolution CT can aid in accurately determining the location of the leak (Fig. 4.27).

Once a CSF leak has been identified, treatment options include observation; CSF diversion via a lumbar drain; subcranial, transnasal endoscopic surgical repair; or direct transcranial repair. If neurosurgical or craniofacial intervention is not planned, then observation with bed rest is the first line of therapy. Bell et al.[129] showed that 85% of patients will experience uncomplicated resolution of the leak without treatment in 2 to 10 days. Persistent CSF rhinorrhea, defined by drainage more than 7 days after injury, generally requires more direct intervention, most commonly with use of a lumbar drain. If the leak fails to resolve after several days of lumbar diversion, surgical repair is indicated. Small leaks from the area of the cribriform plate can generally be managed subcranially, utilizing a transnasal endoscopic approach. Larger defects, or defects that are located more laterally within the anterior cranial fossa and orbital roof, are treated via a transcranial approach. A bifrontal craniotomy is required for direct dura repair or skeletal deformity reconstruction. The anterior skull base needs to be lined with vascularized tissue, usually in the form of a pericranial flap. An anteriorly or laterally based pericranial flap rotated into the anterior cranial fossa defect and the nasofrontal recess is commonly used to isolate the splachnocranium from the nasopharynx prior to wound closure. The obstructed duct requires sealing (fibrin glue is a good choice for this purpose). Cranialization of the frontal sinus, allowing the brain to expand and occupy the space, is required while the anterior table fractures are the last to be reconstructed and stabilized with appropriate fixation.

Aesthetic Deformity

Contour deformities of the forehead may occur as a result of inaccurate reconstruction of the frontal bone or frontal bandeaux, or as a result of infection or debridement of necrotic tissue. If the orbit is deformed and not adequately reconstructed, problems with globe projection and/or vision can also occur. Treatment via secondary reconstruction of the forehead and/or orbital units is usually required.

ORBITAL FRACTURES

The orbit is involved in a high percentage of severely injured patients admitted to a trauma service.[132] The vast majority of these injuries occur as a result of blunt trauma, usually motor vehicle collision or interpersonal violence, as well as sporting accidents, industrial accidents, and ground level falls. Fractures involving the orbit may affect the internal orbit, the external orbital frame, or both.

Optimal management of orbital fractures remains challenging and often enigmatic. Orbital anatomy is complex, and various vital structures and highly specialized organs are bundled in a small space. A number of approaches exist and numerous materials are available for reconstruction. No one approach and no one material is best suited for all patients. Primary repair offers injured patients their best chance at functional recovery. Complications related to the injury itself or to the repair, such as persistent enophthalmos or ocular dysmotility, are difficult to predict in the acute setting, and once clinically manifested are challenging to repair due to intraconal or extraconal fibrosis.

Orbital Blowout and Blowin Fractures

Once an internal orbital fracture occurs, the volume occupied by the soft tissue contents (the eye and adnexa) may expand or contract based on the direction of the orbital fracture displacement (i.e., blow in or blow out). Blowin fractures typically occur on the orbital roof and are usually associated with high-velocity injuries involving the anterior skull base.[4] Blowin fractures result in contraction of orbital volume and downward and forward displacement of the globe. Most blowout fractures on the other hand, occur on the inferior or inferomedial aspect of the orbit and result in volumetric expansion with displacement of the globe posterior medial and inferiorly.[133] Fracture displacement, orbital expansion and/or contraction may lead to extraocular muscle imbalance and subjective diplopia, enophthalmos, or proptosis.

It is clear that increased orbital volume alone has the potential to cause enophthalmos or ocular dysmotility in some, but not all patients; enophthalmos may become apparent weeks or months after injury; diplopia or ocular dysmotility can take weeks to resolve; surgical repair is necessary in some but not all patients; and, if indicated, surgical repair is optimally performed within the first 2 weeks of injury due to secondary scarring intraorbitally or within Tenon's capsule. Therefore, the questions that need to be answered by the clinician are (1) which patients with orbital fractures will benefit from surgical repair (i.e., is there a quantitative volumetric or linear threshold that predicts functional or aesthetic complications?); and (2) which patients can be safely observed?

CT imaging has been used to correlate volume of orbital expansion to the degree of enophthalmos in blowout fractures. An increase of orbital volume of $1\,cm^3$ has been shown to correlate with 0.89 mm of enophthalmos.[134] This information has been used to predict the volume of reconstructive material grafted or implanted in a series of patients undergoing reconstruction for late enophthalmos.[135] In a more recent study, Ploder and coworkers[136] found that an orbital floor area defect of $3.38\,cm^2$ and volumetric displacement of 1.62 cc was associated with 2 mm of enophthalmos (Fig. 4.28). By convention, 2 mm of enophthalmos is thought to be clinically detectable and has been used by some authors as a threshold for undertaking repair of an orbital fracture.

Limitation of Extraocular Muscle Movements

Extraocular muscle imbalance and diplopia are generally the result of muscle contusion. Less commonly, however, they can be the result of incarceration of either the extraocular muscles (e.g., inferior rectus

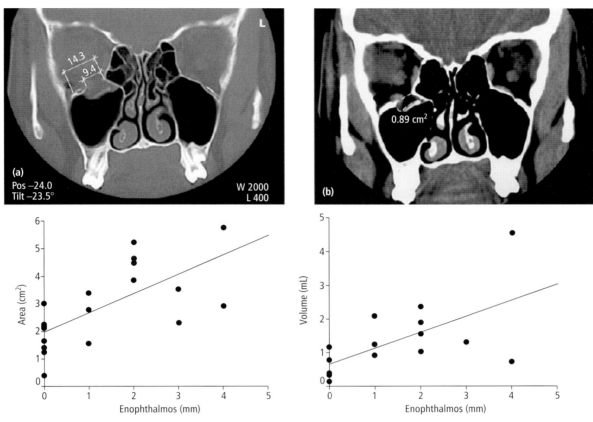

Fig. 4.28. Evaluation of computer based area and volume measurement from coronal CT scans in isolated blowout fractures of the orbital floor. (Ploder O, et al. 2002. *J Oral Maxillofac Surg* 60: 1267–1272).

muscle) or the soft tissue adjacent to the muscles, cranial neuropathy (third, fourth, or fifth cranial nerves), or deviation of the visual axes. True entrapment in adult patients is very unusual. In children, however, blowout fractures may produce complete immobility of the ocular globe with enophthalmos [Figs. 4.29(a), (b)]. Such severe loss of motion implies actual muscle incarceration, which is an indication for immediate orbital exploration with release of the entrapped extraocular muscle system. It is typically accompanied by pain on attempted rotation of the globe, nausea, and vomiting, all of which are unusual in the adult patient with blowout fractures.

Enophthalmos

Enophthalmos is the second major potential complication of orbital injuries, the primary etiology of which is increase in orbital volume (Fig. 4.30). Other mechanisms for enophthalmos are possible, including entrapment of extraocular muscles or periocular soft tissues, fat atrophy, or decrease in vitreous volume. For many years, fat atrophy was thought to be a major etiologic factor of enophthalmos; however, studies by Manson et al.[137] suggest that this is indeed not the case. It has been shown that much of the globe support and position within the orbit is due to intramuscular (intraconal) fat. In the anterior orbit fat is primarily extraconal; however, posteriorly, where support is required, most of the fat is intraconal. It is thought that this intraconal fat is extruded into an extraconal location and that combined with post-traumatic scarring leads to clinically significant enophthalmos.

The most common errors related to internal orbital reconstruction are failure to adequately restore the critical orbital bulges at the posterior inferior portion of the orbit (antral bulge) and posterior medial orbit (ethmoidal bulge) [Figs. 4.31(a)–(c)]. The typical error is placement of the orbital implant flush with the

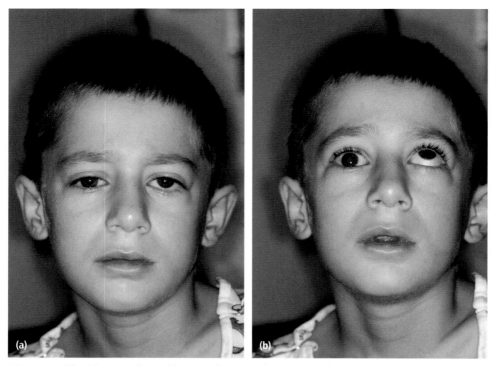

Fig. 4.29. Nine-year-old with "trap door" blow-out fracture of the orbital floor with entrapment of the inferior rectus muscle. This injury represents a surgical emergency and the orbit must be explored and the muscle released expeditiously. (a) Frontal gaze. (b) Upward gaze.

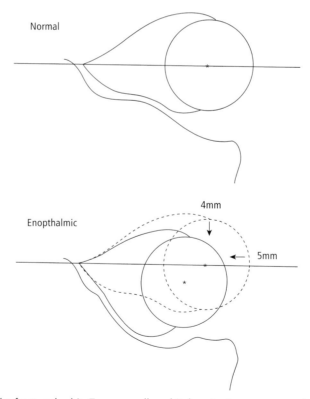

Fig. 4.30. Configuration in the fractured orbit. Top: normally, orbital contents assume a conical shape with a mid-posterior bulge behind the globe. Bottom: spherical configuration in the post-traumatic orbit with concave orbital floor, resulting in enophthalmos and vertical dystopia.

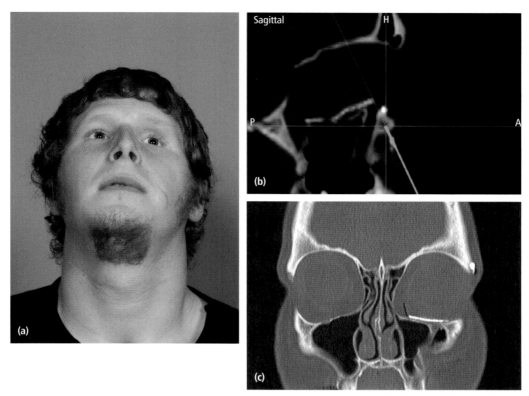

Fig. 4.31. Importance of reconstructing the critical orbital bulges. (a) Enophthalmos following inaccurate reconstruction of the medial ethmoidal and posterior antral bulges. (b) Sagittal CT image demonstrating common error of placing the orbital implant into the maxillary antrum along the posterior antral wall, rather than superiorly in the orbit. (c) Coronal CT image of the same patient demonstrating the lack of restoration of the medial bulge.

anterior portion of the orbit and extending it directly back to the posterior wall of the maxillary sinus. A similar error is made in the medial orbit by inaccurate position of the implant into the ethmoidal labyrinth [Figs. 4.32(a), (b)]. Radiographic assessment of accurate implant placement is essential. This can be provided by either postoperative CT scan in the axial, coronal, and sagittal views, as well as by modern intraoperative CT scanning.

Eyelid Malposition

Lower lid entropion or ectropion can be challenging and frustrating for both surgeon and the patient. The risk of entropion can be minimized by avoiding the use of a lateral canthotomy combined with transconjunctival incisions. Additionally, the placement of the transconjunctival incision at the conjunctival fornix appears to minimize the risk of postoperative entropion. Ectropion can be avoided by performing a so-called midlid incision and avoiding the subciliary approach, which is prone to postoperative scarring and malposition. Finally, infraorbital or malar ptosis is almost unavoidable in some patients in whom the malar eminence and infraorbital rim are completely skeletonized. However, every effort should be made following reduction, stabilization, and fixation of the fractures to resuspend the infraorbital soft tissues to either bone or hardware.

Approaches to the orbital floor should, in most cases, be done with a transconjunctival incision placed at the fornix. Previously popular, the preseptal approach is an elegant dissection, however, that is prone to ectropion, which is particularly true if combined with a lateral canthotomy. Lateral canthotomy is occasionally necessary but care should be taken to resuspend the periorbital musculature and perform an accurate lateral canthopexy upon closure. When wide access is required to the infraorbital rim, particularly in a post-traumatic patient where edema persists, a midlid incision is a predictable means

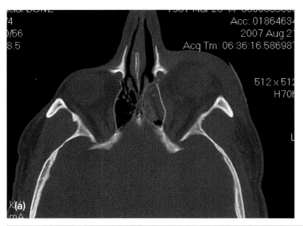

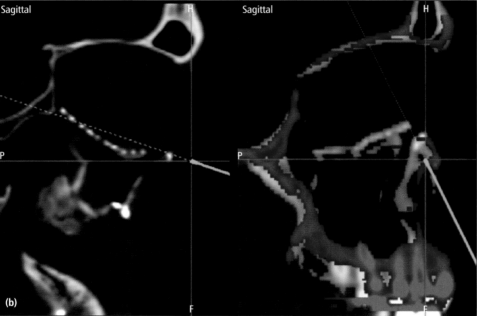

Fig. 4.32. Factors leading to difficulty identifying and accurately reconstructing orbital bony landmarks. (a) Axial CT scan demonstrating the normal postero-medial orbital bulge (left, red), and the common surgical error (right, red) of inadequate restoration of the postero-medial bulge; the green line represents optimal orbital contour. (b) Sagittal CT scan demonstrating the normal ascending slope of the posterior orbit (left) and the common surgical error (right) of inadequate restoration of the height of the posterior orbit.

providing a good balance between cosmesis and minimizing the complications of increased scleral show (Fig. 4.33).

With regard to morbidity of surgical approaches to the orbit, the subtarsal approach has been associated with a lower rate of sclera show than the subciliary approach.[138] The use of the subciliary and subtarsal approach have been associated with a higher rate of ectropion than the transconjunctival approach, though study results vary.[139–142] Some surgeons recommend the subtarsal appoarch for zygomaticomaxillary fractures and the transconjunctival incision for isolated orbital floor fractures, due to the reduction in complications with each incision, respectively. More recently, a transantral endoscopic approach to isolated orbital floor fractures has been reported as an alternative method in order to avoid the potential morbidity of a lower lid incision.[142]

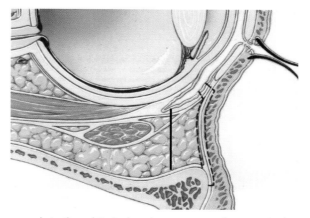

Fig. 4.33. Transconjunctival approach to the orbit. Rather than a preseptal or standard postseptal approach, the incision is preferentially placed toward the conjuntival fornix in order to minimize the risk of entropion. (Modified from: Ellis E III, Zide MF, eds. 2006. *Surgical Approaches to the Facial Skeleton.* Philadelphia: LWW, p. 42.).

Cranio-Orbital Fractures

Complex cranio-orbital fractures are some of the most challenging injuries to manage. High-velocity trauma typically produces defects that affect two, three, or all four walls of the orbit. Such "shattered orbits" produce large volumetric increases, with massive herniation of periorbital contents into the surrounding anatomic spaces, and occasional cranial neuropathies. Typically these defects extend into the orbital cone and may involve the optic canal. Their complex patterns and loss of support in the posterior medial and posterior inferior bulges make restoration of normal orbital anatomy challenging. Although refinements of surgical approaches and the development of new biological materials have improved our ability to more predictably restore these patients' form and function, a significant number of these individuals will still require revision surgery despite the best efforts [Figs. 4.34(a), (b)].[143,144]

Four-walled fractures that involve the anterior skull base may require transcranial approaches, with the assistance of a neurosurgeon, and often involve management of the frontal sinus and occasionally the orbital apex. As the frontotemporal components are repositioned, the orbital roof must be restored with either titanium mesh or calvarial bone grafts, and the anterior skull base lined to prevent CSF leak.

When the entire orbit is disrupted and there are no posterior landmarks to guide the reconstruction, accurate positioning of bone grafts or titanium mesh becomes problematic. There is difficulty in establishing proper orbital contour, volume and medial bulge projection, and there is risk of encroachment upon the orbital apex and optic nerve. Presurgical computer planning to virtually reconstruct the affected orbit or orbits, stereolithographic models to establish proper plate contour, and the use of intraoperative navigation to ensure accurate and safe positioning of the plate in a poorly visualized anatomic region affords the surgeon greater confidence and predictability in the deep orbit.[145]

ORBITO-ZYGOMATICOMAXILLARY COMPLEX FRACTURES

The goal of orbito-zygomaticomaxillary reconstruction is to return the patient to form and function by restoring external and internal orbital anatomy to their premorbid form and to prepare or reposition entrapped or injured soft tissues. Various approaches, techniques, and materials are utilized to achieve these purposes, and there is no universal acceptance as to which combination is best in all instances[146–154]

A good general approach to orbital injuries involves a multistep assessment of whether or not the patient's injury will result in either a functional or aesthetic problem. If the external orbital injury is such that an aesthetic deformity, such as cheek flattening, will be clinically apparent, then treatment is warranted. Once the external orbital frame is reduced into normal anatomic position and stabilized, rigid

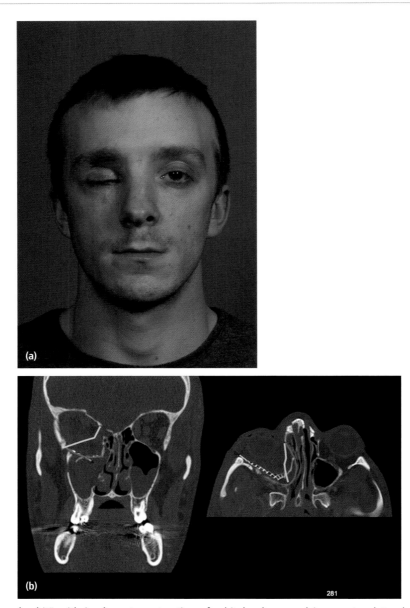

Fig. 4.34. "Shattered orbit" with inadequate restoration of orbital volume and inaccurate plate placement resulting in enophthalmos, further complicated by orbital apex syndrome. (a) Postoperative appearance (note ptosis, ophthalmoplegia, and profound enophthalmos). (b) Inaccurately placed orbital plate (red) and ideal location (yellow).

internal fixation should be applied via the fewest approaches necessary. Internal orbital injuries should likewise be assessed for ocular dysmotility or the potential to result in enophthalmos. If the orbital floor defect is greater than $3\,cm^2$ or $1.5\,cc$ displaced volume as demonstrated on CT images, then treatment of the internal orbit is deemed necessary. Furthermore, internal orbital disruptions posterior and/or medial to the equator of the globe are typically addressed unless the patient is completely devoid of symptoms.

In general, most patients with low-velocity injuries involving the external orbital frame (e.g., bare-fisted assault or ground level falls) can be adequately restored to form and function without exploration or treatment of the internal orbit. Conversely, most high-velocity injuries, such as those occurring in motor vehicle collisions, result in a displacement of energy that causes significant internal orbital disruption and usually necessitate repair of the internal orbit. A selective approach to the repair of the internal orbit takes into consideration the patient's subjective symptoms (e.g., blurred vision, diplopia), physical findings (e.g., entrapment of the inferior rectus muscle), limitation and extraocular muscle movements, radiographic findings (linear defect greater than 3.5 cm^2 and volumetric displacement greater than 1.6 cc), and mechanism of injury (i.e., low velocity versus high velocity).

Minimal to moderately displaced, low-velocity orbito-zygomaticomaxillary complex fractures can often be managed with simple one-point fixation at the maxillary buttress providing that no significant intraorbital component exists. More commonly, moderately displaced fractures of both low and high velocity can be managed with simple two-point fixation provided at the maxillary buttress via a Keen incision, and the zygomaticofrontal suture (ZF suture) is approached via an upper lid blepharoplasty incision. If, following reduction and stabilization with these two points, the complex is not adequately reduced or the infraorbital rim remains displaced, the transverse component of the orbital frame can then be stabilized at the infraorbital rim via a transconjunctival incision. Skeletonization of the infraorbital rim is avoided if at all possible.

Fractures that are the result of a high-velocity injury with severe fragmentation or comminution, or those associated with panfacial fractures, are typically repaired with four-point stabilization. This includes a coronal approach to expose the zygomatic arch and reestablish facial/malar projection. Care must be taken to restore the arch to its normal flat contour rather than creating a rounded arch that will result in deprojection of the zygoma and widening of the face.

Malar Flattening

Gruss et al.[155] recognized the importance of the zygomatic arch in complex midfacial fractures repair and correction of post-traumatic orbitozygomatic deformities. There is a reciprocal relationship between anteroposterior projection and facial width [Figs. 4.35(a), (b)]. As projection of the zygoma decreases, facial width increases. The zygoma, therefore, is key to restoring facial/orbital projection in severely displaced and comminuted fractures and should be returned to its natural "flat" contour. The most common error in reestablishing zygomatic projection is failure to reduce the segments out of a displaced "arch" into a flat zygoma (Fig. 4.36). Failure to adequately flatten the zygomatic arch and achieve optimal rotation of

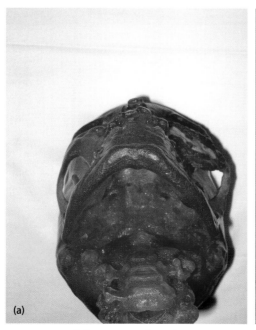
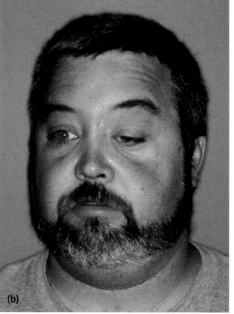

Fig. 4.35. Importance of the zygoma for achieving normal facial width and symmetry. As facial/zygomatic projection decreases, facial width increases. (a) Stereolithographic model of a patient following open reduction and internal fixation of severely comminuted facial factures with improperly restored projection of the zygoma; the zygoma should be "straight" not "arched," and is one of the most common mistakes in restoring external orbital anatomy. (b) Postoperative appearance (note the facial widening).

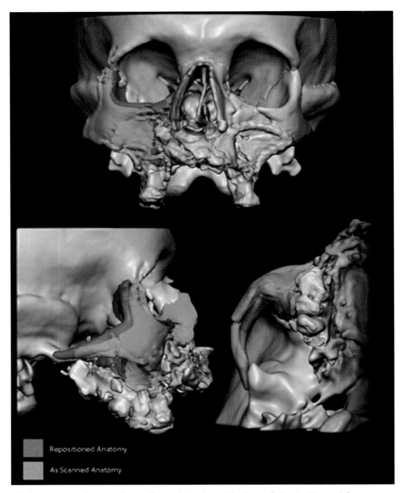

Reposibioned Anatomy

As Scanned Anatomy

Fig. 4.36. "Bowing" of the zygomatic arch (green) resulting in widening of the ipsilateral face compared to the ideal arch contour (blue).

the zygomaticomaxillary complex will result in flattening of the malar eminence and widening of the ipsilateral face. If a coronal incision is not performed, accurate rotation of the zygomaticomaxillary complex can be assessed by inspecting the sphenozygomatic suture region via an upper lid blepharoplasty approach.

Neurosensory Complications

The infraorbital canal and foramen are often disrupted as a result of zygomaticomaxillary complex (ZMC) fractures often causing damage to the infraorbital nerve. Damage to the zygomaticomaxillary and zygomaticofacial nerves is less common.[156] Patients will often complain of anesthesia or parathesisa to the lower eyelid, malar, and upper lip areas. Though usually transient, permanent altered sensation is not uncommon. Anatomic reduction will generally minimize the risk of permanent symptoms, although surgical decompression is occasionally indicated in the delayed setting.[157]

Since the greater wing of the sphenoid makes up the lateral wall of the orbital apex, function of cranial nerves II, IV, V, and VI must be assessed for bone impingement and the presence of orbital apex or superior orbital fissure syndromes. Superior orbital fissure syndrome is manifested by diplopia, ophthalmoplegia, exophthalmos, and ptosis. Orbital apex syndrome is distinguished from superior orbital fissure syndrome by the presence of blindness, caused by the injury to cranial nerve I.[158]

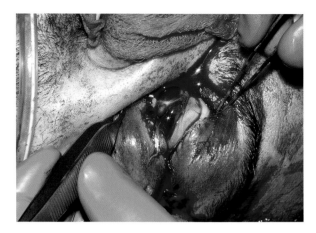

Fig. 4.37. Globe rupture.

1. Vision decreasing despite steroids
2. Visual loss with CT evidence of fracture compressing optic nerve
3. Increasing edema of nerve or hematoma with decreasing vision
4. No light perception with fracture of optic canal
5. CT evidence of optic nerve compression in comatose patient

Fig. 4.38. Relative indications for surgical decompression of the optic nerve.

VI. OCULAR TRAUMA

The majority of eye injuries consist of corneal abrasion, hyphema, and globe rupture (Fig. 4.37). Compressive neuropathy, superior orbital fissure syndrome, and orbital apex syndrome are rare, but functionally and aesthetically devastating injuries.

The preponderance of scientific evidence suggests that progressive visual loss, optic canal fracture, retrobulbar hematoma with increased intraocular pressure, or perineural edema warrants urgent surgical exploration and/or decompression (Fig. 4.38). In one study by Rajiniganth et al.,[159] 70% of patients with visual deterioration and CT evidence of compressive neuropathy responded favorably to surgical intervention, if the operation was performed within the first 7 days after injury. The success rate decreased to 24% when decompression was performed more than 7 days after the injury. Transnasal and/or transorbital endoscopic surgery is an option for some patients with displacement of the optic canal and delayed visual deterioration. However, open surgery is often necessary and facilitated by transcranial neurosurgical repair of concomitant intracranial injuries. It is important to coordinate all disciplines in a trauma center so that all treatment options, both medical and surgical are available.

NASO-ORBITAL-ETHMOIDAL FRACTURES

Treatment of nasal orbital ethmoidal (NOE) fractures is one of the most challenging of all procedures in craniomaxillofacial surgery. Failure to adequately restore nasal projection, normal canthal width, and orbital volume will result in highly unfavorable functional or aesthetic outcomes.

Severe telescoping or combination of the nasal bones must be reduced, stabilized, and fixated to reestablish normal nasal projection. Although strut calvarial bone grafts have been advocated for this purpose and are occasionally necessary, adequate anatomic reduction of the nasal bones with stable fixation is often

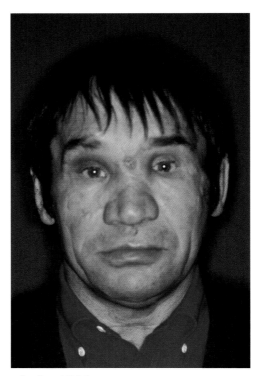

Fig. 4.39. Telecanthus following repair of an NOE fracture.

all that is necessary as long as the frontal bandeau is adequately restored. Once the internal orbital frame has been reduced and stabilized with miniplates and nasal projection reestablished, attention must be directed to the management of the central fragment. Medial canthopexy is facilitated utilizing a commercially available titanium barbed wire.

Traumatic Telecanthus

The importance of reestablishing the central component of NOE fractures is of paramount importance in achieving optimal functional and aesthetic results (Fig. 4.39). In addition, it is important to avoid the unrecognized NOE fracture that occasionally accompanies fractures of the lateral orbit. In this instance, the operating surgeon will repair the orbitozygomaticomaxillary complex (OZMC) component and neglect the NOE component, which results in unilateral telecanthus.

Nasolacrimal Duct Obstruction

Injury to the nasolacrimal apparatus is often associated with NOE fractures, and may occur as often as 20% of the time following open reduction and internal fixation. These injuries occur by either blunt or penetrating trauma to the pump system created by the medial canthal ligament and orbicularis oculi muscle.

The most common symptom and sign of nasolacrimal duct obstruction is epiphora, although this is rarely recognized in the acute setting due to associated periorbital edema. Diagnosis may be facilitated by injecting fluorescein via the Jones technique, using methylene blue, or by introducing a lacrimal probe into the duct under loupe magnification.

Once identified, the lacrimal duct may be intubated and stented open with Crawford lacrimal tubes, although this may not prevent later obstruction. Secondary correction typically requires formal dacrocystorhinostomy (DCR). DCR is performed by creating a window bone between the lacrimal sac and the lateral aspect of the nasal bones. The nasal mucosa is then sewn to the mucosa of the lacrimal sac, creating a fistula.

Cosmetic Deformity/Saddle Nose Deformity

Massive comminution of the NOE complex is classically associated with a saddle nose deformity, due to difficulty restoring the three-dimensional anatomy of the small, thin bones of the NOE region. A number of authors have emphasized the need for calvarial bone grafting in most patients with significant NOE fractures to aid in establishing nasal projection, symmetry, and contour. However, it is more important to restore the frontal bandeaux (if disrupted) and anatomically reduce the nasal bone fractures using very small (1.0 mm or 1.2 mm) miniplates.

NASAL FRACTURES

Nasal fractures are one of the most common injuries. The vast majority of nasal fractures can be successfully managed with either observation (nondisplaced nasal bone fractures) or with closed reduction, with or without internal/external splints. Approximately 50% of patients undergoing closed treatment, however, will benefit from secondary nasal surgery to optimize functional or aesthetic outcomes. Complications do occur, but can be minimized by thorough physical examination at initial presentation.

Septal Hematoma

Intranasal examination of each maxillofacial trauma patient is essential because the occult nasal septal hematoma may be present in the absence of external nasal deformities. The patient will present with pain on palpation of the nasal tip, and unilateral or bilateral fluctuant swelling of the nasal septum.[160] The pathogenesis of these lesions is suspected to result from fracture of the septal cartilage, bleeding from the damaged perichondrial vessels without drainage, and subsequent reflection of the perichondrium off of the cartilage such that the cartilage has no blood supply.[160,161] Pressure from the extravasated blood results in avascular necrosis of the cartilage. This same pathogenic process has rarely been reported in the alar cartilages and the nasal tip.[162–164]

The extravasated blood and necrotic tissue in undiagnosed nasal septal hematomas form a perfect nidus for infection. Nasal septal abscesses have the same presentation as nasal septal hematomas, with inflamed overlying mucosa, with or without an inflammatory exudate.[160] If untreated, septal abscesses can result in the same saddle deformities caused by septal hematomas,[164] as well as life-threatening bacterial meningitis infections via drainage from the septum to the emissary veins and into the cavernous sinus.[165]

Epistaxis

Intractable epistaxis may result from nasal trauma, or from skull base trauma. Cranial computed tomography, combined with selective angiography and subsequent embolization may be necessary to treat the most severe cases.[166]

Cosmetic Deformities/Saddle Nose Deformity

Saddle nose deformity is derived from the similarity of the deficiency in dorsal projection on lateral view to a horse's saddle (Fig. 4.40). Traumatic causes for this deformity involve dorsal cartilage and bone destruction from septal hematoma, septal abscess, or fracture of septal cartilage or bone.[164] The extent of the deformity should guide the reconstructive surgical plan. Minor deformities, such as supratip depression, may be corrected with cartilage onlay grafts taken from the ear, or the posterior nasal septum. Moderate defects may be treated with upper lateral cartilage pedicled flaps. More severe defects, often a result of childhood nasal trauma and future growth disturbance, will need more tissue, either with bone or cartilage grafting or nasal implants.[164] In the past, anterior iliac crest grafts were used, with note of resorption problems long-term. Onlay calvarial bone grafts may afford better long-term results,[167] but experience shows that they also will resorb over time. The costochondral rib grafts shaped to a "keel" have the theoretical advantage of less long-term resorption.

Nasal Airway Obstruction/Septal Deviation

Septal deviation is often the underlying cause for external nasal asymmetries due to the tight fibrous attachments of the upper and lower lateral cartilages to the septum. Careful inspection of the nasal tip, nasal

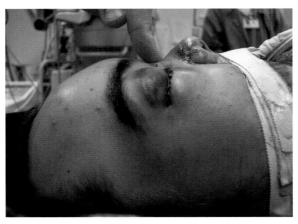

Fig. 4.40. "Saddle nose" deformity prior to repair of an NOE fracture.

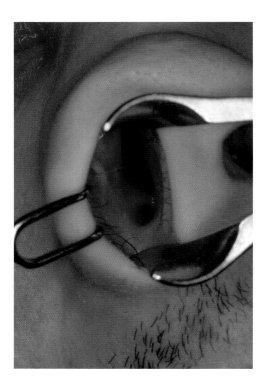

Fig. 4.41. Endonasal synechiae.

base, dorsal line deficiency, the entire septum, and the inferior nasal turbinates is necessary prior to forming a surgical plan. Direct septal visualization via the open rhinoplasty approach is preferred for correction of these defects.[168]

The residual deviated bony nasal vault may result from inadequate closed reduction or bony migration after adequate closed reduction. Internal splints and an external cast with tape will help prevent this problem. The preferred treatment for residual deviations from old nasal fractures is open reduction with controlled osteotomies.[168]

Nasal Scarring

Scarring, both endonasal and extranasal, can cause significant problems for the patient if untreated (Fig. 4.41). Gunshot wounds can produce significant soft tissue and bony destruction within the nasal

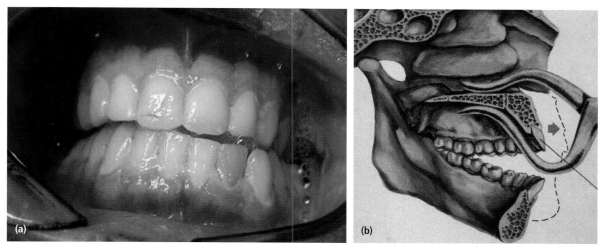

Fig. 4.42. Inadequate reduction of Le Fort I fracture resulting in anterior open bite. (a) Occlusal appearance. (b) Use of a Rowe disimpaction forceps to fully mobilize an impacted fracture at the Le Fort I level.

cavity. When nasal packing or stents are not placed, epithelialization of the wound edges can result in synechia, or adhesions, which may be severe enough to preclude nasal respiration. In such cases, a multiteam approach with a maxillofacial prosthodontist making custom nasal stents will present restenosis.[169]

Scar contracture after alar trauma can result in both cosmetic and functional deformities. Hard palate mucosal grafts to correct these defects have been suggested as good alternatives to auricular composite grafts because of the limited donor site morbidity and increased patient acceptance.[170]

MAXILLARY FRACTURES

Fractures involving the maxilla may be isolated or as part of a pattern of fractures commonly referred to as Le Fort I, II, or III. In contrast to the mandible and zygoma, most of these fractures occur as the result of high-velocity motor vehicle collisions and therefore are associated with a high degree of kinetic energy dispersal. This factor, more than any other, may lead to severe complications.

The same principles of anatomic reduction, stabilization, and fixation that are utilized to guide open reduction and internal fixation of the mandible are also applied to the midface. Most isolated maxillary fractures that do not propagate through the pterygoid plates (at the Le Fort I level) do not require surgical treatment. Le Fort I fractures should be managed using interdental wires, arch bars, or intermaxillary fixation screws to aid in restoring the occlusion. Care should be taken to "disimpact" the maxilla if it has been impacted posteriorly and superiorly—a pattern that causes an anterior open bite. Once reduced, and with the patient in intermaxillary fixation, rigid internal fixation is applied via a circumvestibular incision to the anterior and posterior maxillary buttresses (Fig. 4.42).

For fractures at the Le Fort II or III levels, the lateral external orbital component is repositioned and stabilized at the zygomatico-frontal suture. Following this, proper projection of the zygoma is achieved by reducing and stabilizing the zygomatic arch. The maxillary buttress is then stabilized via a transoral approach, and finally the infraorbital rim connects the lateral skeletal components to the medial nasal orbital ethmoidal complex. Once the external orbital frame is reconstructed, attention is directed toward repairing the central skeletal components, if disrupted.

Severe telescoping or comminution of the nasal bones must be reduced, stabilized, and fixated to reestablish normal nasal projection. Although strut calvarial bone grafts have been advocated for this purpose and are occasionally necessary, the author finds that adequate anatomic reduction of the nasal bones with stable fixation is often all that is necessary as long as the frontal bandeau is adequately restored. Once the internal orbital frame has been reduced and stabilized with miniplates and nasal projection reestablished, attention must be directed to management of the central fragment. Medial canthopexy is facilitated utilizing a commercially available titanium barbed wire and titanium miniscrews placed in a posterior–superior position within the medial orbit behind the lacrimal crest.

Malocclusion

Typical management of fractures of the maxilla involves placing the maxillary dentition in proper occlusion with the integral or reconstructed mandible. Once the maxillomandibular complex is properly rotated superiorly and once maximum boney interface is obtained, the fractured maxilla is then fixated together. However, malocclusion may ensue following treatment and usually follows an anterior open bite and/or a Class III pattern. While malocclusion may occur from improper rigid fixation, it is most likely a result of insufficient mobilization during surgery. Occasionally, manual manipulation of the maxilla into the correct position in relation to the mandible may not be possible, at which time formal osteotomy of the maxilla at the Le Fort I level may be helpful in the primary setting (Fig. 4.43).[171]

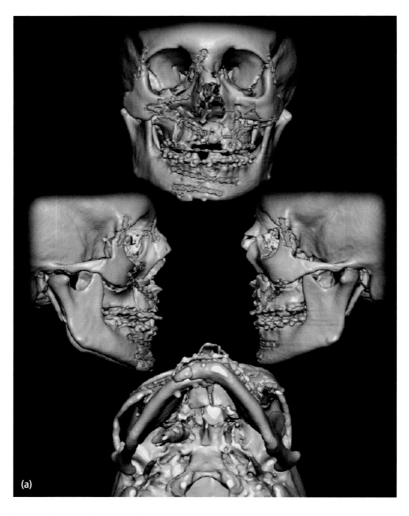

(a)

Fig. 4.43. Facial widening after inadequate reduction, stabilization, and fixation of panfacial fractures. (a) Pre-revision CT reconstruction [note widening of the mandible (condyles lateral to the articular fossa) and retrodisplaced maxillomandibular complex resulting in facial widening and flattening]. (b) Virtual reconstruction (note restoration of facial width and projection).

Sinusitis

The effect of trauma that results in fractures of the paranasal sinuses is not known with certainty. Clinical and experimental evidence suggest that the sinus mucosal lining predictably regenerates after injury and that the bony walls completely or partially regenerate. Complications, however, can occur and include chronic sinusitis, polyps, and mucocele formation and occasionally acute infection leading to a vital area, as discussed previously. The incidence of symptomatic sinus complications resulting from maxillofacial trauma has been estimated to be 1.7%.[172] If more objective criteria of sinus disease are employed, such as radiographic evidence of mucosal thickening or endoscopic evidence of mucositis, hyperplasia, or polyposis, the incidence of sinus complications has been estimated at 8.4% to 35%.[173,174] Most studies, however, were completed in the years prior to the routine practice of open reduction and internal fixation. It is conceivable that with proper anatomic reduction, normal sinus function can be restored predictably.

Hemorrhage

A potentially fatal complication of Le Fort fractures is hemorrhage from branches of the external carotid artery system, most often the posterior superior alveolar artery of the internal maxillary artery,[175] and in rare cases the ascending pharyngeal artery.[176] It should be suspected when perfuse nasal or oral bleeding refractory to local measures is present following a Le Fort fracture. In particular, hemorrhage of the posterior superior alveolar artery (PSA) should be suspected with perfuse bleeding following any fracture of the posterior alveolar wall. Other signs include a rapid decrease in blood pressure, hemoglobin, and

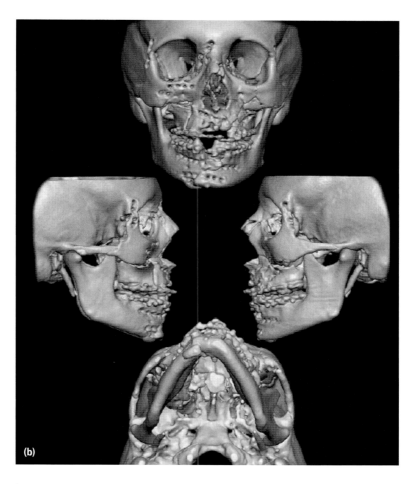

(b)

Fig. 4.43. *Continued*

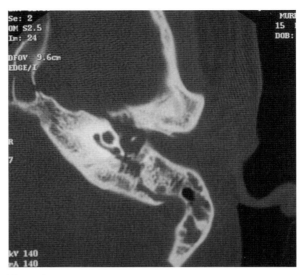

Fig. 4.44. Transverse temporal bone fracture.

hematocrit. If manual ligation of the artery cannot be performed, then selective contrast enhanced angiography should be performed. The area of hemorrhage is identified by extravasated pooling of contrast material. Transcatheter arterial embolization of the offending area of the vessel, usually the distal third of the internal maxillary artery is then performed.[177]

TEMPORAL BONE FRACTURES

Twenty-two percent of skull fractures result in temporal bone fracture that may cause significant compression of the facial nerve.[178] Transverse temporal bone fractures most likely result in injury along the labyrinthine segment and/or the geniculate ganglion, while longitudinal temporal bone fractures result in injury along the geniculate ganglion (Fig. 4.44), and injuries that are nonidentifiable on imaging often result in injury along the mastoid and/or tympanic segments There exists ambiguity of whether early surgical exploration and decompression of facial nerve injuries secondary to temporal bone fractures results in a better prognosis, though early repair seems to produce the most favorable outcomes.[178–180]

TRACHEOSTOMY COMPLICATIONS

When sustaining trauma to the head and neck, standard endotracheal intubation is not always possible, and a tracheostomy is often necessary to create an airway and maintain adequate ventilation. With regard to site placement, the surgeon must be careful of the paratracheal or pretracheal placement of the tracheostomy tube. It may not be apparent, and without careful observation, may only be associated with the lack of end-tidal CO_2.[181] In addition, if breath sounds are not heard on auscultation and when the surgeon passes a suction catheter there is no cough from the lightly anesthetized patient, the tracheostomy tube is malpositioned. Bleeding is the most common complication encountered during the procedure (Fig. 4.45). Bleeding after the initial skin incision is most likely due to trauma to the anterior jugular vein. If bleeding is encountered from the deep tissues, the thyroid gland is most likely the culprit. If encountered, the highly vascular gland may be divided by elevating the isthmus from the trachea, and the stumps should be sutured and ligated. Careful electrocauterization can be used for bleeding lateral to the trachea, and attention must be made to not compromise the recurrent laryngeal nerve that is seen running through the tracheoesophageal groove.

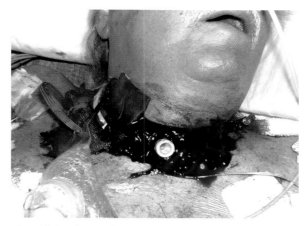

Fig. 4.45. Postoperative hemorrhage following tracheostomy.

A chest film should be performed following the procedure to confirm tube placement and the absence of a pneumothorax or hemothorax, which are uncommon complications but may occur when more lateral dissection takes place. In the postoperative period, granulation tissue buds may appear around the tracheostomy site and can be a potential source of bleeding. When encountered, silver nitrate may be helpful. Infection surrounding the tracheotomy site may occur and can usually be managed with good wound hygiene and wet-to-dry packing placement at the site. These infections may be associated with necrosis of adjacent tissues and may heal by secondary intention, producing an abundance of granulation tissue. Tracheocutaneous fistulas (TCFs) may occur after long-standing tracheostomy tube placement.[182,183] In children they may resolve following electrocauterization of fistula walls. Adults, however, may need more aggressive layered closure of the wounds with interpositional closure of adjacent strap muscles.

A tracheoinnominate fistula (TIF) may develop months after initial tracheostomy and results from attrition of the anterior tracheal wall by the tube tip. It extends to the posterior wall of the innominate artery where it crosses the trachea in the upper mediastinum. Incision near the second and third tracheal rings places the tube tip near where the innominate artery crosses the trachea. Initially this may be managed by inflating the tracheostomy tube cuff or by passing an endotracheal tube adjacent to the tracheostomy tube. If this does not work, the Utley maneuver may be used where the inferior aspect of the tracheostomy site may be opened and, after blunt finger dissection, pressure may be put on the innominate artery against the manubrium. Definitive treatment is thoracotomy. Prolonged tracheal intubation may result in tracheal stenosis or tracheomalacia, the latter prevented with the use of high-volume, low-pressure tracheotomy tubes. Tracheostomy tube displacement into the peritracheal tissues may occur and can be divided into two types.[181] Type I is due to an increase in the distance from the anterior tracheal wall to pretracheal skin, and is usually due to postoperative edema. It usually occurs in the first few postoperative days. Type II displacement occurs in the absence of increase in the distance from the anterior tracheal wall to neck skin. Both types will result in difficulty in passing a suction tube through the tracheostomy tube to the trachea.

The obese patient presents with a special set of complications. In this subset of patients, accidental decannulation can be prevented by using an anthropometric tape measure and selecting the appropriate tracheostomy tube size.[184] Alternatively, some obese patients may benefit from excision of fat from the tracheotomy site and construction of a tracheal stoma via an inferiorly based Bjork flap to form the inferior wall of the stoma, combined with a superiorly based skin flap to form the superior wall.[184–187]

Scarring is an unaesthetic result of tracheostomy. Persistent TCF may result in pneumothorax, bronchitis, chronic aspiration, and patients are more likely to have side effects such as excessive tracheal secretions, dysphagia, phonation difficulties, an ineffective cough, and local skin irritation.[188] Early on, management of TCF fistulas include using a lined bipedicle flap supported by conchal cartilage to excise the TCF. The inferior edge of the flap is left open for provisional air run off to decompress the suture line. This line would then heal by secondary intention. Excision and primary closure is also a simple and reliable option. Several other techniques have been described to revise tracheostomy scars with good success.[188–193]

SUGGESTED READINGS

1. Oehler RL, Velez AP, Mizrachi M, et al. 2009. "Bite-related and septic syndromes caused by cats and dogs." *Lancet Infect Dis* 9: 439.
2. Dire DJ. 1992. "Emergency management of dog and cat bite wounds." *Emerg Med Clin North Am* 10: 719.
3. Villalbi JR, Cleries M, Bouis S, et al. 2010. "Decline in hospitalisations due to dog bite injuries in Catalonia, 1997–2008. An effect of government regulation?" *Inj Prev* 16: 408.
4. Pomara C, D'Errico S, Jarussi V, et al. 2010. "Cave Canem: Bite mark analysis in a fatal dog pack attack." *Am J Forensic Med Pathol* 32: 50.
5. Benfield R, Plurad DS, Lam L, et al. 2010. "The epidemiology of dog attacks in an urban environment and the risk of vascular injury." *Am Surg* 76: 203.
6. Shuler CM, DeBess EE, Lapidus JA, and Hedberg K. 2008. "Canine and human factors related to dog bite injuries." *J Am Vet Med Assoc* 232: 542.
7. Boyce JD, and Adler B. 2006. "How does Pasteurella multocida respond to the host environment?" *Curr Opin Microbiol* 9: 117.
8. Talan DA, Citron DM, Abrahamian FM, et al. 1999. "Bacteriologic analysis of infected dog and cat bites. Emergency Medicine Animal Bite Infection Study Group." *N Engl J Med* 340: 85.
9. Ostanello F, Gherardi A, Caprioli A, et al. 2005. "Incidence of injuries caused by dogs and cats treated in emergency departments in a major Italian city." *Emerg Med J* 22: 260.
10. Kravetz JD, and Federman DG. 2002. "Cat-associated zoonoses." *Arch Intern Med* 162: 1945.
11. Lindsey D, Christopher M, Hollenbach J, et al. 1987. "Natural course of the human bite wound: Incidence of infection and complications in 434 bites and 803 lacerations in the same group of patients." *J Trauma* 27: 45.
12. Agrawal K, Mishra S, and Panda KN. 1992. "Primary reconstruction of major human bite wounds of the face." *Plast Reconstr Surg* 90: 394.
13. Donkor P, and Bankas DO. 1997. "A study of primary closure of human bite injuries to the face." *J Oral Maxillofac Surg* 55: 479.
14. Goldstein EJ, Citron DM, Merriam CV, et al. 2001. "Comparative in vitro activity of ertapenem and 11 other antimicrobial agents against aerobic and anaerobic pathogens isolated from skin and soft tissue animal and human bite wound infections." *J Antimicrob Chemother* 48: 641.
15. Van Sickels JE. 1981. "Parotid duct injuries." *Oral Surg Oral Med Oral Pathol* 52: 364.
16. Stevenson JH. 1983. "Parotid duct transection associated with facial trauma: Experience with 10 cases." *Br J Plast Surg* 36: 81.
17. Epker BN, and Burnette JC. 1970. "Trauma to the parotid gland and duct: Primary treatment and management of complications." *J Oral Surg* 28: 657.
18. Steinberg MJ, and Herrera AF. 2005. "Management of parotid duct injuries." *Oral Surg Oral Med Oral Pathol Oral Radiol Endod* 99: 136.
19. Sparkman RS. 1950. "Laceration of parotid duct further experiences." *Ann Surg* 131: 743.
20. Lewis G, and Knottenbelt JD. 1991. "Parotid duct injury: Is immediate surgical repair necessary?" *Injury* 22: 407.
21. Arnaud S, Batifol D, Goudot P, and Yachouh J. 2006. "Nonsurgical management of traumatic injuries of the parotid gland and duct using type a botulinum toxin." *Plast Reconstr Surg* 117: 2426.
22. Meningaud JP, Pitak-Arnnop P, Chikhani L, and Bertrand JC. 2006. "Drooling of saliva: A review of the etiology and management options." *Oral Surg Oral Med Oral Pathol Oral Radiol Endod* 101: 48.
23. Roland JT, Jr., Lin K, Klausner LM, and Miller PJ. 2006. "Direct facial-to-hypoglossal neurorrhaphy with parotid release." *Skull Base* 16: 101.
24. Sleilati FH, Nasr MW, Stephan HA, et al. 2010. "Treating facial nerve palsy by true termino-lateral hypoglossal-facial nerve anastomosis." *J Plast Reconstr Aesthet Surg* 63: 1087.
25. Tucker HM. 1978. "The management of facial paralysis due to extracranial injuries." *Laryngoscope* 88: 348.
26. Zaldivar RA, Buerger DE, Buerger DG, and Woog JJ. 2006. "Office evaluation of lacrimal and orbital disease. *Otolaryngol Clin North Am* 39: 911.
27. Tao JP, Luppens D, and McCord CD. 2010. "Buccal mucous membrane graft-assisted lacrimal drainage surgery." *Ophthal Plast Reconstr Surg* 26: 39.
28. Onerci M. 2002. "Dacryocystorhinostomy. Diagnosis and treatment of nasolacrimal canal obstructions." *Rhinology* 40: 49.
29. Montandon D. 1991. "Extrinsic eyelid ectropion." *Annals of Plastic Surgery* 26(4): 353.
30. Converse JM, and Smith B. 1959. "Repair of severe burn ectropion of the eyelids." *Plastic & Reconstructive Surgery & the Transplantation Bulletin* 23(1): 21.
31. Ivy RH. 1971. "Who originated the Z-plasty? (Charles Pierre Denonvilliers)." *Plastic & Reconstructive Surgery* 47(1): 67.
32. Levin ML, and Leone CR, Jr. 1990. "Bipedicle myocutaneous flap repair of cicatricial ectropion." *Ophthalmic Plastic & Reconstructive Surgery* 6(2): 119.
33. Xu JH, Tan WQ, and Yao JM. 2007. "Bipedicle orbicularis oculi flap in the reconstruction of the lower eyelid ectropion." *Aesthetic Plastic Surgery* 31(2): 161.

34. Wozniak K, and Sommer F. 2010. "[Surgical management of entropion]." *Ophthalmologe* 107: 905.

35. Pereira MG, Rodrigues MA, and Rodrigues SA. 2010. "Eyelid entropion." *Semin Ophthalmol* 25: 52.

36. Swamy BN, Benger R, and Taylor S. 2008. "Cicatricial entropion repair with hard palate mucous membrane graft: Surgical technique and outcomes." *Clin Experiment Ophthalmol* 36: 348.

37. Leibovitch I. 2010. "Lateral wedge resection: A simple technique for repairing involutional lower eyelid entropion." *Dermatol Surg* 36: 1412.

38. Champy M. 1983. "Biomechanische grundlagen der strassburger miniplattenosteosynthese." *Dtsch Zahnarztl Z* 38: 358.

39. Shetty V, and Freymiller E. 1989. "Teeth in the line of fracture: A review." *J Oral Maxillofac Surg* 47: 1303.

40. Neal DC, Wayne F, and Alpert B. 1978. "Morbidity associated with teeth in the line of mandibular fractures." *J Oral Surg* 36: 859.

41. Amaratunga NA. 1987. "The effect of teeth in the line of mandibular fractures on healing." *J Oral Maxillofac Surg* 45: 312.

42. Thaller SR, and Mabourakh S. 1994. "Teeth located in the line of mandibular fracture." *J Craniofac Surg* 5: 16.

43. Muller W. 1964. "Zur Frage des Versuchs der Erhaltung de rim bruchspalt sthenden zahne unter antibiotischem Schutz." *Dtsch Zahn Mund Kieferheilk* 41: 360.

44. Greenburg RN, James RB, Marier RL, et al. 1979. "Microbiologic and antibiotic aspects of infections in the oral and maxillofacial region." *Journal of Oral Surgery* 37: 873.

45. Kahnberg KE, and Ridell A. 1979. "Prognosis of teeth involved in the line of mandibular fractures." *International Journal of Oral Surgery* 8: 163.

46. Ellis E. 2002. "Outcomes of patients with teeth in the line of mandibular angle fractures treated with stable internal fixation." *Journal of Oral and Maxillofacial Surgery* 60: 863.

47. Bell RB, and Wilson DM. 2008. "Is the use of arch bars or interdental wire fixation necessary for successful outcomes in the open reduction and internal fixation of mandibular angle fractures?" *J Oral Maxillofac Surg* 66(10): 2116.

48. Chacon GE, and Larson PE. 2004. "Principles of management of mandibular fractures." In: *Peterson's Principles of Oral and Maxillofacial Surgery*, 2nd ed. Miloro M, Ghali GE, Larson PE, et al., eds., 401–431. Hamilton: BC Decker Inc.

49. Ellis E, and Walker LR. 1996. "Treatment of mandibular angle fractures using one non-compression miniplate." *Journal of Oral and Maxillofacial Surgery* 54: 864.

50. Passeri LA, Ellis E, and Sinn DP. 1993. "Complications of non-rigid fixation of mandibular angle fractures." *Journal of Oral and Maxillofacial Surgery* 51: 382.

51. Ellis E, and Ghali GE. 1991. "Lag screw fixation of mandibular angle fractures." *Journal of Oral and Maxillofacial Surgery* 49: 334.

52. Ellis E, and Karas N. 1992. "Treatment of mandibular angle fractures using two mini dynamic compression plates." *Journal of Oral and Maxillofacial Surgery* 50: 958.

53. Ellis E. 1993. "Treatment of mandibular angle fractures using the AO reconstruction plate." *Journal of Oral and Maxillofacial Surgery* 51: 250.

54. Ellis E, and Sinn DP. 1993. "Treatment of mandibular angle fractures using two 2.4 millimeter dynamic compression plates." *Journal of Oral and Maxillofacial Surgery* 51: 969.

55. Ellis E, and Walker L. 1994. "Treatment of mandibular angle fractures using two non-compression mini plates." *Journal of Oral and Maxillofacial Surgery* 52: 1032.

56. Potter JK, and Ellis E. 1999. "Treatment of mandibular angle fractures with a malleable non-compression miniplate." *J Oral Maxillofac Surg* 57: 288.

57. Ellis E. 1999. "Treatment methods for fractures of the mandibular angle." *International Journal of Oral and Maxillofacial Surgery* 28: 243.

58. Ellis E, and Miles BA. 2007. "Fractures of the mandible: A technical prospective." *Plastic and Reconstructive Surgery* 120(Supplement 2): 76S.

59. Buchbinder D. 1993. "Treatment of fractures of the edentulous mandible, 1943–1993: A review of the literature." *J Oral Maxillofac Surg* 51: 1174.

60. Zallen RD, and Curry JT. 1975. "A study of antibiotic usage in compound mandibular fractures." *J Oral Surg* 33: 431.

61. Chole RA, and Yee J. 1987. "Antibiotic prophylaxis for facial fractures. A prospective, randomized clinical trial." *Arch Otolaryngol Head Neck Surg* 113: 1055.

62. Abubaker AO, and Rollert MK. 2001. "Postoperative antibiotic prophylaxis in mandibular fractures: A preliminary randomized, double-blind, and placebo-controlled clinical study." *J Oral Maxillofac Surg* 59: 1415.

63. Miles BA, Potter JK, and Ellis E, 3rd. 2006. "The efficacy of postoperative antibiotic regimens in the open treatment of mandibular fractures: A prospective randomized trial." *J Oral Maxillofac Surg* 64: 576.

64. Tuovinen V, Norholt SE, Sindet-Pedersen S, and Jensen J. 1994. "A retrospective analysis of 279 patients with isolated mandibular fractures treated with titanium miniplates." *J Oral Maxillofac Surg* 52: 931.

65. Smith WP. 1991. "Delayed miniplate osteosynthesis for mandibular fractures." *Br J Oral Maxillofac Surg* 29: 73.

66. Ellis E, 3rd, and Walker L. 1994. "Treatment of mandibular angle fractures using two noncompression miniplates." *J Oral Maxillofac Surg* 52: 1032.

67. Marker P, Eckerdal A, and Smith-Sivertsen C. 1994. "Incompletely erupted third molars in the line of mandibular fractures. A retrospective analysis of 57 cases." *Oral Surg Oral Med Oral Pathol* 78: 426.

68. Ellis E, 3rd, and Walker LR. 1996. "Treatment of mandibular angle fractures using one noncompression miniplate." *J Oral Maxillofac Surg* 54: 864.

69. Hermund NU, Hillerup S, Kofod T, Schwartz O, and Andreasen JO. 2008. "Effect of early or delayed treatment upon healing of mandibular fractures: A systematic literature review." *Dent Traumatol* 24: 22.

70. Benson PD, Marshall MK, Engelstad ME, Kushner GM, and Alpert B. 2006. "The use of immediate bone grafting in reconstruction of clinically infected mandibular fractures: Bone grafts in the presence of pus." *J Oral Maxillofac Surg* 64: 122.

71. James RB, Frederickson C, and Kent J. 1981. "Prospective study of mandibular fractures." *Journal of Oral Surgery* 39: 275.

72. Chuong R, Donoff RB, and Guralnick WC. 1988. "A retrospective analysis of 327 mandibular fractures." *Journal of Oral and Maxillofacial Surgery* 41: 305.

73. Tiwana PS, Abraham MS, Kushner GM, and Alpert B. 2009. "Management of atrophic edentulous mandibular fractures: The case for primary reconstruction with immediate bone grafting." *J Oral Maxillofac Surg* 67: 882.

74. Van Sickels JE, and Cunningham LL. 2010. "Management of atrophic mandible fractures: Are bone grafts necessary?" *J Oral Maxillofac Surg* 68: 1392.

75. Carter TG, Brar PS, Tolas A, et al. 2008. "Off-label use of recombinant human bone morphogenetic protein-2 (rh-BMP-2)." *J Oral Maxillofac Surg* 66: 1417.

76. Cillo JE, Ellis E, 3rd. 2007. "Treatment of patient with double unilateral fractures of the mandible." *J Oral Maxillofac Surg* 65(8): 1461.

77. Amaratunga NA de S. 1987. "A study of condylar fractures in Sri Lankan patients with special reference to the recent views on treatment, healing and sequelae." *British Journal of Oral and Maxillofacial Surgery* 25: 391.

78. Beekler DM, and Walker RB. 1969. "Condyle fractures." *Journal of Oral Surgery* 27: 563.

79. Blevins C, and Gores RJ. 1961. "Fractures of the mandibular condylar process: The results of conservative treatment in 140 cases." *Journal of Oral Surgery* 19: 393.

80. Dahlstrom L, Kahnberg KE, and Lindhahl L. 1989. "Fifteen years follow-up on condylar fractures." *International Journal of Oral and Maxillofacial Surgery* 18: 18.

81. Hayward JR. 1990. "Discussion: Comparison of functional recovery after non-surgical and surgical treatment of condylar fractures." *Journal of Oral and Maxillofacial Surgery* 48: 1195.

82. Chalmers J Lyons Club. 1947. "Fractures involving the mandibular condyles: A posttreatment survey of 120 cases." *Journal of Oral Surgery* 5: 45.

83. MacLennan WD. 1952. "Consideration of 180 cases of typical fractures of the mandibular condylar process. *British Journal of Plastic Surgery* 5: 122.

84. Hawitschka M, and Eckelt U. 2002. "Assessment of patients treated for intracapsular fractures of the mandibular condyle by closed techniques." *J Oral Maxillofac Surg* 60: 784.

85. Lieberman DE, Pearson OM, Polk JD, Demes B, and Crompton AW. 2003. "Optimization of bone growth and remodeling in response to loading in tapered mammalian limbs." *J Exp Biol* 206: 3125.

86. Ellis E, and Throckmorton GS. 2000. "Facial symmetry after closed and open treatment of fractures of the mandibular condylar process." *Journal of Oral and Maxillofacial Surgery* 58: 719.

87. Kleinheinz J, Anastassov GE, and Joos U. 1999. "Indications for treatment of subcondylar mandibular fractures." *Journal of Craniomaxillofacial Trauma* 5(2): 17.

88. Dingman RO, and Grabb WC. 1962. "Surgical anatomy of the mandibular ramus of the facial nerve based on the dissection of 100 facial halves." *Plast Reconstr Surg Transplant Bull* 29: 266.

89. Kanno T, Mitsugi M, Sukegawa S, et al. 2010. "Submandibular approach through the submandibular gland fascia for treating mandibular fractures without identifying the facial nerve." *J Trauma* 68: 641.

90. Lutz JC, Clavert P, Wolfram-Gabel R, et al. 2010. "Is the high submandibular transmasseteric approach to the mandibular condyle safe for the inferior buccal branch?" *Surg Radiol Anat* 32: 963.

91. Schmelzeisen R, Cienfuegos-Monroy R, Schon R, et al. 2009. "Patient benefit from endoscopically assisted fixation of condylar neck fractures—a randomized controlled trial." *J Oral Maxillofac Surg* 67: 147.

92. Bagheri SC, Meyer RA, Khan HA, and Steed MB. 2009. "Microsurgical repair of peripheral trigeminal nerve injuries from maxillofacial trauma." *J Oral Maxillofac Surg* 67: 1791.

93. Boyne PJ. 1982. "Postexodontia osseous repair involving the mandibular canal." *J Oral Maxillofac Surg* 40: 69.

94. Bell RB, Dierks EJ, Brar P, Potter JK, and Potter BE. 2007. "A protocol for the management of frontal sinus injuries emphasizing sinus preservation." *J Oral Maxillofac Surg* 65(5): 825.

95. Chuang SK, and Dodson TB. 2004. "Evaluation and management of frontal sinus injuries." In: *Oral and Maxillofacial Trauma*, Vol. 2, 3rd ed., Fonseca RJ, Walker RV, Betts N, Powers MP, Barber HD, eds., 721–735. Philadelphia: WB Saunders Co.

96. Donald PJ, and Bernstein L. 1978. "Compound frontal sinus injuries with intracranial penetration." *Laryngoscope* 88(2): 225.

97. Larrabee WF, Travis LW, and Tabb HG. 1980. "Frontal sinus fractures: Their suppurative complications and surgical management." *Laryngoscope* 90: 1810.

98. Wolfe SA, and Johnson P. 1988. "Frontal sinus injuries: Primary care and management of late complications." *Plast Reconstr Surg* 82: 781.

99. Wallis A, and Donald PJ. 1988. "Frontal sinus fractures: A review of 72 cases." *Laryngoscope* 98: 593.

100. Gonty AA, Marciani RD, and Adornato DC. 1999. "Management of frontal sinus fractures: A review of 33 cases." *J Oral Maxillofac Surg* 57: 372.

101. Ioannides C, and Freihofer HP. 1999. "Fractures of the frontal sinus: Classification and its implications for surgical treatment." *Am J Otolaryngol* 20(5): 273.

102. Gerbino G, Roccia F, Benech A, and Caldarelli C. 2000. "Analysis of 158 frontal sinus fractures: Current surgical management and complications." *J Cranio Maxillofac Surg* 28: 133.

103. Ioannides C, Freihofer HP, and Friens. 1993. "Fractures of the frontal sinus: A rationale of treatment." *Br J Plast Surg* 46: 208.

104. Sailer HF, Gratz KW, and Kalavreezos ND. 1998. "Frontal sinus fractures: Principles of treatment and long-term results after sinus obliteration with the use of lyophilized cartilage." *J Craniomaxillofac Surg* 26: 235.

105. Levine SB, et al. 1986. "Evaluation and treatment of frontal sinus fractures." *Otolaryngol Head Neck Surg* 95: 19.

106. Ducic Y, and Stone TL. 1999. "Frontal sinus obliteration using a laterally based pedicled pericranial flap." *Laryngoscope* 109: 541.

107. Disa JJ, et al. 1996. "Transverse glabellar flap for obliteration/isolation of the nasofrontal duct from the anterior cranial base." *Ann Plast Surg* 36: 453.

108. Duvall AJ, III, et al. 1987. "Frontal sinus fractures: Analysis of treatment results." *Arch Otolaryngol Head Neck Surg* 113: 933.

109. Lakhani RS, et al. 2001. "Titanium mesh repair of the severely comminuted frontal sinus fracture." *Arch Otolaryngol Head Neck Surg* 127: 665.

110. Lee TT, et al. 1998. "Early combined management of frontal sinus and orbital and facial fractures." *J Trauma* 44: 665.

111. Parhiscar A, and Har-El G. 2001. "Frontal sinus obliteration with the pericranial flap." *Otolaryngol Head Neck Surg* 124: 304.

112. Raveh J, and Vuillemin T. 1988. "The surgical one-stage management of combined cranio-maxillo-facial and frontobasal fractures: Advantages of the subcranial approach in 374 cases." *J Craniomaxillofac Surg* 16: 160.

113. Rosen G, and Nachtigal D. 1995. "The use of hydroxyapatite for obliteration of the human frontal sinus." *Laryngoscope* 105: 553.

114. Thaller SR, and Donald P. 1994. "The use of pericranial flaps in frontal sinus fractures." *Ann Plast Surg* 32: 284.

115. Petruzzelli GJ, and Stankiewicz JA. 2002. "Frontal sinus obliteration with hydroxyapatite cement." *Laryngoscope* 112: 32.

116. Shockley WW, et al. 1988. "Frontal sinus fractures: Some problems and some solutions." *Laryngoscope* 98: 18.

117. Stanley RB, Jr, and Schwartz MS. 1989. "Immediate reconstruction of contaminated central craniofacial injuries with free autogenous grafts." *Laryngoscope* 99: 1011.

118. Snyderman CH, et al. 2001. "Hydroxyapatite: An alternative method of frontal sinus obliteration." *Otolaryngol Clin North Am* 34: 179.

119. Wilson BC, et al. 1988. "Comparison of complications following frontal sinus fractures managede with exploration with or without obliteration over 10 years." *Laryngoscope* 98: 516.

120. David DJ, and Sheen R. 1990. "Surgical correction of Crouzon's syndrome." *Plast Reconstr Surg* 85: 344.

121. Fearon JA, and Whitaker LA. 1993. "Complications with facial advancement: A comparison between the Le Fort II and mono-bloc advancements." *Plast Reconstr Surg* 91: 990.

122. Krastinova-Lolov D, and Hamza F. 1996. "The surgical management of cranio-orbital neurofibromatosis." *Ann Plast Surg* 36: 263.

123. Manson PN, Crawley WA, and Hoopes JE. 1986. "Frontal cranioplasty: Risk factors and choice of cranial vault reconstructive material." *Plast Reconstr Surg* 77: 888.

124. Posnick JC, al-Oattan MM, and Armstrong D. 1996. "Monobloc and facial bipartition osteotomies for reconstruction of craniofacial malformations: A study of extradural dead space and morbidity." *Plast Reconstr Surg* 97(6): 1118.

125. Shons AR, et al. 1983. "The use of methyl methacrylate in a two-stage correction of Crouzon's/Apert's deformity." *Ann Plast Surg* 10: 147.

126. Spinelli HM, et al. 1994. "An analysis of extradural dead space after fronto-orbital surgery." *Plast Reconstr Surg* 93: 1372.

127. Whitaker LA, et al. 1987. "Craniosynostosis: An analysis of the timing, treatment, and complications in 164 consecutive patients." *Plast Reconstr Surg* 80: 195.

128. Wolfe SA, et al. 1993. "The monobloc frontofacial advancement: Do the pluses outweigh the minuses?" *Plast Reconstr Surg* 91: 977.

129. Bell RB, Dierks EJ, Homer L, and Potter BE. 2004. "Management of cerebrospinal fluid leaks associated with craniomaxillofacial trauma." *J Oral Maxillofac Surg* 62: 676.

130. Bell RB. 2009. "Management of frontal sinus fractures." *Oral Maxillofac Surg Clin North Am* 21(2): 227.

131. Bell RB, and Chen J. 2010. "Frontobasilar fractures: Contemporary management." *Atlas Oral Maxillofac Surg Clin North Am* 18(2): 181.

132. Bell RB. 2007. "The role of oral and maxillofacial surgery in the trauma care center." *J Oral Maxillofac Surg* 65(12): 2544.

133. Manson PN. 1999. "Pure orbital blowout fracture: New concepts and importance of the medial orbital blowout fracture." *Plastic & Reconstructive Surgery* 104(3): 878.

134. Fan X, Li J, Zhu J, Li H, and Zhang D. 2003. "Computer-assisted orbital volume measurement in the surgical correction of late enophthalmos caused by blowout fractures." *Ophthalmic Plastic & Reconstructive Surgery* 19(3): 207.

135. Whitehouse RW, Batterbury M, Jackson A, and Noble JL. 1994. "Prediction of enophthalmos by computed tomography after 'blow out' orbital fracture." *British Journal of Ophthalmology* 78(8): 618.

136. Ploder O, Klug C, Voracek M, Burggasser G, and Czerny C. 2002. "Evaluation of computer-based area and volume measurement from coronal computed tomography scans in isolated blowout fractures of the orbital floor." *Journal of Oral & Maxillofacial Surgery* 60(11): 1267; discussion 1273.

137. Manson PN, Clifford CM, Su CT, Iliff NT, and Morgan R. 1986. "Mechanisms of global support and posttraumatic enophthalmos: I. The anatomy of the ligament sling and its relation to intramuscular cone orbital fat." *Plastic & Reconstructive Surgery* 77(2): 193.

138. Rohrich RJ, Janis JE, and Adams WP, Jr. 2003. "Subciliary versus subtarsal approaches to orbitozygomatic fractures." *Plast Reconstr Surg* 111: 1708.

139. Converse J. 1944. "Two plastic operations for repair of orbit following severe trauma and extensive comminuted fracture." *Arch Ophthalmol* 31: 323.

140. Ridgway EB, Chen C, and Lee BT. 2009. "Acquired entropion associated with the transconjunctival incision for facial fracture management." *J Craniofac Surg* 20: 1412.

141. Tessier P. 1973. "The conjunctival approach to the orbital floor and maxilla in congenital malformation and trauma." *J Maxillofac Surg* 1: 3.

142. Kim JH, Kook MS, Ryu SY, et al. 2008. "A simple technique for the treatment of inferior orbital blow-out fracture: A transantral approach, open reduction, and internal fixation with miniplate and screws." *J Oral Maxillofac Surg* 66: 2488.

143. Kawamoto HK, Jr. 1982. "Late posttraumatic enophthalmos: A correctable deformity?" *Plastic & Reconstructive Surgery* 69(3): 431.

144. Manson PN, Ruas EJ, and Iliff NT. 1987. "Deep orbital reconstruction for correction of post-traumatic enophthalmos." *Clinics in Plastic Surgery* 14(1): 113.

145. Bell RB, and Markiewicz MR. 2009. "Computer assisted planning, stereolithographic modeling, and intraoperative navigation for complex orbital reconstruction: A descriptive study on a preliminary cohort." *J Oral Maxillofac Surg* 67(12): 2559.

146. Converse JM, Smith B, Obear MF, and Wood-Smith D. 1967. "Orbital blowout fractures: A ten-year survey." *Plastic & Reconstructive Surgery* 39(1): 20.

147. Manson PN, Grivas A, Rosenbaum A, Vannier M, Zinreich J, and Iliff N. 1986. "Studies on enophthalmos: II. The measurement of orbital injuries and their treatment by quantitative computed tomography." *Plastic & Reconstructive Surgery* 77(2): 203.

148. Schon R, Metzger MC, Zizelmann C, Weyer N, and Schmelzeisen R. 2006. "Individually preformed titanium mesh implants for a true-to-original repair of orbital fractures." *International Journal of Oral & Maxillofacial Surgery* 35(11): 990.

149. Glassman RD, Manson PN, Vanderkolk CA, Iliff NT, Yaremchuk MJ, Petty P, Defresne CR, and Markowitz BL. 1990. "Rigid fixation of internal orbital fractures." *Plastic & Reconstructive Surgery* 86(6): 1103; discussion 1110.

150. Romano JJ, Iliff NT, and Manson PN. 1993. "Use of Medpor porous polyethylene implants in 140 patients with facial fractures." *Journal of Craniofacial Surgery* 4(3): 142.

151. Ellis E, 3rd, and Tan Y. 2003. "Assessment of internal orbital reconstructions for pure blowout fractures: Cranial bone grafts versus titanium mesh." *Journal of Oral & Maxillofacial Surgery* 61(4): 442.

152. Metzger MC, Schon R, Zizelmann C, Weyer N, Gutwald R, and Schmelzeisen R. 2007. "Semiautomatic procedure for individual preforming of titanium meshes for orbital fractures." *Plastic & Reconstructive Surgery* 119(3): 969.

153. Metzger MC, Schon R, Weyer N, Rafii A, Gellrich NC, Schmelzeisen R, and Strong BE. 2006. "Anatomical 3-dimensional pre-bent titanium implant for orbital floor fractures." *Ophthalmology* 113(10): 1863.

154. Scolozzi P, Momjian R, Heuberger J, Andersen E, Broome M, Terzic A, and Jaques B. 2009. "Accuracy and predictability in use of AO three-dimensionally preformed titanium mesh plates for posttraumatic orbital reconstruction: A pilot study." *The Journal of Craniofacial Surgery* 20(4): 1108.

155. Gruss JS, Van Wyck L, Phillips JH, and Antonyshyn O. 1990. "The importance of the zygomatic arch in complex midfacial fracture repair and correction of posttraumatic orbitozygomatic deformities." *Plast Reconstr Surg* 85(6): 878.

156. Govsa F, Celik S, and Ozer MA. 2009. "Orbital restoration surgery in the zygomaticotemporal and zygomaticofacial nerves and important anatomic landmarks." *J Craniofac Surg* 20: 540.

157. Peltomaa J, and Rihkanen H. 2000. "Infraorbital nerve recovery after minimally dislocated facial fractures." *European Archives of Oto-Rhino-Laryngology* 257: 449.

158. Reymond J, Kwiatkowski J, and Wysocki J. 2008. "Clinical anatomy of the superior orbital fissure and the orbital apex." *J Craniomaxillofac Surg* 36: 346.

159. Rajiniganth MG, Bupta AK, Bupta A, and Bapuraj JR. 2003. "Traumatic optic neuropathy: Visual outcome following combined therapy protocol." *Arch Otolaryngol Head Neck Surg* 129(11): 1203.

160. Ginsburg CM. 1995. "Infected nasal septal hematoma." *Pediatric Infectious Disease Journal* 14: 1012.

161. Leon MA, et al. 2004. "Deforming posttraumatic hematoma of the nasal tip: An infrequent lesion." *Plast Reconstr Surg* 113: 641.

162. Meehan T, et al. 1994. "Alar cartilage hematoma." *J Laryngol Otol* 108: 500.

163. Green KM. 1999. "Alar hematoma." *J Laryngol Otol* 113: 1104.

164. Sessions DG, and Stallings JO. 1972. "Correction of saddle nose deformity." *Laryngoscope* 82: 2000.

165. Eavey RD, et al. 1977. "Bacterial meningitis secondary to abscess of the nasal septum." *Pediatrics* 60: 102.

166. Borden NM, et al. 1996. "Posttraumatic epistaxis from injury to the pterygovaginal artery." *Amer J Neuroradiol* 17: 1148.

167. Schipchandler TZ, et al. 2008. "Saddle nose deformity reconstruction with a split calvarial bone L-shaped strut." *Arch Facial Plast Surg* 10: 305.

168. Kim DW, et al. 2004. "Management of posttraumatic nasal deformities: The crooked nose and the saddle nose." *Facial Plast Surg Clin N Am* 12: 111.

169. Savion I, et al. 2005. "Construction of a surgical stent for posttraumatic nasal synechiae." *J Prosth Dent* 94: 462.

170. Hatoko M, et al. 2000. "Correction of a posttraumatic nasal deformity using a hard palate mucosa graft." *Aesth Plast Surg* 24: 34.

171. Ellis E. 2004. "Passive repositioning of maxillary fractures: An occasional impossibility without osteotomy." *J Oral Maxillofac Surg* 62: 1477.

172. Steidler NE, Cook RM, and Reade PC. 1980. "Residual complications in patients with major middle third facial fractures." *Int J Oral Surg* 9: 259.

173. Ellis E, and Potter JK. 1999. "The effects of trauma on the maxillary sinus." *Oral Maxillofac Surg Clin No Am* 11: 165.

174. Top H, Aygit C, Sarikaya A, et al. 2004. "Evaluation of maxillary sinus after treatment of midfacial fractures." *J Oral Maxillofac Surg* 62: 1229.

175. Hwang K, and Choi HG. 2009. "Bleeding from posterior superior alveolar artery in Le Fort I fracture." *J Craniofac Surg* 20: 1610.

176. Kurata A, Kitahara T, Miyasaka Y, et al. 1993. "Superselective embolization for severe traumatic epistaxis caused by fracture of the skull base." *AJNR Am J Neuroradiol* 14: 343.

177. Murakami R, Kumazaki T, Tajima H, et al. 1996. "Transcatheter arterial embolization as treatment for life-threatening maxillofacial injury." *Radiat Med* 14: 197.

178. Jongkees LB. 1968. "Surgery of the facial nerve." *J Laryngol Otol* 82: 575.

179. Alford BR, Sessions RB, and Weber SC. 1971. "Indications for surgical decompression of the facial nerve." *Laryngoscope* 81: 620.

180. Tucker HM. 1978. "The management of facial paralysis due to extracranial injuries." *Laryngoscope* 88: 348.

181. Dierks EJ. 2008. "Tracheotomy: Elective and emergent." *Oral Maxillofac Surg Clin North Am* 20: 513.

182. Yavas S, Yagar S, Mavioglu L, et al. 2009. "Tracheostomy: How and when should it be done in cardiovascular surgery ICU?" *J Card Surg* 24: 11.

183. Colman KL, Mandell DL, and Simons JP. 2010. "Impact of stoma maturation on pediatric tracheostomy-related complications." *Arch Otolaryngol Head Neck Surg* 136: 471.

184. Waldron J, Padgham ND, and Hurley SE. 1990. "Complications of emergency and elective tracheostomy: A retrospective study of 150 consecutive cases." *Ann R Coll Surg Engl* 72: 218.

185. Szeto C, Kost K, Hanley JA, et al. 2010. "A simple method to predict pretracheal tissue thickness to prevent accidental decannulation in the obese." *Otolaryngol Head Neck Surg* 143: 223.

186. Gross ND, Cohen JI, Andersen PE, and Wax MK. 2002. "'Defatting' tracheotomy in morbidly obese patients." *Laryngoscope* 112: 1940.

187. Malata CM, Foo IT, Simpson KH, and Batchelor AG. 1996. "An audit of Bjork flap tracheostomies in head and neck plastic surgery." *Br J Oral Maxillofac Surg* 34: 42.

188. Stanton DC, Kademani D, Patel C, and Foote JW. 2004. "Management of post-tracheotomy scars and persistent tracheocutaneous fistulas with dermal interpositional fat graft." *J Oral Maxillofac Surg* 62: 514.

189. Jackson C, and Babcock WM. 1934. "Plastic closure of tracheocutaneous fistula." 14: 199.

190. Goldsmith AJ, Abramson AL, and Myssiorek D. 1993. "Closure of tracheocutaneous fistula using a modified cutaneous Z-plasty." *Am J Otolaryngol* 14: 240.

191. Lee UJ, Goh EK, Wang SG, and Hwang SM. 2002. "Closure of large tracheocutaneous fistula using turn-over hinge flap and V-Y advancement flap." *J Laryngol Otol* 116: 627.

192. Fisher SR. 1991. "Closure of tracheocutaneous fistula with perichondrial flap following cricothyroidotomy." *Laryngoscope* 101: 684.

193. Carlson ER, Marx RE, and Jones GM. 1991. "Tracheostomy scar revision using allogenic dura." *J Oral Maxillofac Surg* 49: 315.

5

Orthognathic Surgery

Stephanie J. Drew, DMD

Complications may occur at any point in time along the course of treating the patient undergoing orthognathic surgery. From diagnosis to discharge, the list is extensive, and, for the most part, preventable. Preparation is the key. Careful treatment planning and excellent technical training to manage these potential risks are paramount to the success of orthognathic surgery. Multiple reviews of the incidence and types of complications have been reported in the literature.[1-10] A Medline search in early 2011 of "orthognathic surgery complications" revealed 479 articles. The majority of these articles focus on the incidence of complications related to a specific osteotomy (Fig. 5.1).

A list of complications from orthognathic surgery can be divided into three main sections: preoperative complications, perioperative complications, and postoperative complications. For the purposes of this chapter, the preoperative complications will be considered if they have occurred before the actual surgery has started. Perioperative complications are those that take place in the operating room during the surgical procedure, and postoperative complications occur anytime after the surgery is completed until patient discharge from the practice (see Fig. 5.2).

PREOPERATIVE COMPLICATIONS

Diagnosis

Accurate diagnosis of the skeletal facial deformity is the beginning of the time line for the orthognathic surgical patient. The diagnosis will dictate which osteotomies will be necessary to align the facial skeletal components into a functional, aesthetic, and orthognathic position. Cephalometric analysis, face-bow mounted dental models and/or computer generated models, photographs, and clinical measurements must be accurate and reproducible.

The accurate gathering of this data is essential to the outcome of the surgical plan.[11] If the patient's head position is not correct during record taking, the dental models not mounted with the right occlusion, or the facial measurement not correct, the skeletal components will not be surgically moved into the correct predicted position. To insure that data collection is consistent, protocols must be established by the practitioner so that the information can be consistently utilized with minimal margin of error while transferring the data from the patient to the laboratory and the computer, and then the operating room. From the use of light-cured acrylic splints to stereolithographic biomodeling generated splints from computer tomography technology, the accuracy of obtaining the predicted occlusion continues to improve.[12-14]

Management of Complications in Oral and Maxillofacial Surgery, First Edition. Edited by Michael Miloro, Antonia Kolokythas.
© 2012 John Wiley & Sons, Inc. Published 2012 by John Wiley & Sons, Inc.

MAXILLARY OSTEOTOMIES	MANDIBULAR OSTEOTOMIES	GENIOPLASTY
• Hemorrhage • Dental Trauma • Poor Down fracture • Mobilization • Soft Tissue Injury • Positioning problems • Stabilization • Unaesthetic Soft Tissue Changes • Nerve injury • Airway Compromises	• Nerve Injury • Poor Osteotomy splitting • Poor segment alignment • Bleeding • Impacted Wisdom Teeth • Condylar Positioning • Dental Trauma • Stabilization • Mobilization	• Nerve Injury • Dental Trauma • Mobilization • Stabilization • Mandible Fracture • Unaesthetic Soft Tissue Changes • Bleeding

Fig. 5.1. Complications by osteotomy location.

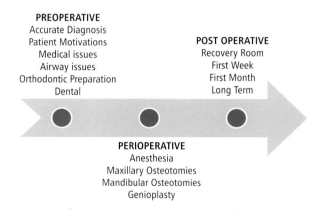

PREOPERATIVE
Accurate Diagnosis
Patient Motivations
Medical issues
Airway issues
Orthodontic Preparation
Dental

POST OPERATIVE
Recovery Room
First Week
First Month
Long Term

PERIOPERATIVE
Anesthesia
Maxillary Osteotomies
Mandibular Osteotomies
Genioplasty

Fig. 5.2. Preoperative, perioperative, and postoperative complication time frames.

Patient Motivation

During the initial phases of treatment, finding out the reason why a patient is motivated to seek treatment is another key component to successful outcome.[15–18] If patient expectations cannot be met or if they are unrealistic, then no matter what type of accuracy is obtained with the workup or surgery, the patient will not be satisfied. This is not only a disappointment to the surgeon but a true failure to the patient. The use of patient preoperative questionnaires may elucidate the patient's initial motivation and understanding of why they are seeking surgical consultation. If the patient's expectations are not realistic and cannot be met then it may be best to defer treatment.

Time spent educating the patient and family until they are able to understand what the surgery can realistically accomplish will enable for better emotional and physical outcomes. There are many resources available to help the surgeon in this regard from written materials to Web-based teaching tools to video imaging of the surgical procedures. The type of teaching tools can be customized for each patient and family. This is the beginning of the informed consent process.

Medical Issues

Medical issues that may be associated with or create skeletal facial deformities may also be an undiagnosed "monster in the closet." Diseases such as pituitary adenomas; bleeding dyscrasias; sleep apnea; myotonias; temporomandibuar joint disorders, including tumors; idiopathic condylar lysis; arthritis; and psychological diseases are to name a few. The majority of these problems not only affect the intraoperative anesthesia and medical management of patients but the long-term function and stability of the results as well. The impact of several medical conditions on perioperative planning can be found in other texts and is not the focus of this work.

Airway Issues

The initial airway evaluation of the orthognathic patient includes not only looking at the anatomic issues that the patient has preoperatively, but how the postoperative changes in the skeletal support of the airway will affect the airway patency.[19,20] The presence of large tonsillar tissues, deviated nasal septum, chronic sinus disease, large tongue, or even pulmonary diseases such as asthma will affect the patient's perioperative airway and postoperative management. Therefore, patients who are undergoing orthognathic surgery should be screened for signs of airway issues as well as possible obstructive sleep apnea (OSA). This includes excessive daytime somnolence, snoring, increased body mass index (BMI), and medical conditions related to OSA. If these findings are positive then further investigation for sleep disorders with appropriate studies including a polysomnography (PFG) should be undertaken. If sleep apnea is diagnosed, then the proposed treatment plan may require modifications according to the risk of potential airway compromise from moving the skeletal bases and a plan can be developed instead to improve the airway.[21,22]

Speech may also be affected by movement of the jaws.[23,24] Changes in speech are best managed by involving a specialist in speech therapy from the beginning of treatment planning. Those patients that present with large skeletal discrepancies, especially those with apertognathia, may have learned to compensate with lip and tongue habits that will need to be addressed in the pre- and postoperative periods. Having a formal speech evaluation preoperatively will help the team provide good speech therapy in the postoperative period.

Another area where a speech pathologist's evaluation will be valuable is velopharyngeal incompetence pre- and postoperatively.[25,26] A formal nasopharyngoscopy is necessary to document the movement of the posterior pharyngeal walls and soft palate when evaluating for velopharyngeal incompetence. Special consideration and careful planning during intubation for orthognathic surgery are required for patients who had correction of velopharyngeal incompetence with pharyngeal flaps. Flap release and secondary reconstruction at a later time once tissue revascularization is complete may be required.

Orthodontic Preparation

Communication mishaps with the orthodontist are also an area where complications may occur preoperatively. Once the initial diagnosis and treatment plan is established, it is important for the surgeon to follow along as the orthodontic preparation of these patients is progressing. Taking periodic study models will enable the treating team to discuss progression and identify potential problems that may impact on the ability to execute the planned surgical movements and achieve the desirable results.[27–32]

Accurate diagnosis of the skeletal discrepancy to be corrected is paramount for appropriate orthodontic preparation and avoidance of perioperative complications and future relapses. Such is the case of transverse deficiencies that will lead to relapse if not recognized and addressed appropriately early in the treatment. When segmental osteotomies are required, their position should be clearly communicated so adequate spaces between the roots can be created orthodontically and the bony cuts can be safely performed. Furthermore, appropriate leveling and alignment of the dentition will allow for spaces to be created accommodating both the surgical movements and the postoperative final orthodontic manipulations for case completion. Finally, details such as the position of the orthodontic appliances, utilization of the appropriate arch wire, and no manipulation whatsoever once impressions for surgical planning are obtained require clear understanding.

Dental Issues

For many dental issues such as the extraction of impacted thirds, space preparation for congenitally missing teeth must be addressed in the preoperative period.

The presence of impacted mandibular third molars, for example, increases the risk of an unfavorable osteotomy (bad split). It appears that this may be an age-dependent event. The younger the patient the more likely that the split will be "bad" if the tooth is taken at the time of the split. It has been recommended that if the teeth are going to be removed prior to surgery, extractions should be performed between 6 and

9 months prior to the osteotomy. This may decrease the risk of a "bad split" due to an impacted tooth in the osteotomy site.[33–36]

If the patient is missing teeth that are to be replaced with dental implants, the timing of when implants and bone grafting to prepare implant sites is of importance.[37–39] Soft tissue grafting and bone grafting require flap designs that may compromise the blood supply to the alveolus of the maxilla if a Le Fort I osteotomy is expected. Adequate time should be allowed for these tissues to revascularize. Typically, at least 6 months should be allowed before Le Fort I surgery to insure adequate revascvariztion.

Congenitally missing teeth pose a problem related to arch length and also the prosthetic rehabilitation of these cases. If the congenitally missing tooth is going to be replaced with a dental implant then two issues must be addressed. First, how will enough room be achieved in three dimensions to place the fixture? Is there a need to expand the arch surgically to gain length? Or can simple orthodontic movement create enough room?

Second, once spacing is achieved, is there enough bone there to support an implant? If not, then when should bone grafting be done? For instance, the incisions that are created to access the osteotomies may impact on local soft tissue healing when placing onlay grafts to the alveolus and potentially lead to vascularity issues and wound healing problems. It is also possible to graft at the time of orthognathic surgical positioning. However, care at these alveolar sites related to the ability to maintain vascularity of the soft tissues over these grafts is important. Modifying the incisions to provide maximum coverage of these grafts and thus vascularity is essential to survival of these grafts.

INTRAOPERATIVE COMPLICATIONS

Proper communication between the surgeon, nursing, and anesthesia staff is essential (Fig. 5.3).

It is essential to control blood loss with an excellent technique and understanding of surgical anatomy; however, using hypotensive anesthetic techniques may also help.[40] The most common use of this technique is during the Le Fort I osteotomy downfracture. This process is not without its own potential complications of circulatory and vascularity issues to the maxilla. Return to a normotensive stage should be accomplished as soon as the downfracture is completed.[40–43]

MAXILLARY SURGERY: INTRAOPERATIVE COMPLICATIONS

The work horse of maxillary orthognathic surgery is the Le Fort I osteotomy. Hemorrhage is the most well known complication and has been well documented as a complication of this osteotomy.[44–47] However, errors in execution of this procedure can lead to compromises in the dentition, bone healing, and soft

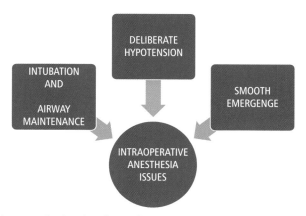

Fig. 5.3. Possible intraoperative anesthesia-related complications.

tissue healing. Other issues that have been reported as a result of poor intraoperative technique include neural deficits; nasal airway obstruction; ocular issues, including blindness; and sinus pathology.[48–54]

Dental Trauma

Dental trauma from Le Fort osteotomy is usually a result of improper osteotomy placement. For example, if the horizontal maxillary osteotomy is positioned too inferiorly there is a risk of transection of the root apices.[55] It is generally recommended that these osteotomies are planned at least 5 mm above the apices of the maxillary roots.[56–58] Other complications that arise are related to maxillary segmental osteotomies that are used to either level the occlusal plane or for correction of transverse discrepancies.[59,60] Adequate space is required between the roots of the teeth at the sites of the planned vertical osteotomies to allow for bony coverage of the roots. When preparing the space orthodontically care should be taken to not tip the teeth but rather achieve bodily movement. Careful radiographic examination of the root length and adequacy of space in cases of segmental osteotomies are essential in avoiding dental injuries perioperatively. Drawing the root surfaces on the casts or utilization of three-dimensional software for osteotomy planning may also help in decreasing these potential complications.

Although pulp necrosis post Le Fort osteotomy is unusual, it does occur. The pulp tissues will heal spontaneously despite an impaired blood supply.[61] Vitality testing is not a reliable indicator of pulpal necrosis because between 6% and 29% of all teeth remain insensate up to 54 months post osteotomy.[62] Endodontic treatment should only be indicated once the clinical symptoms or radiographic evidence is demonstrated that it is clearly necessary. One may notice a darkening of the maxillary incisor or pink color. It is best at the initial postoperative visits to wait for at least 8 weeks before embarking on endodontic treatment. This will allow for possible revascularization and vitalization that is often the case with these teeth. However, if the teeth remain nonvital then endodontic treatment is essential.

Intraoperative complications specific to the maxillary bone itself include poor fracture of the maxilla, inability to mobilize the segments to gain anterior movement or width, and difficulty posteriorly or superiorly positioning the maxilla.

Soft Tissue Issues

The gingival and palatal tissues at these sites can also be injured by lacerating it from sharp instruments or rotary burs and during the osteotomies as well as by crushing of the tissues when the segments are collapsed during a segmental osteotomy. Attention to these details will prevent injury in these sites and the use of segmental surgery can be done in a predictable manner with good results.[63]

Lacerations to the soft tissues of the hard palate or alveolar mucosa may also occur with improper use of cutting instruments. This soft tissue injury may lead to necrosis of the soft tissues and possibly vascular compromise of the bone in these areas (Fig. 5.4).[64] Clinically, the vascular compromise may lead to the formation of oral-antral or oro-nasal fistula formation or sequestrum formation (Fig. 5.5). The patient may even lose an entire segment of teeth. These soft tissue injuries are best managed very conservatively in the operating room. Raising flaps to close these defects may further compromise the blood supply to the underlying maxillary bone and lead to avascular necrosis. In the postoperative period these communications are best managed conservatively with irrigation and covering the tissues with a noncompressive splint to allow for mucosal healing. Consideration must be given toward adjunctive hyperbaric oxygen therapy to limit the extent and degree of necrosis. Formal closure, if required, may be achieved at a later time with local or distant flaps once vascularization of the maxilla and healing of the bone segments has occurred.

Fixation Issues

Other complications arise when there is either instability from the fixation used in the operating room or inherent problems with dysplastic or hypoplastic bone. Since the most unstable movement of the maxilla is downward and forward simultaneously, rigid fixation, along with bone grafting, may theoretically help increase stability and allow the bone heal.[65,66] However, direct bone contact seems to be the key to maintaining stability. This has been reported to be accomplished by modifying the osteotomy design to ensure bone contact. However, the downward movement is limited by the length of vertical cuts made to approximately a total of 6 mm.[67]

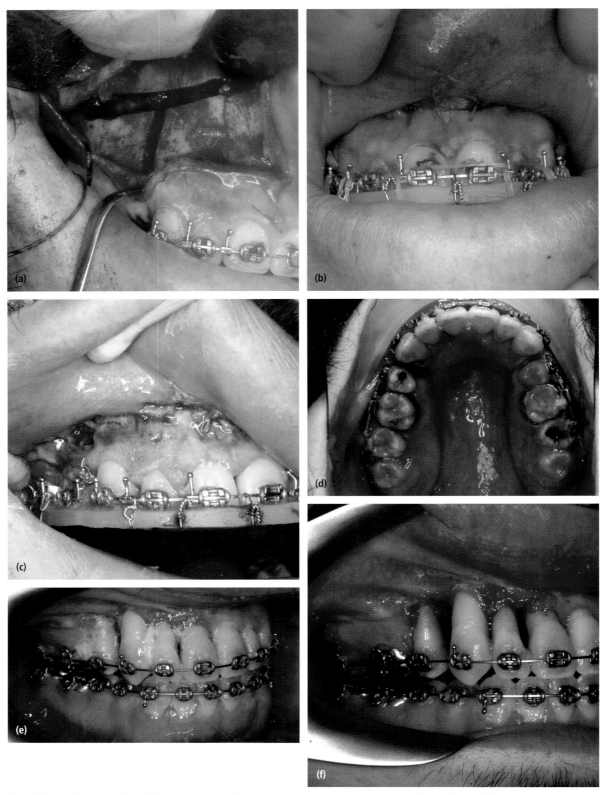

Fig. 5.4. (a) Segmental maxillary osteotomy. (b) Intraoperative dusky appearance of anterior maxillary gingiva indicating vascular compromise. (c) 1-week appearance of necrotic gingival tissues. (d) 1-week appearance of palate without significant vascular compromise. (e) 3-week appearance prior to HBO therapy. (f) 2-month appearance after HBO therapy. Tooth loss and bone grafting is required.

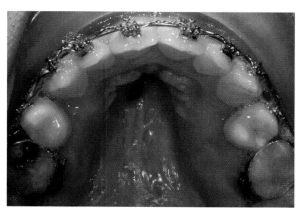

Fig. 5.5. Persistent oronasal fistula following segmental maxillary surgery.

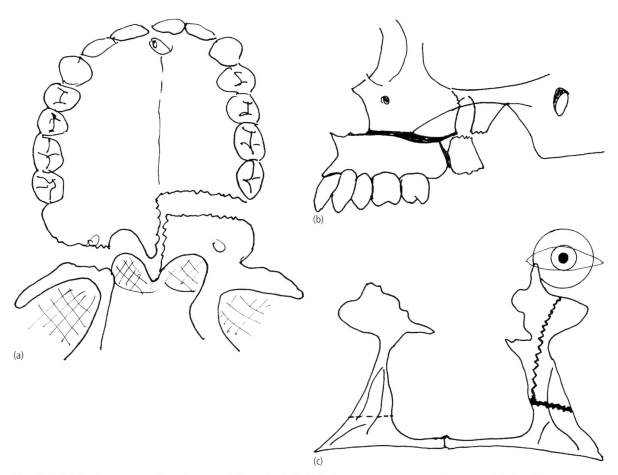

Fig. 5.6. (a) Inadvertent maxillary fracture of the palatal shelf during Le Fort osteotomy. (b) Pterygoid plate fracture during Le Fort osteotomy. (c) Pyramidal fracture of maxillary extending to inferior orbital fissure.

The Downfracture

Downfracture of the maxilla will occur predictably only if the osteotomies are properly executed. The process of downfracturing the maxilla should require minimal force if all osteotomies are complete. Inadequate osteotomies will lead to atypical fracture patterns and can create unfavorable fracture lines that can lead up to the skull base or the orbit (Fig. 5.6).[68] These unfavorable fractures may also create tears in the soft tissues and lead to bleeding and hematoma formation within the orbit or posterior maxilla.

If the maxilla is not separated properly, incomplete osteotomies when forced can also create unfavorable fractures across the palatal shelves. Fracture at the junction of the horizontal process of the palatine bone with the palatal process of the maxilla occurs when the plates are not separated. High horizontal fracture of the pyramidal process of the palatine bone occurs when the medial osteotomy is not completed to the pyramidal process. Horizontal fracture of the pterygoid plates with or without separation of the tuberosity is also due to incomplete separation along with a horizontal cut into the plates from the saw or chisels. The palatal shelves remain attached to the pterygoid plates, and it may then be difficult to mobilize, advance, or position the maxilla.

Intraoperative attempts to correct these problems predispose the patient to possible damage to adjacent vascular or neural structures and if not released in the long term, relapse may occur.

Another issue that may arise with improper osteotomy is damage to the nasolacrimal duct as it exits the inferior meatus area causing scarring thus leading to epiphora. The nacolacrimal duct is approximately 11–14 mm posterior to the pyriform rim and 11–17 mm superior to the nasal floor.[69–71]

Maxillary Mobilization and Positioning

Mobilizing the maxilla and getting it into its final position may also be a challenge if the patient has had multiple surgeries in the past. This would include patients with cleft lip and palate or those with history of trauma. The scar tissues may inhibit the maxilla from anterior or inferior positioning, especially over a large distance. The scar tissue will put strain on the rigid fixation and possibly have a higher potential to relapse. In cases where the maxilla may have to move more than its "biologic soft tissue envelope" will allow, consideration to using tissue expansion with distraction osteogenesis or palatal expansion should be considered.[72]

Positioning issues arise intraoperatively during the movement of the maxilla in the superior, posterior, or inferior directions. Superior movement must take into account the upper airway structures that may inhibit the required or planned movements. The nasal septum and the inferior turbinate may prevent planned maxillary impaction. These structures in turn may be damaged, torqued, or bent, resulting in aesthetic and functional problems. Obstruction of the opening of the nasolacrimal ducts when manipulating and recontouring tissues in this region may also occur. Posterior positioning issues arise when the bone contact is not relieved either from a thick tuberosity/pterygoid plate region or poorly downfractured Le Fort I, leaving multiple bone interferences.

Intraoperative attention to possible unaesthetic soft tissue changes that may occur from the proposed movements is also important. As the maxilla is moved in any direction, the nasal tip and the nasal apertures will change shape and position. Poor aesthetic results frequently occur from anterior and superior maxillary movement, creating excessive tip rise and widening of the alar bases. Poor nasal function results from septal deviation, changing the nasal valves and thus increasing the potential for obstruction of the airway.[73–76] The upper lip will also change shape and shorten after movement of the maxilla and closure of the incisions should be planned to address these alterations. The V to Y closure technique and its modifications is the commonest way of controlling for these changes. Although this may help preventing unaesthetic results, the V to Y closure will also thin the lateral aspects of the upper lip and should be taken into consideration.[77]

The final position of the maxilla must be verified once it is stabilized.[78–80] If the model surgery was accurate, this is accomplished by checking the occlusion and evaluating the patient's vertical incisor position. To properly hold the maxilla while applying rigid fixation requires special attention. Excess force while rotating the maxillomandibular complex or inappropriate direction of the force can displace the condyles. This will result in an open bite once maxillomandibular fixation is released and will require removal and replacement of fixation. In addition, if the complex does not move smoothly into its new position, either soft tissue or bony interferences exist and should be addressed.

Inability to stabilize the maxilla with current rigid fixation is rare. If stability is not obtained, the osteotomies will heal with fibrous union formation.[81] Alternative means of fixation need to be utilized when current bone plating systems cannot be employed effectively. Older techniques of wire suspension and external fixation must not be forgotten as well as the "newer" techniques with intermaxillary fixation screws.

BLEEDING AND HEMORRHAGE

Bleeding is a part of any operation; hemorrhage is not. The causes of hemorrhage from Le Fort I surgery arise from multiple etiologies. Improper use of osteotomes, chisels, the reciprocating saw or retracting instruments can create tears in the vasculature around the osteotomy site.[82] Excessive force may lead to poor fractures and possible bone fragments that may create lacerations in blood vessels and bleeding. Previously operated maxillas and patients with traumatic injuries to the midface may be at higher risk for bleeding perioperatively. Patients with unusual skeletal deformities and severe maxillary hypoplasia with anomalous anatomy are also at risk if the altered anatomy is not considered. Decisions as to how alter the approach to the suture line for disjunction must be considered in these special cases, such as directing the osteotomies into the tuberosity region thus avoiding inadvertent injury to the vasculature.[83]

The blood vessels most likely to be injured during the downfracture process are the lateral and medial pterygoid vessels, the posterior superior alveolar artery, the greater palatine artery, the terminal branches of the maxillary artery, the pterygoid venous plexus, and the internal carotid artery. The internal maxillary artery is normally positioned approximately 23–25 mm superior to the base of the junction of the maxilla with the ptyergoid plates, and its average diameter is 2.5 mm. When appropriately placing a pterygoid osteotome (average 10 mm wide) into the fissure, which is on average 14.5 mm in length, and directing it anteriorly, medially, and inferiorly the vessel can be easily avoided. These average measurements allow for a 10-mm space between the instrument and the vessel. The greater palatine artery is located approximately 20–25 mm posterior to the pyriform rim. It can be avoided by utilizing the measurements usually present on the lateral nasal wall osteotomes and stopping the osteotomies, thus not severing the vessel.

If brisk bleeding does occur, it will most likely originate in order of frequency from the posterior superior alveolar artery, the greater palatine, the pterygoid plexus, pterygoid muscles, or in rare occasions, the terminal branches of the maxillary and/or internal carotid. Completion of the osteotomies and downfracture of the maxilla is required in order to visualize the source and control brisk arterial bleeding.

If the source is identified, ligation with hemoclips (or sutures) is required, especially for the descending palatine artery, as the vessel can retract into the bony canal and become a source of delayed bleeding. Alternatively, bleeding of venous or muscular origin may be controlled with careful use of electrocautery. Packing the wound, using microfibrillar collagen or a similar material, and reassessing may help with establishing a clot, especially in cases of venous origin bleeding or when the source is not easily identifiable. Hypotensive anesthesia can also assist in reducing bleeding and enabling visualization until control is achieved. Ligation of the external carotid artery has not been proven to be a successful way of achieving hemostasis due to collateral circulation in the head and neck. Additionally, there is the risk of injury to adjacent cranial nerves, accidental ligation of the internal carotid or delay in accessing the vessel while brisk bleeding continuous, all associated with serious consequences. By far the most effective means of controlling severe hemorrhage from the high pressure vessels of the head and neck is through interventional radiology and angiographic embolization (Fig. 5.7).[84–88]

Nerve Injury During Le Fort Osteotomy

Cranial nerves II, III, IV, V, VI, and VII may all be traumatized by the Le Fort I osteotomy. Essentially, these nerves are found in the pterygomaxillary fissure and the inferior or superior orbital fissure. Most of the nerves mentioned, if injured, will go unnoticed until the postoperative period. However, during surgical manipulation of the maxilla at the time of downfracture, if a decrease in the pulse rate is noted this may be due to the effect of pressure on the cranial nerve V. The trigeminocardiac reflex will cause sudden bradycardia that may be severe and even lead to asystole if not corrected. If sudden bradycardia is noted during manipulation or downfracture of the maxilla, the procedure should be stopped and the jaw returned to its original position until the heart rate returns to normal. Consultation with the anesthesiologists for use of atropine or glycopyrolate in cases of persistent or severe bradycardia may be needed to allow for completion of the procedure. In addition, use of local anesthetic in the soft tissues to decrease the sensitivity of the nerve to manipulation in this area maybe beneficial.[87,88]

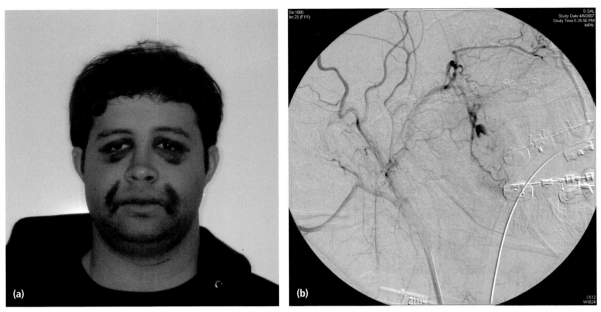

Fig. 5.7. (a) Postoperative persistent ecchymosis and bleeding requiring angiographic diagnosis and embolization. (b) Maxillary artery angiogram showing extravasation prior to embolization.

Airway Compromise

Laceration of the endotracheal tube may occur as sharp instruments are being used for the maxillary osteotomies.[89–92] If this occurs and adequate ventilation cannot be maintained, the tube must be exchanged. Appropriate measurements are necessary to ensure that this will be done safe and atraumatically. Ideally, bleeding should be controlled first and fiberoptic instruments should be readily available in case difficulties with visualization arise during the process. The surgeon should be prepared to establish a surgical airway should attempts to reintubate or maintain a patent airway fail.[93]

GENIOPLASTY

Preoperative

The choices of genial augmentation are to use the sliding genioplasty or an alloplastic implant. The aesthetic results desired and amount of bone stock available will dictate the procedure of choice for genial augmentation.[94–98]

   The relationship of the lower lip to soft tissue pogonion in the horizontal plane should be carefully evaluated when treatment planning the correction of the chin position. Advancement beyond the soft tissue envelope tolerance could result in unacceptable aesthetics. The chin may appear too big or even create a "witch's" chin with a very deep mentolabial groove. Facial balance in the vertical dimension is also important. The height of the lower incisor to menton must be addressed so that the lower facial third is in harmony with the remainder of the face. It is imperative to recognize that occasionally a chin deficit that is due to mandibular position, retrognathia, or apertognathia may be corrected once these deformities are addressed. In cases of inadequate bone stock, an appropriate size alloplastic chin implant should be considered instead.

Perioperative

Perioperatively, the most common complication is injury to the mental nerve or of less importance the mylohyoid nerve. Identification of the mental foramen and keeping the osteotomies at least 5–6 mm

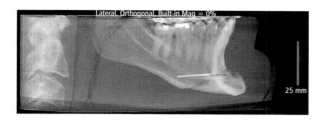

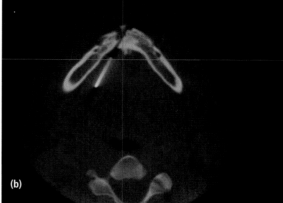

(a)

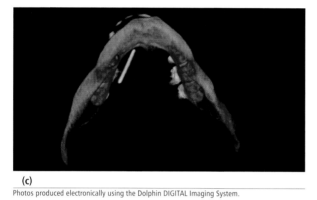

(c)

Fig. 5.8. (a) Lateral cephalograph showing overpenetration of genioplasty pins. (b) CT scan showing genioplasty pins beyond the lingual plate of the mandible. (c) 3D CT showing genioplasty pin overpenetration into the floor of the mouth.

below the foramen decreases the risk of nerve damage by avoiding the nerve as it loops in the mandible in this region.[99] Laceration of the soft tissues and blood vessels in the floor of the mouth is also a possibility, either from the drill or saw used for the osteotomy, or from the hardware used for fixation of the genial segment (Fig. 5.8). This can lead to hematoma formation in the floor of mouth and possible airway compromise. The inability to advance the genial segment, inability to stabilize the genial segment, and inadvertent asymmetrical placement of the segment are also possible complications. Fracture of the mandible can be a potential complication of the genioplasty osteotomy if inadequate bone is maintained superiorly or if sharp angles create weak points. Damage to the teeth is another potential complication, and careful evaluation of the root lengths in preoperative radiographs is essential.

Postoperative

Postoperative complications are related to wound healing issues at the incision site, instability of the segments and hardware failure, infection, numbness of the lower lip and unaesthetic result due to poor positioning.[100-102] Necrosis of the genial segment "wings" with formation of deep depressions at the junction with the native mandible distally can occur. This is usually the result of poorly planned and executed osteotomies with inadequate bone stock. Finally, improper handling of the soft tissues and failure to approximate the mentalis muscle will cause lip ptosis.

MANDIBLE: INTRAOPERATIVE COMPLICATIONS

Whereas the work horse of the maxilla is the Le Fort I osteotomy, the mandible can be moved into position with many different types of osteotomy designs. These include the vertical ramus osteotomy, sagittal split ramus osteotomy, inverted L osteotomies, midline osteotomies, and various anterior segmental osteotomies. Choices depend upon bone stock, movement required, effect on the temporomandibular joint, and anatomic vital structures. The various complications associated with these osteotomies vary from poor osteotomy design to vascular and neural issues to wound healing problems.[103]

INTRAORAL VERTICAL RAMUS OSTEOTOMY (IVRO)

Complications with intraoral vertical ramus osteotomies arise when this procedure is employed for mandibular advancement or lengthening of posterior facial height. Bone healing, without grafting, at the osteotomy site is not possible due to lack of bony contact between the proximal and distal segments. The pterygomasseteric sling will interfere with planned movements, especially in cases of advancement, even if the muscles are stripped from the mandible. Stable occlusion may not be possible and will result in an anterior open bite once maxillomandibular fixation is released.

The intraoral vertical ramus osteotomy is performed under limited visibility and special instrumentation is designed to assist in overcoming this problem.[104–109] Special retractors that engage the posterior border of the mandible, the sigmoid, and the antegonial notch can be utilized to improve exposure. In addition, the instruments can accommodate fiberoptic cables and thus improve visibility in the field.

Trauma to the tissues, however, such as laceration of periosteum and risk of injury to surrounding vessels, is possible from inappropriate or careless use of these retractors. The masseteric vessels in the sigmoid notch, the facial vessels in the antegonial notch, and the retromandibular vein at the posterior border are at risk from the misuse of the instruments. Furthermore, these vessels are at risk from the micro-oscillating saw during the osteotomy if not appropriately protected.

Appropriate positioning of the osteotomy at the ramus is essential to avoid injury to the inferior alveolar neurovascular bundle while ensuring that the proximal segment is of appropriate size to avoid condylar sag. The micro-oscillating saw blade specially designed for execution of the IVRO osteotomy is available in two lengths: short and long. Using the appropriate size blade based on the width of the ramus is essential to avoid injury to the lingual tissues or create incomplete osteotomies. It is essential when performing the osteotomy to avoid excess force that may cause breakage of the saw blade. The blade is difficult to retrieve from the medial surface of the mandible once it is lost in the cut. Endoscopic surgical techniques to better visualize the osteotomy during this procedure have been described. In addition, with the endoscopic approach use of rigid fixation is possible, thus eliminating need for maxillomandibular fixation. Endoscopic techniques necessitate an extraoral incision that requires care in placement and closure in order to avoid visible scars.

Distal segment positioning may cause undesired torque on the condyle or even displacement of the proximal segment distally that may lead to intra-articular problems or occlusal discrepancies postoperatively (Fig. 5.9). Rigid fixation is not usually employed with IVRO, thus adequate bone overlapping and stability is required for healing. Bone segment stability is achieved by a period of maxillomandibular fixation. It is advisable to place the patient in maxillomandibular fixation, ensure that the segments are appropriately positioned, and then close the incisions. As with all orthognathic procedures, careful preoperative workup will allow for anticipation of potential problems and choice of the appropriate osteotomy to use.

SAGITTAL SPLIT RAMUS OSTEOTOMY

This osteotomy is the most versatile of the mandibular osteotomies. It can be used to lengthen or shorten the mandible as well as correct asymmetries. It can also be used in combination with IVRO surgery to correct asymmetry that requires length only on one side and setback on the other.

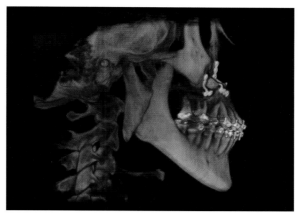

Fig. 5.9. Vertical ramus osteotomy with overrotation of the proximal segment that may lead to postoperative malocclusion.

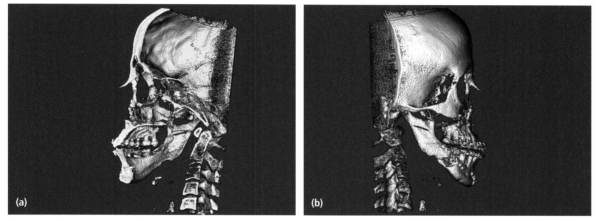

Fig. 5.10. (a) 3D CT scan showing the medial horizontal osteotomy of a sagittal split osteotomy procedure. (b) 3D CT scan showing overextension of the medial SSO cut through the lateral ramus.

The sagittal split, however, has been shown to have the highest complication rate of any procedure that we do.[110–112] The complications associated with this osteotomy are related to the design of the cuts.[113] The medial cut is placed just above the lingula. Instruments are placed here to "protect" the soft tissues and the inferior alveolar neurovascular bundle. These, if not carefully managed (including the cutting instrument used to create the medial surface cut), can cause nerve injury. Continuing along the external oblique ridge, the dentition can be damaged by either the saw blades or burs used to create the cut. The anterior portion of the osteotomy, if too deep, can cut the inferior alveolar nerve in this region, and the inferior border osteotomy can also transect the nerve if the depth is not controlled (Fig. 5.10). The retractors improperly used at the inferior border can endanger the facial vessels or injure the marginal mandibular branch of the facial nerve by impinging on the soft tissues.[113]

A common complication associated with the sagittal split osteotomy (SSO) is a "bad split" that can occur in any type of mandible.[114] This complication must be dealt with to avoid poor healing at the osteotomy sites and malocclusion. The usual cause of a bad split is too much force applied during the separation of the proximal and distal segments while having incomplete or improperly placed osteotomies. This will create poor fracture lines, thus leading to the improper separation of the proximal and distal segments. An incomplete cut at the inferior border often causes proximal buccal plate fractures, and these can range in size and extent and sometimes include the condyle (Fig. 5.11). Additionally, this can lead to distal segment

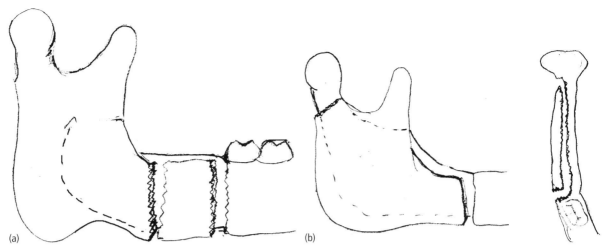

Fig. 5.11. (a) Buccal plate fracture of the proximal segment. (b) High buccal plate fracture involving the subcondylar region.

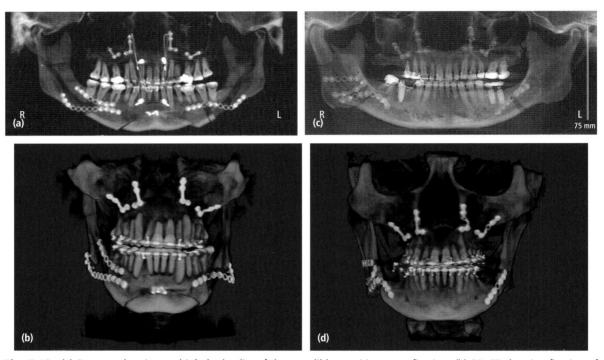

Fig. 5.12. (a) Panorex showing multiple bad splits of the mandible requiring extra fixation. (b) 3D CT showing fixation of multiple bad splits. (c) Panorex showing bad splits of the mandible including the condyle, fixated with plates and screws. (d) 3D CT showing the fixation of bad splits of the mandible.

fracture that causes the inferior border to remain on this segment. Presence of an impacted third molar or a thin edentulous area increases the risk of this complication. Cuts that are too high on the medial can cause the coronoid process to fracture. The final goal of managing a bad split is to create stability and continuity of the bone segments (Fig. 5.12).[115]

Clearly, avoiding unfavorable splits before separation occurs is essential. A minimal amount of pressure is needed to separate the proximal and distal segments if osteotomies are properly done. The marrow space can be seen peeling open as the spreaders or chisels are used properly. If resistance is encountered or a buccal plate fracture develops, the cuts need to be rechecked and retracted before proceeding. Buccal plate fractures are the most common unfavorable occurrences encountered. The buccal segment becomes a free bone graft as it is usually stripped of its periosteum during the dissection for access to perform the SSO. The sagittal osteotomy needs to be completed to separate the proximal from the distal segments in order to establish a functional result. Converting this nonseparation problem by using an IVRO, thereby separating off the condyle, is the best choice to manage this mishap if the sagittal split cannot be completed. This is true especially if the mandible is being set back. This type of IVRO cut still allows bone contact, and the condyle stays in the fossa. However, if the completion of the cuts will create bony segments that cannot be aligned, perhaps it is best to abandon the procedure until the mandible is consolidated and try again.

When mandibular advancement surgery and anterior movement of the distal segment is necessary to achieve a functional occlusion, IVRO can also be used to salvage a bad split, but the gap created by the anterior separation of the proximal and distal segments must be grafted in order to obtain continuity. Plans for using rigid fixation may be compromised when this happens and the patient will need to be placed into maxillomandibular fixation until the osteotomies heal. Airway compromise, especially if preexisting conditions exist, is a serious potential risk every time maxillomandibular fixation is required; appropriate measures should be in place.

Once the mandible is split properly the position of the inferior alveolar nerve is in the distal segment. However, as the mandible is being split open the surgeon may observe the nerve being caught in the proximal side buccal segment marrow space; the nerve must be freed before it can become injured. If the nerve is transected, it should be repaired immediately for the best chance of healing. Even with careful osteotomy design and execution, immediate postoperative neurosensory deficits occur even in the absence of direct nerve trauma.

Rigid fixation is typically used to stabilize the proximal and distal segments in the sagittal split osteotomy. Again, condylar torquing may occur if the proximal segment is not able to lie passively against the distal segment when aligning the bones to place the fixation (Fig. 5.13). This issue can be anticipated from preoperative planning and bone removal in critical areas can be performed. Control of the proximal segment is the most important aspect of stability and prevention of relapse and loss of gonial angle projection after sagittal split osteotomy (Fig. 5.14).

Impacted wisdom teeth in the area of the osteotomy site may be an issue related to the control of the segments splitting properly as well as possible damage to the inferior alveolar nerve.[116,117] The amount of tooth development at the position of the impaction and its impact on the thickness of the lingual plate of bone can be visualized preoperatively with CT technology and may help in decision making when planning to remove these teeth in preparation for surgery.

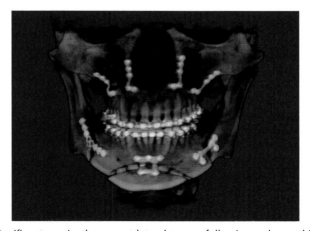

Fig. 5.13. 3D CT showing significant proximal segment lateral torque following orthognathic surgery.

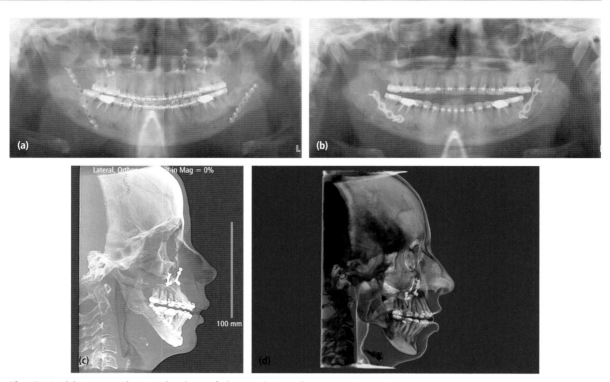

Fig. 5.14. (a) Panorex showing hardware failure with plate fracture on the right side due to the use of improper hardware. (b) Panorex showing improper use of fixation, one screw in each segment, with significant postoperative segment mobility. (c) lateral cephalograph showing counterclockwise rotation of the proximal segment after SSO surgery. (d) 3D CT showing counterclockwise rotation of the proximal segment with loss of the gonial angle projection.

RECOVERY ROOM	FIRST WEEK	FIRST MONTH	LONG TERM
• Airway	• Malocclusion	• Hardware Failure	• Stability
• Bleeding	• Pain	• Bleeding	• Permanent Nerve
• Nausea	• Swelling	• Nasal and Sinus	Damage
• Pain	• Nausea	• Hearing	• Temporomandibular
• Malocclusion	• Psychological	• Devitalized teeth	Joint
	• Neurological	• Range of Motion	
	• Nutritional	• Splints	
	• Wound Healing	• Transverse Stability	
	• Bleeding	• Sequestrum	
	• Hardware Failure	• Hardware	
		• Neural changes	
		• Orthodontic issues	
		• Patient Satisfaction	
		• Sleep Apnea	

Fig. 5.15. Postoperative complications based upon time frame following orthognathic surgery.

POSTOPERATIVE COMPLICATIONS OF ORTHOGNATHIC SURGERY

Postoperative complications can be divided into short- and long-term problems (Fig. 5.15).

Short-Term Complications

The short-term complications may arise in the first few minutes to weeks after surgery. Airway compromise secondary to changes in airway size can be due to the use of intermaxillary fixation or the actual movements of the skeletal bases related to the surgery. Pain management with narcotic or anxiolytic meds used to keep the patients at ease can impact respiratory efforts. Medication-related apneas must be monitored closely in the immediate postoperative period.

Patients with a known history of obstructive sleep apnea will need special monitoring postoperatively and this is discussed elsewhere in this text.

Bleeding

Continued bleeding postoperatively can be expected during the normal recovery room time. However, brisk bleeding from the mouth or nose requires special attention. Uncontrolled bleeding that cannot be managed with pressure and/or packing may require return to the operating room for identification of the source and control. This may not be always possible and use of interventional radiology, when available, for identification and selective embolization may be a better alternative. Bleeding can occur days to weeks or even months after orthognathic surgery and thus the patients should be adequately informed. Minimal nasal bleeding usually consistent of dark blood accumulated in the maxillary sinuses is expected and usually of no concern. Sudden brisk bright red blood from the nose or the incisions or a sudden facial swelling that is expanding, require immediate attention. Patients should be adequately informed and given detailed instructions should these issues occur.

Malocclusion

Gross malocclusion should be noted immediately in the operating room once intermaxillary fixation is released upon placement of rigid fixation and should be addressed at that time by resetting the fixation.

During the first week post surgery, however, swelling is usually the primary culprit of malocclusions. Hardware failure is next and will be verified with segmental mobility and appropriate imaging. Swelling and occlusal control can be managed with gentle traction from orthodontic elastics. Hardware failure requires a return to the operating room. Not setting the occlusion correctly at the time of surgery, segmental procedures, or ill-fitting splints are potential reasons for malocclusion and should be examined.

A poorly positioned proximal segment of the IVRO osteotomy may lead to changes in ramus height with "condylar sagging" that may cause anterior open bite once the fixation is released. The malocclusion may need to be corrected surgically.

Pain

Complications from use of pain medications and pain management from jaw surgery are nausea induced by narcotic use as well as respiratory depression. The use of anxiolytic medications pre- and postoperatively may assist in reducing the amount of narcotic needed.[118] The use of NSAIDS or aspirin should be used with caution if the patient had a bleeding issue in the operating room or history of gastric ulcer. Pain management should be tailored to the individual patient.

Swelling

While swelling is an expected part of any surgical intervention, complications arise when swelling is due to hematoma formation or infection. Swelling must be monitored for resolution progress over the initial weeks post surgery. The use of systemic steroids is advocated to help with decreasing the amount of post-operative edema. However, these patients must be monitored for possible side effects of these drugs.[119–122] If hematoma formation or infection are the reasons for the swelling incision and drainage along with appropriate antibiotic coverage may be required.[123,124]

Nausea

Postoperative nausea and vomiting after orthognathic surgery is a very common complication in this patient population.[125] Evaluation of more than 500 orthognathic patients revealed a 40% risk of having nausea, and most patients experience this problem within the first 24 hours. The risk factors identified were female patients, young age, nonsmokers, prior history of motion sickness or migraine headaches, use of volatile anesthesia agents, maxillary surgery, increased pain, and use of opioid medications.

Intravenous antiemetics seem to work the best for this patient population, as well as leaving in the nasogastric tube in place postoperatively to ensure that swallowed blood is evacuated from the stomach.

Psychological

Steroid-induced psychosis post surgically is a known entity. Changes in behavior and mood swings are noted in patients that have no psychiatric history. Depression that lasts or aggressive behaviors need to be addressed quickly with the patients, their families, and psychiatrist if they are reported to be of new onset.

Dramatic changes in facial appearance and patient satisfaction are also areas that can affect the patient's overall postoperative experience.[126–128] Understanding the aesthetic goals of the patient prior to surgery and education of the patient to the facial changes they can expect to experience with surgery is essential to having a good emotional outcome. Educational tools such as a photo journal of previous patients' surgical courses with similar surgical problems are helpful for the right patients. The support of families and friends during this time period is important as well. Have these people involved from the preoperative discussions to prepare all of them for immediate and long-term postoperative expectations and outcomes.

Neurologic

Cranial nerve dysfunction after orthognathic surgery is documented to affect the inferior alveolar nerve primarily from the sagittal split technique.[112] The facial nerve may have transient palsy secondary compression during mandibular surgery.[113] This is noted from soft tissue swelling and retraction at the mandibular osteotomy sites.

Blindness has been reported as a very rare but devastating complication after orthognathic surgery. Specifically, patients undergoing Le Fort I osteotomies may have unusual fracture lines generated that may travel up to the skull base and create deformation or bleeding in the optic canal region and compress the optic nerve. Any patient with a complaint of visual acuity changes or eye pain should be evaluated immediately.[68]

Nutrition

Diet modifications may be required for the patient who undergoes orthognathic surgery and has difficulties adapting to the changes that may be encountered. Inadequate oral intake may lead to dehydration, weakness, dizziness, and potentially prolonged recovery with poor wound healing. High-calorie liquid supplements may be required and should be encouraged. Appropriate education and preparedness for the patient and family should assist in overcoming these issues. Meal suggestions and recipes for the orthognathic patient on a liquid or soft diet could be developed and included in the postoperative instructions package.[129–131]

Wound Healing

Mucosal dehiscence problems may be noted with either maxillary or mandibular surgery. Mandibular wounds that may open postoperatively may be managed conservatively with irrigations and allowed to heal by secondary intention. Maxillary mucosal issues along the incision line or osteotomy sites, however, may be due to devascularization of the underlying bone segments either from segmental surgery or the Le Fort osteotomy. These patients must be monitored for potential loss of a devascularized segment of bone or tooth. The use of hyperbaric oxygen therapy (HBO) may help with increasing angiogenesis and oxygen in these compromised tissues once they are injured.

Patients with medical issues that compromise the immune system—such as diabetic patients or patients with arthritis who are on immunosuppressive medications—are of special concern in this category as they may be more likely to exhibit slow wound healing and postoperative infections.

Hardware Failure

Patients returning for normal postoperative visits that exhibit malocclusions must be checked for hardware failure. A history of trauma to the surgical sites or chewing hard foods can lead to fracture of bone plates or loosening of the screws. Often what will be noted is the formation of soft tissue breakdown overlying the loose hardware and/or the loose osteotomy site. In either case this requires surgical exploration.

Bleeding/Hemorrhage

Patients who have had maxillary surgery have been reported to develop hemorrhagic bleeding up to 2 weeks post surgery. Other vascular anomalies such as false aneurysms and arteriovenous fistulas, and the development of AV malformations of the branches of the carotid artery have been reported.

Nasal and Sinus Complications

Most patients intubated nasally for jaw surgery have some degree of nasal discharge post surgery. Crusting of mucous and blood also decrease the nasal aperture opening and decrease nasal airflow until cleared. These issues are usually temporary and resolve with the use of oral decongestants, nasal sprays if necessary, and humidified air. The sinuses fill with blood post Le Fort surgery. This blood will drain and be absorbed over time in a healthy sinus that can drain properly. Patients may develop infections of the sinus or chronic sinusitis when the ostea become blocked, bone grafting whether autogenous or allogeneic are sequestered in the sinus, or the nasal septum is deviated from compression of the maxilla during impaction surgery.[132-134]

Unnoticed effects of the maxillary movements on the nasal aesthetic may be noticed only after facial swelling decreases postoperatively. Nasal aesthetic concerns arise when the nasal tip moves in the vertical vector too much or too little leading to tip rise or droop. The alar width also changes with the Le Fort osteotomy as the maxilla advances the shape changes and the width increases. This may not be the desired outcome aesthetically and must be planned for when making these skeletal movements.

Hearing

Eustachian tube dysfunction after maxillary orthognathic surgery has been reported as a temporary complication usually due to the swelling of the soft tissues around this anatomic structure as it passes the posterior maxilla.[135-139]

Range of Jaw Motion

All patients should be expected to experience a decreased range of motion of the mandible after corrective jaw surgery.[139-145] This range of motion issue is expected to increase as the tissue swelling decreases and the joints regain mobility. However, persistent musculoskeletal complaints of decreased range of motion and pain of the jaw upon movement are complications of jaw surgery that need to be further evaluated and treated. Poorly positioned osteotomy segments and condyle positions may create painful function of the muscles of mastication as well as the temporomandibular joints. Scar tissue formation along the incision line may limit the mandibular range of motion. Hemorrhage into the joint space and subsequent traumatic calcifications may lead to ankylosis or pseudoankylosis of the joints especially if the patient is wired into maxillomandibular fixation for an extended period of time. Even the use of heavy elastic traction for a couple of months may lead to decreased range of motion.

Treatment of this issue if primarily muscular should begin with passive range of motion exercises and progress to physical therapy as needed.

True temporomandibular joint (TMJ) issues that develop post orthognathic surgery must be evaluated and treated as necessary. These include disk displacement, condylar sag, avascular necrosis, or idiopathic condylar resorption. Patients presenting with presurgical TMJ pathology or prior history of TMJ surgery may have special needs postoperatively as well. They are more prone to TMJ pain and symptoms post orthognathic surgery.[146] These patients typically have had physical therapy already as part of their treatment. Some patients may also require different pain management techniques or even a pain specialist, especially if they have been in chronic pain. If there is an acute closed lock problem following orthognathic surgery and a disc displacement is the etiology, then consideration should be given toward immediate arthrocentesis to attempt to release a stuck disc.

Splints

Acrylic splints used in the postoperative period are typically secured to the maxillary dentition with small wires. This is often done for segmental surgery of the maxilla to maintain the width and arch form and improve on the stability of the segments and allow for osseous healing to occur. Splints may fracture or loosen over time. These splints may need to be removed "early" due to occlusal issues. Once this occurs the orthodontist needs to be on board to help to change the segmented arch wire to a continuous wire as well as plan for the possible placement of transpalatal arches to maintain width and stability and allow for bone to heal.

Transverse Issues

Loss of maxillary width post segmental Le Fort osteotomy will lead to malocclusion and healing in poor osteotomy position. The need for preplanning skeletal width expansion prior to formal Le Fort I surgery is key to preventing the need to try to expand the maxilla past its biologic limit of tolerance at the time of segmental surgery. The use of surgically assisted rapid palatal expansion (SARPE) surgery is a powerful tool in the orthognathic surgeon's armamentarium.[147–150]

Sequestrum Formation

Sequestra may form as a result of several issues of vascular compromise of the osteotomy sites.

In maxillary surgery, sequestra may form within the maxillary sinuses post surgery because it was not noticed that part of the walls of the maxilla may have fractured off during downfracture and were removed before placing the maxilla into fixation.

In the mandible the tip of the IVRO osteotomy may sequester as it is very thin and may become devascularized instead of healing. These patients present with buccal space swelling and sometimes abscess formation. The bilateral sagittal split osteotomy (BSSO)patient may also sequester bone. Using bone plates along the thin edge of the superior border of the proximal segment may lead to pathologic fracture of this sequestered segment once the sequestrum forms. These patients also present with pain and swelling in the region of the sequestered bone.

In all cases the sequestered pieces of bone need to be debrided to allow the wounds to heal properly.

Loss of the gonial angle of the mandible secondary to remodeling of a poorly positioned proximal segment is also a known complication of the sagittal split ramus osteotomy.[151] This is usually seen postoperatively during the healing process when the proximal segment was not positioned and stabilized properly. Once this occurs, the angle soft tissue defect created usually will need a graft to augment this region into an acceptable aesthetic result.

Hardware

Hardware failure due to screw loosening over the long term is seen once the patient has healed and the bone tissues have remodeled around the bone plates. If the patient presents with discomfort overlying the hardware, consideration to exploration of these plates and removing the hardware should be given. A loose screw may not be noted on radiograph if it is not displaced.[152–154]

Taste Alteration

Taste function of the hard palate is reduced for at least 6–9 months post Le Fort I. This surgery may impair the function of the greater superficial petrosal branch of the facial nerve. Taste function of the tongue is reduced for 1–2 months post BSSO. This is due to impairment of the chorda tympani nerve, which may be traumatized with the lingual nerve during a BSSO procedure. This impairment was transient and improved over 6–9 months.[155]

Orthodontic Issues

Complications that arise in the first month postoperatively related to orthodontic care fall into several of areas. First is loss of brackets during surgery and the need to replace the hardware here so that there is no movement of teeth into a poor position. Second is the need to change arch wires or add transpalatal support in a timely fashion after surgery to maintain the skeletal stability of a width change. These visits should be prearranged with the orthodontist and they must alert their staff that appointments cannot wait for surgical patients. The surgeon must follow through to make sure these wire changes take place at the correct time. Third is tooth movement that creates unwanted forces on the occlusal scheme that may open a bite, create transverse collapse, or stripping of gingival tissues. It is extremely important to follow patients closely as the orthodontic treatment is finished postoperatively. Excellent communication between the surgeon and orthodontic colleague are essential to a stable long-term result.

Patient Satisfaction

Even if the most technically perfect surgery and orthodontic treatment are done for the patient, if the patient perceives that they do not like the result, then this is, at least in the eyes of the patient, a failure.[16,156–158] The failure arises from poor communication between the surgeon, the patient, and the orthodontist. Why the patient is seeking treatment is paramount in understanding how to achieve good results.

Long-Term Complications

Issues that arise after the first year are considered long-term complications. These may be related to function, hardware failure, and skeletal stability.

Stability

Stability of jaw surgery depends upon several factors. The direction of the surgical movements, type of fixation used, and surgical technique have been discussed predictors for long-term stability.[65,66,159–166] However, the primary issue is correct diagnosis appropriate orthodontic set up for the proposed movements necessary to correct the deformity while not violating the biologic limits of tissue tolerance. Secondary concerns are in planning the osteotomies. There is a limit of soft tissue tolerance versus bone advancement. When faced with severe deformities consideration of other means or techniques such as distraction osteogenesis, which may allow slow movement of the bones along with some tissue expansion, may give a more stable long-term result.[167]

While rigid fixation techniques have improved overall stability of orthognathic surgery, the types of movements planned still impact long-term outcomes. Adequate planning, with incorporation of bone grafts, for example, when movements with high relapse rates are undertaken, will assist in better long-term results.

The direction of mandibular movement also impacts on long-term stability; mandibular advancement is more stable than setback surgery even with rigid fixation.

Occlusal plane alteration with double jaw surgery will also impact long-term stability of movements. Increasing or decreasing the plane has to be judged along with the actual movements of the maxilla and mandible to understand how much post surgical change can be expected.

The next issue is to carefully plan surgery around the skeletal growth of the patient. Unless a growing child is severely functionally compromised and a plan to perform multiple surgical interventions is developed, surgery to correct skeletal facial deformities has traditionally been done in the "nongrowing" or skeletally mature patient population.

Last are the issues related to systemic diseases that may lead to changes in the occlusion due to secondary skeletal changes from their underlying disease. Neuromuscular diseases that have either hypotonia or hypertonia or marrow-expanding diseases such as thalassemia will contribute to the long-term stability of the jaw deformity correction.

Permanent Cranial Nerve Damage

Sensory nerve loss or poorly functioning sensory nerves are a well-documented complication of corrective jaw surgery. The sagittal split osteotomy is the most common osteotomy to have hypofunctioning of the sensory branches of the third division of the fifth cranial nerve. However, the incidence of this complication varies from 5% to 70% in the literature. The intraoral vertical ramus osteotomy has less incidence of this complication in the long term. However, when ramus osteotomies are combined with genioplasty, the incidence of nerve damage increases. Regardless of which osteotomy is used, complete anesthesia of this nerve rarely occurs and is a consequence of direct nerve injury via hardware impingement or transection. Neuroma formation is rare but a reported complication and may require surgical intervention if becomes symptomatic.[168]

Cranial Nerve VII

Permanent seventh nerve damage has not been reported in our literature from an intraoral approach to the maxillary or mandibular skeleton. All injuries to this nerve have been reported to be transient in nature unless direct injury to the nerve had occurred from most likely an extraoral dissection to access the jaw.[169,170] What is most important to recognize is the early intervention necessary when treating a traumatized motor nerve.

TMJ Issues

The TMJ problems that can result following orthognathic surgery include pain, internal derangements, and idiopathic condylar resorption. The occurrence of pain and TMJ sounds in the first few months postoperatively are highly suspicious for condylar changes that might occur in the following months. Patients with preexisting TMJ dysfunction who undergo orthognathic surgery, particularly mandibular advancement, are likely to have significant worsening of the TMJ dysfunction post surgically. Regaining range of motion and bite forces post corrective jaw surgery is important in improving overall functional correction of the patient. Postoperative physical therapy may be necessary to augment the patient's normal postoperative course. However, persistent pain and lack of range of motion may be an indication of continued or developing internal derangements of the joint or the musculature. Lack of range of motion may also be attributed to scar contracture formation from poorly placed incisions at the time of mandibular osteotomy.

Mandibular ramus height decrease as a consequence of a dissolving condylar head will lead to a slowly opening skeletal-based anterior open bite post surgically. Idiopathic condylar resorption has no known etiology. It can occur before or after jaw surgery. It is usually noted in young women between the ages of 15 and 35. It is progressive until the process resorbs to the sigmoid notch. TMJ dysfunction must be closely evaluated, treated if necessary, and monitored in the orthognathic surgery patient.[171–176] Risk factors have been identified that may predispose a patient to this potential complication. Risk factors include: female patient with mandibular retrognathia associated with an increased mandibular plane angle, presence of pretreatment condylar atrophy, and undergoing posterior condylar displacement and upward and forward rotation of the mandible at the time of surgery. Condyles with preexisting radiological signs of osteoarthrosis or having a posterior inclination were at high risk for progressive resorption.

This patient should be surgically managed if at all possible once the process burns out to give the best chance of surgical stability. The condyles can be monitored for active disease with Technitium 99 bone scans. The choice of timing and method of reconstruction will be determined as always by the severity of the remaining deformity and its impact on function.

CONCLUSIONS

Orthognathic surgery has a rich history of triumphs and failures. The giants who led the field of corrective jaw surgery into the 21st century have laid the ground work for future oral and maxillofacial surgeons to continue their work by providing patients with safe and predictable reconstructive surgery of the maxillofacial region. The basic principles of understanding the limitations of our surgical procedures, coupled with an expert understanding of surgical anatomy and skills needed to accomplish our task, enables the modern surgeon to not only manage their potential risks in "rough seas" but to potentially navigate around them all together.

SUGGESTED READINGS

1. Kim SG, and Park SS. 2007. "Incidence of complications and problems related to orthognathic surgery." *J Oral Maxillofac Surg* 65: 2438.
2. Patel PK, Morris DE, and Gassman A. 2007. "Complications of orthognathic surgery." *J Craniofac Surg* 18: 975.
3. Mahy P, Siciliano S, and Reychler H. 2002. "Complications and failures in orthognathic surgery." *Rev Belge Med Dent* 57: 71.

4. Panula K, Finne K, and Oikarinen K. 2001. "Incidence of complications and problems related to orthognathic surgery: A review of 655 patients." *J Oral Maxollofac Surg* 59: 1128.
5. Dimitroulis G. 1998. "A simple classification of orthognathic surgery complications." *Int J Adult Orthod Orthognath Surg* 13: 79.
6. Van de Perre JPA, Stoelinga PJW, Blijdorp PA, et al. 1996. "Perioperative morbidity in maxillofacial orthopaedic surgery: A retrospective study." *J Craniomaxillofac Surg* 24: 263.
7. O'Ryan FS. 1990. "Complications of orthognathic surgery." *Oral and Maxillofac Surg Clin North Am* 2: 593.
8. El Deeb M, Wolford L, and Bevis R. 1989. "Complications of orthognathic surgery." *Clin Plast Surg* 16: 825.
9. Phillips C, Blakey G, 3rd, and Jaskolka M. 2008. "Recovery after orthognathic surgery: Short-term health r-related quality of life outcomes." *J Oral Maxillofac Surg* 66(10): 2110.
10. Bays RA, and Boulous GF. 2003. "Complications of orthognathic surgery." *Oral Maxillofac Surg Clin North Am* 15(2): 229.
11. Shariffi A, Jones R, Ayoub A, Moos K, Walker F, Khanbay B, and McHugh S. 2008. "How accurate is model planning for orthognathic surgery?" *Int J Oral Maxillofac Surg* 37(12): 1089.
12. Danesh G. Lippold C, Joos U, and Meyer U. 2006. "Technical and clinical assessment of the use of a new material-based splint in orthognathic surgery." *Int J oral Maxillofac Surg* 35(9): 96.
13. Mavili ME, Canter HI, Saglam-Aydinatay B, Kiamaci S, and Kocadereli I. 2007. "Use of three-dimensional medical modeling methods for precise planning of orthognathic surgery." *J Craniofac Surg* 18(4): 740.
14. Swennen GR, Mollemans W, and Schutyser F. 2009. "Three-dimensional treatment planning of orthognathic surgery in the era of virtual imaging." *J Oral Maxillofac Surg* 67(10): 2080.
15. Meade EA, and Inglehart MR. 2010. "Young patients' treatment motivation and satisfaction with orthognathic surgery outcomes: The role of 'possible selves.'" *Am J orthod Dentofacial Orthop* 137(1): 26.
16. Narayanan V, Guhan S, Sreekumar K, and Ramadorai A. 2008. "Self-assessment of facial form oral function and psychosocial function before and after orthognathic surgery: A retrospective study." *Indian J Dent Res* 19(1): 12.
17. Espeland L, Hogevold HE, and Stenvik A. 2008. "A 3-year patient-centered follow-up of 516 consecutively treated orthognathic surgery patients." *Eur J orthod* 30(1): 24.
18. Benumof JL. 1997. *Anesthesia and Uncommon Diseases*, 4th ed. Philadelphia: Elsevier.
19. Ghoreishian M, and Gheisari R. 2009. "The effect of maxillary multidirectional movement on nasal respiration." *J Oral Maxillofac Surg* 67(10): 2283.
20. Lye KW. 2008. "Effect of orthognathic surgery on posterior airway space (PAS)." *Ann Acad Med Singapore* 37(8): 677.
21. Goodday R. 2009. "Diagnosis, treatment planning and surgical correction of obstructive sleep apnea." *J Oral Maxillofac Surg* 67(10): 2183.
22. Gilon V, Raskin S, Heymans O, and Poirrier R. 2001. "Surgical management of maxillomandibular advancement of sleep apnea patients: Specific technical considerations." *Int J Adult Orthodon Orthognath Surg* 16(4): 305.
23. Ruscello DM, Tekieli ME, Jakomis T, Cook L, and Van Sickles JE. 1986. "The effects of orthognathic surgery on speech production." *Am J Orthod* 89(3): 237.
24. Jorge TM, Brasolottoa G, Goncales ES, Filho HN, Berretin L, and Felix G. 2009. "Influence of orthognathic surgery on voice fundamental frequency." *J Craniofacial Surg* 20(1): 161.
25. O'Gara M, and Wilson K. 2007. "The effects of maxillofacial surgery on speech and velopharyngeal function." *Clin Plast Surg* 34(3): 395.
26. Vallino LD. 1990. "Speech, velopharyngeal function, and hearing before and after orthognathic surgery." *J Oral Maxillofac Surg* 48(12): 1274.
27. Bousaba S, Delatte M, Barbarin V, Faes J, and DeClerck H. 2002. "Pre- and post-surgical orthodontic objectives and orthodontic preparation." *Rev Belge Med Dent* 57(1): 37.
28. Sarver DM, and Sample LB. 1999. "How to avoid surgical failures." *Semin Orthod* 5(4): 257.
29. Sabri R. 2006. "Orthodontic objectives in orthognathic surgery: State of the art today." *World J Orthod* 7(2): 177.
30. Herford AS, and Stella JP. 2000. "An algorithm for determination of ideal location of interdental osteotomies in presurgical orthodontic treatment planning." *Int J Adult Orthodon Orthognath Surg* 15(4): 299.
31. Ueki K, Marukawa K, Shimada M, Alam S, Nakagawa K, and Yamamoto E. 2006. "The prevention of periodontal bone loss at the osteotomy site after anterior segmental and dento-osseous osteoeomy." *J Oral Maxillofac Surg* 64(10): 1526.
32. Burford D, and Noar JH. 2003. "The causes, diagnosis and treatment of anterior open bite." *Dent Update* 30: 235.
33. Kriwalsky MS, Maurer P, Veras RB, Eckert AW, and Schubert J. 2008. "Risk factors for a bad split during sagittal split osteotomy." *Br J OMS* 46(3): 177.
34. Precious DS, Lung KE, Pynn BR, and Goodday RH. 1998. "Presence of impacted teeth as a determining factor of unfavorable splits in 1256 sagittal split osteotomies." *Oral Surg Oral Med Oral Path Oral Radiol Endod* 85(4): 362.
35. Mehra P, Castro V, Freitas RZ, and Wolford LM. 2001. "Complications of the mandibular sagittal split ramus osteoeomy associated with the presence or absence of third molars." *J Oral Maxillof Surg* 59(8): 854.
36. Reyneke JP, Tsakiris P, and Becker P. 2002. "Age as a factor in the complication rate after removal of unerupted/impacted third molars at the time of mandibular sagittal split osteotomy." *J Oral Masillofac Surg* 60(6): 654.
37. Worsaae N, Jensen BN, Holm B, and Holsko J. 2007. "Treatment of severe hypodontia-oligodontia—An interdisciplinary concept." *Int J Oral Maxillofac Surg* 36(6): 473.
38. Baralle MM, Ferri J, Maes JM, Mercier J, Ovaert I, and Pellerin P. 1995. "Orthognathic surgery with missing teeth." *Rev Stomatol Chir Maxillofac* 96(4): 201.

39. Kim Y, Park JU, and Kook YA. 2009. "Alveolar bone loss around incisors in surgical skeletal Class III patients." *Angle Orthod* 79(4): 676.

40. Choi WS, and Samman N. 2008. "Risks and benefits of deliberate hypotension in anaesthesia: A systematic review." *Int J Oral Maxillofac Surg* 37(8): 687.

41. Varol A, Basa S, and Ozturk S. 2010. "The role of controlled hypotension upon transfusion requirement during maxillary downfracture in double-jaw surgery." *J Craniomaxillofac Surg* 38(5): 345.

42. Rodrigo C. 2000. "Anesthetic considerations for orthognathic surgery with evaluation of difficult intubation and technique for hypotensive anesthesia." *Anesth Prog* 47(4): 151.

43. Teeples TJ, Rallis DJ, Rieck KL, and Viozzi CF. 2010. "Lower extremity compartment syndrome associated with hypotensive general anesthesia for orthognathic surgery: A case report and review of the disease." *J Oral Maxillofac Surg* 68(5): 1166.

44. Tiner BD, Van Sickels JE, and Schmitz JP. 1997. "Life-threatening delayed hemorrhage after LeFort I osteotomy requiring surgical intervention: Report of two cases." *J Oral Maxillofac Surg* 55(1): 91.

45. Lanigan DT, and West RA. 1984. "Management of postoperative hemorrhage following the Le Fort I maxillary osteoeomy." *J Oral Maxillofac Surg* 42(6): 367.

46. Newhouse RF, Schow SR, Kraut RA, and Price JC. 1982. "Life-threatening hemorrhage from a Le Fort I osteotomy." *J Oral Maxillofac Surg* 40(2): 117.

47. Mehra P, Cottrell DA, Calazzo A., et al. 1999. "Life-threatening, delayed epistaxis after surgically assisted rapid palatal expansion: A case report." *J Oral Maxillofac Surg* 57: 201.

48. Nannini V, and Sachs SA. 1986. "Mediastinal emphysema following LeFort I osteotomy: Report of a case." *Oral Surg Oral Med Oral Pathol* 62(5): 508.

49. St. Hilaire H, Montazem AH, and Diamond J. 2004. "Pneumomediastinum after orthognathic surgery." *J Oral Maxillofac Surg* 62(7): 892.

50. Chebel NA, Ziade D, and Achkouty R. 2010. "Bilateral pneumothorax and pneumomediastinum after treatment with continuous positive airway pressure after orthognathic surgery." *Br J Oral Maxillofac Surg* 48(4): e14.

51. Lai JP, Hsieh CH, Chen YR, and Liang CC. 2005. "Unusual late vascular complications of sagittal split osteoeomy of the mandibular ramus." *J Craniofac Surg* 16(4): 664.

52. Bradley JP, Elahi M, and Kawamoto HK. 2002. "Delayed presentation of pseudoaneurysm after LeFort I osteotomy." *J Craniofac Surg* 13(6): 746.

53. Li KK, Meara JG, and Rubin PA. 1995. "Orbital compartment syndrome following orthognathic surgery." *J Oral Maxillofac Surg* 53(8): 964.

54. Phillips C. Blakely G, 3rd, and Jaskolka M. 2008. "Recovery after orthognathic surgery: Short term health-related quality of life outcomes." *J Oral Maxillofac Surg* 66(10): 2110.

55. Kahnberg KE, Vannas-Lofqvist L, and Zellin G. 2005. "Complications associated with segmentation of the maxilla: A retrospective radiographic follow up of 82 patients." *Int J Oral Maxillofac Surg* 34: 840.

56. Bell WH, and Levy BM. 1971. "Revascularization and bone healing after posterior maxillary osteotomy" *J Oral Surg* 29: 313.

57. Bell WH. 1973. "Biologic basis for maxillary osteotomies." *Am J Phys Anthropol* 38: 279.

58. Bell WH, Fonseca RJ, Kennedy JW, et al. 1975. "Bone healing and revascularization after total maxillary osteotomy." *J Oral Surg* 33: 253.

59. Ueki K, Marukawa K, Shimada M, et al. 2006. "The prevention of periodontal bone loss at the osteotomy site after anterior segmental and dento-osseous osteotomy." *J Oral Maxillofac Surg* 64: 1526.

60. Mordenfeld A, and Andersson L. 1999. "Periodontal and pulpal condition of the central incisors after midline osteotomy of the maxilla." *J Oral Maxillofac Surg* 57(5): 523.

61. Harada K, Sato M, and Omura K. 2004. "Blood-flow and neurosensory changes in the maxillary dental pulp after differing Le Fort I osteoeomies." *Oral Surg Oral Med Oral Pathol Radiol Endod* 97(1): 12.

62. Vedtofte P, and Nattestad A. 1989. "Pulp sensibility and pulp necrosis after LeFort I osteotomy." *J Craniomaxillofac Surg* 17(4): 167.

63. Morgan TA, and Fridrich KL. 2001. "Effects of the multiple-piece maxillary osteotomy on the periodontium." *Int J Adult Orthodon Orthognath Surg* 16(4): 255.

64. Lanigan DT, Hey JW, and West RA. 1990. "Aseptic necrosis following maxillary osteotomies: Report of 36 cases." *J Oral Maxillofac Surg* 48(2): 142.

65. Proffit WR, Turvey TA, and Phillips C. 1996. "Orthognathic surgery: A hierarchy of stability." *Int J Adult Orthodon Orthognath Surg* 11(3): 191.

66. Proffit WR, Turvey TA, and Phillips C. 2007. "The hierarchy of stability and predictability in orthognathic surgery with rigid fixation: An update and extension." *Head Face Med* 3: 21.

67. Junger TH, Krenkel C, and Howaldt HP. 2003. "Lefort I sliding osteotomy—A procedure for stable inferior repositioning of the maxilla." *J Craniomaxillofac Surg* 131(2): 82.

68. Girotto JA, Davidson J, Wheatly M, Redett R, et al. 1998. "Blindness as a complication of Le Fort osteotomies: Role of atypical fracture patterns and distortion of the optic canal." *Plast Reconstru Surg* 102(5): 1409.

69. Demas PN, and Sotereanos GC. 1989. "Incidence of nasolacrimal injury and turbinectomy-associated atrophic rhinitis with Lefort I osteotomies." *J Craniomaxillofac Surg* 17: 116.

70. You ZH, Bell WH, and Finn RA. 1992. "Location of the nasolacrimal canal in relation to the high LeFort I osteotomy." *J Oral Maxillofacial Surg* 50: 1075.

71. Shoshani Y, Samet N, Ardekian L, et al. 1994. "Nasolacrimal Duct injury after LeFort I osteoeomy." *J Oral Maxillofac Surg* 52: 406.

72. Drew SJ. 2008. "Clinical controversies in oral and maxillofacial surgery: Part One. Maxillary distraction osteogenesis for advancement in cleft patients, internal devices." *J Oral Maxillofac Surg* 66(12): 2592.

73. Mitchell C, Oeltjen J, Panthaki Z, and Thaller SR. "Nasolabial aesthetics." 2007. *J Craniofac Surg* 18(4): 75.

74. O'Ryan F, and Schendel S. 1989. "Nasal anatomy and maxillary surgery. I. Esthetic and anatomic principles." *Int J Adult Orthodon Orthognath Surg* 4(1): 27.

75. O'Ryan F, and Schendel S. 1989. "Nasal anatomy and maxillary surgery. II. Unfavorable nasolabial esthetics following the LeFort I osteotomy." *Int J Adult Orthodon Orthognath Surg* 4(2): 75.

76. O'Ryan F, and Carlotti A. 1989. "Nasal anatomy and maxillary surgery. III. Surgical techniques for correction of nasal deformities in patient undergoing maxillary surgery." *Int J Adult Orthodon Orthognath Surg* 4(3): 157.

77. Stella JP, Streater MR, Epker BN, and Sinn DP. 1989. "Predictability of upper lip soft tissue changes with maxillary advancement." *J Oral Maxillofac Surg* 47(7): 697.

78. Polido WD, Ellis E, 3rd, and Sinn DP. 1991. "An assessment of the predictability of maxillary repositioning." *Int J Oral Maxillofac Surg* 20(6): 349.

79. Gil JN, Claus JD, Manfro R, and Lima SM, Jr. 2007. "Predictability of maxillary repositioning during bimaxillary surgery: Accuracy of a new technique." *Int J Oral Maxillofac Surg* 36(4): 296.

80. Kretschmer WB, Zoder W, Baciut G, and Wangerin K. 2009. "Accuracy of maxillary positioning in bimaxillary surgery." *Br J Oral Maxillofac Surg* 47(6): 446.

81. Kramer FJ, Baethge C, Swennen G, Teltzrow T, et al. 2004. "Intra- and perioperative complications of the LeFort I Osteotomy: A prospective evaluation of 1000 patients." *J Craniofac Surg* 15(6): 971.

82. Turvey TA, and Fonseca RJ. 1980. "The anatomy of the internal maxillary artery in the ptyergopalatine fossa: Its relationship to maxillary surgery." *J Oral Surg* 38: 92.

83. Trimbel LD, Tideman H, and Stoelinga PJW. 1983. "A modification of the ptyergoid plate separation in low-level maxillary osteotomies." *J Oral Maxillofac Surg* 41: 544.

84. Lanigan DT, Hey, JH, and West RA. 1990. "Major vascular complications of orthognathic surgery: Hemorrhage associated with Le Fort I osteotomies." *J Oral Maxillofac Surg* 48(6): 561.

85. Manafi A, Ghenaait H, Dezham F, and Arshad M. 2007. "Massive repeated nose bleeding after bimaxillary osteotomy." *J Craniofac Surg* 18(6): 1491.

86. Lanigan DT, Hey JH, and West RA. 1991. "Major vascular complications of orthognathic surgery: False aneurysms and arteriovenous fistulas following orthognathic surgery." *J Oral Maxillofac Surg* 49(6): 571.

87. Campbell R, Rodrigo D, and Cheung L. 1994. "Asystole and bradycardia during maxillofacial surgery." *Anesth Prog* 41: 13.

88. Schaller B, Cornelius JF, Prabhakar H, Koerbel A, et al. 2009. "Trigemino-cardiac reflex: An update of the current knowledge." *J Neruosurg Anesthesiol* 21(3): 187.

89. Ketzler JT, and Landers DF. 1992. "Management of a severed endotracheal tube during Lefort OSteoeomy." *J Clin Anesth* 4(2): 144.

90. Valentine DJ, and Kaban LB. 1992. "Unusual nasoendotracheal tube damage during Le Fort I Osteotomy. Case report." *Int J Oral Maxillofac Surg* 21(6): 333.

91. Davies JR, and Dyer PV. 2003. "Preventing damage to the tracheal tube during maxillary osteotomy." *Anaesthesia* 59(9): 914.

92. Peskin RM, and Sachs SA. 1986. "Intraoperative management of a partially severed endotracheal tube during orthognathic surgery." *Anesth Prog* 33(5): 247.

93. Huang TT, Tseng CE, Lee TM, Yeh JY, and Lai YY. 2009. "Preventing pressure sores of the nasal ala after nasotracheal tube intubatin: From animal model to clinical application." *J Oral Maxillofac Surg* 67(3): 543.

94. O'Ferrara JJ, Cheynet F, Guyot L, Thiery G, and Blanc JL. 2001. "Complications of genioplasty." *Rev Stomatol Chir Maxillofac* 102(1): 34.

95. Van Butsele B, Neyt L, Abeloos J, De Clercq C, et al. 1993. "Mandibular fracture: An unusual complication following osteotomy of the chin." *Acat Stomatol Belg* 90(3): 189.

96. Clark CL, and Baur DA. 2004. "Management of mentalis muscle dysfunction after advancement genioplasty: A case report." *J Oral Maxillofac Surg* 62(5): 611.

97. Jones BM, and Vesely MJ. 2006. "Osseous genioplasty in facial aesthetic surgery–A personal perspective reviewing 54 patients." *J Plast Reconstr Aesthet Surg* 59(11): 1177.

98. Guyot L, Layoun W, Richard O, Chenynet F, and Gola R. 2002. "Alteration of chin sensibility due to damage of the cutaneous branchj of the mylohyoid nerve during genioplasty." *J Oral Maxillofac Surg* 60(11): 1371.

99. Ritter EF, Moelleken BR, Mathes SJ, and Ousterhout DK. 1992. "The course of the inferior alveolar neurovascular canal in relation to sliding genioplasty." *J Craniofac Surg* 13(1): 20.

100. Varol A, Sencimen M, Kicabiyik N, Gilses A, and Ozan H. 2009. "Clinical and anatomical aspects of possible mylohyoid nerve injury during genioplasties." *Int J Oral Maxillofac Surg* 38(10): 1084.

101. Shaughnessy S, Mobarak KA, Hogevold HE, and Espeland L. 2006. "Long-term skeletal and soft tissue responses after advancement genioplasty." *Am J Orthodon Dentofacial Orthop* 130(1): 8.

102. Hwang K, Lee WJ, Song YB, and Chung IH. 2005. "Vulnerability of the inferior alveolar nerve and mental nerve during genioplasty: An anatomic study." *J Craniofac Surg* 16(1): 10.

103. Van Merkesteyn JP, Groot RH, van Leeuwaarden R, and Kroon FH. 1987. "Intra-operative complications in sagittal and vertical ramus osteoeomies." *Int J Oral Maxillofac Surg* 16(6): 665.

104. Tuinzing DB, and Greebe RB. 1985. "Complications related to the intraoral vertical ramus osteotomy." *Int J Oral Surg* 14(4): 319.
105. Hall HD, and McKenna SJ. 1987. "Further refinement and evaluation of intraoral vertical ramus ostoeotmy." *J Oral Maxillofac Surg* 45(8): 684.
106. Blinder D, Peleg O, Yoffe T, and Taicher S. 2010. "Intraoral vertical ramus osteotomy: A simple method to prevent medial trapping of the proximal fragment. *Int J Roal Maxillofac Surg* 39(3): 289.
107. Calderon S, Gal G, Anavi Y, and Gonshorowitz M. 1992. "Techniques for ensuring the lateral position of the proximal segment following intraoral vertical ramus osteotomy." *J Oral Maxillofac Surg* 50(10): 1044.
108. Ueki K, Hashiba Y, Marukawa K, Nakagawa K, et al. 2009. "The effects of changing position and angle of the proximal segment after intraoral vertical ramus osteotomy." *Int J Oral Maxillofac Surg* 38(10): 1041.
109. Lanigan DT, Hey J, and West RA. 1991. "Hemorrhage following mandibular osteotomies: A report of 2 cases." *J Oral Maxillofac Surg* 49(7): 713.
110. Resnick CM, Kaban LB, and Troulis MJ. 2009. "Minimally invasive orthognathic surgery." *Facial Plast Surg* 25(1): 49.
111. Teltzrow T, Kramer FJ, Schulze A, Baethge C, and Brachvogel P. 2005. "Perioperative complications following sagittal split osteotomy of the mandible." *J Craniomaxillofac Surg* 33(5): 307.
112. Hwang K, Nam YS, and Han SH. 2009. "Vunerable structures during intraoral sagittal split ramus osteotomy." *J Craniofac Surg* 20(1): 229.
113. Jones JK, and Van Sickels JE. 1991. "Facial nerve injuries associated with orthognathic surgery: A review of incidence and management." *J Oral Maxillofac Surg* 49(7): 740.
114. Kriwalsky MS, Maurer P, Veras RB, Eckert AW, and Schubert J. 2008. "Risk factors for bad split during sagittal split osteotomy." *Br J Oral Maxillofac Surg* 46(3): 177.
115. Patterson AL, and Bagby SK. 1999. "Posterior vertical body osteotomy (PVBO): A predictable rescue procedure for proximal segment fracture during sagittal split ramus osteotomy of the mandible." *J Oral Maxillofac Surg* 57(4): 475.
116. Mehra P, Castro V, Freitas RZ, and Wolford LM. 2001. "Complications of the mandibular sagittal split ramus osteoeomy associated with the presence or absence of third molars." *J Oral Maxillofac Surg* 59(8): 854.
117. Marquez IM, and Setella JP. 1998. "Modification of sagittal split ramus osteotomy to avoid unfavorable fracture around impacted third molars." *Int J Adult Orthodon Orthognath Surg* 13(3): 183.
118. Geha H, Nimeskern N, and Beziat JL. 2009. "Patient-controlled analgesia in orthognathic surgery: Evaluation of the relationship to anxiety and anxiolytics." *Oral Surg Oral Med Oral Pathol Oral Radiol Endod* 108(3): e33.
119. Schaberg SJ, Stuller CB, and Edwards SM. 1984. "Effect of methyoprednisolone on swelling after orthognathic surgery." *J Oral Maxillofac Surg* 42(6): 356.
120. Weber CR, and Griffin JM. 1994. "Evaluation of dexamethasone for reducing postoperative edema and inflammatory response after orthognathic surgery." *J Oral Maxillofac Surg* 52(1): 35.
121. Precious DS, Hoffman CD, and Miller R. 1992. "Steroid acne after orthognathic surgery." *Oral Surg Oral Med Oral Path* 74(3): 279.
122. Fleming PS, and Flood TR. 2005. "Steroid-induced psychosis complicating orthognathic surgery: A case report." *Br Dent J* 2005 199(10): 647.
123. Barrier A, Breton P, Girard R, Dubost J, and Bouletreau P. 2009. "Surgical site infections in orthognathic surgery and risk factors associated." *Rev Stomatol Chir Maxillofac* 110(3): 127.
124. Spaey YJ, Bettens RM, Mommaerts MY, et al. 2005. "A prospective study on infections complications in orthognathic surgery." *J Craniomaxillofac Surg* 33(1): 24.
125. Silva AC, O'Ryan F, and Poor DB. 2006. "Postoperative nausea and vomiting (PONV) after orthognathic surgery: A retrospective study and literature review." *J Oral Maxillofac Surg* 64: 1385.
126. Flanary CM, Barnwell GM, VanSickels JE, Littlefield JH, and Rugh Al. 1990. "Impact of orthognathic surgery on normal and abnormal personality dimensions: A 2-year follow-up study of 61 patients." *Am J Orthod Dentofacial Orthop* 98(4): 313.
127. Pogrel MA, and Scott P. 1994. "Is it possible to identify the psychologically 'bad risk' orthognathic surgery patient preoperatively?" *Int J Adult Orthodon Orthognath Surg* 9(2): 105.
128. Cunningham SJ, Hunt NP, and Feinmann C. 1995. "Psychological aspects of orthognathic surgery: A review of the literature." *Int J Adult Orthodon Orthognath Surg* 10(3): 159.
129. Olejki TD, and Fonseca RJ. 1984. "Preoperative nutritional supplementation for the orthognathic surgery patient." *J Oal Maxillofac Surg* 42(9): 573.
130. Kendell BD, Fonseca RJ, and Lee M. 1982. "Postoperative nutritional supplementation for the orthognathic surgery patient." *J Oral Maxillofac Surg* 40(4): 205.
131. Connor AM. 1982. "A diet for orthognathic surgery patients." *J Clin Orthod* 16(1): 33.
132. Moses JJ, Lange CR, and Arredondo A. 2000. "Endoscopic treatment of sinonasal disease in patients who have had orthognathic surgery." *Br J Oral Maxillofac Surg* 38(3): 177.
133. Cano J, Campo J, Alobera MA, and Baca R. 2009. "Surgical ciliated cyst of the maxilla. Clinical case." *Med Oral Patol Oral Cir Buccal* 14(7): 361.
134. Bell CS, Thrash WJ, and Zysset MK. 1986. "Incidence of maxillary sinusitis following LeFort I maxillary osteotomy." *J Oral Maxillofac Surg* 44(2): 100.
135. Yaghmaei M, Ghoujeghi A, Sadeghinejad A, Aberoumand D, Seifi M, and Saffarshahroudi A. 2009. "Auditory changes in patients undergoing orthognathic surgery." *Int J Oral Maxillofac Surg* 38(11): 1148.

136. Barker GR. 1987. "Auditory tube function and audiogram changes following corrective orthognathic maxillary and mandibular surgery in cleft and non-cleft patients." *Scand J Plast Reconstr Surg Hand Surg* 21(1): 133.

137. Ellingsen RH, and Artun J. 1993. "Pulpal response to orthognathic surgery: A long term radiographic study." *Am J Orthod Dentorfacial Orthop* 103(3): 338.

138. Justus T, Chang BL, Bloomquist D, and Ramsay DS. 2001. "Human gingival and pulpal blood flow during healing after Le Fort I osteotomy." *J Oral Maxillofac Surg* 59(1): 2.

139. Hatch JP, Van Sickels JE, Rugh JD, Dolce C, et al. 2001. "Mandibular range of motion after bilateral sagittal split ramus osteotomy with wire osteosynthesis or rigid fixation." *Oral Surg Oral Med Oral Pathol Oral Radiol Endod* 91(3): 274.

140. Zarrinkelk HM, Throckmorton GS, Ellis E, 3rd, and Sinn DP. 1996. "Functional and morphologic changes after combined maxillary intrusion and mandibular advancement surgery." *J Oral Maxillofac Surg* 54(7): 828.

141. Athanasiou AE, Elefteriadis JN, and Dre E. 1996. "Short term functional alterations in the stomatognathic system after orthodonti-surgical management of skeletal vertical excess problems." *Int J Adult Orthodon Orthogn Surg* 11(4): 339.

142. Storum KA, and Bell WH. 1984. "Hypomobility after maxillary and mandibular osteotomies." *Oral Surg Oral Med Oral Pathol* 57(1): 7.

143. Boyd SB, Karas ND, and Sinn DP. 1991. "Recovery of mandibular mobility following orthognathic surgery." *J Oral Maxillofac Surg* 49(9): 924.

144. Ueki K, Marukawa K, Hashiba Y, Nakagawa K, et al. 2008. "Assessment of the relationship between the recovery of maximum mandibular opening and maxillomandibular fixation period after orthognathic surgery." *J Oral Maxillofac Surg* 66(3): 485.

145. Ueki K, Marukawa K, Shimada M, Nakagawa K, Yamamoto E. 2007. "Changes in occlusal force after mandibular ramus osteotomy with and without Le Fort I osteotomy." *Int J Oral Maxillofac Surg* 36(4): 301.

146. Wolford LM, Reiche-Fischel O, and Mehra P. 2003. "Changes in TMJ dysfunction after orthognathic surgery." *J Oral Maxillofac Surg* 61(6): 655.

147. Bailey LJ, Wite RP, Jr, Proffit WR, and Turvey TA. 1997. "Segmental Lefort I osteotomy for management of transverse maxillary deficiency." *J Oral Maxillofac Surg* 55(7): 728.

148. Vandersea BA, Ruvo AT, and Frost DE. 2007. "Maxillary transverse deficiency-surgical alternatives to management." *Oral Maxillofac Surg Clin North Am* 19(3): 351.

149. Chrcanovic BR, and Custodio AL. 2009. "Orthodontic or surgically assisted rapid maxillary expansion." *Oral Maxillofac Surg* 13(3): 123.

150. Baek SH, AHN HE, Kwon YH, and Choi JY. 2010. "Surgery-first approach in skeletal Class III malocclusion treated with 2-jaw surgery: Evaluation of surgical movement and post operative orthodontic treatment. *J Craniofac Surg* 21(2): 332.

151. Leyder P, Lahbabi M, and Panajotopuoulos A. 2001. "Unfavorable effects induced by mandibular surgery in Class III malocclusions." *Rev Stomatol Chir Maxillofac* 102(1): 12.

152. Moenning JE, Garrison BT, Lapp TH, and Bussard DA. 1990. "Early screw removal for correction of occlusal discrepancies following rigid internal fixation in orthognathic surgery." *Int J Adult Orthodon Orthognath Surg* 5(4): 225.

153. Khulefelt M, Laine P, Suominen-Taipale L, Ingman T, et al. 2010. "Risk factors contributing to symptomatic miniplate removal: A retrospective study of 153 bilateral sagittal split osteotomy patients." *Int J Oral Maxillofac Surg* 39(5): 430.

154. O'Connell J, Murphy C, Ikeagwuani O, Adley C, and Kearns G. 2009. "The fate of titanium miniplates and screws used in maxillofacial surgery: A 10 year retrospective study." *Int J Oral Maxillofac Surg* 38(7): 731.

155. Gent JF, Shafer DM, and Frank ME. 2003. "The effect of orthognathic surgery on taste function on the palate and tongue." *J Oral Maxillofac Surg* 61(7): 766.

156. Kim S, Shin SW, Han I, Joe SH, et al. 2009. "Clinical review of factors leading to perioperative dissatisfaction related to orthognathic surgery." *J Oral Maxillofac Surg* 67(10): 2217.

157. Al-Ahmad HT, Al-Omari IK, Eldurini LN, and Suleiman AA. 2008. "Factors affecting satisfaction of patients after orthognathic surgery at a university hospital." *Saudi Med J* 29(7): 998.

158. Bock JJ, Maurer P, and Furhmann RA. 2007. "The importance of temporomandibular function for patient satisfaction following orthognathic surgery." *J Orofac Orthop* 68(4): 299.

159. Costa F, Robinoy M, and Politi M. 2000. "Stability of LeFort I osteotomy in maxillary inferior repositioning: Review of the literature." *Int J Adult Orthod Orthognath Surg* 15(3): 197.

160. Dowling PA, Espeland L, Sandvik L, Mobarak KA, and Hegevold HE. 2005. "Lefort I maxillary advancement: 3-year stability risk factors for relapse." *Am J Orthod Dentofac Orthop* 128(5): 560.

161. Ianetti G, Fadda MT, Marianetti TM, Terenzi V, and Cassoni A. 2007. "Long-term skeletal stability after surgical correction in class III open-bite patients: A retrospective study of 40 patients treated with mono- or bimaxillary surgery." *J Craniofac Surg* 18(2): 350.

162. Chemello PD, Wolford LM, and Buschang PH. 1994. "Occlusal plane alteration in orthognathic surgery. Part II: Long-term stability of results." *Am J Orthod Dentofacial Orthop* 106(4): 434.

163. Silvestri A, Cascone P, Natali G, and Iaquaniello M. 1994. "Long-term control of the stability of skeletal structures in Class II dentoskeletal deformities after surgical-orthodontic therapy." *Am J Orthod Dentofacial Orthop* 105(4): 375.

164. Hack GA, De Mol van Otterloo JJ, and Nanda R. 1993. "Long-term stability and prediction of soft tissue changes after LeFort I surgery." *Am J Orthodon Dentofacial Orthop* 104(6): 544.

165. Yosano A, Kaktakura A, Takaki T, and Shibahara T. 2009. "Influence of mandibular fixation method on stability of the maxillary occlusal plane after occlusal plane alteration." *Bull Tokyo Dent Coll* 50(2): 71.

166. Kitahara T, Nakasima A, Kurahara S, and Shiratsuchi Y. 2009. "Hard and soft tissue stability of orthognathic surgery." *Angle Orthod* 79(1): 158.

167. Serafin B, Perciaccante VJ, and Cunningham LL. 2007. "Stability of orthognathic surgery and distraction osteogenesis: Options and alternatives." *Oral Maxillofac Surg Clin North Am* 19(3): 311.

168. Kallal RH, Ritto FG, Almeida LE, Crofton DJ, and Thomas GP. 2007. "Traumatic neuroma following sagittal split osteotomy of the mandible." *Int J Oral Maxillofac Surg* 36(5): 453.

169. Phillips C, Kim SH, Essick G, Tucker M, and Turvey TA. 2009. "Sensory retraining after orthognathic surgery: Effect on patient report of altered sensations." *Am J Orthodon Dentofacial Orthop* 136(6): 788.

170. Rai KK, Shivakumar HR, and Sonar MD. 2008. "Transient facial nerve palsy following bilateral sagittal split ramus osteotomy for setback of the mandible: A review of incidence and management." *J Oral Maxillofac Surg* 66(2): 373.

171. Wolford LM, and Cardenas L. 1999. "Idiopathic condylar resorption: Diagnosis, treatment protocol, and outcomes." *Am J Orthod Dentofacial Orthop* 116(6): 667.

172. Troulis MJ, Tayebaty FT, Papadaki M, Williams WB, and Kaban LB. 2008. "Condylectomy and costochondral graft reconstruction for treatment of active idiopathic condylar resorption." *J Oral Maxillofac Surg* 66(1): 65.

173. Gill DS, El Maaytah M, Maini FB. 2008. "Risk factors for post-orthognathic condylar resorption: A review." *World J Orthod* 9(1): 21.

174. Posnick JC, and Fantuzzo JJ. 2007. "Idiopathic condylar resorption: Current clinical perspectives." *J Oral Maxillofac Surg* 65(8): 1617.

175. Mercuri LG. 2008. "Osteoarthritis, osteoarthrosis, and idiopathic condylar resorption." *Oral Maxillofac Surg Clin North Am* 20(2): 169.

176. Papadaki ME, Tayebaty F, Kaban LB, and Troulis MJ. 2007. "Condylar resorption." *Oral Maxillofac Surg Clin North Am* 19(2): 223.

6

Distraction Osteogenesis

Maria J. Troulis, DDS, MSc
Alexander Katsnelson, DMD, MS
Carl Bouchard, DMD, MSc, FRCD(C)
Bonnie L. Padwa, DMD, MD
Leonard B. Kaban, DMD, MD

INTRODUCTION

Distraction osteogenesis (DO) was first described by Codivilla in 1905 for the treatment of a short femur.[1] It was later popularized by Ilizarov, an orthopedic surgeon, who formulated and applied the principles of DO for limb lengthening to a large number of patients. As a result of his pioneering work, Ilizarov is recognized as the "father of distraction osteogenesis."[2] McCarthy was the first to use the technique of distraction for treatment of craniofacial deformities.[3] Distraction osteogenesis is now part of the standard surgical armamentarium for skeletal expansion in the craniomaxillofacial region.[4]

Distraction osteogenesis offers many advantages over traditional techniques, including gradual lengthening of the soft tissue envelope[5] and the potential elimination of the need for bone grafting.[6] However, as with any technique, limitations and disadvantages exist. Some of the shortcomings include difficulties in establishing the correct distraction vector, need for patient cooperation, and prolonged treatment time. As with most procedures, complications may be avoided by careful patient selection and proper surgical planning and technique.[6] Complications can be divided into three phases: preoperative (planning), intraoperative, and postoperative.[7,8]

In this chapter, complications associated with distraction will be described. This chapter is based on two other chapters of complications of DO.[7,8]

PREOPERATIVE PLANNING PHASE

The best strategy is to prevent complications by careful preoperative planning, which includes appropriate patient selection, accurate assessment of the anatomy and planning of the vector of distraction, and osteotomy location and placement of the distraction device.[7,8]

Patient Selection

Distraction osteogenesisis a treatment that demands significant commitment from the patient, family, and surgeon. Whether distraction devices are intraoral or extraoral, pin borne or bone borne, they can be bulky and complicated to use.[7,8]

Management of Complications in Oral and Maxillofacial Surgery, First Edition. Edited by Michael Miloro, Antonia Kolokythas.
© 2012 John Wiley & Sons, Inc. Published 2012 by John Wiley & Sons, Inc.

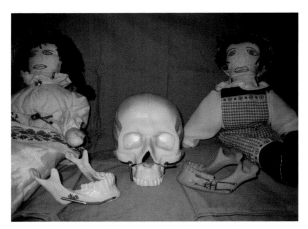

Fig. 6.1. Dolls and skull models with distraction devices used for demonstration.

Primrose et al. reported a series of pediatric patients who underwent distraction with either an intraoral or extraoral device.[9] Patients who had extraoral devices reported sleep disturbances because of the bulkiness of the distractor. They also complained of limited ability to engage in recreational activities. Older patients who had extraoral devices felt "abnormal." Patients with intraoral devices reported speech, eating, and oral hygiene difficulties but felt the devices had less of an effect on social activities.[9] Modfid et al. reported that 4.7% of all DO patients displayed poor compliance regardless of the type of device.[6] This is a clinical observation, which multiple authors have reported.[6–9]

The preoperative interview with the family should include a discussion of the impact that this technique will have on the patient's social life and the possible disruption of participating in educational and recreational activities. The diet should be reviewed with the patient in advance because it will be limited to soft or blenderized foods throughout the distraction and fixation periods. The patient and family should be familiarized with the appliance and verify that they will be able to activate it as needed. The use of educational tools including models and dolls with distraction devices can be helpful (Fig. 6.1). Additionally, the patient and family should be made aware that a number of postoperative visits are necessary with DO (usually more than with conventional procedures).[7,8] As with all surgical procedures, alternative treatments, risks and benefits of DO (including possible reoperation) need to be clearly outlined.

Distraction Vector Planning

An accurate distraction vector is necessary to obtain the desired final position of the distracted segment. Mofid et al. reported an incorrect distraction vector in 8.8% of patients who had a single vector distractor and in 7.2% who had a multivector distractor.[6] The wrong vector of distraction can cause malocclusion and/or facial asymmetry, and may require additional procedures for correction (Fig. 6.2).

In order to accurately obtain the correct distraction vector across the osteotomy, development of the appropriate preoperative treatment plan is required and correct transfer of this information to the operating room is necessary. Preoperative treatment preparation is based on clinical and radiographic examination [lateral and anteroposterior cephalograms, orthopantograms, and computer tomography (CT) with three-dimensional (3D) reconstruction].[7,8] Treatment planning software can assist with developing the movement of the distractor, analyzing interferences, and fabricating the accurate device or choosing the correct distractor from a set of existing devices.[7,8,10,11]

A surgical guide can help transfer the preoperative plan to the operating room.[11] After establishing a treatment plan that includes the osteotomy and distractor position, this information can then be entered into a virtual computer environment that allows envisioning the surgical outcome based on the treatment plan. This treatment plan is then transformed to stereolithographic models, and surgical guides are made according to these models (Fig. 6.3). This preparation minimizes the risk of an inaccurate direction of distraction.[8] Intraoperative surgical navigation is a developing field and can be a useful tool to use to correctly perform osteotomies and position devices.

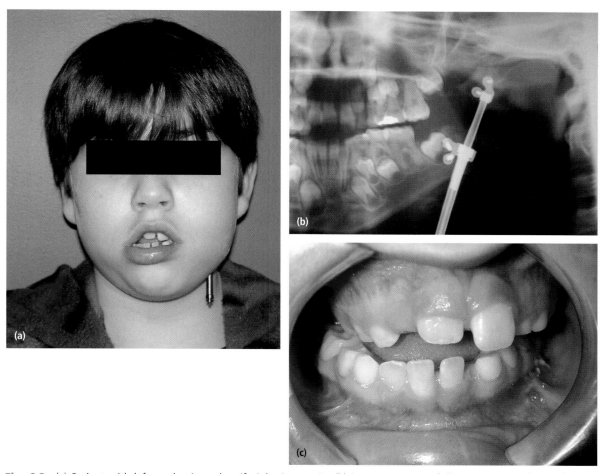

Fig. 6.2. (a) Patient with left predominant hemifacial microsomia; (b) incorrect vector of distraction caused cross bite on the right side and (c) did not create the desired open bite on the left side. (All images printed with permission from PMPH-USA.)

INTRAOPERATIVE PHASE

Neurologic and Dental Injury

Distraction osteogenesis requires a complete osteotomy and placement of the appliance that can result in damage to adjacent structures such as teeth and nerves.[7,8] Mofid et al. reported a review of 3,278 cases. There were 81 (3.6%) cases of damage to the inferior alveolar nerve, 69 (1.9%) had tooth bud injury, and 12 (0.4%) had facial nerve injury.[6] Swennen et al. found tooth damage in 2.3% of cases.[12] Most of the damage to adjacent structures can be reduced during the osteotomy by careful analysis of preoperative radiographs and accurate execution of the planned osteotomy. In most cases, the paresthesia of the inferior alveolar nerve is transient; typically, younger patients spontaneously recover sensation more quickly and to a higher degree than older patients.[7,8]

Incomplete Osteotomy and Improper Device Placement

The correct vector of distraction requires a precise osteotomy in the proper location and accurate device placement.[7,8] The osteotomy and placement of the distractor is sometimes limited by adjacent anatomical structures. Intraoperatively, a surgical guide (or navigation) based on preoperative planning can help avoid this complication by assisting with accurate positioning of the osteotomy and device placement.

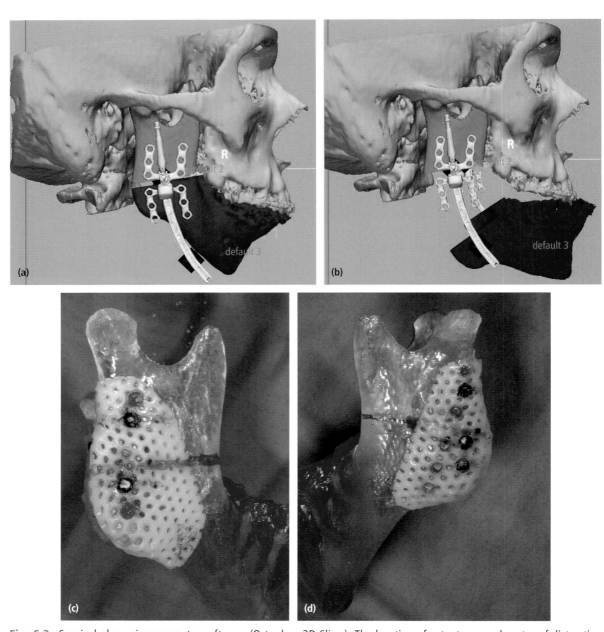

Fig. 6.3. Surgical plan using computer software (Ostoplan, 3D Slicer). The location of osteotomy and vector of distraction can be determined. (a), (b) The surgical guide can be made using stereolytic model. (c), (d) The location of osteotomy and position of the distractor can be marked on the surgical guide. (e), (f) Accurate osteotomies and (g), (h) correct placement of distractors can be achieved intraoperatively using surgical guides. (All images printed with permission from PMPH-USA.)

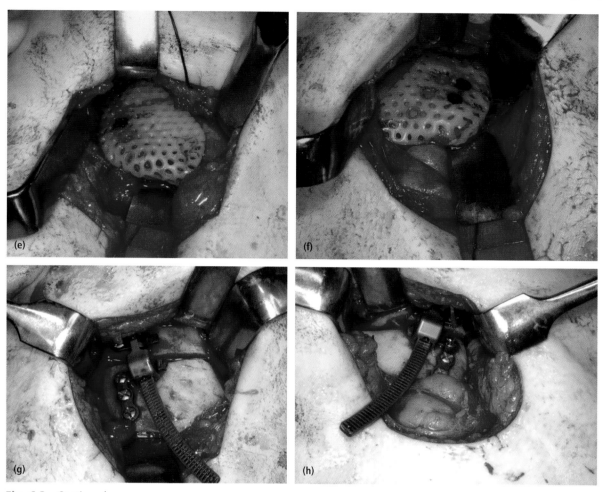

Fig. 6.3. *Continued*

Another complication that can occur intraoperatively is an incomplete osteotomy. This leads to inadequate movement of the bony segments, malfunction of the distractor, bending, or breakage of the device (Fig. 6.4).[7,8] An incomplete osteotomy can also result in pain and/or pressure at the distraction site upon activation. This can affect patient compliance.

A sign of inadequate distraction (either because of incomplete osteotomy, interferences, or device failure) is a discrepancy between the number of days of distraction and the measured bony gap. The device may appear activated on radiographs (gap between activation arms), but there will be no bony gap, no gap between foot plates, and no change in the occlusion. As a result, premature consolidation can occur. Examination of the surgical site along with careful evaluation of the radiographs when such discrepancies are found will assist in identification of the problem. The device should be removed the osteotomy recreated and the process restarted.

To avoid incomplete osteotomy and subsequent inadequate distraction, the distractor should be activated intraoperatively and the resultant gap examined for separation between the segments. Then the device should be reversed to its natural inactivated position. However, when using detachable footplates, care should be taken not to disengage the device from the footplate. Postoperatively, appropriate and adequate images should be obtained to evaluate the position of the distractor, as well as its components (i.e., position of the rod in the detachable foot plate, position of screws, gap, etc.).[7,8]

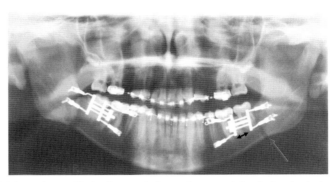

Fig. 6.4. Patient who had bilateral mandibular intraoral distraction complained of pain during activation. Panorex shows the distraction device on the left side was fully open (black arrow) but there was only a small bony gap (red arrow). An inadequate osteotomy caused bending of the foot plates, and failure of the distraction. (Printed with permission from PMPH-USA.)

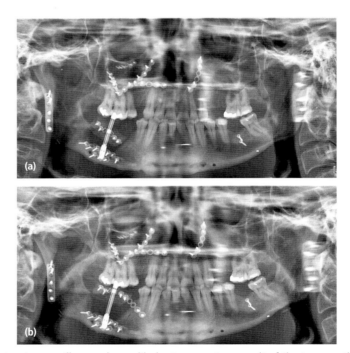

Fig. 6.5. Patient after extensive maxillary and mandibular trauma. As a result of the trauma, the patient had a deficient mandible on the right side. (a) During alveolar distraction, the device broke and was distracting at an angle. (b) The transport segment was stabilized with a plate during the consolidation phase.

POSTOPERATIVE PHASE

Device Failure

As with every surgical technique, familiarity with the components of the device and clear understanding of their functions are essential. Any component of the distraction device can experience hardware failure during the placement, activation, and consolidation phases of distraction (Fig. 6.5). Mofid et al. reported a rate of 4.5% for hardware failure and 3% for hardware dislodgement.[6] Swennen et al. reported 33.1% of patients had a device with mechanical problems (including pin loosening).[12] In a review by van Strijen, there were five distraction device failures in 70 patients (7.1%).[13]

Extraoral distraction devices have additional complications such as pin loosening, infection of the skin at the pin site, instability of fixation, unacceptable scarring, risk for osteomyelitis, bicortical skull penetration, cerebrospinal fluid leakage, and intracranial infection (abscess and meningitis).[14] Nout et al. reported that maxillary distraction using RED devices (KLS Martin, Jacksonville, FL) had a 42.9% occurrence of pin loosening and a 28.6% incidence of pin migration.[15] Extra care while inserting the pins should be exercised to avoid injury to branches of the facial nerve or adjacent vessels. Furthermore, strict adherence to sterile techniques and basic surgical principles taking into account the local anatomy are essential when stabilizing the DO device to the skull or inserting the pins.[14,15] Extreme care must be used when performing the osteotomies and when placing the pins to the cranium to avoid neurologic complications. Adequate tissue protection, adequate irrigation while preparing the pin sites, stabilizing the device, or creating the osteotomy are basic principles that should be adhered to.[14,15]

Inadequate Distraction

Anatomic interferences, device failure, lack of patient compliance, and premature fixation or consolidation of the regenerate can limit the amount of skeletal movement from distraction (Fig. 6.6).

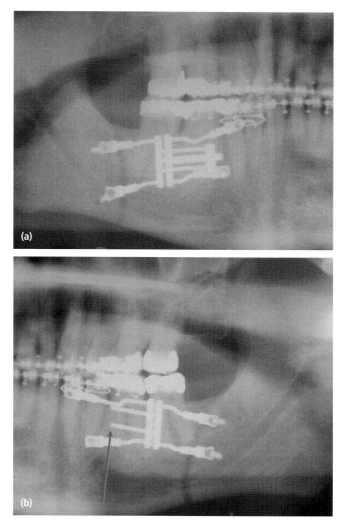

Fig. 6.6. Patient after bilateral mandibular distraction. (a) On the right side, he turned the distractor in the correct direction. (b) On the left side, he activated the device in the incorrect direction, which caused the distractor to dismantle (red arrow). (All images printed with permission from PMPH-USA.)

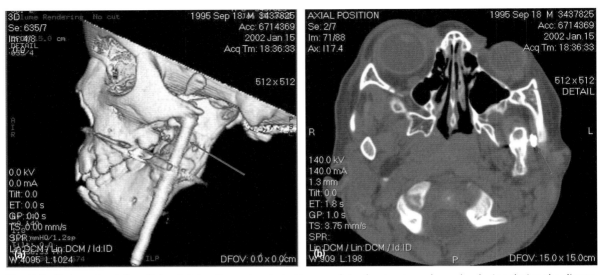

Fig. 6.7. Patient after left unilateral distraction, who started to complain about pain and a malocclusion during the distraction phase. (a), (b) The 3D CT shows the distraction device was abutting with the zygomatic arch (red arrows). (All images printed with permission from PMPH-USA.)

Anatomic interferences can prevent distraction. The coronoid process can interfere with the skull base and prohibit elongation of the proximal segment (Fig. 6.7).

A preoperative CT scan and an analysis of the movement, as well as a planning software system that recognizes interferences and collisions, are most useful.[10,11] For example, if the coronoid touches the skull base prior to the completion of the planned distraction, a coronoidectomy is performed prior to distractor placement in order to avoid anatomic interference.[10,11]

Inadequate distraction occurs when distraction is used instead of a bilateral sagittal split osteotomy and it appears that the desired occlusion has been achieved but the patient is posturing forward. To avoid this problem, careful evaluation of a panorex needs to be preformed to ensure that the temporomandibular joint space is not enlarged and clinically a centric relation/centric occlusion (CR/CO) discrepancy is not elicited. Class II elastics placed for a few days are useful to ensure proper jaw position. Distraction can concurrently continue to complete the desired advancement.[7,8]

Another common limitation of DO is premature consolidation of the bony regenerate. This complication varies from study to study but has been reported to be in the range of 1.9% to 7.6%. [6,12] The complication can occur if the latency period is too long or the rate of distraction is too slow.[16] When the rate of the distraction is too fast, degenerative changes can occur in the inferior alveolar nerve[17] and joint[18] or a fibrous nonunion can develop. The rate of distraction depends on the age of the patient, area of distraction (i.e., cortical vs. alveolar bone) and type of distraction.

Infection

Typically, there may be minor infections (e.g., at the pin sites) or minor soft tissue dehiscences, which respond well to local wound care. The infection rate varies (0.5–2.9%) depending on the type of distractor and anatomic area of placement (Fig. 6.8).[6,12,13] The incidence of infection in craniomaxillofacial distraction osteogenesis is lower than with extremity distraction due to the vast and collateral blood supply in the head and neck region. Also, distraction increases the blood supply to the area. Perioperative systemic antibiotic prophylaxis should be considered during the placement and removal of the distractor. Also, excellent oral hygiene can decrease the risk of minor infections associated with intraoral DO sites.[7,8]

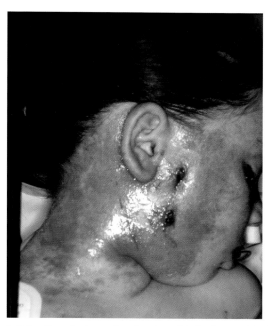

Fig. 6.8. Patient with an extraoral distraction device, who developed infection and facial cellulitis during the distraction phase. The device was removed and the patient had an aggressive course of antibiotic treatment. (All images printed with permission from PMPH-USA.)

Inadequate Bony Regenerate

Cope and Aronson point out that an incorrect rate of distraction, abnormal displacement of bone segments, excessive initial bony gap, damage to bone marrow and periosteum, and instability of the distraction device can result in inadequate healing of the regenerate.[19,20] The risk of inadequate regenerate is higher in patients who have undergone multiple previous surgeries, those who smoke, and in older individuals.

Generally, an inadequate regenerate has deficient mineralization in the distraction gap, as seen on radiographs.[8] The best way to resolve the problem is to decrease the rate of distraction, temporarily stop the distraction, or even compress the regenerate by activating the distractor in the opposite direction.[7,16] In cases where the distraction device has to be removed prior to consolidation, a rigid fixation plate can be used for stabilizing the segments (Fig. 6.9).

Interestingly, of all the applications of distraction osteogenesis, alveolar distraction shows the highest rate of inadequate bone formation (as high as 8%).[21] The type of device used and a distraction rate of more than 0.5 mm/24 h were found to be significantly related to insufficient bone formation at the site.[21]

CONCLUSIONS

Distraction osteogenesis is a unique and innovative technique for maxillofacial surgery. It has many advantages that make it a valuable alternative to the traditional osteotomies for skeletal expansion. However, DO requires accurate planning, is technically demanding, and involves intense patient and surgeon participation. Surgeons are continuing to try to minimize the risks and complications associated with this technique.

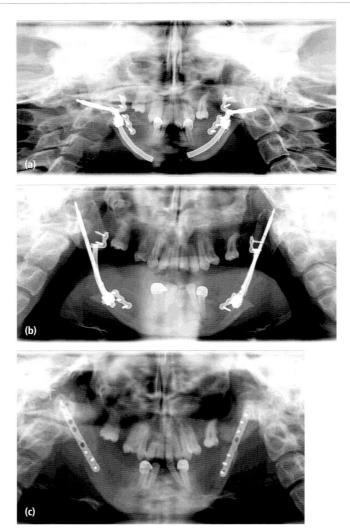

Fig. 6.9. Patient with Nager syndrome, who underwent bilateral mandibular distraction (a) before and (b) after the distraction phase. The distraction was done at a rate of 2 mm per day, which caused inadequate regenerate. (c) Therefore, bilateral rigid fixation plates were placed in order to avoid collapse of the expanded skeleton. (All images printed with permission from PMPH-USA.)

SUGGESTED READINGS

1. Codivilla A. 1905. "On the means of lengthening, in the lower limbs, the muscle and tissues which are shortened through deformity." *Am J Orthop Surg* 2: 353–369.
2. Ilizarov GA. 1988. "The principles of the Ilizarov method." *Bull Hosp Jt Dis Orthop Inst* 48: 1–11.
3. McCarthy JG, Schreiber J, Karp N, Thorne CH, and Grayson BH. 1992. "Lengthening the human mandible by gradual distraction." *Plast Reconstr Surg* 89: 1–8; discussion 9–10.
4. Thomas DJ, and Rees MJ. 2001. "Fibrous ankylosis after distraction osteogenesis of a costochondral neomandible in a patient with grade III hemifacial microsomia." *J Craniofac Surg* 12(5): 469–474.
5. Alkan A, Inal S, Baş B, and Ozer M. 2007. "Incomplete mobilization of the maxilla resulting in failed maxillary distraction: A case report." *Oral Surg Oral Med Oral Pathol Oral Radiol Endod* 104(6): e5–11.
6. Mofid MM, Manson PN, Robertson BC, Tufaro AP, Elias JJ, and Vander Kolk CA. 2001. "Craniofacial distraction osteogenesis: A review of 3278 cases." *Plast Reconstr Surg* 108: 1103–1114; discussion 1115–1117.
7. Troulis MJ, and Kaban LB. 2003. "Complications of mandibular distraction osteogenesis." *Oral Maxillofac Surg Clin North Am* 15(2): 251–264.

8. Bouchard C, Sharaf BA, Smart RJ, Troulis MJ, Padwa BL, and Kaban LB. 2011. "Complications with distraction osteogenesis of the craniofacial skeleton." In: *Minimally Invasive Maxillofacial Surgery*, Troulis M, and Kaban L, eds. Sheldon, CT: PmPh-USA.

9. Primrose AC, Broadfoot E, Diner PA, Molina F, Moos KF, and Ayoub AF. 2005. "Patients' responses to distraction osteogenesis: A multi-centre study." *Int J Oral Maxillofac Surg* 34: 238–242.

10. Yeshwant K, Seldin EB, Gateno J, Everett P, White CL, Kikinis R, Kaban LB, and Troulis MJ. 2005. "Analysis of skeletal movements in mandibular distraction osteogenesis." *J Oral Maxillofac Surg* 63(3): 335–340.

11. Troulis MJ, Everett P, Seldin EB, Kikinis R, and Kaban LB. 2002. "Development of a three-dimensional treatment planning system based on computed tomographic data." *Int J Oral Maxillofac Surg* 31: 349–357.

12. Swennen G, Schliephake H, Dempf R, Schierle H, and Malevez C. 2001. "Craniofacial distraction osteogenesis: A review of the literature: Part 1: Clinical studies." *Int J Oral Maxillofac Surg* 30: 89–103.

13. Van Strijen PJ, Breuning KH, Becking AG, Perdijk FB, and Tuinzing DB. 2003. "Complications in bilateral mandibular distraction osteogenesis using internal devices." *Oral Surg Oral Med Oral Pathol Oral Radiol Endod* 96: 392–397.

14. Van der Meulen J, Wolvius E, van der Wal K, Prahl B, and Vaandrager M. 2005. "Prevention of halo pin complications in postcranioplasty patients." *J Craniomaxillofac Surg* 33(3): 145–149.

15. Nout E, Wolvius EB, van Adrichem LN, Ongkosuwito EM, and van der Wal KG. 2006. "Complications in maxillary distraction using the RED II device: A retrospective analysis of 21 patients." *Int J Oral Maxillofac Surg* 35(10): 897–902.

16. Ilizarov GA. 1989. "The tension-stress effect on the genesis and growth of tissues: Part II. The influence of the rate and frequency of distraction." *Clin Orthop Relat Res* 239: 263–285.

17. Hu J, Tang Z, Wang D, and Buckley MJ. 2001. "Changes in the inferior alveolar nerve after mandibular lengthening with different rates of distraction." *J Oral Maxillofac Surg* 59: 1041–1045; discussion 1046.

18. Thurmüller P, Troulis MJ, Rosenberg A, Chuang SK, and Kaban LB. 2006. "Microscopic changes in the condyle and disc in response to distraction osteogenesis of the minipig mandible." *J Oral Maxillofac Surg* 64(2): 249–258.

19. Cope JB, and Samchukov ML. 2001. "Mineralization dynamics of regenerate bone during mandibular osteodistraction." *Int J Oral Maxillofac Surg* 30: 234–242.

20. Aronson J. 1994. "Temporal and spatial increases in blood flow during distraction osteogenesis." *Clin Orthop Relat Res* 301: 124–131.

21. Saulacic N, Zix J, and Iizuka T. 2009. "Complication rates and associated factors in alveolar distraction osteogenesis: A comprehensive review." *Int J Oral Maxillofac Surg* 38(3): 210–217.

7

Obstructive Sleep Apnea

Peter D. Waite, MPH, DDS, MD
Kenneth C. Guffey, DMD, MD

INTRODUCTION

Obstructive sleep apnea (OSA) is a condition characterized by repetitive partial or complete upper airway obstruction during sleep. It is the result of inspiratory negative pressure overcoming the intrinsic ability of the pharyngeal soft tissues to maintain a patent airway, either through anatomical factors, hypotonic musculature, or a combination of both. This leads to episodes of hypoxia and multiple sleep arousals and subsequent sleep deprivation. As a result, OSA patients often experience reduction in quality of life, poor social function, and neurocognitive underperformance. Depression, fatigue, snoring, personality changes, and poor sexual performance are also frequent symptoms. OSA has also been associated with medical morbidity including obesity, hypertension, cardiovascular disease, stroke, metabolic syndrome, polycythemia, cor pulmonale, cardiac arrhythmias, and even early mortality. It is a highly prevalent disease affecting approximately 20% of adults using a criteria on the apnea hypopnea index (AHI) of AHI ≥5/h, with up to 10% being defined as moderate to severe disease (AHI ≥15/h).[1,2] When symptoms of sleepiness are included as part of the definition, approximately 4% of men and 2% of women meet the criteria.[3,4] Risk factors include obesity, male gender, advancing age, and craniofacial abnormalities such as mandibular insufficiency.

The most common and effective nonsurgical means of treatment for OSA is positive airway pressure (PAP), either continuous (CPAP) or bilevel (BiPAP). It is considered first-line treatment and works by stenting open the upper airway during sleep, thereby reducing apneic events. It has been shown to be highly effective at improving subjective measure such as quality of life and daytime sleepiness, as well as reducing cardiovascular mortality. However, long-term acceptance and adherence is low. Patients often complain of chest discomfort, dry mucous membranes, mask discomfort, congestion, and claustrophobia, among others. Ultimately, more than 50% reject CPAP therapy. Other nonsurgical methods include weight loss, oxygen therapy, pharmacological management, and a variety of oral appliances. Weight loss has been shown to be effective but is seldom sustained. Other methods have had variable results.

Given the poor adherence to CPAP therapy, many seek surgical treatment for correction of their sleep apnea. To be successful, surgery must bypass the obstructed area or prevent its collapse. Tracheostomy was the first surgical treatment for OSA, introduced by Kuhlo and colleagues in 1969.[5] Ikematsu described uvulopalatopharyngoplasty (UPPP) for treatment of snoring in 1964,[6] which was later adapted in the late 1970s for the treatment of sleep apnea. Kuo and colleagues first described mandibular advancement for the treatment of OSA in 1979.[7] Since the early description of these surgical procedures, multiple modifications have been described and new procedures introduced. Each procedure is unique in regard to the level of obstruction it addresses, as well as its potential complications. In addition, these procedures are often combined as part of a multimodality approach, which must be considered, as this will influence the type and incidence of complications.

Management of Complications in Oral and Maxillofacial Surgery, First Edition. Edited by Michael Miloro, Antonia Kolokythas.
© 2012 John Wiley & Sons, Inc. Published 2012 by John Wiley & Sons, Inc.

Full understanding of these potential complications is vital to the success of surgical treatment in the OSA patient as it facilitates not only proper management but anticipation in order to prevent their occurrence. The preoperative, intraoperative, and postoperative periods are all critical time points that can negatively affect surgical success if not managed appropriately. The goal of this chapter is to provide guidance concerning each of these time periods in regard to potential complications and their management, as well as an overview of some of the most common surgical procedures performed today for correction of OSA.

PREOPERATIVE PHASE

Medical History Considerations

Obstructive sleep apnea is associated with a multitude of comorbidities (Table 7.1). A full understanding of these associations and their management is important to the practitioner treating the OSA patient. While many of these associations are well established and have the advantage of strong clinical research that supports their relationship, others remain less clear. Regardless, when performing a thorough history, an awareness of these conditions should alert the surgeon of the possibility of their association and help direct appropriate care.

The initial evaluation of a patient with OSA begins with a history and physical exam, with particular emphasis on certain key elements. A thorough history is critical to the preoperative planning and prevention of surgical complications. Patients should be questioned regarding the severity of their OSA and subjective symptoms such as daytime sleepiness and level of function. Standard questionnaires filled out by the patient prior to the appointment are helpful to assess symptoms and subjective sequelae of their disease. Previous successful and unsuccessful surgical and nonsurgical treatments, including oral appliances and PAP therapy, should be reviewed. Adherence and response to PAP should also be discussed. The patient's bed partner should be included for history of observed apneic events and snoring, and any available laboratory studies including recent sleep studies reviewed. A thorough cardiovascular and pulmonary history should be performed, and any patient with a positive history should be further questioned regarding their current level of function and about any symptoms such as shortness of breath and chest pain. Any recent studies including stress tests and echocardiograms should be requested. Vitals should be obtained and any previously undiagnosed hypertension or other finding should be dealt with prior to surgery. Any concerning findings during the patient history should be considered for further medical workup prior to surgery. This may involve the patient's primary physician, a specialist, or the anesthesia team and will be considered in a subsequent section.

Table 7.1. Comorbidities Associated with OSA

Obesity
Cognitive impairment
Hypertension
Congestive heart failure
Ischemic heart disease
Cardiac arrhythmias
Cerebral vascular accidents
Metabolic syndrome
Diabetes
Pulmonary hypertension
Hypothyroidism
GERD
Depression

Preoperative Consultation and Medical Clearance

Patients with complex medical histories and multiple comorbid conditions should have preoperative evaluation by a primary care physician or appropriate specialist prior to surgery. Hypertension should be adequately controlled before any surgical procedure. Hypertension is often undiagnosed in OSA patients, and it is therefore important to screen patients on evaluation. Poorly controlled blood pressure preoperatively will make hypertension more difficult to manage in the perioperative period. It should be noted that many of these patients can have difficult to treat or treatment-resistant hypertension.[8] Patients with diabetes should have optimization of glucose control prior to surgery. The patient's primary care physician or cardiologist should assess the patient's level of function and provide clearance for surgery in patients with known cardiovascular disease. The patient should be educated about the risks of surgery with full disclosure about how their medical conditions may affect outcome. Any other information concerning medical comorbidities should be managed prior to surgery to optimize outcomes and reduce the risk of surgical complications.

Patients with OSA should also have a preoperative evaluation by an anesthesiologist. Open communication between the anesthesia and surgical teams facilitates appropriate treatment planning. While OSA patients generally are assumed to have more difficult airways, those who present with particularly challenging airways may require a more well-developed plan. Indicators of difficult ventilation and intubation revealed in the physical exam must be communicated and contingency plans discussed. The anesthesiologist should be made aware if more invasive techniques are anticipated such as elective tracheostomy.

Anesthesia Considerations

The next decision involves the selection of the type of anesthesia to be used. Whenever possible, surgical procedures should be performed with local or regional anesthesia. Care should be exercised when conscious sedation is employed in this patient population. American Society of Anesthesiology (ASA) status and comorbid conditions only represent part of the problem when discussing anesthetic risk in OSA patients. Their narrow and easily collapsible airways may be compounded by anesthetic-induced relaxation on the pharyngeal musculature. Surgery on the airway results in varying levels of edema and resultant narrowing. Sleep deprivation secondary to their disease as well as anxiety about the upcoming procedure may result in accidental oversedation. Additionally, if airway obstruction does occur, it is not uncommon to encounter difficulty with ventilation and intubation in these patients. Conscious sedation, therefore, should be used sparingly and only in select nonsevere cases under supervision of a practitioner experienced in airway management. Sedatives should be titrated slowly to effect to avoid oversedation. Deep sedation is rarely indicated due to the risk of airway loss. General anesthesia with a secure airway is preferred over moderate or deep sedation, even in closely monitored situations such as in the operating room.

Preoperative Medications

It is common practice to provide sedatives, anxiolytics, or narcotics prior to transport to the operating room in many surgical centers. These medications serve to alleviate patient anxiety and improve the transition to the operating suite. While safe in most instances, it should be practiced with caution in OSA patients. While the most common agents, benzodiazepines, depress respiratory drive less than most narcotics, the potential for ventilatory compromise in these patients may have serious consequences. Death in the preoperative area has been reported.[9] This practice may be used in certain centers with appropriately trained personnel and well-established protocols including one-on-one supervision and continuous vital sign monitoring. In the absence of these provisions, it is generally best to avoid preoperative sedatives in OSA patients.

Obesity, GERD, and the potential for difficult, prolonged intubation may increase the risk of aspiration in OSA patients. The use of a combination of proton pump inhibitor, H2 blocker, antacid, or esophageal motility stimulant has been advocated to help prevent aspiration on induction. These patients are also at increased risk upon extubation and gastric suctioning is advised at the end of the procedure.

Preoperative CPAP

As mentioned previously, patients are often sleep deprived prior to surgery. This sleep deprivation is a result of OSA-related extreme daytime sleepiness (EDS) and anxiety about the upcoming procedure. After surgery and general anesthesia, the patient is more likely to enter deep sleep and may be predisposed to more severe sleep apnea.[10] The goal of CPAP therapy prior to surgery is to limit the accumulation of sleep debt and reduce deep sleep rebound in the perioperative period. Some recommend the CPAP be worn for 2 weeks prior to any planned surgical procedure.[11] One potential hurdle is that patients who are undergoing surgery for OSA are often CPAP noncompliant. Even modest use before surgery may be beneficial, however, and should be encouraged.[12]

INTRAOPERATIVE PHASE

Airway Management

OSA patients are generally believed to produce more challenging airways and may present difficulty in ventilation and intubation. OSA patients are often obese, male, have increased neck circumference, higher Mallampati scores, and other craniofacial abnormalities that may be associated with a more difficult airway. They may also have excessive, floppy oral and pharyngeal airway tissues, or significant obstructions anywhere along the upper airway. The patients should be evaluated by an anesthesia provider preoperatively and communication with the surgical team should be provided to reduce the incidence of postoperative complications through proper planning. Important physical exam findings that may predict difficult intubation include mouth opening, protrusion of teeth, Mallampati scores, jaw protrusion, mandibular length, neck circumference, and neck length and mobility.

Excess saliva production and aspiration risk should be reduced preoperatively with an antireflux agent and antisialagogue.[13] Before induction, a 3- to 5-minute period of 100% oxygen administration should be employed to maximize oxygen reserves in preparation for a potentially prolonged intubation. The risk of inability to ventilate should always be anticipated, and preoxygenation allows for increased working time for airway establishment. Induction should be accomplished with short-acting intravenous anesthetic such as propofol. Additionally, if a neuromuscular blockade is used, preference should be given to an agent with quick onset and short duration of action, such as succinylcholine. The use of short-acting agents is important in case ventilation and intubation are unsuccessful. Ventilation success begins with proper positioning and preparation for a difficult airway. The patient should be positioned with a head-tilt, chin-lift, or jaw-thrust technique to open the airway. Reverse Trendelenberg position may be used to relieve intrathoracic pressure and improve ventilation. An oropharyngeal or nasopharyngeal airway of appropriate length to extend past the hypopharyngeal obstruction should be used. A two-person ventilation technique may be required in order to provide adequate mask seal and jaw positioning. A laryngeal mask airway (LMA) can also be placed for ventilation and used later to intubate through.[14] LMA allows ventilation while overcoming the soft tissue obstruction and provides a portal for suctioning and intubation. Patients that are unable to be ventilated using these techniques may require more advanced procedures such as percutaneous transtracheal jet ventilation or cricothyrotomy until a definitive airway can be established.

While intubation may be accomplished in a standard fashion with direct laryngoscopy, alternative methods are available and are frequently utilized (Table 7.2). The selection of one particular method

Table 7.2. Techniques for Difficult Intubation

Awake oral or nasal traditional intubation

Blind nasal intubation

Intubating LMA

Awake or asleep fiberoptic intubation

Retrograde intubation

Light wand technique

Video laryngoscope

Transnasal jet ventilation assisted fiberoptic intubation

often depends on preoperative exam findings and the anticipation of a difficult airway. Options for intubation include awake oral or nasal, awake or asleep fiberoptic, and intubation through an LMA. Newer techniques include utilization of a light wand or video laryngoscopy and are growing in popularity. Awake procedures may be preferred in the incidence of preoperative exam findings consistent with difficult intubation. Boyce and colleagues described the use of transnasal jet ventilation-assisted fiberoptic intubation. In this technique, a transnasal jet is used through a nasopharyngeal airway to provide intermittent flow of pressurized air to the upper airway. The purported advantages are improved visualization and simultaneous ventilation of the patient during fiberoptic intubation. They reported no incidences of serious complications and high intubation success rates.[15,16] In their prospective study of 180 morbidly obese patients undergoing bariatric surgery, Neligan and colleagues used direct laryngoscopy after standard induction with the patient in the "ramped" position, with the head and shoulders above the chest. The incidence of OSA in this population was 68%. They found this technique to be very successful and had no incidences of rescue airway use. The difficult intubation rate was only 3.3% (defined as three or more intubation attempts). Interestingly, they found no relationship between body mass index (BMI), neck circumference, or presence of OSA and the difficulty of intubation. They did note male gender and higher Mallampati scores to be predictive, however.[17] Finally, in select cases of patients with severe disease and significant medical comorbidity, such as life-threatening arrhythmia, and failed intubation attempts, an elective tracheostomy may be considered. The surgeon may also be required to perform a tracheostomy or cricothyrotomy emergently if the patient cannot be ventilated.

Extubation is best performed in the operating room in a controlled setting. The patient should be extubated awake, once spontaneous ventilation, the ability to follow commands, and ability to sustain a head lift have returned. Full reversal of neuromuscular blockade should be verified. In patients who were easy to ventilate prior to intubation whose surgery did not affect the airway, deep extubation may be considered. It is advised to allow the patient to awake sufficiently as is needed to protect their airway and avoid suspending extubation until the patient is in the recovery room or ICU. This practice will hopefully minimize complications secondary to airway compromise.

Blood Pressure Control

Hypotensive anesthesia, particularly during maxillary osteotomies, may be used to help control blood loss. This may be difficult to achieve intraoperatively if adequate control has not been obtained prior to the procedure. This underscores the importance of appropriate management and consultation preoperatively. The need for hypotensive anesthesia, however, must be weighed against the risk of inadequate organ perfusion. In patients at risk for ischemic heart disease or stroke, hypotensive anesthesia may need to be abandoned to reduce surgical events.

The proper application of the technique involves communication between the anesthesia and surgical team. The anesthesia team must be given adequate time prior to the osteotomy to safely lower the blood pressure in a slow, controlled fashion to minimize the risk of an unsafe drop and inadequate perfusion. In addition, blood pressure should be allowed to return to normal as soon as possible. This will allow minimum time under hypotensive anesthesia and hopefully reduce cardiovascular or neurologic complications. In patients felt to be inadequate to withstand anesthesia-induced hypotension, preparations should be made and the patient educated about the possibility of blood transfusion.

Additional Considerations

Proper patient positioning and adequate padding are important to reduce pressure ischemia. Obesity, long procedures, and hypotensive anesthesia can all potentially exacerbate its occurrence and must be taken into consideration. Both steroids and the judicious use of intravenous fluids intraoperatively may help reduce the risk of airway edema and respiratory compromise. Additionally, narcotics should be used sparingly whenever possible in this patient population during the procedure. When needed, it is better to use shorter-acting agents. Postoperatively, the cumulative effect of excessive narcotic administration may contribute to respiratory compromise.

SURGICAL PROCEDURES

After diagnostic evaluation of the OSA patient and identification of the level of obstruction, a surgical procedure must be selected. Surgical treatment of OSA involves a variety of procedures that address the obstruction at multiple levels. Properly matching the type of obstruction to the procedure is paramount to success. The nasal cavity, nasopharynx, oropharynx, and hypopharyx are all potential sites of obstruction that may contribute to the pathogenesis of OSA. Surgical procedures for OSA can be classified by the types of structures being modified (soft tissue, hard tissue, or both) or by anatomical location (nasal airway, nasopharynx, oropharynx, hypopharynx, or a combination) (Table 7.3). As mentioned previously, there have been many procedures described for the treatment of OSA. It is important that any practitioner performing these procedures be well educated on the potential complications. For those procedures not described here, they have been extensively covered in other texts. The following is a review of the most common procedures used to treat OSA by anatomic location, and a discussion of associated complications and their management.

Nasal Cavity

The role of nasal obstruction in OSA is different from that which occurs at other levels. It does not cause the primary obstruction central to the pathology of sleep apnea, but may contribute to the disease process. Increased resistance to nasal airflow can lead to turbulent flow and increase the incidence of mouth breathing. Oral breathing alters upper airway dynamics and can predispose to obstruction. Obstruction can occur by a variety of mechanisms including septal deviation, turbinate hypertrophy, polyps, and valve collapse.

Surgical procedures directed at the cause of the obstruction include septoplasty, turbinate reduction, polypectomy, and valve reconstruction. They are generally not curative but may improve AHI and CPAP pressure requirements. They have also been linked to improvement in subjective outcomes such as daytime energy levels.[18] It is often performed as part of a multimodality approach as opposed to a stand-alone procedure for the treatment of sleep apnea.

Deviation of the nasal septum may cause obstruction along any portion, and it is important to identify the area responsible prior to surgery. High deflections may mimic a weak or collapsed internal nasal valve and should be treated appropriately.[19] Septal hematoma is a potential complication and can be minimized with the use of septal splints for 1 week or mattress sutures. Mattress suturing through the mucosa and septum is accomplished with 4-0 chromic gut suture on a straight needle. Mucosal tears may be observed

Table 7.3. Location of Upper Airway Obstruction and Common Surgical Procedures

Anatomic Location of Obstruction	Tissue Type	Procedure
Nasal	Soft	Turbinectomy, polypectomy
	Hard	Septoplasty, alar base reconstruction, nasal valve reconstruction
Oropharyngeal	Soft	Tonsillectomy, UPPP, LAUP, radio-frequency palate tissue reduction (somnoplasty), Pillar palatal implants, transpalatal advancement, pharyngoplasty
	Hard/soft	Maxillary expansion, maxillary advancement
Hypopharyngeal	Soft	Glossectomy, radio-frequency tongue base ablation, mandibular distraction
	Hard/soft	Genioglossus advancement, hyoid advancement
Oropharyngeal and hypopharyngeal	Hard/soft	MMA
Bypass procedures		Tracheostomy

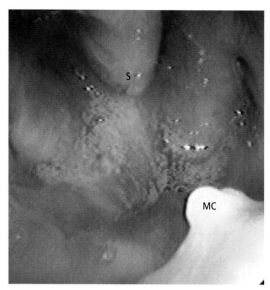

Fig. 7.1. Septal defects after MMA. Perforations of the posterior septum are incidental findings by nasopharyngoscopy. Septoplasty combined with Le Fort I osteotomy often causes asymptomatic septal defects. S: septum, MC: maxillary crest.

if they occur on one side of the mucosa. For through-and-through tears, closure of at least one side with 5-0 chromic gut should be completed. Often, septoplasty is performed simultaneously with maxillary advancement. The amount of removal varies and may range from minor trimming when the septum is straight but subject to deflection with movement of the maxilla, to formal septoplasty when concomitant septal deviation contributes to the obstruction. During postoperative nasopharyngolaryngoscopy, it is common to encounter a defect in the posterior portion of the septum after maxillomandibular advancement (MMA) with combined septoplasty (Fig. 7.1). It should be noted that this is often of little clinical consequence, and should require no intervention. As long as an anterior septal strut is maintained, changes in the nasal morphology such as nasal tip deprojection should not occur.

Turbinate hypertrophy may be addressed with a variety of techniques. Submucosal radiofrequency and electrocautery turbinate reduction, laser turbinate excision, partial or total inferior turbinate removal, turbinate outfracture, and submocosal turbinoplasty are all frequently employed methods. Postoperative bleeding, tissue edema and subsequent worsening of obstructive symptoms, atrophic rhinitis, and nasal crusting are all potential complications. Rhinitis sicca (excessive dryness) may occur and lead to additional crusting and bleeding. It should be noted that opening of the nasal passages may lead to worsening of this condition if presented preoperatively. The use of submucosal techniques may decrease crusting and maintain ciliary function. Radiofrequency submucosal reduction has the advantage of producing little edema and does not generally require nasal packing. It takes 8 weeks to produce maximum effect, however, and multiple procedures may be required to achieve optimal result. For any nasal surgery, nasal packing should generally be avoided, as obstruction can worsen in the postoperative period. Nasal stents or tubes that allow patency of the airway are.[19]

Oropharynx

Tonsillectomy

Adenotonsillectomy is the procedure of choice for OSA in children, and tonsillectomy may be useful in the treatment of adult patients with enlarged tonsils and without other major airway abnormalities.[20] A meta-analysis of pediatric patients with uncomplicated disease revealed a reduction in AHI of 13.9 events per hour and normalization of AHI in 80% of patients.[21] Outcomes are affected by upper airway anatomy, nasal inflammatory disease, obesity, and general medical condition. Pain, swelling, and bleeding are the most common complications. Electrocautery and ultrasonic blades have been used to reduce bleeding but are still associated with postoperative pain. Other methods include the use of serial reduction with a carbon-dioxide laser in the outpatient setting aimed at reducing postoperative pain and bleeding, though this has been associated with tissue regrowth and recurrent infection.[22] Radiofrequency ablation may be performed in a single setting or serially and has been associated with decreased pain, but some have expressed concern with increased chance of hemorrhage. Life-threatening complications are rare, but postoperative respiratory failure requiring mechanical ventilation can occur in up to 30% of children.[23,24]

Palatal Procedures

UPPP is a common surgical procedure designed to reduce obstruction by selective removal of pharyngeal tissue to enlarge the oropharyngeal airway lumen. It was first described as a technique to treat snoring,[6] and later adapted by Fujita and colleagues for the correction of sleep apnea.[25] Generally it involves the removal of redundant tissues of the soft palate, tonsils, tonsillar pillars, and uvula. Since it was initially described, many technical variations have been proposed. Despite variations in technique, the ultimate goal is to widen the posterior airway space. Despite reports of low success rates of 40–60% and cure rate (defined as an AHI of <5%) of 16% in several meta-analyses, it remains the most widely performed OSA pharyngeal surgical procedure today.[26] Evaluation of candidates for the procedure has evolved, and thus development of more sophisticated methods has led to improved results. The Friedman staging system of the oropharyngeal airway is based on the tonsil size, a modified Mallampati classification, presence or absence of severe obesity, and craniofacial abnormalities. It helps identify patients at risk for sleep apnea who present with snoring symptoms and also has positive and negative predictive values for UPPP. Higher success rates for Friedman stage I have been demonstrated over stage III for palatal surgery alone. Performance of UPPP blindly without proper identification of the level of obstruction has likely contributed, historically, to poor success.

Complications are common and include bleeding, severe pain, dysphagia, pharyngeal discomfort, mucosal dryness, wound infections, and taste and speech disturbances. Dysphagia can be persistent in up to 30%, though it is generally mild. Major complications are rare and include velopharyngeal insufficiency, acute respiratory distress, nasopharyngeal stenosis, and hemorrhage. As previously discussed, early reports indicated high frequency complications associated with UPPP, including serious events such as respiratory compromise and death.[9,27] More recent reports, however demonstrate a trend towards lower rates.[28] One systematic review reported serious complications with an incidence of 2.5% (with 0.2% mortality). However, persistent side effects were high at 58% (31% nasal regurgitation, 13% voice changes, and 5% taste disturbances).[29] Complications such as dysphagia, discomfort, and pain may be difficult to avoid. Management generally involves proper patient education and expectant management. Care should be taken in administration of postoperative narcotics and strategies to minimize their use. This is particularly important after upper airway procedures where the potential for respiratory compromise exists secondary to pharyngeal edema. The use of steroids, tissue coolants, and blood pressure control also may decrease edema and will be discussed later. The patient should also be properly informed about the risk of failure and possibility for additional procedures. The majority of avoidable complications, however, are due to aggressive tissue removal. Management generally involves judicious excision followed by meticulous tissue rearrangement and closure.[30] Additionally, nasal CPAP tolerance may be decreased due to mouth leak from excessive tissue removal, further justifying the need for conservative surgery.

Generally performed in the office under local anesthesia, laser-assisted uvulopalatoplasty (LAUP) involves the partial removal of the palate and uvula via laser. Usually indicated for the treatment of snoring, its utilization for surgical management of sleep apnea is controversial. Two randomized clinical trials found no change in the AHI after surgery when used as a treatment for OSA.[31,32] Additionally, other concerns include studies that have suggested no statistical significance in daytime sleepiness, and possible worsening of OSA after undergoing the procedure.[26] Complications are similar to those for UPPP, and include severe pain, bleeding, infection, globus sensation, velopharyngeal insufficiency (VPI), and taste changes. Globus sensation may require a secondary procedure to break up scar banding. Staged or "titrated" surgeries with reevaluation prior to each step reduce occurrence of VPI.[20]

Hypopharynx

Soft tissue procedures

Glossectomy

Designed to eliminate hypopharyngeal obstruction, midline glossectomy and linguoplasty are partial glossectomies performed usually via laser. Surgical success rates have been reported from 25% to 83%, with an average of approximately 50%.[33] Complications approach 25% and include bleeding, severe odynophagia, tongue edema, and taste changes. Due to morbidity and poor success of the procedure, glossectomy has been relegated to a limited population of patients who are not candidates for other procedures. Additionally, historically perioperative tracheostomies were often performed due to risk of postoperative airway obstruction resulting in high morbidity.[20]

Radiofrequency Ablation of the Tongue Base

Radiofrequency ablation of the tongue base is often performed in the office setting under local anesthesia. It may be either performed as a single-modality treatment or often in conjunction with other airway procedures. Randomized controlled studies have demonstrated effectiveness of the procedure in reducing OSA severity and improving quality of life. This has also been demonstrated in the long term. Complications include abscess, tongue base weakness, alteration of speech and swallowing, cellulitis, and airway obstruction and edema. Fortunately, these complications are rare.[20] Mucosal ulcerations can be avoided by not placing the electrodes too superficially. Abscesses and infections can be reduced with preoperative antibiotics, but may require surgical drainage. The middle third of the tongue should be treated to avoid the major branches of the hypoglossal nerve, which may result in tongue paralysis. By this same reasoning, avoiding the lateral neurovascular bundles by central electrode placement may prevent significant postoperative bleeding.[34]

Skeletal/Soft Tissue

Hyoid Advancement

Hyoid myotomy and advancement is designed to enlarge the hypopharyngeal space by advancement of retrolingual soft tissues.[35] The hyoid is isolated, and transection of the infrahyoid muscles is performed to allow advancement and fixation anteriorly. Suspension to the mandible and thyroid cartilage has been described. It is often performed in conjunction with other airway procedures such as genioglossus advancement or UPPP. Results have been varied, and a review of four studies documenting results with hyoid suspension alone has shown they demonstrated success rates of only approximately 50%. This only marginally improved with the addition of genioglossus advancement.[33] Careful transecton of the infrahyoid muscles while staying on the hyoid bone must be performed to avoid injury to the superior laryngeal nerves. Severe aspiration has been reported secondary to transection of the thyrohyoid membrane. One author advocates the use of suspension to the superior thyroid cartilage and reports complications as minor in nature and include seroma, transient aspiration, and relapse. Major complications are rarely reported. They suggest placement of surgical drains for prevention of seroma formation. Additionally, they advocate placement of multiple sutures between the thyroid cartilage and hyoid to reduce relapse secondary to suture destabilization. Aspiration and dysphagia are usually transient and should resolve in approximately 10 days. Significant persistent dysphagia can be managed with removal of suspension sutures.[30]

Genioglossus Advancement

Genioglossus muscle advancement is a technique used to open the retrolingual space by advancement of the genial tubercle. Genial tubercle advancement (GTA) is accomplished with an anterior rectangular mandibular osteotomy that incorporates the genial tubercle, and the bony fragment with attached muscle is advanced and stabilized. Superior and posterior bone struts remain, and as the chin point is not changed, the aesthetic impact is minimal. Standard, mortised, and circle genioplasty have been described (Fig. 7.2).

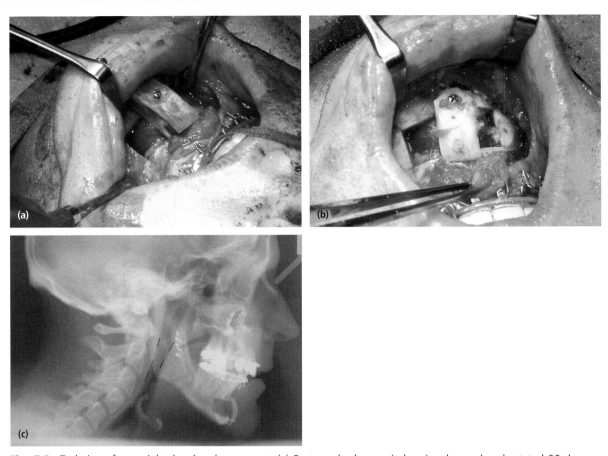

Fig. 7.2. Technique for genial tubercle advancement. (a) Rectangular bone window is advanced and rotated 90 degrees to prevent posterior movement. The screw is used for holding the segment while it is advanced. (b) The outer cortex is removed to reduce the profile of the segment. The first screw is removed and a securing screw is placed in the inferior strut of bone. (c) Lateral cephalogram demonstrates the advanced segment.

Table 7.4. Complications of Genial Tubercle Advancement

Dehiscence
Bone necrosis
Infection
Tooth root damage
Fracture
Parasthesia
Hematoma
Chin ptosis
Failure to incorporate muscle
Genioglossus muscle avulsion

It is often performed as a multimodality approach in conjunction with other procedures. As a sole procedure, success rates have been reported at 38–78% (average 67%).[33]

Complications are usually minor (Table 7.4). Poor osteotomy design is responsible for most of the complications associated with this procedure. Understanding the surgical anatomy is paramount. Damage to the roots of the teeth or devitalization can occur and may require extraction or endodontic therapy. The design of the osteotomy must allow adequate room between the roots of the teeth and superior portion of the osteotomy (usually 5 mm). Failure to incorporate the genioglossus muscle in the osteotomy design can also occur. This can be prevented by careful palpation of the genioglossus prior to osteotomies and evaluation of preoperative radiographs. Genioglossus muscle avulsion can occur if a robust segment of muscle is not incorporated in the segment or if too much traction is placed. Failure to incorporate the muscle into the bony segment or muscle avulsion may result in an unusable segment. The muscle may be salvaged, however, by using a strong, slowly resorbable suture such as a 2-0 Vicryl, and securing it to the fixation plate or to the bone through an osteotomy created with a surgical drill. Placing the osteotomy too inferiorly can lead to a small strut of inferior border bone that may fracture. In addition, small remaining bone struts superiorly and inferiorly to the osteotomy can weaken the mandible and may result in a symphyseal or parasymphyseal fracture. Fracture may require open reduction and internal fixation or a short period of maxillomandibular fixation (MMF).

Excessive bleeding and postoperative hematoma formation are also a concern in these patients. Carefully performing the osteotomy without excessive extension past the lingual cortical plate can help minimize lingual tissue damage and excessive bleeding. Despite proper technique, however, damage to small vessels and the lingual muscular bed can occur. This can be exacerbated by the high concordance of hypertension in OSA patients. Therefore, meticulous hemostasis, careful clinical monitoring for hematoma formation postoperatively, and aggressive hypertension management are all indicated.[30] The occurrence of postoperative hematoma formation must be monitored closely in this subset of patients for potential airway compromise. Nasal CPAP or intubation may be indicated.

In patients who would benefit aesthetically from chin advancement, a high geniotomy with advancement is the procedure of choice. One advantage to this technique over GTA, aside from the impact on facial aesthetics, is that the digastric muscles are incorporated in the advanced segment, resulting in anterior repositioning of the hyoid and associated hypopharyngeal tissues. Complications are similar to GTA, with a few special considerations (Table 7.5). Care should be taken in the osteotomy design, as without the benefit of an inferior strut of bone, the superior portion will provide the entirety of the support. Placing the central portion of the osteotomy too high will make the mandible weak and may damage teeth. When accomplished as part of a stage I protocol, the risk of fracture increases as the structurally weak parasymphysis may not withstand the strong rotational forces of an unoperated ramus. This situation is much different when performed simultaneously with routine orthognathic surgery or MMA where ramus osteotomies are performed. The authors use prebent titanium plates to provide strength and allow for maximum, predictable advancement to the segment (Fig. 7.3). These are the same plates the authors use in the maxilla, which will be discussed further in the section on maxillomandibular advancement.

Table 7.5. Complications of Geniotomy Advancement

Dehiscence

Bone necrosis

Infection

Tooth root damage

Parasymphysis fracture

Parasthesia

Hematoma

Chin ptosis

Failure to incorporate muscle

Poor facial aesthetic results

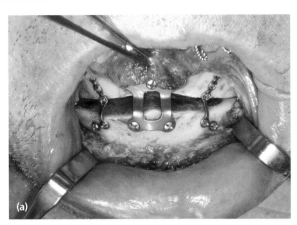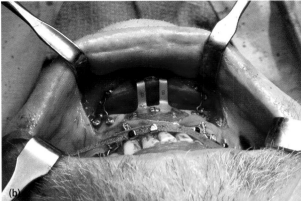

Fig. 7.3. Prebent advancement plate for sliding genioplasty.

Oropharynx and Hypopharyx

Maxillomandibular Advancement

Maxillomandibular advancement (MMA) involves a maxillary Le Fort I osteotomy and bilateral sagittal split osteotomy (BSSO) of the mandible with advancement. It enlarges the pharyngeal space by expanding the skeletal framework and associated attached oropharyngeal and hypopharygeal soft tissues. By placing tension on the soft tissue, it also reduces their collapsibility during negative pressure inspiration. MMA is widely considered as the most effective surgical method for treatment of sleep apnea, apart from tracheostomy. A systematic review and meta-analysis by Holty and Guilleminault demonstrated a success rate of 86% defined as AHI <20/h and ≥50% reduction in AHI post surgery. Additionally, a cure rate of 43.2%, defined as AHI ≤5%, was found.[36] Also demonstrated was long-term stability of the results with surgical success rates of 89% and no difference between short- and long-term AHI.

Controversy exists regarding the timing of MMA. One popular protocol is a staged approach to therapy. In this method, patients diagnosed with OSA undergo a phase I therapy consisting of UPPP and possibly adjunctive procedures such as genioglossus advancement. MMA is considered as a phase II surgery if phase I fails. Part of the rationale behind the staging is the assumed morbidity and the view of MMA as an aggressive procedure when compared to phase I surgeries. Another contributing factor is the initial referral pattern of some institutions to surgeons who may be adept at phase I surgeries, but not be trained to perform MMA. The dissatisfaction with poor success rates and associated morbidity for UPPP and other procedures, coupled with the high success rates of MMA, has lead some practitioners to offer MMA as the initial procedure of choice, depending on the level of obstruction. One advantage of MMA over other procedures is the addressing of the obstruction at multiple levels from the nasal passages to the hypopharynx. It is important to consider the staging of these procedures because the complication pattern differs between those who had previous phase I surgery and those for whom MMA was the only surgical procedure to address their sleep apnea.

In the meta-analysis previously mentioned, major complications were rare and consisted of two cardiac arrests, one dysrhythmia, and one mandible fracture. Most complications were minor and included malocclusion, paresthesia, infection, and minor hemorrhage. However, nonunion, VPI, hardware failure, unacceptable aesthetic changes, significant relapse, and vascular compromise are all potential untoward events associated with this procedure that must be recognized and managed appropriately (Table 7.6). When excluding parasthesia and malocclusion, minor complications occur at an incidence of approximately 3%.[36]

Parasthesia of the inferior alveolar nerve is the most common complication following MMA. Transient neurosensory disturbance can be found in up to 100% of patients, though 86% resolve in 1 year.[36,37] It is important that slow, controlled split of the mandible with adequate visualization of the nerve be

Table 7.6. MMA Complications

Parethesia
Infection
Malocclusion
Hardware failure
Bleeding
Vascular compromise
Relapse
Malunion/nonunion
Fracture
VPI
Unacceptable aesthetic changes
Respiratory compromise

undertaken to minimize trauma. The nerve should then be adequately freed from its bony canal with an elevator or rotary instrument. Minimizing surgical trauma is especially important in this patient population as most OSA patients are middle-aged or older, and their ability to recover from injury diminished. Despite careful dissection, manipulation and stretch on the nerve will often result in transient paresthesia in almost all cases. It is therefore important to discuss this with patients prior to surgery, as it is not likely to be avoided. Given the high satisfaction rates with the surgery, this consequence is acceptable to most patients. Despite adequate education, however, some patients will be dissatisfied with this outcome. In these cases routine nerve injury protocol may be considered.

In addition to inferior alveolar nerve paresthesia, injury to the lingual nerve may occur as well, and with a large mandibular advancement, the chance of spontaneous recovery is significantly diminished. This is due to the increased distance between the proximal and distal nerve stumps with a transection injury, or significant traction that can be placed on the lingual nerve with advancement of the distal segment of the mandible. If microneurosurgical intervention is warranted in nonresolving cases of paresthesia, most likely a significant nerve gap will be encountered that will require consideration for nerve grafting (autogenous or allogeneic) or conduit repair.

Malocclusion has a variable reported incidence, though it is reasonable to assume that minor occlusal discrepancies are fairly common. It can be potentially increased in this population by a variety of patient- and procedure-related factors, when compared to traditional orthognathic surgery. Skeletal relapse can lead to malocclusion and is a concern due to the large amount of advancement that places tension on oral and pharyngeal tissues as well as the hardware. Also, the higher incidence of obesity may place additional forces on fixation devices that may change the end-treatment position of the maxilla and mandible. Patient non-compliance and early excessive loading may also contribute to poor occlusal relationship. Often, these patients are managed without preoperative orthodontics so it is prudent to establish ideal occlusion from the outset, since small orthodontic movements will not be available to correct minor discrepancies post-operatively. Most malocclusions, when they do occur, are mild. Waite and colleagues reported 44% incidence of premature contacts that were all treated with equilibration and prosthetics.[38,39] In a large series of 175 patients, Li and colleagues reported no major malocclusions, and all cases were managed by dental adjustments.[37] No incidence was reported in this study. In cases of major discrepancy not amenable to occlusal adjustment, a surgical revision may be considered (Fig. 7.4). Early recognition and correction is important in these cases to avoid the increased difficulty associated with late revision after bony healing has occurred. For some patients, postoperative orthodontics should be considered, particularly in those who are not candidates for a second surgery and who cannot be corrected by equilibration or prosthetic rehabilitation.

The rate of infection after orthognathic surgery has been reported to range from 1% to 33%,[40] though it is generally considered lower with contemporary antibiotic use. Orthognathic surgery is a clean

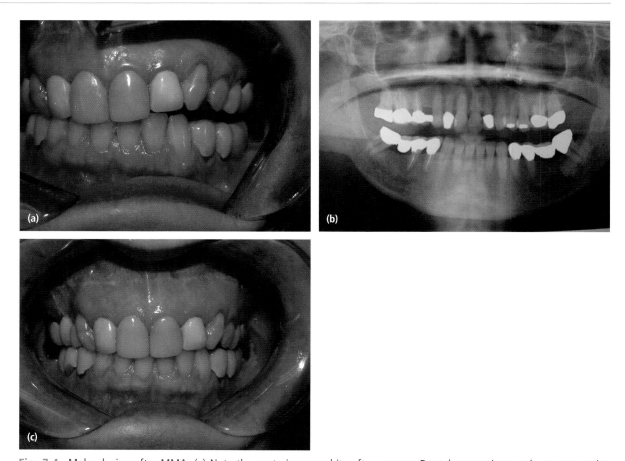

Fig. 7.4. Malocclusion after MMA. (a) Note the posterior open bite after surgery. Dental restorations make postoperative orthodontics difficult, and the patient did not want replacement of her existing prosthesis. This patient was treated with a surgical revision. (b) Postoperative radiograph after Le Fort I osteotomy for correction of her malocclusion. (c) Postoperative occlusion.

contaminated procedure, and thus an inherent risk of infection is accepted. Factors that may influence these rates include age of the patient, length of surgery, type of procedure, and method of antibiotic prophylaxis. Increased age and longer procedures have been associated with increased risk of infection and plate removal.[41] The use of prophylactic antibiotics in the prevention of surgical site infections is widely accepted. Debate exists, however, regarding the type and duration of prophylaxis that should be used. Most consider a minimum of preoperative administration to be standard of care, and studies have shown an increased incidence of infection in orthognathic surgery patients when antibiotics are withheld.[42] When discussing the duration of antibiotic administration, however, conflicting reports have made a consensus difficult to establish. While many advocate short-term antibiotics involving single or multiple perioperative doses, others support extending prophylaxis for 5–7 days postoperatively. Several reports have indicated no difference in infection rates when short-term dosing schedules are compared to extended protocols.[43–47] Interestingly, several of these reports did indicate increased infection rates in the short-term group, though no statistical significance was reached.[43,44,47] Additionally, one of these studies demonstrated statistically significant higher morbidity scores and degree of swelling with short-term administration.[43] In a randomized, double-blind clinical trial comparing 1- and 5-day prophylaxis regimens, Bently and colleagues demonstrated significantly higher infection rates in the short-term group (6.7% vs. 60%).[48] A retrospective review of 1,294 orthognathic surgery patients by Chow and colleagues found similar results.[40]

In regard to prevention of infection, the authors advocate a conservative approach. We routinely use preoperative antibiotics, followed by a 5- to 7-day postoperative course. While the literature is insufficient to support a single protocol, we feel it is necessary to provide the best possible chance of avoiding this complication. Postoperative infection can lead to considerable morbidity including pain, swelling, non-union, and malocclusion, and may require the removal of hardware. In addition, OSA patients have multiple factors that may increase the risk of infection when compared to traditional orthognathic patients, in whom the majority of infection studies have been performed. They are older, often require longer procedures, and may be immunocompromised secondary to their medical condition or medications. Their medical comorbidities may make the clinical sequelae or procedures required in the management of postoperative infections undesirable. In the event that a postoperative infection presents, similar conservative management is recommended. Simple infections may be managed by local measures including opening the wound and possible drain placement. Antibiotics should be extended and close monitoring is warranted. Removal of hardware should be avoided until bony healing across the osteotomy has occurred. Keep in mind that this may be delayed in the presence of infection. In the incidence of chronic or recurrent infection requiring long-term antibiotic administration, waiting 4–6 months before plate removal may allow for stability of the fragments to occur. Cases of early infection that are poorly controlled with local measures and antibiotics, however, may require hardware removal. If this is required prior to healing, stabilization can be achieved with alternative methods. For the mandible, the patient should be placed in MMF if adequate dentition exists and reduction of the segments is achieved. This is not advised for maxillary infections requiring plate removal, as the pull of the mandible may increase the osteotomy gap, resulting in change in the maxillary position and nonunion. For these cases, wiring to a stable buttress such as the zygoma or piriform may be used. The dentition or a maxillary splint can serve as a second point of fixation. External fixation is another option and is most often used in the mandible. Hopefully, utilizing one of these methods will allow for proper union and circumvent the need for a secondary revision procedure.

The correction of sleep apnea generally requires a larger advancement than traditional orthognathic movements. Most advocate at least 10 mm of mandibular advancement to maximize airway expansion. This can place considerable strain on internal fixation, particularly when traditional methods are used, resulting in fixation failure and nonunion or malunion. While traditional BSSO advancement may be successfully managed in many cases with minimal fixation, such as a single superior border non-load-bearing plate, often increased support is needed in these patients. One must also keep in mind that many of these patients are obese, which may call for stronger fixation as a factor independent of the amount of advancement. In the mandible, some advocate the use of miniplates along with bicortical screws, whereas others may use multiple bicortical screws alone or even skeletal suspension wires with a short course of MMF. Other methods may include the use of two miniplates or single 2-mm titanium plate for increased stability (Figs. 7.5, 7.6, and 7.7). The size of the advancement may alter the internal fixation protocol in other ways.

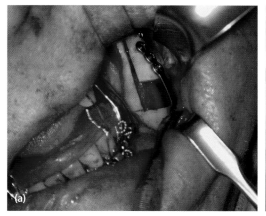 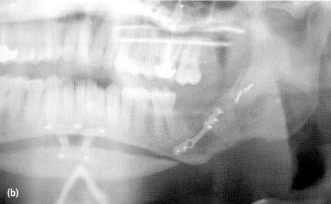

Fig. 7.5. Plating the mandible. (a) A mandibular plate spanning the large gap is augmented by the use of bicortical screws posteriorly. (b) Panoramic image showing the use of two bicortical screws posterior to the osteotomy.

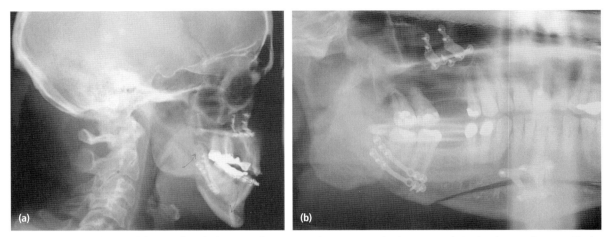

Fig. 7.6. <u>Fixation failure.</u> (a) Lateral cephalogram of a patient after MMA with placement of single plate at the mandibular osteotomy. Note the proximal segment rotation and anterior open bite. (b) In OSA patients and large mandibular advancements, standard orthognathic plating systems may not provide adequate fixation. In this case two strong monocortical plates are used per side.

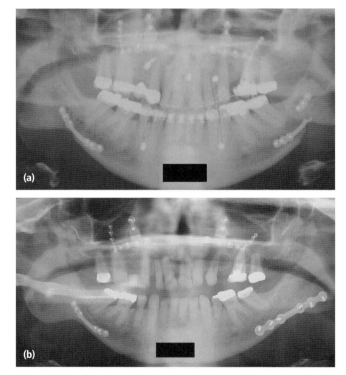

Fig. 7.7. <u>Plate fracture.</u> (a) After MMA, placement of a routine monocortical plate resulted in fracture. Note the superior rotation of the proximal segment. (b) After hardware removal, the left mandibular malunion was corrected by realigning the proximal segment and placement of a stronger plate.

While standard plates for orthognathic surgery have been developed, with the amount of advancement required for MMA for OSA management, longer plates may have to be selected. It is important to remember, however, that as the length of the plate increases, its ability to withstand bite forces decreases, and additional fixation may be required. Bicortical screws, while frequently used in orthognathic surgery, may be difficult to place or inadequate for fixation. As the amount of advancement increases, the amount of

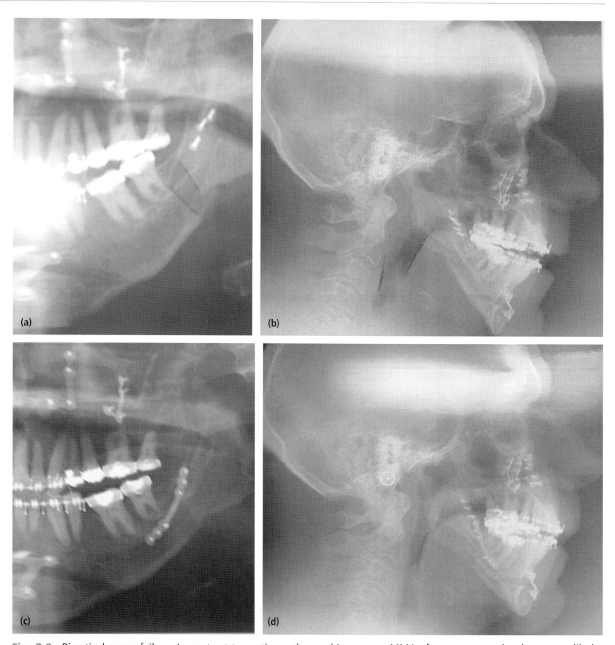

Fig. 7.8. Bicortical screw failure. In contrast to routine orthognathic surgery, MMA often creates such a large mandibular advancement with minimal bone apposition that standard bicortical screw fixation above and below the nerve is not possible. (a) Two weeks post-op proximal segment rotation and poor bony alignment is noted on panoramic X-ray. (b) Lateral cephalogram demonstrating anterior open bite. (c) Left side bicortical screws replaced with plate with realignment of the segments. Though poor alignment of the right side was also noted, the segments were stable. (d) Lateral cephalogram demonstrating satisfactory occlusion.

bony overlap decreases. Also, since the mandible is shaped like a "V," with its widest portion posterior, as the distal segment is advanced the width of the mandible between the two proximal segments increases. This may result in pushing of the proximal segments laterally with decreased bony adaptation (Fig. 7.8). This may be overcome by recontouring of the segments with a rotary instrument. In situations where this is not successful, additional methods of fixation may have to be used.

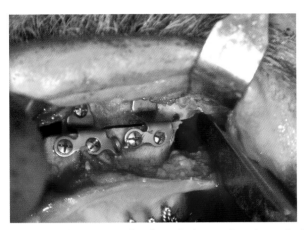

Fig. 7.9. Maxillary prebent plates. These plates are easily adapted. The number "8" marked on the superior portion of the plate may be visible, which indicates the amount of advancement in millimeters.

In the maxilla, four 2-mm L-shaped plates are commonly used.[49] The authors advocate the use of 2-mm prebent maxillary advancement plates. They are available in different sizes depending on the amount of advancement needed and require minimal manipulation for adaptation. The decrease in the amount of bending required reduces weakening of the hardware, and presumably helps maintain strength under cyclical loading. An additional advantage is that these plates provide accurate advancement while eliminating the need for measurements and thus reducing operative time (Fig. 7.9). This method has shown good initial results.[50]

For reasons previously mentioned, namely the excess external forces on the advanced maxillomandibular apparatus and the amount of advancement, skeletal relapse is another concern in these patients. This may adversely affect the postoperative occlusion, but in itself has not been shown to adversely affect treatment outcomes. A 10–20% surgical relapse has been documented in up to 15% of patients after MMA; however, no apparent increase in AHI or subjective worsening of symptoms has occurred.[37,51,52] Additionally, surgical relapse has not been shown to correlate with the amount of mandibular advancement.[51] In a study by Louis and colleagues, the amount of maxillary advancement also did not correlate with long-term skeletal relapse. Though a small increase in relapse was observed in the large advancement group (1.9 ± 1.8 mm in those advanced 12.3 ± 2.8 mm), it did not achieve statistical significance.[53] No studies are known to the authors comparing fixation techniques for the maxilla and mandible for MMA, so considerable variation is assumed between surgeons. Additionally, modifications in surgical technique exist, including step designs for the maxillary osteotomy to enhance bony interface and long-term stability.[49] Regardless of technique, major skeletal relapse with recurrence of symptomatic OSA, though rare, should be considered for a reoperation. In these patients, alteration of the previous technique and addition of increased fixation or even a period of MMF should be used. Relapse without recurrence of clinically significant OSA may be managed by observation.

Nonunion is a potential complication with any orthognathic surgical procedure. Controversy exists regarding the use of bone grafting, particularly in the maxillary advancement. It generally results in contact only in the piriform aperture and zygomatic buttresses, producing a large gap in the lateral wall. Bone harvested from the chin, ramus, iliac crest, or any autogenous site may be used. Disadvantages include the increased operative time and donor site morbidity. For this reason, many advocate modified steps and strong fixation techniques to maximize bony interface and maxillary stability, obviating the need for bone grafts. In a review of 131 patients treated without bone grafting, only 4 (3%) developed nonunion that required iliac crest bone grafting as a second procedure.[49,54,55] In our opinion, patients with large gaps are managed best by cadaveric tibial bone graft shaped to mortise into the lateral wall defect. The wedge effect also presumably adds to maxillary stability. A single screw can be used to secure the graft if adequate wedging is not obtained (Figs. 7.10 and 7.11). There have been no known incidences of nonunion, though a comprehensive review has not been undertaken. Advantages include lack of donor site morbidity and

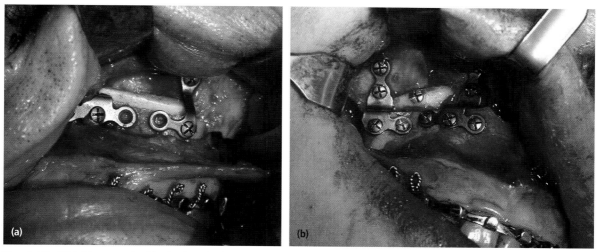

Fig. 7.10. Tibial bone graft. (a) Tibial graft shaped and set into the lateral wall defect. The wedge effect provides stability and prevents dislodgement. (b) In cases where adequate wedge is not achieved, a single screw can be used to enhance stability.

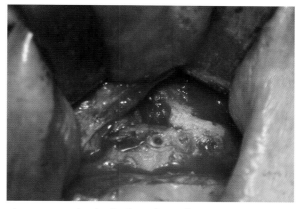

Fig. 7.11. Osseus union. Note the osseus union in the lateral maxillary wall. This patient was treated with banked tibial bone shaped to fit the defect. It has been completely replaced by the patient's bone. The holes adjacent to the union represent the previous location of the plate.

decreased operative time over autogenous bone grafting. The disadvantages of this technique are increased cost and operative time when compared to no bone grafting. Occasionally, infection of the bone graft may occur or it may become dislodged into the maxillary sinus. Patients complaining of sinus symptoms who have radiographs demonstrating a radiopaque foreign body in the sinus should be explored to remove the graft. It may be then refixated or consideration should be given to an alternative technique such as autogenous grafting.

Ischemic necrosis of the maxilla is a feared but fortunately rare complication of MMA. In their review of 22 studies describing 627 patients undergoing MMA, Holty and Guilleminault reported no incidences of this potentially devastating complication.[36] The occurrence of necrosis is of particular concern in this patient population because of the amount of advancement required. This places excess stretch on the soft tissue envelope and arterial blood supply, leading to decreased perfusion. Management involves careful monitoring of maxillary perfusion intra- and postoperatively and prompt management should it occur. Poor perfusion noted during the procedure can be managed by decreasing the amount of planned advancement and observing for a return of perfusion. Some advocate replating the maxilla to its preoperative position and discontinuation of the procedure completely. In more than 400 cases performed at a single center, Li and colleagues reported only two cases requiring discontinuation for this reason. They reported no incidences of necrosis using this protocol, which includes routine preservation of the greater palatine arteries.[30] One important point is that hypotensive anesthesia is often used during this portion of the procedure, and that simply allowing return of normal blood pressure may alleviate signs of decreased perfusion. One preventative measure that can be taken is a modification in the standard Le Fort incision to maximize the size of the vascular pedicle. Shorter length incisions may be used, but this will compromise visibility. The authors use a standard length incision with superior releases at the distal ends, which are created at an approximately 45-degree angle along the body of the zygoma. This effectively increases the pedicle width while not sacrificing incision length and maintaining adequate visibility. It is prudent to monitor these patients closely postoperatively as well, and any signs of hypoperfusion should be dealt with immediately. A return to the operating room should not be delayed. Some have advocated the use of nitroglycerin paste along the mucosa to increase perfusion, and though this is not done routinely, anecdotal reports have been favorable. A potential adverse outcome of this method is a drop in blood pressure.

Unlike traditional orthognathic surgery, aesthetic outcome is not a primary goal in maxillomandibular advancement for OSA. As a result, advancement of the maxilla and mandible could potentially result in unaesthetic facial changes in the pursuit of expanding the parapharyngeal airway. Subjective outcome studies have attempted to explore the magnitude of these facial changes based on patient's perception. In a study of 44 patients undergoing MMA, 96% reported a change in facial appearance.[56] Twenty-four (55%) patients found these changes favorable, 14 were neutral, and only 3 found the changes to be unfavorable. Interestingly, 40 of these patients were found have maxillomandibular protrusion by cephalometric parameters postoperatively.[35] In another study of 70 MMA patients, 67% reported improved facial appearance, 20% were indifferent, and only 3 patients (4%) were unsatisfied with their results. In this study, 9% of patients did not even notice a change.[55] Other smaller studies have substantiated these results, some reporting no changes in facial appearance after MMA.[57] Most subjective studies have reported overall low incidence of unacceptable aesthetics. These findings are perhaps due to the fact that most patients undergoing MMA are middle-aged and have more facial aging and soft tissue laxity. Advancing the maxilla and mandible increases skeletal support of these tissues and can result in facial rejuvenation. Due to the large amount of advancement, most patients will demonstrate bimaxillary protrusion after surgery. It is hard to predict which patients will find these changes unfavorable, which makes it difficult to avoid poor aesthetic outcome. The main tenant of management in these patients is proper patient education and expectant management. A report by Blumen and colleagues demonstrated much higher poor outcomes where 18% were either disappointed or unsatisfied with their appearance.[58] However, in this same study, 94% stated they would recommend this operation to friends and family. This is perhaps due to the high tolerance patients have of poor facial aesthetic outcome in the setting of a highly successful treatment of their sleep apnea. Regardless, patients must be made aware of possible poor results. Some recommend caution in younger patients, those with preexisting maxillomandibular protrusion, and in nonobese patients with thinner soft tissues. Advancement in these patients may lead to poor results.[30] Computer-aided simulated surgery can be used for patient education, though the accuracy of these methods has not been validated. However, tools such as these may increase patient acceptance. In patients with preexisting protrusion or proclined teeth, one may consider total or segmental subapical osteotomy with setback simultaneously with advancement. This will increase the amount of advancement that can be obtained while staying in an acceptable aesthetic window. One must keep in mind, however, that the potential for increased complications exists, including damage to the teeth within the osteotomized segment. Also, it often requires the extraction of teeth to make room for the vertical portion of the osteotomy that increases the potential for complications and adds to the treatment time.

The advancement of the maxilla enlarges the oropharyngeal space and theoretically could lead to incompetence of the soft palate and resultant VPI. This complication is fortunately rarely reported after MMA.[26] The incidence increases, however, in patients with a previous history of UPPP. Subjective changes in speech (24%) and swallowing (12%) were noted in 42 patients who received sequential phase I and phase II surgery.[56] All symptoms resolved in 1 year. This same group in a larger series reported a much lower incidence (approximately 10%) after MMA following UPPP.[59] Though less frequency has been reported, Bettega and colleagues reported all patients with previous UPPP experienced VPI after MMA.[60] Patients should be informed of this complication, especially those with previous UPPP, but be reassured that it will be most likely transient. Special consideration should be given to those with a history of cleft lip and palate or other surgical procedures resulting in velopharyngeal scarring, as the likelihood is presumably increased. Additionally, careful history is warranted as some research suggests those who experience significant VPI postoperatively likely exhibited this tendency preoperatively.[22]

One concern for patients undergoing MMA is the potential for respiratory complications following MMA. Anesthetists at many surgical centers are particularly concerned about postoperative obstruction after extubation in this patient population. In a study of 70 consecutive patients, Li and colleagues performed nasopharyngolaryngoscopy before and 48 hours after surgery. They noted lateral pharyngeal wall edema in all patients, 20% incidence of edema and eccymosis of the piriform sinus and aryepiglottic fold, and a 6% incidence of hematoma of the hypopharyngeal region resulting in partial airway obstruction. None of their patients, however, developed respiratory complications or required intervention. Additionally, none of the patients treated at their surgical center prior to this study experienced acute airway obstruction requiring tracheostomy or intubation. Based on these results, they advocated the use of postoperative nasopharyngolaryngoscopy in all patients following MMA.[61] In another study of 25 consecutive MMA patients, cephalometric data immediately postoperatively during the period of maximum edema demonstrated an increase in the posterior airway space from preoperative values.[62] Another study demonstrated significant reduction in pre- and postoperative desaturations (15.2/h to 1.3/h) immediately after surgery.[63] In light of these findings and clinical experience, in all reality the airway is most likely significantly improved in the immediate postoperative period. Given the nature of the disease, however, and the concern for potential complications, these patients are usually best managed conservatively. As discussed previously, extubation in the operating room with the surgeon and anesthesia team present is advised. In the rare event of respiratory distress, it is best to be in a controlled setting with experienced personnel and proper equipment that is easily accessible. Inpatient management with at least overnight stay in an ICU or other closely monitored unit with one-on-one care is advised. Our protocol involves an overnight ICU stay with transfer to a step-down unit on postoperative day 2 with close nursing supervision. Continuous pulse oximetry is used, with supplemental oxygen as needed to maintain adequate saturation. This is particularly important in the immediate postoperative period where narcotic analgesics are often required in patients with a propensity for respiratory depression. Postoperative CPAP can also be considered in patients not responsive to oxygen administration, though this is rarely needed.

Distraction Osteogenesis

Distraction osteogenesis (DO) may be used in conjunction with, or as an alternative to MMA. Distraction involves osteotomy of the maxilla or mandible followed by placement of external or internal distraction devices that are turned slowly. The surgically created gap fills in with bone as the segments are advanced. DO has been used to successfully treat children with craniofacial abnormalities and concomitant OSA. Its use in adults has been limited due to the high success of MMA, but it is a viable alternative, particularly in patients with severely limited bone and soft tissue such as those with craniofacial abnormalities. In such cases it may be difficult or impossible to surgically lengthen the facial skeleton with a single advancement. It therefore may be used alone or prior to MMA, which may then be performed after an adequate period of healing. Poor patient satisfaction, particularly with the length of treatment (often 3–6 months) and cumbersome internal or external hardware make paramount proper patient education prior to treatment. A full disclosure of the length of treatment and educational materials demonstrating device pictures will help to increase patient acceptance and satisfaction with the procedure. The application of the device and control of the vector during the activation phase can be technically difficult, and postoperative malocclusion can be common. Occlusal adjustments or postoperative orthodontics may be required, and the patient must be educated preoperatively to this possibility. Distractor loosening or failure may occur and require reapplication. Removal of the device may be required if infection occurs. It may be replaced after an appropriate course of antibiotics, and if bony healing occurs during this time frame, a revision osteotomy will be required.

Bypass Procedures

Tracheostomy

Perhaps the most effective means of treatment, tracheotomy was the first surgical intervention for the treatment of sleep apnea. Today it is reserved for select cases of severe apnea in patients not tolerant of CPAP who are not candidates for other procedures. It is associated with a high incidence of complications including social morbidity, poor patient acceptance, wound infections, tissue necrosis, granulation tissue formation, tracheomalacia, and trachea-innominate fistula. Complications are generally higher in obese patients. It is occasionally indicated as a temporary measure for patients undergoing other airway and nonairway procedures. Additionally, long-term use can lead to hyperplastic pharyngeal tissue that can result in OSA after decannulation. The surgical complications of tracheostomy have been extensively covered in other texts and are beyond the scope of this chapter.

POSTOPERATIVE CONSIDERATIONS

Monitoring

The goal of postoperative monitoring is the early detection of surgical complications. OSA patients are at risk for respiratory compromise postoperatively, which may be exacerbated by narcotic use and sleep deprivation. Additionally, sleep apnea may be unchanged or worse immediately after surgery.[64] As discussed previously, controversy exists regarding the type of postoperative care required after OSA surgery. The appropriate level of monitoring should be tailored to the patient and procedure being performed.

In those patients who require inpatient monitoring, continuous pulse oximetry is an easy and reliable method to detect hypoxemia. This may be performed in a closely supervised area such as a step-up unit or in a regular floor bed with alarms. It may also be linked to telemetry with electrocardiography. Electro-cardiographic monitoring should be considered in patients with a history of cardiac disease. Routine vital signs including pain and blood pressure should be recorded, and consideration for increase frequency over standard practices should be given due to their frequent difficulty in management. Historically, it was often advocated that OSA patients should be managed in an ICU setting early postoperatively. Recent improvements in reported complication rates, improved techniques, and patient management protocols have led some to recommend less acute care. While many still advocate early monitoring of MMA patients in an ICU setting, recent reports of many soft tissue procedures successfully managed in closely monitored nursing units or even as an outpatient has made the necessity questionable. The literature does not clearly support one management scenario over another.

One important consideration when deciding the level of postoperative care required is the amount of narcotic pain management required postsurgically. The managing practitioner should assess the level of anticipated pain management required as a factor when deciding the amount of monitoring needed. While some procedure may be associated with little pain, others such as UPPP and MMA may require stronger pain management and thus closer supervision.

Pain Management and Sedatives

Narcotic pain medications are frequently required after OSA surgery. They should be used with caution, however, in this patient population. Opiate medications can cause dose-dependent reduction of respiratory drive leading to hypoventilation, hypoxemia, and hypercarbia. This may lead to an increased incidence of respiratory events after surgery. The use of non-narcotic medications should be maximized prior to the administration of opiate pain medications. Nonsteroidal anti-inflammatory agents such as ibuprofen, ketoralac, or naproxen may be used with caution due to the increased chance of bleeding. Acetaminophen and tramadol are additional options without respiratory side effects or increased risk of bleeding. When this is not sufficient to alleviate the pain, narcotics may be used. They should be administered by trained staff members, and when the patient requests them. It is best to avoid scheduling these medications and important that they not be given until the patient's level of consciousness has been assessed. Patient-administered IV narcotics should be used with caution, and family members should be educated on their proper use. Smaller doses and longer lock-out intervals should be used initially until the patient's threshold has been assessed. Oral narcotics may provide longer-acting baseline pain control with fewer respiratory side effects and may be preferred once the patient is able to take oral medications. It is important to establish protocols for administration of any medication that may affect the respiratory drive in these patients and that they are administered only by appropriately trained personnel. Following such an established protocol will help to minimize complications.

Insomnia is a common problem compounded in the hospital setting due to stimulating environment and alterations in the sleep-wake cycle. Patients who have difficulty sleeping are commonly prescribed sedatives after surgery. This practice should be used with caution or avoided altogether in sleep apnea patients. Sedative hypnotics have been shown to have adverse effects on arousal thresholds, apnea duration and frequency, and oxygen saturation. Two short-acting nonbenzodiazepine hypnotic agents with minimal effect on sleep apnea severity—Zaleplon and Zolpidem—may be used if necessary.[65] It should be noted, however, that any sedative hypnotic has the potential for adverse respiratory effects and may be potentiated by their use simultaneously with narcotics.

Reducing Airway Edema and Obstruction

Airway edema is a concern in the OSA patient after surgery and may be the result of the surgical procedure or difficult or traumatic intubation. After surgery, the head of the bed should be elevated and the supine position avoided. This helps reduce venous congestion and edema in the head and neck. In addition to worsened edema, the supine position tends to worsen sleep apnea as the oral soft tissues collapse on the posterior pharyngeal wall.

Airway edema may also be improved by the use of steroids or cooling agents. The preferred steroid protocol of the authors is dexamethasone 10 mg every 8 hours for three doses after surgery. This, in conjunction with a preoperative steroid dose, helps to reduce surgical edema and protect the airway in the postoperative period. Cooling of the soft tissues may also be used, usually through sucking on ice chips or encouraging the drinking of cool liquids. The use of cooling agents has also been shown to reduce pain.

Antibiotics may also reduce swelling by preventing infection. They may be given as a single perioperative dose or may be used for a short period after surgery, as is common practice after upper airway procedures. Topical agents such as chlorhexidine rinse are commonly used before and after surgery and help reduce oral bacterial counts.

In addition, the use of systemic or topical decongestants may improve the patient's airway, particularly when nasal surgery has been performed. Improving the nasal airway may improve sleep apnea and CPAP compliance postoperatively.

Maintaining Adequate Oxygenation

In the immediate postoperative period, patients should be monitored closely for adequate oxygenation. OSA patients commonly have baseline low oxygen saturation secondary to their disease. Additionally, anesthesia and narcotic use cause respiratory depression due to hypoventilation, and the patient may have postsurgical atelectasis leading to hypoxemia. Patients should be monitored with continuous pulse oximetry postoperatively and oxygen administered until baseline levels of oxygen saturation are maintained. The patient should be alert and able to maintain his or her airway without assistance. Oxygen may be administered by nasal cannula, but patients who have had nasal surgery or who have inherent difficulty with nasal breathing may require an open face mask. Humidified oxygen can help prevent drying of the mucous membranes. It should be noted that for OSA patients, oxygen saturation may drop during sleep, and an alternate protocol may be required. Those patients may benefit from CPAP use during this period.

It is important that patients who use CPAP at home bring their device to the hospital when inpatient management is expected. Some recommend that CPAP be readily available throughout any hospitalization and routinely use it post surgery.[11] Others recommend having the CPAP available and only using it as needed. In their prospective study of OSA patients in the postsurgical period, only 4 of 131 patients required administration of nasal CPAP for oxygen desaturation when a strict protocol was used.[66] Regardless of individual protocol, it is important that the device is available to be used if required. The patient's preoperative settings can be used as a starting point but may require adjusting after surgery. Airway improvements may result in lower pressure settings while temporary edema and airway narrowing may require higher settings. Caution should be used in patients who undergo MMA as the potential for subcutaneous emphysema may limit the use of CPAP. After nasal surgery, those who used nasal CPAP preoperatively may require full face mask.

Blood Pressure Control

Hypertension is commonly seen postoperatively in the OSA patient and must be managed appropriately. Hypertension in this patient population is directly linked to sympathetic activation secondary to arousals and hypoxia and therefore may be difficult to manage in the setting of ongoing disease. There may be some improvement in blood pressure control, however, in the postsurgical patient if immediate improvement in sleep apnea is seen. CPAP has been shown to normalize blood pressure and can be an effective adjunct to antihypertensives to lower blood pressure in patients with OSA and hypertension in some cases.[67] Given that many patients have worsened or unchanged disease after surgery, though, strict monitoring and treatment are warranted. Poorly controlled blood pressure can lead to increased tissue swelling, ongoing blood loss, or even end-organ damage. After surgical osteotomies, blood loss is pressure dependent and cannot be controlled intraoperatively with cautery or ligatures. Home medications should be restarted if proven effective prior to surgery, keeping in mind that lower doses may be needed in the postoperative setting. Additional protocols for as needed dosing should be instituted and adjusted accordingly.

Deep Venous Thrombosis Prophylaxis

All patients undergoing OSA surgery admitted to the hospital should have deep venous thrombosis (DVT) prophylaxis. Obesity, long procedures, bed rest, and advanced age predispose the patient to DVTs and pulmonary embolism. Pneumatic compression hose, compression stockings, and early ambulation are all minimally invasive methods to prevent DVTs and should be used regularly. Anticoagulants such as enoxaparin or heparin sodium should be used with caution after surgery, particularly after osteotomies or in the setting of uncontrolled blood pressure when the risk of bleeding may be higher.

CONCLUSIONS

The management of complications in obstructive sleep apnea requires a thorough understanding of the procedures to be performed as well as the medical comorbidities that are frequently associated with this condition. The preoperative, intraoperative, and postoperative periods are all critical time points with special considerations that must be anticipated for successful outcome. When implemented properly, proper surgical technique in combination with appropriate perioperative management can result in significantly improved quality of life with minimal morbidity.[68]

SUGGESTED READINGS

1. Duran J, Esnaola S, Rubio R, and Iztueta A. 2001. "Obstructive sleep apnea-hypopnea and related clinical features in a population-based sample of subjects aged 30 to 70 yr." *Am J Respir Crit Care Med* 163: 685–689.
2. Young T, Finn L, Peppard PE, Szklo-Coxe M, Austin D, Nieto FJ, Stubbs R, and Hla KM. 2008. "Sleep disordered breathing and mortality: Eighteen-year follow-up of the Wisconsin sleep cohort." *Sleep* 31: 1071–1078.
3. Yaggi HK, and Strohl KP. 2010. "Adult obstructive sleep apnea/hypopnea syndrome: Definitions, risk factors, and pathogenesis." *Clin Chest Med* 31: 179–186.
4. Hirshkowitz M. 2008. "The clinical consequences of obstructive sleep apnea and associated excessive sleepiness." *J Fam Pract* 57: S9–16.
5. Kuhlo W, Doll E, and Franck MC. 1969. "[Successful management of Pickwickian syndrome using long-term tracheostomy]." *Dtsch Med Wochenschr* 94: 1286–1290.
6. Ikematsu T. 1964. "Study of snoring, 4th report." *J Jpn Otol Rhino Laryngol Soc* 64: 434–435.
7. Kuo PC, West RA, Bloomquist DS, and McNeil RW. 1979. "The effect of mandibular osteotomy in three patients with hypersomnia sleep apnea." *Oral Surg Oral Med Oral Pathol* 48: 385–392.

8. Worsnop CJ, Naughton MT, Barter CE, Morgan TO, Anderson AI, and Pierce RJ. 1998. "The prevalence of obstructive sleep apnea in hypertensives." *Am J Respir Crit Care Med* 157: 111–115.

9. Fairbanks DN. 1990. "Uvulopalatopharyngoplasty complications and avoidance strategies." *Otolaryngol Head Neck Surg* 102: 239–245.

10. Cullen, DJ. 2001. "Obstructive sleep apnea and postoperative analgesia—a potentially dangerous combination." *J Clin Anesth* 13: 83–85.

11. Li KK, Powell N, and Riley R. 2002. "Postoperative management of the obstructive sleep apnea patient." Oral Maxillofac *Surg Clin North Am* 14: 401–404.

12. Mickelson SA. 2007. "Preoperative and postoperative management of obstructive sleep apnea patients." *Otolaryngol Clin North Am* 40: 877–889.

13. Dodds C, and Ryall DM. 1992. "Tonsils, obesity and obstructive sleep apnoea." *Br J Hosp Med* 47: 62–66.

14. Meoli AL, Rosen CL, Kristo D, et al. 2003. "Upper airway management of the adult patient with obstructive sleep apnea in the perioperative period–avoiding complications." *Sleep* 26: 1060–1065.

15. Boyce JR, Waite PD, Louis PJ, and Ness TJ. 2003. "Transnasal jet ventilation is a useful adjunct to teach fibreoptic intubation: A preliminary report." *Can J Anaesth* 50: 1056–1060.

16. Lai JB, Boyce JR, Sittitavornwong S, and Waite PD. 2010. "Use of transnasal jet ventilation-assisted fiberoptic intubation in obstructive sleep apnea patients undergoing orthognathic surgery: A new technique." *J Oral Maxillofac Surg* 68: 2025–2027.

17. Neligan PJ, Porter S, Max B, et al. 2009. "Obstructive sleep apnea is not a risk factor for difficult intubation in morbidly obese patients." *Anesth Analg* 109: 1182–1186.

18. Friedman M, Tanyeri H, Lim JW, Landsberg R, Vaidyanathan K, and Caldarelli D. 2000. "Effect of improved nasal breathing on obstructive sleep apnea." *Otolaryngol Head Neck Surg* 122: 71–74.

19. Goode R. 2005. "Nasal surgery for sleep apnea patients." In: *Surgical Management of Sleep Apnea and Snoring*, Terris DJ, and Goode RL, eds. Boca Raton, FL: Taylor and Francis Group.

20. Woodson BT, and O'Connor PD. 2009. "Reconstruction of airway soft tissues in obstructive sleep apnea." *Oral Maxillofac Surg Clin North Am* 21: 435–445.

21. Brietzke SE, and Gallagher D. 2006. "The effectiveness of tonsillectomy and adenoidectomy in the treatment of pediatric obstructive sleep apnea/hypopnea syndrome: A meta-analysis." *Otolaryngol Head Neck Surg* 134: 979–984.

22. Ephros HD, Madani M, and Yalamanchili SC. 2010. "Surgical treatment of snoring & obstructive sleep apnoea." *Indian J Med Res* 131: 267–276.

23. McColley SA, April MM, Carroll JL, Naclerio RM, and Loughlin GM. 1992. "Respiratory compromise after adenotonsillectomy in children with obstructive sleep apnea." *Arch Otolaryngol Head Neck Surg* 118: 940–943.

24. Rosen GM, Muckle RP, Mahowald MW, Goding GS, and Ullevig C. 1994. "Postoperative respiratory compromise in children with obstructive sleep apnea syndrome: Can it be anticipated?" *Pediatrics* 93: 784–788.

25. Fujita S, Conway W, Zorick F, and Roth T. 1981. "Surgical correction of anatomic abnormalities in obstructive sleep apnea syndrome: uvulopalatopharyngoplasty." *Otolaryngol Head Neck Surg* 89: 923–934.

26. Holty JE, and Guilleminault C. 2010. "Surgical options for the treatment of obstructive sleep apnea." *Med Clin North Am* 94: 479–515.

27. Esclamado RM, Glenn MG, McCulloch, TM, and Cummings CW. 1989. "Perioperative complications and risk factors in the surgical treatment of obstructive sleep apnea syndrome." *Laryngoscope* 99: 1125–1129.

28. Terris DJ, Fincher EF, Hanasono MM, Fee WE, Jr., and Adachi K. 1998. "Conservation of resources: Indications for intensive care monitoring after upper airway surgery on patients with obstructive sleep apnea." *Laryngoscope* 108: 784–788.

29. Franklin KA, Anttila H, Axelsson S, Gislason T, Maasilta P, Myhre KI, and Rehnqvist N. 2009. "Effects and side-effects of surgery for snoring and obstructive sleep apnea—a systematic review." *Sleep* 32: 27–36.

30. Li KK, Riley R, and Powell N. 2003. "Complications of obstructive sleep apnea surgery." *Oral Maxillofac Surg Clin North Am* 15: 297–304.

31. Ferguson KA, Heighway K, and Ruby RR. 2003. "A randomized trial of laser-assisted uvulopalatoplasty in the treatment of mild obstructive sleep apnea." *Am J Respir Crit Care Med* 167: 15–19.

32. Larrosa F, Hernandez L, Morello A, Ballester E, Quinto L, and Montserrat JM. 2004. "Laser-assisted uvulopalatoplasty for snoring: Does it meet the expectations?" *Eur Respir J* 24: 66–70.

33. Kezirian EJ, and Goldberg AN. 2006. "Hypopharyngeal surgery in obstructive sleep apnea: An evidence-based medicine review." *Arch Otolaryngol Head Neck Surg* 132: 206–213.

34. Mickelson S. 2005. *Radiofrequency Tissue Volume Reduction of the Tongue*. Boca Raton, FL: Taylor and Francis Group.

35. Riley RW, Powell NB, and Guilleminault C. 1990. "Maxillary, mandibular, and hyoid advancement for treatment of obstructive sleep apnea: A review of 40 patients." *J Oral Maxillofac Surg* 48: 20–26.

36. Holty JE, and Guilleminault C. 2010. "Maxillomandibular advancement for the treatment of obstructive sleep apnea: A systematic review and meta-analysis." *Sleep Med Rev* 14: 287–297.

37. Li KK, Powell NB, Riley RW, Troell RJ, and Guilleminault C. 2000. "Long-term results of maxillomandibular advancement surgery." *Sleep Breath* 4: 137–140.

38. Waite PD, Wooten V, Lachner J, and Guyette RF. 1989. "Maxillomandibular advancement surgery in 23 patients with obstructive sleep apnea syndrome." *J Oral Maxillofac Surg* 47: 1256–1261; discussion 1262.

39. Waite PD, and Vilos GA. 2002. "Surgical changes of posterior airway space in obstructive sleep apnea." *Oral Maxillofac Surg Clin North Am* 14: 385–399.

40. Chow LK, Singh B, Chiu WK, and Samman N. 2007. "Prevalence of postoperative complications after orthognathic surgery: A 15-year review." *J Oral Maxillofac Surg* 65: 984–992.

41. Theodossy T, Jackson O, Petrie A, and Lloyd T. 2006. "Risk factors contributing to symptomatic plate removal following sagittal split osteotomy." *Int J Oral Maxillofac Surg* 35: 598–601.

42. Zijderveld SA, Smeele LE, Kostense PJ, and Tuinzing DB. 1999. "Preoperative antibiotic prophylaxis in orthognathic surgery: A randomized, double-blind, and placebo-controlled clinical study." *J Oral Maxillofac Surg* 57: 1403–6; discussion 1406–1407.

43. Baqain ZH, Hyde N, Patrikidou A, and Harris M. 2004. "Antibiotic prophylaxis for orthognathic surgery: A prospective, randomised clinical trial." *Br J Oral Maxillofac Surg* 42: 506–510.

44. Bystedt H, Josefsson, K, and Nord CE. 1987. "Ecological effects of penicillin prophylaxis in orthognatic surgery." *Int J Oral Maxillofac Surg* 16: 559–565.

45. Fridrich KL, Partnoy BE, and Zeitler DL. 1994. "Prospective analysis of antibiotic prophylaxis for orthognathic surgery." *Int J Adult Orthodon Orthognath Surg* 9: 129–131.

46. Kang SH, Yoo JH, and Yi CK. 2009. "The efficacy of postoperative prophylactic antibiotics in orthognathic surgery: A prospective study in Le Fort I osteotomy and bilateral intraoral vertical ramus osteotomy." *Yonsei Med J* 50: 55–59.

47. Ruggles JE, and Hann JR. 1984. "Antibiotic prophylaxis in intraoral orthognathic surgery." *J Oral Maxillofac Surg* 42: 797–801.

48. Bentley KC, Head TW, and Aiello GA. 1999. "Antibiotic prophylaxis in orthognathic surgery: A 1-day versus 5-day regimen." *J Oral Maxillofac Surg* 57: 226–230; discussion 230–232.

49. Boyd, SB. 2009. "Management of obstructive sleep apnea by maxillomandibular advancement." *Oral Maxillofac Surg Clin North Am* 21: 447–457.

50. Lye KW, Waite PD, Wang D, and Sittitavornwong S. 2008. "Predictability of prebent advancement plates for use in maxillomandibular advancement surgery." *J Oral Maxillofac Surg* 66: 1625–1629.

51. Nimkarn Y, Miles PG, and Waite PD. 1995. "Maxillomandibular advancement surgery in obstructive sleep apnea syndrome patients: Long-term surgical stability." *J Oral Maxillofac Surg* 53: 1414–1418; discussion 1418–1419.

52. Riley RW, Powell NB, and Guilleminault C. 1990. "Maxillofacial surgery and nasal CPAP. A comparison of treatment for obstructive sleep apnea syndrome." *Chest* 98: 1421–1425.

53. Louis PJ, Waite PD, and Austin RB. 1993. "Long-term skeletal stability after rigid fixation of Le Fort I osteotomies with advancements." *Int J Oral Maxillofac Surg* 22: 82–86.

54. Goodday R. 2009. "Diagnosis, treatment planning, and surgical correction of obstructive sleep apnea." *J Oral Maxillofac Surg* 67: 2183–2196.

55. Gregoire C. 2008. "Patient outcomes following maxillomandibular advancement surgery to treat obstructive sleep apnea syndrome." Master's thesis. Dalhoise University, Halifax, Nova Scotia.

56. Li KK, Riley RW, Powell NB, and Guilleminault C. 2001. "Patient's perception of the facial appearance after maxillomandibular advancement for obstructive sleep apnea syndrome." *J Oral Maxillofac Surg* 59: 377–380; discussion 380–381.

57. Smatt Y, and Ferri J. 2005. "Retrospective study of 18 patients treated by maxillomandibular advancement with adjunctive procedures for obstructive sleep apnea syndrome." *J Craniofac Surg* 16: 770–777.

58. Blumen MB, Buchet I, Meulien P, Hausser Hauw C, Neveu H, and Chabolle F. 2009. "Complications/adverse effects of maxillomandibular advancement for the treatment of OSA in regard to outcome." *Otolaryngol Head Neck Surg* 141: 591–597.

59. Li KK, Troell RJ, Riley RW, Powell NB, Koester U, and Guilleminault C. 2001. "Uvulopalatopharyngoplasty, maxillomandibular advancement, and the velopharynx." *Laryngoscope* 111: 1075–1078.

60. Bettega G, Pepin JL, Veale D, Deschaux C, Raphael B, and Levy P. 2000. "Obstructive sleep apnea syndrome. Fifty-one consecutive patients treated by maxillofacial surgery." *Am J Respir Crit Care Med* 162: 641–649.

61. Li KK, Riley RW, Powell NB, Zonato A, Troell R, and Guilleminault C. 2000. "Postoperative airway findings after maxillomandibular advancement for obstructive sleep apnea syndrome." *Laryngoscope* 110: 325–327.

62. Robertson C, Goodday RH, Rajda DS, Precious DS, and Morrison A. 2003. "Subjective and objective treatment outcomes of maxillomandibular advancement for the treatment of obstructive sleep apnea syndrome." *Journal of Oral and Maxillofacial Surgery* 61(Suppl 1): 76.

63. Powell JE, Yim D, Morrison A, and Godday RH. 2004. "Oxygen saturations in patients undergoing maxillomandibular advancement surgery for obstructive sleep apnea: A preoperative to postoperative comparison." *Journal of Oral and Maxillofacial Surgery* 62(Suppl 1): 57–58.

64. Johnson JT, and Sanders MH. 1986. "Breathing during sleep immediately after uvulopalatopharyngoplasty." *Laryngoscope* 96: 1236–1238.

65. Mickelson SA. 2009. "Anesthetic and postoperative management of the obstructive sleep apnea patient." *Oral Maxillofac Surg Clin North Am* 21: 425–434.

66. Rotenberg B, Hu A, Fuller J, Bureau Y, Arra I, and Sen M. 2010. "The early postoperative course of surgical sleep apnea patients." *Laryngoscope* 120: 1063–1068.

67. Campos-Rodriguez F, Perez-Ronchel J, Grilo-Reina A, Lima-Alvarez J, Benitez MA, and Almeida-Gonzalez C. 2007. "Long-term effect of continuous positive airway pressure on BP in patients with hypertension and sleep apnea." *Chest* 132: 1847–1852.

68. Gross JB, Bachenberg KL, Benumof JL, et al. 2006. "Practice guidelines for the perioperative management of patients with obstructive sleep apnea: A report by the American Society of Anesthesiologists Task Force on Perioperative Management of patients with obstructive sleep apnea." *Anesthesiology* 104: 1081–1093; quiz 1117–1118.

8

Cleft and Craniofacial Surgery

Bernard J. Costello, DMD, MD, FACS
John F. Caccamese, Jr., DMD, MD, FACS
Ramon L. Ruiz, DMD, MD

INTRODUCTION

Cleft lip with or without cleft palate occurs with a frequency of 1 in 600 live births, making it one of the most common congenital malformations. The functional and aesthetic consequences associated with both syndromic and nonsyndromic facial clefting are well understood and are routinely addressed in an interdisciplinary fashion to optimize the care of the patient. Despite well-established treatment pathways, significant variation still exists in the surgical techniques used to repair the cleft, though many have shown to have excellent results.[1] Fortunately, a patient's age and the anatomic site of their problem contribute to excellent healing with rare complications so long as the surgery is well executed. Early complications range from wound-specific issues and infection to perioperative and anesthetic problems, while late complications can be best categorized as to their effect on appearance, function, and growth.

It has long been held as a general rule that infants are age appropriate for lip repair according to the "rule of 10's," or at roughly 3 months of age. Some studies suggest that acceptable perioperative morbidity can be achieved by 1 week of life. In 2007, Fillies et al. retrospectively examined a cohort of 174 cleft lip and palate patients and were able to correlate anesthetic complication risk with body weight at the time of surgery. Interestingly, their work is reflective of results seen in Wilhelmsen's 1966 review of morbidity of and mortality in cleft surgery.[2,3] Given the possibility of syndromic association with clefts and the lack of data supporting early repair, it is generally recommended that sufficient time be allowed for comprehensive workup and weight gain before definitive repair is accomplished. In most centers, this is somewhere between 3 and 6 months of age.

The preoperative evaluation for a cleft patient is fairly standard and is dictated largely by the requirements to undergo a general anesthetic at a given age and by the comorbidities of a specific patient. At the author's institution, no blood work (CBC or type and screen) is performed for healthy babies undergoing this procedure. The lip repair itself has little systemic impact to the physiology of the child, and blood loss is minimal during surgery. In fact, many institutions routinely perform cleft lip repair as an outpatient procedure and have demonstrated comparable outcome data with those institutions where these children are admitted as inpatients.[1,2,4–7]

COMPLICATIONS IN CLEFT LIP REPAIR

Early Complications

Early surgical site complications are uncommon. Despite a relative paucity in the literature of reported early lip repair complications, those most frequently reported include infection, lip dehiscence, flap necrosis, and nasal airway obstruction.[8–10]

Management of Complications in Oral and Maxillofacial Surgery, First Edition. Edited by Michael Miloro, Antonia Kolokythas.
© 2012 John Wiley & Sons, Inc. Published 2012 by John Wiley & Sons, Inc.

Despite being performed as a clean contaminated surgery, cleft lip repair is generally performed in edentulous patients where the typical oral flora has not yet evolved to contain the multiple anaerobic aerodigestive pathogens seen in adult patients. In fact, the flora in this patient population is considerably more limited as demonstrated by Chuo's retrospective review of swab culture data in 250 patients with clefts.[11] In this study, the predominant pathogens were *S. aureus* and β-hemolytic *streptococcus*. They chose to administer prophylactic perioperative antibiotics and/or postpone surgery based on culture-positive data and in patients with other comorbidities (e.g., failure to thrive, malnutrition). Unfortunately, they did not list their infection rate in this cohort despite these measures. One has to weigh cost, risk, and available outcome data when deciding on best practices in the absence of a prospective randomized study. At the author's institution, perioperative antibiotics are used. While others report the additional use of postoperative antibiotics in noninfected patients, we believe that this is difficult to justify routinely in an era of increasing antibiotic resistance and in a surgery that already carries with it a very low risk of infection.[9]

Lip dehiscence in the acute setting is rarely a problem with the careful and tension-free construction of all tissue layers in the unilateral or bilateral cleft lip patient. Dehiscence has been attributed to both tension and trauma. Reinisch observed traumatic lip dehiscence in 7 of his 123 reviewed cleft patients (all of these were bilateral but one). Five of these patients were older than 9 months of age and age-related mobility and activity was felt to be the cause of this unfortunate outcome.[9] Some surgeons opt to use the Logan bow or arm restraints, though there are no substantive data that demonstrate their effectiveness.[12,13]

Infants are obligate nasal breathers and in the acute postoperative time period, nasal obstruction can occur due to edema or simply the presence of tissue where there was none previously. This can be further exacerbated in the postoperative period by upper respiratory tract infections. Some of these obstruction issues can be ameliorated by the use of nostril conformers or cut-to-fit cannulae made from endotracheal tubes. This not only helps to prevent obstruction, but the conformer or stent can help to support the redraping of the nasal skin/vestibular tissue when a primary rhinoplasty has been performed.[14,15,16] These tubes must be routinely cared for with bulb suction and saline drops, lest they clog with dried mucus themselves.

Clinically, significant postoperative hemorrhage is very uncommon in cleft lip repair. Bleeding can be avoided with meticulous dissection, hemostasis, and closure. Care is taken during surgery to perform the operation with the assistance of infiltrated local anesthetic and vasoconstrictors along with the judicious use of electrocautery. Many perform the surgery with loupe or microscope magnification, making any small bleeding points readily identifiable, and layered closure of mucosa, muscle and skin should all but assure a dry field. A small amount of bleeding is to be expected, especially when a mucosal field is involved in the surgery. This can take place for 1–2 days after surgery and might appear somewhat magnified as it mixes with oral and nasal secretions. A small amount of perinasal, perioral, and periorbital bruising is not uncommon either, depending on the surgical techniques utilized for repair.

Flap necrosis has been reported in bilateral cleft lip and palate patients due to excessive thinning of the prolabial skin in efforts to refine the philtral dimple.[8] Interestingly, however, as more aggressive nasal surgery has been reported in the recent past to address the nasal tip and the columella at the time of bilateral cleft lip repair, one would expect that the prolabium is even more at risk. For example, Cutting has described a prolabial unwinding technique to reposition the lower lateral cartilages, and Mulliken described marginal incisions paired with extensive tip undermining and suturing despite reporting the use of an extremely narrow prolabial pedicle and flap.[17,18,19] No complications have been reported in any detailed manner using these techniques. This should not imply that these maneuvers are without risk. They should simply be undertaken with a thorough understanding of the local anatomy and the techniques described.

Late Complications

The appearance and function of the repaired cleft lip are greatly impacted by the initial surgery (Fig. 8.1). The simultaneous construction of functional nasal and labial muscles influence the growth and development of the underlying facial skeleton as well as the appearance of the lip.[20,21] The eventual form of the lip is the result of both the choice of skin incision and the muscle repair at the initial surgery. Of the various skin incisions that have been used, several, such as the geometric triangular and quadrangular incisions violate the subunits of the upper lip, while modifications of the advancement rotation most accurately replicate normal anatomic structures.[22,23,24] While complications classified as "early," such as infection or

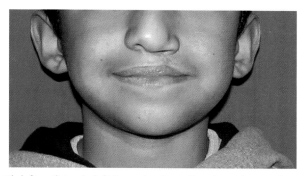

Fig. 8.1. Nine-year-old boy with left unilateral cleft lip and palate. Note how the nasal asymmetry and vertical deficiency of the lip on the cleft side are part of the same problem. In this case, a muscle reconstruction was not performed at the level of the nose, the medial element was under-rotated, and the lip was left short. A revision here would require recreation of the initial defect and complete reconstruction.

dehiscence often lead to sequelae that could be categorized as "late," many late complications or secondary deformities are the result of avoidable errors in technique or judgment. The end result is suboptimal lip aesthetics that can be difficult to correct.

The surgical correction of cleft lip and palate consists of a series of procedures where timing is dependent on both chronological and developmental milestones. The lip repair, consequently, is critical to all procedures that follow it. It is also important to keep in mind that the staged reconstruction of these patients is a stepwise process and that careful consideration must be given to each procedure and its downstream effects including growth.

While the construction of the labial and nasal muscular rings guides the eventual appearance and symmetry of the lip and nose, the individual's innate ability to heal and scarring tendencies also play key roles in the aesthetic appearance of the repair.[20,21] Certain technical shortcomings in the repair can also lead to less than optimal results. The underlying skeletal platform must be considered when evaluating secondary lip deformities, as the presence or absence of a bony alveolar cleft or maxillary hypoplasia greatly impacts the appearance of the nasolabial structures as the child grows. Despite best efforts with soft tissue correction and camouflaging techniques, facial harmony can only be accomplished when these hard tissue problems have been addressed as well. Therefore, it is recommended that, depending on the age of the child and the degree of skeletal dysplasia, soft tissue revisions are sometimes deferred until maxillary bone grafting and/or Le Fort osteotomy have been accomplished.

When evaluating a secondary lip/nose deformity, an understanding of the initial malformation and the goals of primary surgery are important. Understanding the true underlying cause of the secondary deformity and its global functional and aesthetic shortcomings are also crucial. For example, lesser procedures can be used to address minor height mismatches of the white roll, vermilion notching, or vermilion fullness when the muscle is otherwise noted to be functional and united across the cleft. When applied inappropriately, however, these "minor" procedures might only serve to amplify defects, increase scarring, or leave the patient well short of a complete correction. However, a complete takedown of the lip should be considered if there are significant issues with lip height or symmetry, nasal symmetry, substantial vermilion/white roll mismatches, or a dehiscent orbicularis oris. Lastly, when there is significant damage and scarring to the cleft adjacent tissue, especially in the case of the bilateral cleft lip, one may have to recruit nearby tissue to reconstitute the philtral complex and the orbicularis muscular ring.

Cutaneous Lip Problems

Long Upper Lip

The long upper lip is infrequently seen in patients with unilateral cleft lip given the predominance of advancement rotation repairs performed today. Excessive lip length was primarily a problem of the triangular and quadrangular repairs but can be encountered as a result of overzealous rotation in an

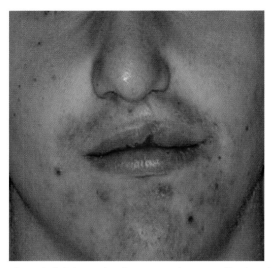

Fig. 8.2. Teenage boy with left unilateral cleft lip and palate. Note the vertically short lip on the cleft side, the vermilion notch, and the wet-dry line mismatch. This is best approached with complete takedown and reconstruction.

advancement rotation technique. The long upper lip, however, continues to plague the bilateral patient. While this is somewhat a function of postoperative lip animation and function, the aesthetic result can be visible as a long upper lip. The long lip can be a difficult problem to correct, frequently requiring the horizontal excision of tissue at the supravermilion level or in the subalar region. The scars left by these revisions, though reasonably well camouflaged by the white roll and the alar crease, respectively, are often less than optimal in appearance.

Tight Upper Lip

The tight upper lip can stem from aggressive soft tissue excision at the time of primary or secondary repair, inadequate mobilization of the soft tissues, or be the result of a protuberant premaxilla. The appearance of tissue deficiency can be further mimicked or accentuated by maxillary hypoplasia, or a full lower lip. Further lip revision that includes soft tissue excision might only serve to worsen the problem unless nearby tissue in the form of an Abbé flap is utilized. This pedicled cross-lip flap, based on the labial artery, will add width and appropriate bulk, while decreasing the width differential between the upper and lower lip. The Abbé flap may also be of value when the prolabial tissue has been severely damaged by scar. This technique often has less than desirable aesthetic results, but provides more tissue to the upper lip.

Short Upper Lip

The short upper lip may be the result of several errors in the primary lip repair. Most commonly, it is the result of an under rotated, improperly/incompletely repaired, or dehisced muscle and this will often require a re-repair of the lip (Fig. 8.2). Occasionally, it is the result of exuberant scarring or the sequelae of early infection or dehiscence. In any case, the original repair scar can be used to access the nasal and labial muscles for a more precise functional repair. If conversion to an advancement rotation from a geometric repair is feasible without too much tissue loss, it should be considered, as this places the cutaneous scars in a more natural position. Additionally, Z-plasties can placed at the vermilion-cutaneous junction or at the wet dry line as needed to accomplish aesthetic goals by lengthening the lip.

Philtrum Abnormalities

Obliteration of the philtral dimple and Cupid's bow asymmetries are occasionally seen following primary lip repair. A flat Cupid's bow is sometimes the result of a triangular repair as well. The philtral dimple can often be preserved in unilateral clefts with minimal cutaneous undermining of the noncleft side at the time of initial repair. This dimple should be respected, as a natural-appearing dimple is quite difficult to restore

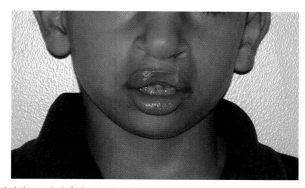

Fig. 8.3. Six-year-old boy with bilateral cleft lip and palate. Note the wide philtral complex and the hypoplastic vermilion in contrast to the robust lateral lip elements. Prolabial vermilion had been utilized in this case for the reconstruction of the red lip. Revision would require recreation of the initial defect, narrowing of the philtrum, and utilization of lateral vermilion flaps to fill out the central lip.

surgically. Additionally, widening of the scar in the philtral column position can occur as a result of early wound tension (due to inadequate muscle reconstruction), poor suturing, or wound breakdown at the initial repair. This can often be treated with simple excision and augmented with other surface treatments such as surface laser or dermabrasion. In bilateral clefts, the philtrum is often left too wide in conservative attempts to preserve tissue or with stretching that occurs with growth. This can yield an overly wide philtrum that will benefit from a re-repair (Fig. 8.3).

The philtral column(s) are also often left flat. This is largely due to the fact that we cannot surgically recreate the dermal insertions of the orbicularis muscle. We are therefore left to provide surgical camouflage, with carefully everted skin edges, dermal grafts, or local subcutaneous, dermal, or muscular flaps. As previously stated, when the philtrum area has sustained significant damage from the primary repair or a complication thereof, an Abbé flap may be considered.

Cutaneous Defects

Isolated unaesthetic cutaneous lip scarring can be managed in a manner similar to other facial scars, by excision, dermabrasion, or laser resurfacing. One must keep in mind the normal anatomic orientation of the philtral column and other local lip structures. For example, the horizontal orientation of a running W-plasty might not suit this area as well as a wavy line excision to re-create the philtral column in a scar excision. One must also be mindful that the skin of the nose and the skin of the lip are of different quality, much as the skin of the white and red lip. If the skin of the nose has migrated down onto the skin of the upper lip or conversely, the skin of the vermilion has elevated into the cutaneous lip, this must be addressed in the revision (Fig. 8.4).

Nostril Stenosis

Nostril stenosis does occur with some frequency on the repaired side (Fig. 8.5). This complication can obscure breathing and impair the normal toileting of the nasal vault and sinuses. A constricted nostril is one of the more difficult secondary deformities to treat. A common strategy is to avoid the complication by leaving the nostril slightly larger than that of the noncleft side at the time of the primary surgery. By the time the wound contracts, the nostrils will become more symmetric. If they do not, it is much easier to reduce a nostril secondarily than to enlarge one. There is rarely a deficiency of tissue, and it is usually the result of over-resection of normal tissue. Additionally, intranasal incisions can contribute to scar contracture. Some have suggested the use of postoperative stents or nasal conformer to combat stenosis. These devices must be used for a prolonged period of time for this purpose and can become somewhat laborious for parents. While most would advocate surgical release with or without grafting and some form of nostril retainer, some have recommended serial dilation with custom stents or secondary Z-plasty procedures.[25,26,27]

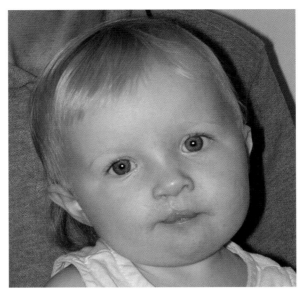

Fig. 8.4. Two-year-old girl with right unilateral complete cleft lip and palate. Note the mild nasal asymmetry as well as the vermilion cutaneous mismatch, in the face of an adequately full and vertically long lip.

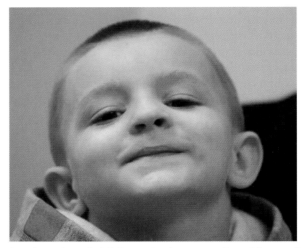

Fig. 8.5. Four-year-old boy with right unilateral cleft lip and palate. Note the mild to moderate right nostril stenosis.

Nasal Asymmetry

Nasal asymmetry can be a challenge in the cleft lip and palate patient and is unique to the initial severity and morphology of the cleft (Fig. 8.6). Primary rhinoplasty can be safe and does not result in growth disturbance. This has been significant in the evolution of the cleft repair as the lip and nose are too intimately related to be considered separately in the malformation. In the initial lip and nasal construction, surgeons must do their best to achieve symmetry in the face of an absent or hypoplastic maxillary bony platform. The lack of support for the nasal base can make absolute symmetry difficult to accomplish, though some techniques offer better solutions to this problem than do others. Many techniques have been able to minimize the depressed ala and nasal sill in the initial repair, and with limited alar, nasal tip, and septal work, excellent results can be obtained. If one has to achieve symmetry in any component of the nose at the primary surgery, it is the author's opinion that this should be the nostril sill, primarily from the standpoint of its vertical position, bulk and shape. This area can be difficult to deal with in revisions, especially if it has not been well cared for in the initial procedure. A common mistake is the use of an

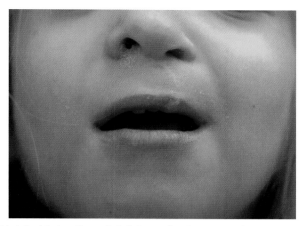

Fig. 8.6. Five-year-old girl with left-sided unilateral cleft lip and palate. Note the nasal asymmetry and smaller nostril on the cleft side. There is also a small amount of hyperplastic tissue/scar along the vermilion. These issues are independent and can be addressed separately when age appropriate according to growth.

overly extensive perialar incision and a repair in which the ala and sill are somewhat left behind laterally or deep in the bony defect, relative to the cleft-side lip element mobilization and advancement. Frequently, insufficient attention is given to the mobilization and repositioning of the perinasal muscles to their proper insertion on the maxilla. Often, the muscles in the lateral lip element are treated as one unit and little attention is given to separating and repositioning specific anatomic components. Tip symmetry can be addressed later if need be, though much of this is best addressed at the primary surgery if possible. Once again, nostril conformers can be used to assist in the healing and redraping of the primary rhinoplasty but should not be solely relied upon to achieve nasal symmetry.

Facial Growth

It has long been debated whether the lip or the palate repair causes the most harm to the growth potential of the maxilla. While there appear to be compelling data that the lip repair might very well be involved, the debate is far from over.[28] Studies implicating gingivoperiosteoplasty and certain forms of presurgical orthopedics have their following as well.[29] Additionally, the timing and the technique of primary palate repair likely have an impact.[29,30] To further muddy the waters, both subperiosteal and supraperiosteal dissection techniques have been advocated in lip repair. Both techniques have had their passionate supporters and detractors, with neither technique having been shown to out- or underperform the other. Approximately 25% or more of adolescents with cleft lips and palates will suffer from the additional stigmata of maxillary hypoplasia, despite the timing of lip/palate repair or the techniques used.[1] This leaves the surgeon with the additional task of restoring the skeletal foundation to a more normal anatomic position at some later date. This is traditionally performed with a Le Fort I osteotomy, either as a single stage procedure or utilizing distraction techniques with various devices. Both techniques have been shown to work well in capable hands and require the assistance of a knowledgeable orthodontist. These techniques are fraught with orthodontic and dental challenges, given the frequent absence of teeth and sometimes deficient bone in the cleft area. Occasionally, the maxillary-alveolar cleft must be grafted or regrafted in conjunction with the orthognathic surgery. Iliac crest grafts are frequently used for added stability in the orthognathic procedures, particularly when the maxilla is deficient both horizontally and vertically.

COMPLICATIONS IN PALATOPLASTY PROCEDURES

To clearly understand complications of palate repair, the cleft surgeon must understand the details of current outcome data regarding cleft palate repair. Velopharyngeal insufficiency (VPI) is a debilitating and unfortunately predictable consequence of a certain percentage of patients who undergo palatoplasty. There are also other complications seen with palatoplasty procedures related to technical aspects of the procedure or particular predispositions with some patients (e.g., airway problems in Pierre Robin sequence). This section discusses some of the more common complications and presents the current data regarding functional outcomes of palatoplasty, particularly as they relate to speech.

Palatoplasty Procedures and Outcome Differences

Le Monnier, a French dentist, reported the first successful cleft palate repair in Paris in 1766.[31,32] Since that time, many surgical techniques for cleft palate closure have been described. There is still debate over which technique produces superior results. A lack of clinical data from prospective trials forces clinical decisions to be made from retrospective studies, cohort studies, and surgeons' experience. Due to the inherent bias and uncontrolled nature associated with this level of evidence, clinicians need to be aware of the shortcomings and incorporate the information appropriately into practice. The primary objective of soft palate closure is the development of normalized speech.[1,33] Outcome measures for palate closure should also include maxillary growth, facial profile, dental occlusion, and presence of a fistula.[1,34,35]

A number of procedures exist for palatoplasty, and their outcome results are complex to evaluate and study with any precision. Bernard von Langenbeck described a palatoplasty technique in 1861, which is the oldest such procedure still in use today. The von Langenbeck palatoplasty involves bipedicled mucoperiosteal flaps with medial repositioning of nasal and oral side mucosa for closure. The technique leaves minimal hard palate exposed but does not lengthen the velum and can impair access for repair of the nasal lining and velar musculature. Subsequently, multiple palate repair techniques incorporated a pushback component designed to lengthen the palate and decrease the incidence of velopharyngeal insufficiency.[36] These include variations of the V–Y pushback described separately by Veau, Wardill, and Kilner in 1937.[37–39] Mucoperiosteal flaps are raised based on the greater palatine vasculature then retropositioned via a V–Y technique, resulting in lengthening of the velum at the expense of denuded anterior hard palate. Poor growth outcomes and anterior fistula formation has limited the use of this technique. The Bardach two-flap palatoplasty was described in 1967 and further refined with excellent anatomical and functional results.[40,41] In the Bardach repair, two mucoperiosteal flaps based on the greater palatine vessels are raised, as the flaps are not pedicled anteriorly (Fig. 8.7). The technique also limits hard palate bone exposure as the flaps are rotated downward at the expense of palatal depth. These cleft palate surgical procedures are now collectively termed the "two-flap palatoplasties."

In 1978 Leonard Furlow introduced a novel technique of repairing palatal clefts using double-opposing Z-plasties of the oral and nasal layers with anatomic orientation of the soft palate musculature (Fig. 8.8) Furlow has reported superior speech results using this procedure as compared with his experience with the two-flap palatoplasty.[42,43] Many centers adopted the Furlow palatoplasty and have reported better outcomes.[44–47] These reports consist mostly of self-reported experiences from a single center or surgeon and limited retrospective comparisons of techniques. They do not provide powerful data sufficient enough to make definitive statements regarding their superiority. Currently, only some level II and mostly level III evidence is currently available to help us make clinical decisions regarding repair techniques. Successful cleft palate repair requires adequate muscular reconstruction of the velum to create a dynamic and functional soft palate. The two-flap and Furlow palatoplasties both reconstruct the velar musculature (i.e., the levator veli palatine or palatopharyngeus) into a dynamic sling but do so in different manners.

One criticism of the Furlow technique relates to the higher fistula rates found in many studies when compared to two-flap techniques. Fistula rates reported in the literature are infamous for reporting bias, differing definitions and classifications of fistulas, and faulty study design. This makes meaningful comparisons nearly impossible, and a number of authors have recommended strategies to decrease fistula rates—particularly with the Furlow technique. The placement of acellular dermis between the oral and nasal flaps is recommended by some, and this has shown a significant reduction in fistula rates comparable to two-flap closures.[48,49,50] Some recent reviews of fistula formation after two-flap palatoplasty revealed low rates of 3%.[51,52] Helling reported a fistula rate of 3.2% when acellular dermis was used in conjunction with the Furlow technique.[50]

The speech outcome data for Furlow palatoplasty technique compared against the two-flap techniques has generally been favorable. Multiple authors have reported their own improved speech results and low

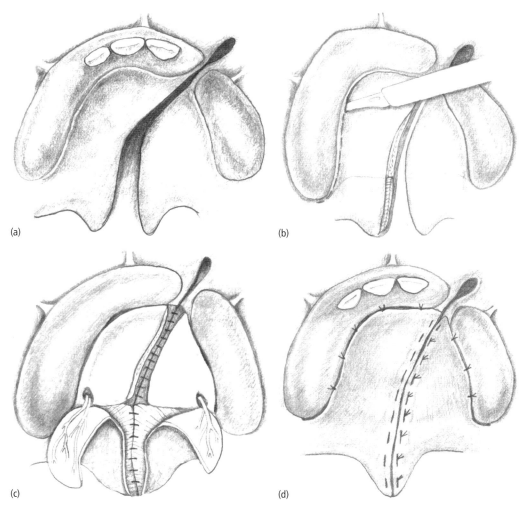

(a)

(b)

(c)

(d)

Fig. 8.7. (a) Unilateral cleft of the primary and secondary palates is shown with the typical involvement from the anterior vestibule to the uvula. (b) The Bardach palatoplasty technique requires two large, full-thickness mucoperiosteal flaps to be elevated from each palate shelf. The anterior portion (anterior to the incisive foramen) of the cleft is not reconstructed until the mixed dentition stage. (c) A layered closure is performed in the Bardach palatoplasty by reapproximating the nasal mucosa. The muscle bellies of the levator palatini are elevated off their abnormal insertions on the posterior palate. They are then reapproximated in the midline to create a dynamic functional sling for speech purposes. (d) Once the nasal mucosa and musculature of the soft palate are approximated, the oral mucosa is closed in the midline. The lateral releasing incisions are quite easily closed primarily because of the length gained from the depth of the palate. In rare cases, in very wide clefts a portion of the lateral incisions may remain open and granulate by secondary intention. (From Fig. 35-12 A–D: Fonseca RJ, ed. 2009. *Oral and Maxillofacial Surgery*, Vol. III. St. Louis: Saunders Elsevier, p. 729.)

rates of VPI with Furlow versus various modifications of two-flap palatoplasties.[46,53–56] These studies consist of single surgeon/center experience prior to and after adoption of the Furlow technique. While compelling, these data represent level III evidence and have not had the statistical power to convincingly provide a wave of change in the surgical community. Despite flaws in the study designs, the reduction in reported rates of VPI is impressive. Randall reported a decrease in VPI from 68% to 25% after instituting the Furlow technique.[57] Williams reports a VPI rate of 13% with the Furlow and 25% with von Langenbeck palatoplasties.[55] A small number of uncontrolled studies have reported no significant difference in speech or VPI outcomes between the Furlow and Veau-Wardill-Kilner or von Langenbeck techniques.[58,59] A study conducted at the University of Florida and Sao Paolo, Brazil, sought to compare outcomes of the Furlow and von Langenbeck

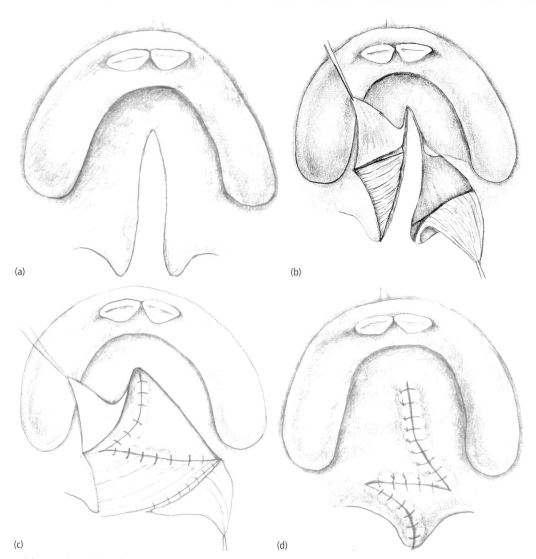

(a)

(b)

(c)

(d)

Fig. 8.8. (a) Complete cleft of the secondary palate (both hard and soft) is shown from the incisive foramen to the uvula. (b) The Furlow double-opposing Z-plasty technique requires that separate Z-plasty flaps be developed on the oral and then nasal side. Note the cutbacks creating the nasal side flaps, highlighted in blue. (c) The flaps are then transposed to theoretically lengthen the soft palate. A nasal side closure is completed in the standard fashion anterior to the junction of the hard and soft palate. In general, this junction is the highest area of tension and can be difficult to close. This contributes to the higher fistula rate in this type of repair at this location. (d) The oral side flaps are then transposed and closed in a similar fashion, completing the palate closure. (From Fig. 35-13: Fonseca 2009, Vol. III, p. 730.)

palatoplasties. The results are unpublished but preliminary findings presented in abstract form have suggested only minor differences in outcome with the exceptions that the Furlow group has a higher fistula rate and the von Langenbeck procedure with increased measurements of hypernasality as only one element of a comprehensive speech evaluation.[60] The available published data have been either weak level II or level III evidence, and as such they are difficult to utilize when deciding between repair techniques. As a result, the data at this time are not convincing enough to advocate the Furlow over the two-flap palatoplasties. As evidenced by the available literature, good results can be obtained with either two-flap or double-opposing Z-plasty techniques.

Perioperative Complications of Cleft Palate Repair

Perioperative complications associated with palatoplasty for cleft palate are generally rare. Experienced surgeons routinely obtain superior results with a variety of standardized techniques. Complications associated with the surgical procedure in the perioperative period include bleeding, airway compromise, infection, and vascular compromise of the flaps. Fistulas may be seen early after repair and are discussed in a separate section below.

Bleeding occurs with the palatoplasty procedure due to the rich vascular supply of the local soft tissue and bone. Since most patients undergo palatoplasty between the ages of 9 and 18 months, their blood volumes are fairly small. Diligent control of bleeding is important to limit the blood loss during the procedure. While it is rare to require transfusion after palatoplasty, those children who have palatoplasties at a young age and that involve the hard and soft palate will have significantly higher transfusion requirements. This requires careful attention with volume status assessments, and occasionally an evaluation of the patient's red blood cell mass intraoperatively and/or postoperatively. Bipolar electrocautery is recommended to avoid conduction of the current down an axial flap and to allow for precise coagulation. Preservation of the greater palatine vasculature is important to avoid vascular compromise of the flaps. Reexploration is quite rare at less than 1%.[61]

Airway compromise can occur at multiple time points associated with the procedure. While many patients can be visualized during intubation with a simple direct laryngoscopy, others require more specialized techniques. Careful planning should be a part of the preoperative process, including the readiness of specialized airway equipment for the difficult airway. Intraoperative loss of the airway is uncommon but can be related to positioning of the endotracheal tube, tape failure, displacement of the mouth gag/retractor, or placement and removal of an oral–gastric suction tube at the end of the procedure. Postoperative airway compromise may occur with extended periods of retractor activation. The tongue should be allowed to revascularize and empty the venous pooling on a regular basis throughout the procedure. If this is not done properly, the result is often a swollen tongue that impedes normal respiration and may compromise the patient's airway significantly either in the postoperative recovery unit or on the floor. Swelling is limited with regular release of the retraction device for several minutes. Placement of a tongue stitch can be helpful in managing the airway during the first postoperative day. The overall incidence of postoperative airway compromise is generally less than 2%.[61]

Infection is an unusual complication but can occur with compromise of the vascular supply of the flaps or with grafted material such as interpositional grafts of freeze-dried dermis. Infection of grafted material occurs more frequently when the material becomes exposed. These materials do best when completely submerged. It is generally recommended to use the thinnest material possible such that it can be integrated quickly, with less of a chance for extrusion or exposure.

Management of Palatal Fistulas

Unfortunately, residual palatal fistulas are occasionally encountered after the initial palate repair. The risk of fistula formation seems to be associated with the size of the original cleft defect and the experience of the surgeon.[62,63] As mentioned above, the type of repair used may also affect the fistula rate. The two-flap palatoplasty technique is typically associated with the lowest rate of palatal fistula formation,[1] while the Furlow double-opposing Z-plasty, is, in most studies, associated with a higher incidence of oronasal fistula.[64] The most common location of residual palatal fistula occurrence after cleft palate repair is the junction of the hard and soft palates. This is followed by the anterior hard palate and incisive foramen region.[64–66] The incidence of palatal fistula after single-stage palatoplasty varies greatly, with the reported rates from zero to higher than 60%.[1,63–67]

Before deciding on a specific management approach to the residual fistula, it is important to define the clinical situation based on the patient's age, previous surgical history, and exact location of the fistula. The goals of cleft palate repair during infancy are twofold: first, to establish complete "watertight" closure of the secondary palate for separation of the oral and nasal cavities, and, second, to repair the levator musculature in order to allow for optimal speech production. Repair of the skeletal maxillary alveolar cleft defect and its associated oronasal communication is not generally attempted at this stage. Many surgeons consider this alveolar defect part of the original cleft deformity that has been purposely left and therefore not a true fistula. Definitive repair of the anterior alveolar aspect of the cleft (or nasolabial fistula) is instead incorporated into the bone graft reconstruction performed during mid-childhood based on dental development.[1,64–69] Ideally, a child with a complete cleft palate will undergo palate repair (successful closure of the hard and soft palates) during infancy, followed by bone graft reconstruction of the maxilla and alveolus (or primary palate) with closure of the residual nasolabial fistula during childhood.

Most fistulas are noted early in the postsurgical period after palate repair. These are the direct result of local wound breakdown secondary to tension, vascular compromise, wound healing problems, or other factors. Another time period when a palatal fistula may be encountered is during phase I (before bone graft) orthodontic treatment, especially if maxillary expansion is undertaken. There is disagreement about the causal relationship of orthodontic expansion and development of palatal fistula. Most experienced cleft surgeons believe that fistula defects discovered during maxillary expansion are small, preexisting oronasal communications and are not caused by orthodontic treatment. Small fistulas present since infancy can be hidden within a narrow palate by collapsed maxillary segments and then become "uncovered" as the maxillary arch form is expanded by orthodontic or orthopedic means. Most are not major functional concerns, and can be addressed at the time of bone grafting.

The recommended timing of fistula closure may vary significantly and remains a controversial topic. Some surgeons and cleft teams may advocate aggressive management with early closure of any fistula present after initial palate repair. We prefer to take a more long-range view of these problems and delay surgery for several years when possible (no functional speech and/or feeding-related issues). In infants, the closure of a small (up to 4 mm), nonfunctional fistula can generally be deferred until later in childhood. In such cases fistula repair may be incorporated into future procedures such as pharyngeal surgery for VPI or bone graft reconstruction of the cleft maxilla and alveolus.

When a larger (>5 mm) fistula is present, there is a greater likelihood that functional concerns will be encountered, such as nasal air escape affecting speech, nasal reflux of food and liquids, and hygiene difficulties. When significant functional issues exist, earlier closure of the persistent fistula is indicated. As part of the decision-making process, surgeons must weigh the benefits of fistula repair against the negative effects of a second palatal surgery (involving stripping of mucoperiosteum) on maxillary growth.

Operative Techniques for Closure of Palatal Fistulas

Repair of residual palatal fistulas using a number of different techniques after cleft palate repair has been described.[1,64–72] Current techniques used for fistula repair include local palatal flaps, modifications of the von Langenbeck and two-flap palatoplasty techniques, palatoplasty with incorporation of a pharyngeal flap, and the use of a tongue flap. Other regional flaps, including the buccal mucosal, buccinator myomucosal, temporalis muscle, and vascularized tissue transfers are less frequently used but have been described.[70,73–77] Recently, the use of an acellular dermal matrix as an interpositional barrier has been used as an adjunct to repairing fistulas.[49,50]

One of the most frequently described procedures for closure of residual fistulas is the use of local soft tissue flaps created within the palatal mucosa and rotated over the defect for closure. The components of this approach are the creation of turnover flaps around the defect for nasal side closure, elevation of a palatal finger flap, and rotation of the flap for coverage of the defect. A significant area of exposed bone is left at the donor site, and this is allowed to heal by secondary intention. Unfortunately, this type of repair is useful only for very small palatal defects and is associated with a relatively high failure rate.[70] Small rotational flaps within palatal tissues that contain extensive scarring from prior surgical procedures are difficult to mobilize without residual tension and may have diminished blood supply, resulting in a less-than-ideal healing capacity and a potentially greater chance of wound breakdown. Our preferred approach to residual palatal fistulas involves the modification of one of the primary palate repair techniques, namely the Bardach (two-flap) or von Langenbeck procedure in conjunction with the use of acellular dermal matrix as an interpositional graft material.[1,64,78] These approaches allow adequate coverage of even large defects with the use of bulky soft tissue flaps, a layered repair of the nasal and oral sides, and a tension-free line of closure. In addition, the amount of bone that is left exposed after the repair is minimal to none. This is because the vertical depth of the palatal vault translates into soft tissue extension medially, and the result is palatal soft tissue flaps that adequately cover the underlying bone with a layer of dead space between the palatal shelves and the oral mucosa lining. The Bardach (two-flap) palatoplasty is our preferred operation in cases in which the fistula defect is 5 mm or larger. The primary advantage of this approach is the ability to raise large soft tissue flaps, which can be mobilized easily and allow for visualization and tension-free closure of the nasal mucosa. By comparison, one of the theoretical advantages of the von Langenbeck procedure is the creation of bipedicled flaps that maintain anterior and posterior blood supplies. Although the anterior pedicles do provide additional perfusion, they also result in less freely movable flaps with limited access and visualization of the nasal side tissues. For this reason we use the von Langenbeck technique only for relatively small defects within the hard palate. When there is a much larger (>1.5 cm) defect, successful closure may dictate that the surgeon recruit additional soft tissue using a regional flap.

Fistula defects within the posterior hard palate or soft palate may be addressed with the use of a modified palatoplasty procedure, as described earlier, in combination with a superiorly based pharyngeal flap. After the palatal flaps are developed and the nasal side dissection is complete, a pharyngeal flap is harvested. The pharyngeal flap soft tissue is then incorporated into the nasal side closure of the area where the fistula was present. With this technique a substantial amount of additional soft tissue can be recruited for tension-free repair of a large palatal defect. When the fistula is located within the anterior two-thirds of the hard palate and cannot be closed using local tissue with an acellular dermal matrix interposed, then the procedure of choice for recruitment of additional soft tissue may be the anteriorly based dorsal tongue flap. First, the nasal side closure of the palatal defect is performed using turnover flaps with multiple interrupted sutures. Next, this technique calls for development of an anteriorly based tongue flap that is approximately 5 cm in length by one- to two-thirds the width of the tongue. The tongue flap is elevated along the underlying musculature and then inset using multiple mattress sutures for closure of the oral side. The recipient bed within the tongue is closed primarily. After the initial surgery, the tongue flap is allowed to heal and primarily vascularize for approximately 2 weeks. After this time the patient is returned to the operating room. Nasal fiberoptic intubation may be indicated for the second-stage procedure because the tongue is still sutured to the palate, restricting normal visualization of the airway. The flap is sectioned and the stump at the donor site is freshened and inset. The use of laterally or posteriorly based tongue flaps has also been presented in the literature.[79,80] In our opinion an anteriorly based flap is better tolerated by most patients and allows for the greatest degree of tongue mobility, decreasing the risk of tearing the flap from its palatal insertion.

Growth After Palatoplasty

Growth outcome is a major area of study in cleft lip and palate care, and an important long-term outcome variable. Outcomes traditionally measured include degree of maxillary horizontal and vertical retrusion, transverse arch restriction, and occlusion. It is generally accepted that the surgical repair (and resultant scarring) of the palate, lip, and other interventions in cleft correction contribute greatly to midface growth restriction. Ross has demonstrated that the final facial form is a result of treatment effects, inherent growth potential and features specific to each deformity.[1,35,53,81–85] He also concluded that surgeons performing the same repairs can have significantly different growth outcomes. With such an integrated mechanism complicated by the myriad of surgical variables growth inhibition continues to be an area of controversy. Among dozens of studies, a minority based their results on a series of consecutively treated patients (e.g., longitudinal analysis). Many of these have related maxillary growth deficiency in adolescents with a decreased SNA (sella-nasion-A point) (an average of 4.5 degrees) compared to noncleft controls.[86,87,88] In order to improve growth outcomes centers have attempted delayed hard palate closure with conflicting results, increased fistula rates, and poor speech outcomes in the short term. A major advantage stated for two-stage repairs is the narrowing of the hard palate cleft after primary veloplasty.[1,21] The reduced defect size then allows for closure later on the growth curve with smaller flaps and presumably less of a negative effect on future growth. Excellent growth results have been reported with this technique.[89,90] However, one-stage palate repair remains the most common protocol in North America. It is well described that scarring of the hard palatal tissues is associated with maxillary growth inhibition.[91] Techniques that minimize the degree of palatal scarring are considered beneficial to overall maxillary growth. In contrast, the pushback palatoplasties leave areas of the anterior hard palate denuded to heal by secondary intention with resultant scarring. Multiple studies have reported greater growth impairment secondary these techniques versus the von Langenbeck palatoplasty with some centers abandoning the push-back for that reason.[35,47,81–85,92]

Whatever the etiology of hypoplastic maxillae, a significant cohort of treated cleft lip and palate patients will require maxillary advancement surgery. The frequency in which Le Fort I surgery is required in the cleft population has a wide range depending on the subgroup treated. A retrospective cohort study of a heterogeneous cleft population by Good and colleagues found an overall need for maxillary advancement of 20.9%. When subgroups were considered, they found a range of 0.0% to 47.7%; no patient with isolated clefting of the lip or secondary palate required Le Fort I advancement, but 47.7% of those with cleft lip and palate required an osteotomy.[93] Posnick states that rates of maxillary advancement range from 25% to 75% in a cleft population depending on the criteria applied.[94] The evidence available on this topic is level III in nature and often does not control for cleft type or the surgical variables. In order to reduce the need for maxillary advancement, consistent team care with a minimum number of surgical procedures and timely orthodontic intervention has been advocated.[95] With roughly one-quarter of the cleft population requiring this additional surgical intervention, growth needs to remain an area of active investigation. More importantly, the concepts of how to potentially alter the current protocols based on the available level III evidence remains a mystery. Given the multiple variables we assess in the long-term outcome of patients with clefts, larger studies are necessary to strongly advocate for one protocol over another.

Management of Velopharyngeal Dysfunction

The exact cause of VPI after "successful" cleft palate repair is a complex problem that remains difficult to define and quantify. Inadequate surgical repair of the musculature is one potential cause of VPI. The role of postsurgical scarring and its impact on muscle function and palatal motion is poorly understood. The theoretic advantages of using a double-opposing Z-plasty procedure for the initial palate repair include better realignment of the palatal muscles and lengthening of the soft palate. These benefits may be negatively balanced by a velum that demonstrates less mobility secondary to scarring associated with two separate Z-plasty incisions. Even muscles that are appropriately realigned and reconstructed may fail to heal normally and function properly because of congenital defects having to do with their innervation. In addition, a repaired cleft palate is only one factor contributing to velopharyngeal function. Nasal airway dynamics and abnormalities related to vocal tract morphology and lateral and posterior pharyngeal wall motion may contribute to velopharyngeal dysfunction. Certainly, these other structures may also play a positive role in compensating for palatal deformity. For example, a short, scarred soft palate that does not elevate very well may be compensated for by recruitment and hypertrophy of muscular tissue within the posterior pharyngeal wall (e.g., activation of Passavant's ridge).[96–99]

A variable number of children with VPI after palatoplasty will go on to require management involving additional palatal and pharyngeal surgery.[25] The percentage is variable and not universally agreed upon, but generally it is 20% to 40% for nonsyndromic patients. Patients with syndromes do have higher rates of VPI, but these are often due to other contributing factors such as cognitive status or neural innervation. Other studies claim much lower rates of VPI, but the measurement and reporting is not uniform or validated in these published studies. Without a truly objective measure of speech in this patient population, it is difficult to know the true incidence of VPI after repair.

Secondary palatal surgery in young children is indicated when VPI causes hypernasal speech on a consistent basis and is related to a defined anatomic problem.[100–103] The timing of surgery for VPI remains controversial. Recommendations typically range from 3 to 5 years of age. In young children, obtaining enough diagnostic information to make a definitive decision regarding treatment is often difficult. In such a young age group, variables such as the child's language and articulation development and a lack of compliance during the speech evaluation compromise the diagnostic accuracy of preoperative assessments.[104–106]

By the time a child reaches 5 years of age, compliance with nasopharyngoscopy is better, and there is enough language development to allow for a more thorough perceptual speech evaluation. These factors allow for more definitive conclusions regarding the status of velopharyngeal function or dysfunction in the child with a repaired cleft palate. It is also important to note that decisions regarding advisability of surgery for VPI are usually made after close collaboration with an experienced speech and language pathologist. The surgeon and speech pathologist should make this decision together and try to tailor the treatment to that particular child's needs.

VPI and hypernasal speech may also be encountered in older patients at the time of orthognathic surgery for treatment of cleft-related maxillary deformity.[107] This usually involves midface advancement at the Le Fort I level with or without mandibular surgery to restore skeletal proportions, treat malocclusion, and improve facial balance. Advancements of the maxilla in patients with a repaired cleft palate may worsen existing VPI or may be the cause of new-onset VPI.[107–110] A minority of patients with borderline velopharyngeal closure preoperatively will develop hypernasal speech even after relatively small degrees of maxillary advancement. Because predicting exactly how each patient will respond to maxillary advancement is difficult, formal speech assessment and detailed counseling of the patient and family regarding the possibility for development of postoperative VPI before any cleft orthognathic surgery is undertaken is recommended. Fortunately, most patients who develop VPI after maxillary advancement will recover adequate velopharyngeal closure without the need for additional palatal surgery within approximately 6 months of the orthognathic procedure.

In a study by Turvey and Frost, pressure-flow studies were used to examine velopharyngeal function after maxillary advancement in patients with repaired cleft palate.[111] In their study group, patients with adequate velopharyngeal closure before surgery demonstrated three differing responses after midfacial advancement: (1) adequate velopharyngeal closure after surgery, (2) deterioration with inadequate velopharyngeal function after surgery followed by a gradual improvement and recovery of normal closure over a 6-month period, and (3) inadequate velopharyngeal closure after surgery without improvement, necessitating pharyngeal flap surgery. It is important to note that no significant difference has been convincingly documented when one looks at the speech outcomes after use of distraction osteogenesis techniques for midface advancement and conventional orthognathic surgery.

Operative Techniques for Treatment of VPI

Contemporary surgical management of VPI generally involves one of three types of procedures: (1) the superiorly based pharyngeal flap, (2) the sphincter pharyngoplasty, and (3) palate re-repair. The use of autogenous and alloplastic implants for augmentation of the posterior pharyngeal wall has been described but is not a commonly used procedure today. The superiorly based pharyngeal flap remains the standard approach for surgical management of VPI after palate repair. The procedure was initially described by Schoenborn in 1876.[112–114] Surgical maneuvers are directed at recruiting tissue by developing a superiorly based soft tissue flap from the posterior pharyngeal wall (Fig. 8.9). The soft palate is then divided along midsagittal plane from the junction of the hard and soft palates to the uvula, and the flap from the posterior pharyngeal wall is inset within the nasal layer of the soft palate. As a result, a large nasopharyngeal opening that cannot be completely closed by the patient's velopharyngeal mechanism is converted into two (right and left) lateral pharyngeal ports. Closure of these ports is easier for the patient to accomplish as long as adequate lateral pharyngeal wall motion is present. When randomly applied to patients with VPI, the superiorly based pharyngeal flap procedure is effective 80% of the time.[1,115] When the flap is applied using careful preoperative objective evaluations, success rates as high as 95–97% have been reported.[116,117] Shprintzen and colleagues have advocated custom tailoring of the pharyngeal flap width and position based on the particular characteristics of each patient as seen on nasopharyngoscopy.[115,118] The high overall success rate and the flexibility to design the dimensions and position of the flap itself are advantages of the superiorly based pharyngeal flap procedure. The disadvantages of the pharyngeal flap procedure are primarily related to the possibility of nasal obstruction resulting in mucous trapping and postoperative obstructive sleep apnea (OSA).

The dynamic sphincter pharyngoplasty is another option for the surgical management of VPI. This procedure was described by Hynes in 1951 and since has been modified by a number of other authors.[119–124] The operative procedure involves the creation of two superiorly based myomucosal flaps created within each posterior tonsillar pillar (Fig. 8.10). Each flap is elevated, with care taken to include as much of the palatopharyngeal muscle as possible. The flaps are then attached and inset within a horizontal incision made high on the posterior pharyngeal wall. The goal of this procedure is the creation of a single nasopharyngeal port (instead of the two ports of the superiorly based pharyngeal flap) that has a contractile ridge posteriorly to improve velopharyngeal valve function. The main advantage of the sphincter pharyngoplasty over the superiorly based flap is the perceived lower rate of complications related to nasal airway obstruction as described earlier.[1,125–127] Despite this perceived advantage, there is no evidence that

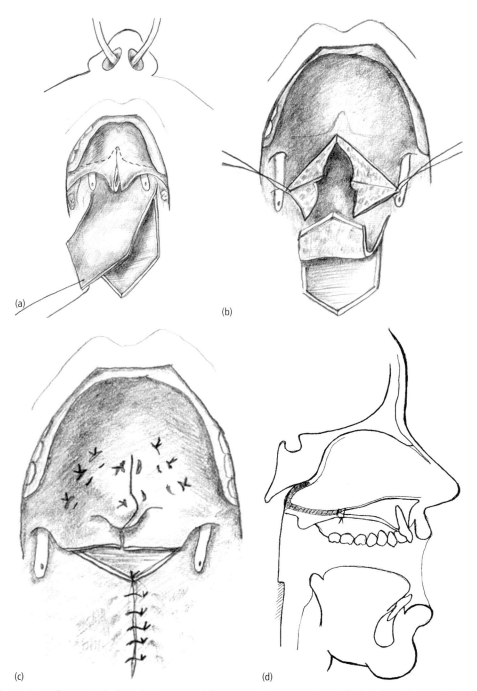

Fig. 8.9. Illustration of superiorly based pharyngeal flap operative procedure. (a) Creation of superiorly based flap of posterior pharyngeal wall soft tissues. The pharyngeal flap is developed and elevated off the prevertebral fascia. The soft palate is divided with a midline incision from the uvula to the junction of the hard and soft palates. (b) Soft palate oral, nasal, and muscle layer dissection in preparation for flap inset. Nasopharyngeal airways are placed in order to help size each lateral pharyngeal port. (c) The flap is sutured into the nasal side of the soft palate before the nasal side is repaired and the oral mucosa and underlying musculature are repaired. (d) Sagittal view demonstrating appropriate vertical level of flap inset. (From Fig. 42-5: Fonesca 2009, Vol. III, p. 838.)

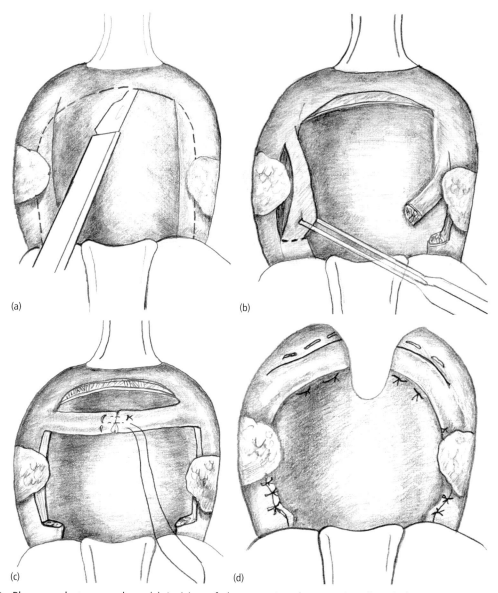

(a)

(b)

(c)

(d)

Fig. 8.10. Pharyngoplasty procedure. (a) Incision of the posterior pharyngeal wall and the posterior tonsillar pillars. (b) Elevation of bilateral myomucosal flaps within the tonsillar pillars. Care is taken to include palatopharyngeus muscle. (c) The mobilized flaps are then sutured to each other at the midline. (d) Closure is then achieved by insetting the joined flaps within the posterior pharyngeal wall incision. The donor site of each flap is also closed with interrupted sutures. (From Fig. 42-6: Fonesca 2009, Vol. III, p. 839.)

pharyngoplasty procedures achieve superior outcomes in the resolution of VPI. Also, the use of a sphincter pharyngoplasty technique may be associated with increased scarring along the tonsillar pillar region. Some advocate its use to avoid the uncommon complication of OSA, but little data exist examining the true incidence of this complication.

Some surgeons advocate the use of a revision palatoplasty or re-repair instead of a pharyngeal flap or pharyngoplasty procedure in the management of patients with VPI after cleft palate repair in infancy.[128] Some initial experience has shown this to be effective in a select group of patients who may have had incomplete or less aggressive muscular repairs. The technique can be performed using either a double-opposing Z-plasty or a two-flap palatoplasty with radical retropositioning of the levator musculature. Unfortunately, the anticipated benefits of these second palatoplasties have not, as of yet, been objectively established. The clinician must consider the disadvantages of this type of surgical procedure and weigh them against potential benefits. The double-opposing Z-plasty procedure requires a more aggressive dismantling of the palate than what is required during a conventional pharyngeal flap procedure. The result may be a slightly longer palate but one with more extensive scarring and less physiologic movement. Another consideration is the significantly higher rate of fistula formation associated with this type of repair. This can be alleviated with the use of an acellular dermal matrix as an interpositional graft material.

Complications Related to Surgical Procedures for VPI

Surgery involving airway structures is associated with the potential for complications related to postoperative hemorrhage and edema. As a result, patients who undergo attachment of a pharyngeal flap benefit from admission to the surgical intensive care unit or other observation setting with continuous airway monitoring during the first day after surgery. This type of setting permits the rapid recognition and prompt management of any complication that may lead to airway compromise. Of all the procedures related to cleft care, the pharyngeal flap and sphincteroplasty operations carry the greatest risk for early airway compromise. Airway compromise is not common but requires swift management in order to avoid life-threatening consequences. Long-term postoperative complications related to the superiorly based pharyngeal flap for correction of VPI are frequently associated with problems related to increased airway resistance. Insertion of a pharyngeal flap is designed to decrease the size of the nasopharyngeal airway, facilitate velopharyngeal closure, decrease nasal air escape, and make speech more intelligible. At the same time, the procedure may create a pathologic level of upper airway obstruction that leads to new problems. Patients who undergo pharyngeal flap surgery may start snoring. Snoring itself does not represent any significant pathophysiology but may concern parents or significant others who observe the patient during sleep. When the degree of upper airway resistance is more severe, the result may be postoperative OSA. OSA is defined as cessation of breathing during sleep secondary to upper airway obstruction. OSA disrupts the sleep cycle, compromises effective oxygenation, and can cause behavioral changes and daytime somnolence in affected individuals. Left untreated, OSA is associated with cardiac and pulmonary consequences. When OSA is suspected in a child who has previously undergone a pharyngeal flap procedure, a formal workup including nasopharyngoscopy and a sleep study (polysomnography) is indicated. Care should be taken to evaluate the entire airway in order to determine the level of the obstruction. Often, a thorough clinical evaluation yields abnormal findings that contribute to the problem of OSA at multiple levels of the upper airway. Because of the potential complexity of the clinical problem, the decision to modify or take down a pharyngeal flap in a child with OSA must be made only after discussions among the surgeon, sleep specialist (e.g., pediatric otolaryngologist, neurologist, or pulmonologist), and speech and language pathologist. Of interest, many patients who have had pharyngeal flap placement during childhood will tolerate surgical division of the flap without a recurrence of severe VPI or hypernasal speech. On the rare occasion when VPI does recur after flap takedown, interval treatment with a prosthetic device such as a palatal lift appliance for a minimum of 6 months should be considered before one embarks on any further palatal surgery. Palate re-repair may be an option in this patient population, but the incidence of sleep apnea after this procedure versus others is not documented convincingly as of yet.

COMPLICATIONS OF CRANIOFACIAL SURGERY

This section will focus on the particular complications encountered in transcranial procedures. The types of complications seen are similar to those seen in other types of craniomaxillofacial procedures such as orthognathic surgery. However, there are a number of particular concerns in the cranio-orbital region that require special attention. A particular emphasis on infant and pediatric congenital procedures is presented due to the high risk associated with these procedures.

Intraoperative Complications of Craniofacial Surgery

Craniofacial surgeons are afforded significant latitude and can expect fairly predictable healing because of the rich blood supply of the region. However, this rich blood supply also can be problematic, as significant bleeding can be seen in craniofacial procedures and must be managed quickly, particularly in children with small blood volumes.[129–131] While there are many factors involved, the technique utilized can have a significant impact on the volume of blood loss. A coronal flap is often associated with significant bleeding because of the rich blood supply within the scalp and the vascular supply to the periosteum through the bone. Dissection superficial to the periosteal plane (e.g., superficial to the pericranium) significantly decreases blood loss. Additionally, it also allows for a large pericranial flap to be raised at the last portion of the flap elevation simplifying meticulous hemostasis. Bone wax, gel foam with thrombin, and other local measures can be utilized to address small bleeding areas of bone while elevating the flap from posterior to anterior, improving hemostasis. The amount of bleeding seen is often more severe with increased intracranial pressure. Even with the best of hemostasis measures and blood conservation measures such as the use of a cellular blood reprocessing machine, over 80% of infant patients who undergo cranial vault surgery will require transfusion.

Additional bleeding can be seen with the craniotomy from the diploic space, dura, and sagittal or sigmoid sinuses. Bleeding along the osteotomy sites can be controlled with bone wax. Sagittal sinus or sigmoid sinus bleeding is a serious complication that requires immediate hemostatic control. Direct suturing of the vessel is often performed. Significant blood loss can be encountered and requires an aggressive approach to resuscitation. Additionally, late effects including intraluminal clotting of the sinus can propagate thrombosis or altered flow of the sinus that can lead to serious neurologic complications including death.[132]

Significant bleeding is also seen during the closure phase of the operation whether clip appliances are used or not. As the flap is turned back for closure, additional bleeding is seen and should be addressed with local measures and quick closure techniques. The anesthesia team should be made aware of this potential, and experienced teams understand this risk. Planning for this blood loss avoids complications near the end of the procedure and prepares the patient for the best recovery in the intensive care unit.

In children, air embolism can be seen with flap elevation or craniotomies. These events are likely due to the rich supply of emissary vessels and venous lakes in the pediatric cranial vault and surrounding area.[133] Patients with a patent foramen ovale are at risk for aberrant travel of this air to the left heart chambers and passage to the cerebral circulation or to the coronary arteries, causing arrest. The outcomes are variable, but some patients who experience a large embolism that causes an effect on the cardiac or central nervous systems do not survive. While less significant venous air embolism occurs with some higher frequency, the event usually does not produce a life-threatening episode. This event contributes significantly to the 1% mortality rate seen in craniofacial procedures. Thankfully, the incidence is likely well under 1%.[134] This complication is in most instances unavoidable.

Electrolyte abnormalities can occur with the extensive fluid shifting that may occur with more complicated craniofacial reconstructions. As such, hyponatremia, hypokalemia, and acid–base imbalances are relatively common. Etiologies of the sodium abnormalities can include syndrome of inappropriate antidiuretic hormone, salt wasting, or aggressive crystalloid replacement. Electrolyte parameters should be monitored carefully and addressed in an expeditious manner to avoid large shifts in electrolytes. Replacement therapies are sometimes needed to address these abnormalities and avoid other complications such as cardiac instability, arrhythmias, or central effects. The central nervous system may be particularly sensitive to sodium shifts if they are rapid.[135]

Infection of the craniofacial bones or in the soft tissue flaps is rare.[136] A subperiosteal abscess is occasionally seen. More significant infections of the bone flaps are thankfully rare, but they do occur. Loss of bone segments occurs most often due to lack of blood supply in compromised areas such as those patients with significant acute soft tissue injury, radiation to the site, or scarred soft tissue from multiple procedures. Even the most biocompatible of implants can become infected and tend to do so in those instances that involve compromised tissue. Patients who have infections with collections should be cultured, particularly those with long histories of revision surgery or extensive hospital visits. The infection rate tends to be higher in those procedures that involve the sinuses such as the monobloc or bipartition osteotomies.[137] Intracranial infections are rare in congenital craniofacial procedures but are seen more commonly after the removal of neoplasms—particularly after adjuvant therapies. They are addressed aggressively with antibiotics and occasionally drainage procedures.

Sometimes, surgical incision sites can open at the scalp due to seroma, abscess formation, or inflammatory reactions. Most wounds of this type are addressed easily with local wound care measures. Occasionally, debridement and reclosure is needed, although most are managed with local measures. In these instances, every effort should be made to address these concerns with a tension-free closure. Allopecia will form in these areas if a large, hypertrophic scar band results due to the secondary intention healing. Excision and a local flap rotation can aid in limiting the area of alopecia once the site has healed for at least 6 months. At times, tissue expansion for recruitment of local tissue may be necessary to close larger defects.

Blindness is a rare complication of craniofacial surgery, but it has been seen with osteotomies that involve the orbit, distraction osteogenesis of the midface, and even in orthognathic procedures.[138,139] Intraoperative misadventure is a possible etiology, as is anatomic variation with unusual fracture patterns of the cranial base—particularly in syndromic or growing patients. An increased incidence of blindness is seen in patients with growing skeletons and syndromic patients with hypoplasia of the cranial base, orbits, and/or midface.[139] On rare occasions, bleeding in the posterior orbit at or near the palatine bone can cause a compressive neuropathy of the optic nerve. Intervention in an expeditious manner is important when this complication can be recognized early. Steroids and possible decompressive approaches to the optic nerve may be helpful depending upon the etiology. Navigation-assisted optic nerve decompression can be utilized by skilled practitioners to relieve pressure.

Cerebrospinal fluid leaks are sometimes encountered with severe cranial base fractures or extensive surgery at the cranial base. They are often limited by careful blockage of the cranial base with various materials including pericranial flaps, fibrin glue, dermal grafts, bone, fat, or others. However, leaks can still occur rarely despite the best intraoperative efforts. Patients can be given a lumbar drain, and precautions can be taken such as elevating the head to limit intracranial pressure. These maneuvers will allow small leaks to heal. Larger leaks can be addressed operatively with navigation-assisted patches from below, or open procedures to readdress the cranial base.[140]

Late Postoperative Complications of Craniofacial Surgery

Once initial healing has occurred, most complications that occur late are a consequence of nonviable tissue (poorly healed bone). For patients with substantial reconstructions of the cranio-orbital region, nonhealing bone segments are a relatively rare occurrence.[129–134] Smaller fragments may have difficulty healing, especially in compromised soft tissue beds. Defects smaller than 15 mm may not require reconstruction, and they pose little risk to the patient. However, even small defects in sensitive areas may present aesthetic concerns, such as the superorbital rim or frontal region. When areas of bone resorb, hardware may become more palpable or mobile. Inflammation may ensue, and removal of hardware may become necessary. Defects larger than 15 mm may require reconstruction with autogenous grafts, titanium mesh, or alloplastic materials. Current alloplasts are generally not recommended in compromised patients who have already failed a primary reconstruction. Titanium mesh is useful for small- to medium-size defects but still carries a lifetime infection risk (Fig. 8.11). Custom computer-aided design/computer-aided manufactured titanium implants are commonly used but have some of the same drawbacks. Regenerative techniques may provide additional options but are currently not approved for most craniofacial indications at this time.[141] Split thickness cranium or titanium mesh still provide the best and most-predictable solution to many cranial vault defects (Fig. 8.12).

Relapse of cranio-orbital advancements occurs occasionally, and it does so most often in instances of large advancements and/or patients with syndromes and poor bone quality. Good fixation is important for retention of advancements in the immediate postoperative time period. Late relapse occurs in patients who have earlier procedures during early phases of growth. Single suture craniosynostosis reconstructions have a reoperation rate of appropriately 5%, but certain dysmorphologies, such as more severe unicoronal synostosis, may predispose to higher rates of revision.[137,142] Syndromic craniosynostosis reconstructions have a higher revision rate, but often require additional procedures for other reasons than relapse (e.g., increased intracranial pressure). Nonetheless, understanding the limits of the soft tissue envelope and the quality of bone are important when deciding the amount of advancement of the frontal bandeau.

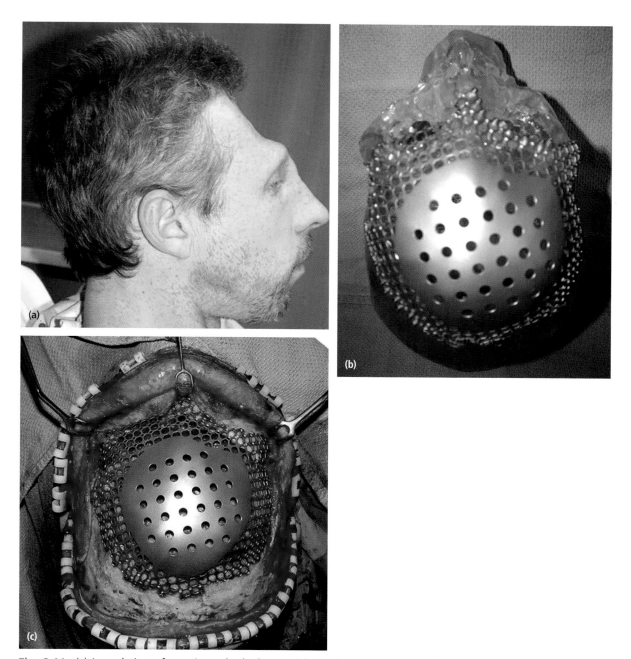

Fig. 8.11. (a) Lateral view of a patient who had an initial anterior cranial vault and bandeau reconstruction by another surgeon after blunt trauma from a baseball bat that became infected and was removed. He is missing his entire frontal bone and supraorbital ridge areas including nasion. (b) A custom titanium computer-aided design and computer-aided manufacturing prosthesis was made to replace the missing components using data from a detailed computed tomography scan and an SLA model. (c) The custom appliance in place, reconstructing the lost components. Unfortunately, this reconstruction carries a lifetime infection risk.

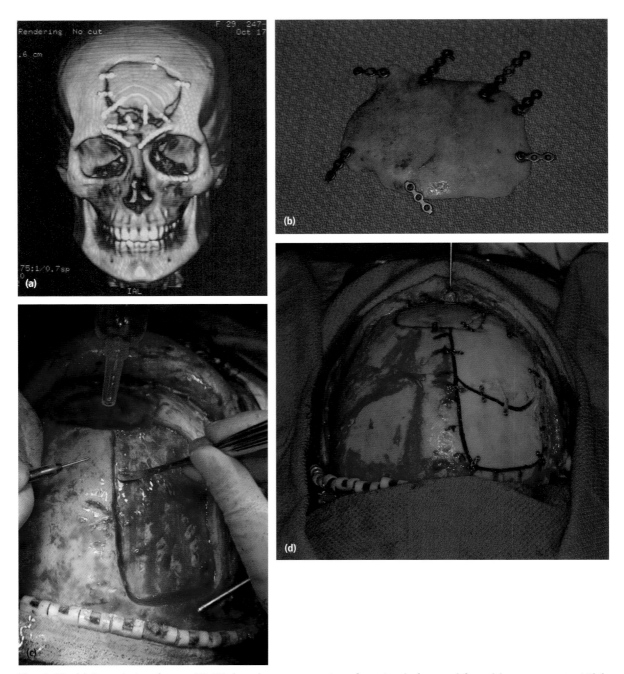

Fig. 8.12. (a) Frontal view from a 3D CT that shows a nonunion of previously fractured frontal bone segments. While nonunions are somewhat unusual, they occur more often when overlying soft tissue is injured severely as in this young woman who sustained severe trauma to the frontal bones from a falling piece of concrete from a bridge. Severe soft tissue injury including the pericranium likely contributed to the inability for this area to heal properly. (b) The nonunion segment is removed easily, and the dura is left intact. (c) The resultant defect is replaced with autogenous bone graft taken from the inner table of the adjacent temporal/parietal bones. (d) The defect is reconstructed with large rather than small pieces, and the outer table is returned to the graft site.

In general, cleft and craniofacial surgery is predictable and successful. A clear understanding of the nuances, optimal outcomes, and complications is important at the highest level in treating patients with these disorders. Management of complications and optimizing outcomes require an awareness of the possibility of these issues as well as the technical ability and experience to address them most effectively.

SUGGESTED READINGS

1. Campbell A, Costello BJ, and Ruiz RL. 2010. "Cleft lip and palate surgery: An update of clinical outcomes for primary repair." *Oral Maxillofac Surg Clin North Am* 22: 43–58.
2. Fillies T, Homann C, Meyer U, et al. 2007. "Perioperative complications in infant cleft repair." *Head Face Med* 3: 9.
3. Wilhelmsen HR, and Musgrave RH. 1966. "Complications of cleft lip surgery." *Cleft Palate J* 3: 223–231.
4. Al-Thunyan AM, Aldekhayel SA, Al-Meshal O, and Al-Qattan MM. 2009. "Ambulatory cleft lip repair." *Plast Reconstr Surg* 124: 2048–2053.
5. Eaton AC, Marsh JL, and Pilgram TK. 1994. "Does reduced hospital stay affect morbidity and mortality rates following cleft lip and palate repair in infancy?" *Plast Reconstr Surg* 94: 911–915; discussion 916–8.
6. Hopper RA, Lewis C, Umbdenstock R, Garrison MM, and Starr JR. 2009. "Discharge practices, readmission, and serious medical complications following primary cleft lip repair in 23 U.S. children's hospitals." *Plast Reconstr Surg* 123: 1553–1559.
7. Rosen H, Barrios LM, Reinisch JF, Macgill K, and Meara JG. 2003. "Outpatient cleft lip repair." *Plast Reconstr Surg* 112: 381–387; discussion 388–9.
8. Reinisch JF, and Sloan GM. 1990. "Secondary surgical treatment of cleft lip/nose." In: *Multidisciplinary Management of Cleft Lip and Palate*, Bardach J, and Huglett MH, eds. Philadelphia: WB Saunders.
9. Reinisch JF, Li W, and Urata M. 2009. "Complications of cleft lip and palate surgery." In: *Comprehensive Cleft Care*, Losee J, and Kirschner R, eds. New York: McGraw-Hill.
10. Schettler D. 1973. "Intra- and postoperative complications in surgical repair of clefts in infancy." *J Maxillofac Surg* 1: 40–44.
11. Chuo CB, and Timmons MJ. 2005. "The bacteriology of children before primary cleft lip and palate surgery." *Cleft Palate Craniofac J* 42: 272–276.
12. Tokioka K, Park S, Sugawara Y, and Nakatsuka T. 2009. "Video recording study of infants undergoing primary cheiloplasty: Are arm restraints really needed?" *Cleft Palate Craniofac J* 46: 494–497.
13. Wilson AD, and Mercer N. 2008. "Dermabond tissue adhesive versus Steri-Strips in unilateral cleft lip repair: An audit of infection and hypertrophic scar rates." *Cleft Palate Craniofac J* 45: 614–619.
14. Precious DS. 2000. "Unilateral cleft lip and palate." *Oral Maxillofac Surg Clin North Am* 12: 399–420.
15. Precious DS. 2009. "Primary bilateral cleft lip/nose repair using the 'Delaire' technique." *Atlas Oral Maxillofac Surg Clin North Am* 17: 137–146.
16. Precious DS. 2009. "Primary unilateral cleft lip/nose repair using the 'Delaire' technique." *Atlas Oral Maxillofac Surg Clin North Am* 17: 125–135.
17. Cutting C, and Grayson B. 1993. "The prolabial unwinding flap method for one-stage repair of bilateral cleft lip, nose, and alveolus." *Plast Reconstr Surg* 91: 37–47.
18. Cutting C, Grayson B, Brecht L, et al. 1998. "Presurgical columellar elongation and primary retrograde nasal reconstruction in one-stage bilateral cleft lip and nose repair." *Plast Reconstr Surg* 101: 630–639.
19. Mulliken JB. 2000. "Repair of bilateral complete cleft lip and nasal deformity–state of the art." *Cleft Palate Craniofac J* 37: 342–347.
20. Markus AF, Delaire J, and Smith WP. 1992. "Facial balance in cleft lip and palate. I. Normal development and cleft palate." *Br J Oral Maxillofac Surg* 30: 287–295.
21. Markus AF, Delaire J, and Smith WP. 1992. "Facial balance in cleft lip and palate. II. Cleft lip and palate and secondary deformities." *Br J Oral Maxillofac Surg* 30: 296–304.
22. Markus AF, and Delaire J. 1993. "Functional primary closure of cleft lip." *Br J Oral Maxillofac Surg* 31: 281–291.
23. Millard D. 1976. *Cleft Craft: The Evolution of its Surgery*. Boston: Little, Brown and Company.
24. Millard DR, Jr. 1958. "A radical rotation in single harelip." *Am J Surg* 95: 318–322.
25. Daya M. 2009. "Nostril stenosis corrected by release and serial stenting." *J Plast Reconstr Aesthet Surg* 62: 1012–1019.
26. Wolfe SA, Podda, S, and Mejia M. 2008. "Correction of nostril stenosis and alteration of nostril shape with an orthonostric device." *Plast Reconstr Surg* 121: 1974–1977.
27. Ziada HM, Gavin D, Allen P, et al. 2005. "Custom made alar stents for nostril stenosis: A 24-month evaluation." *Int J Oral Maxillofac Surg* 34: 605–611.
28. Kapucu MR, Gursu KG, Enacar A, and Aras S. 1996. "The effect of cleft lip repair on maxillary morphology in patients with unilateral complete cleft lip and palate." *Plast Reconstr Surg* 97: 1371–1375; discussion 1376–8.
29. Berkowitz S, Mejia M, and Bystrik A. 2004. "A comparison of the effects of the Latham-Millard procedure with those of a conservative treatment approach for dental occlusion and facial aesthetics in unilateral and bilateral complete cleft lip and palate: Part I. Dental occlusion." *Plast Reconstr Surg* 113: 1–18.
30. Berkowitz S, Duncan R, Evans C, et al. 2005. "Timing of cleft palate closure should be based on the ratio of the area of the cleft to that of the palatal segments and not on age alone." *Plast Reconstr Surg* 115: 1483–1499.

31. Rogers BO. 1964. "Hairlip repair in colonial America: A review of 18th century and earlier surgical techniques." *Plast Reconstr Surg* 34: 142–162.

32. LeMesurier AB. 1949. "Method of cutting and suturing lip in complete unilateral cleft lip." *Plast Reconstr Surg* 4: 1–12.

33. Khosla RK, Mabry K, and Castiglione CL. 2008. "Clinical outcomes of the Furlow Z-plasty for primary cleft palate repair." *Cleft Palate Craniofac J* 45(5): 501–510.

34. LaRossa D. 2000. "The state of the art in cleft palate surgery." *Cleft Palate Craniofac J* 37(3): 225–228.

35. Ross B. 1987. "Treatment variables affecting facial growth in complete unilateral cleft lip and palate. Part 7: An overview of treatment and facial growth." *Cleft Pal J* 24: 71–77.

36. Pantaloni M, and Hollier L. 2001. "Cleft palate and velopharyngeal incompetence." In: *Selected Readings in Plastic Surgery* 9(23): 1–36. Dallas, TX: University of Texas Southwestern.

37. Veau V. 1931. *Division Palantine*. Paris: Masson.

38. Kilner TP. 1937. "Cleft lip and palate repair technique." *St. Thomas Hosp Rep* 2: 127.

39. Wardill WFM. 1937. "The technique of operation for cleft palate." *Br J Surg* 25: 117.

40. Bardach J. 1995. "Two-flap palatoplasty: Bardach's technique." *Oper Tech Plast Reconstr Surg* 2: 211.

41. Salyer KE, Sng KW, and Sperry EE. 2006. "Two-flap palatoplasty: 20-year experience and evolution of a surgical technique." *Plast Reconstr Surg* 118: 193.

42. Furlow LT. "Cleft palate repair: preliminary report on lengthening and muscle transposition by Z-Plasty." Southeastern Society of Plastic and Reconstructive Surgeons, Boca Raton, FL, May 1978.

43. Furlow LT. 1995. "Cleft palate repair by double opposing z-plasty." *Oper Tech Plast Recon Surg* 2: 223.

44. Bardach J, Morris HL, LaRossa D, et al. 1990. "The Furlow double reversing Z-plasty for cleft palate repair: The first 10 years of experience." In: *Multidisciplinary Management of Cleft Lip and Palate*, Bardach J, and Huglett MH, eds. Philadelphia: WB Saunders.

45. Grobbelar AO, Hudson DA, Fernandes DB, and Lentin R. 1985. "Speech results after repair of the cleft soft palate." *Plast Reconstruct Surg* 95: 1150–1154.

46. Kirschner RE, Wang P, Jawad AF, et al. 1999. "Cleft palate repair by modified Furlow double opposing Z-plasty: The Childrens Hospital of Philadelphia experience." *Plast Reconstr Surg* 104: 1998–2010.

47. Pigott RW, Albery EH, Hathorn IS, et al. 2002. "A comparison of three methods of repairing the hard palate." *Cleft Palate Craniofac J* 39: 383–391.

48. Noorchashm N, Duda JR, Ford M, et al. 2006. "Conversion Furlow palatoplasty: Salvage of speech after straight-line palatoplasty and 'incomplete intravelar veloplasty.'" *Ann Plast Surg* 56: 505–510.

49. Seagle MB. 2006. "Palatal fistula repair using acellular dermal matrix: The University of Florida Experience." *Ann Plast Surg* 56: 50–53.

50. Helling ER, Dev VR, Garza J, et al. 2006. "Low fistula rate in palatal clefts closed with the Furlow technique using decellularized dermis." *PRS* 117(7): 2361–2365.

51. Wilhelmi BJ, Appelt EA, Hill L, et al. 2001. "Palatal fistulas: Rare with the two-flap palatoplasty repair." *Plast Reconstr Surg* 107(2): 315–318.

52. Schendel SA. 1999. "A single surgeon's experience with the Delaire palatoplasty." *Plast Reconstr Surg* 104(7): 1993–1997.

53. Ross RB. 1987. "Treatment variables affecting facial growth in complete unilateral cleft lip and palate. Part 2: Presurgical orthopedics." *Cleft Palate J* 24: 24.

54. Yu CC, Chen PK, and Chen YR. 2001. "Comparison of speech results after Furlow palatoplasty and von Langenbeck palatoplasty in incomplete cleft of the secondary palate." *Chang Gung Med J* 24: 628–632.

55. Williams WN, Seagle MB, Nackashi AJ, et al. 1998. "A methodology report of a randomized prospective trial to assess velopharyngeal function for speech following palatal surgery." *Control Clin Trials* 19: 297–312.

56. Gunther E, Wisser JR, Cohen MA, and Brown AS. 1998. "Palatoplasty: Furlow's double reversing z-plasty versus intravelar veloplasty" *CPCJ* 35(6): 546–549.

57. Randall P, La Rossa D, Solomon M, et al. 1986. "Experience with the Furlow double reversing z-plasty for cleft palate repair." *Plast Reconst Surg* 77: 569–576.

58. Brothers DB, Dalston RW, Peterson HD, and Lawrence WT. 1995. "Comparison of the Furlow double opposing z-plasty with the Wardill-Kilner procedure for isolated clefts of the soft palate." *Plast Reconstr Surg* 95(6): 969–977.

59. Spauwen PH, Goorhuis-Brouwer SM, and Schutte HK. 1992. "Cleft palate repair: Furlow versus von Langenbeck." *J Craniomaxillo Surg* 20(1): 18–20.

60. Seagle MB. Abstract presentation. American Cleft Palate-Craniofacial Association, 63rd Annual Meeting, 2006.

61. Moore MD, Lawrence WT, Ptak JJ, and Trier WC. Complications of primary palatoplasty: a twenty-one-year review." *Cleft Palate J* 25(2): 156–156.

62. Cohen SR, Kalinowski J, LaRossa D, and Randall P. 1991. "Cleft palate fistulas: A multivariate statistical analysis of prevalence, etiology, and surgical management." *Plast Reconstr Surg* 87: 1041–1047.

63. Ogle OE. 2002. "The management of oronasal fistulas in the cleft palate patient." *Oral Maxillofacial Surg Clin North Am* 14: 553–562.

64. Posnick JC. 2000. "The staging of cleft lip and palate reconstruction: Infancy through adolescence.": In: *Craniofacial and Maxillofacial Surgery in Children and Young Adults*, Posnick JC, ed. Philadelphia: WB Saunders.

65. Posnick JC, and Ruiz RL. 2002. "*Stages of cleft lip and palate reconstruction: Infancy through adolescence.*" In: *Cleft Lip and Palate: From Origin to Treatment*, Wyszynski DF, ed. New York: Oxford University Press.

66. Stal S, and Spira M. 1984. "Secondary reconstructive procedures for patients with clefts." In: *Pediatric Plastic Surgery*, Serafin D, and Georgiade NG, eds. St Louis: Mosby.

67. Wilhelmi BJ, Appelt EA, Hill L, and Blackwell SJ. 2001. "Palatal fistulas: Rare with the two-flap palatoplasty repair." *Plast Reconstr Surg* 107: 315–318.

68. Abyholm FE, Bergland O, and Semb G. 1981. "Secondary bone grafting of alveolar clefts." *Scand J Reconstr Surg* 15: 127.

69. Turvey TA, Vig K, Moriarty J, and Hoke J. 1984. "Delayed bone grafting in the cleft maxilla and palate: A retrospective multi-disciplinary analysis." *Am J Orthod* 86: 244–256.

70. Lehman JA. 1995. "Closure of palatal fistulas." *Oper Tech Plast Surg* 2: 255.

71. Schendel SA. 1992. "Secondary cleft surgery." *Select Read Oral Maxillofac Surg* 3: 1.

72. Posnick JC. 2000. "Cleft orthognathic surgery: The isolated cleft palate deformity." In: *Craniofacial and Maxillofacial Surgery in Children and Young Adults*, Posnick JC, ed. Philadelphia: WB Saunders.

73. Turvey TA, Vig KWL, and Fonseca RJ. 1996. "Maxillary advancement and contouring in the presence of cleft lip and palate." In *Facial Clefts and Craniosynostosis: Principles and Management*, Turvey TA, Vig KWL, and Fonseca RA, eds. Philadelphia: WB Saunders.

74. Posnick JC, and Ruiz RL. 2000. "[Invited discussion.] Repair of large anterior palatal fistulas using thin tongue flaps: Long-term follow-up of 10 patients." *Ann Plast Surg* 45: 114–117.

75. Bozola AR, and Ribeiro-Garcia ERB. 1995. "Partial buccinator myomucosal flap, posteriorly based." *Oper Tech Plast Surg* 2: 263–269.

76. Ninkovic M, Hubli EH, Schwabegger A, and Anderl H. 1997. "Free flap closure of recurrent palatal fistula in the cleft lip and palate patient." *J Craniofac Surg* 8: 491.

77. Posnick JC. 1997. "The treatment of secondary and residual dentofacial deformities in the cleft patient. Surgical and orthodontic treatment." *Clin Plast Surg* 24: 583–597.

78. Bardach J. 1995. "Two-flap palatoplasty: Bardach's technique." *Oper Tech Plast Surg* 2: 211–214.

79. Johnson PA, Banks P, and Brown AE. 1992. "Use of the posteriorly based lateral tongue flap in the repair of palatal fistula." *Int J Oral Maxillofac Surg* 23: 6–9.

80. Kinnebrew MC, and Malloy RB. 1983. "Posteriorly based, lateral lingual flaps for alveolar cleft bone graft coverage." *J Oral Maxillofac Surg* 41: 555–561.

81. Ross RB. 1987. "Treatment variables affecting facial growth in complete unilateral cleft lip and palate. Part 1: Treatment affecting growth." *Cleft Palate J* 24: 5.

82. Ross RB. 1987. "Treatment variables affecting facial growth in complete unilateral cleft lip and palate. Part 3: Alveolus Repair and bone grafting." *Cleft Palate J* 42: 33.

83. Ross RB. 1987. "Treatment variables affecting facial growth in complete unilateral cleft lip and palate. Part 4: Repair of the cleft lip." *Cleft Palate J* 42: 45.

84. Ross RB. 1987. "Treatment variables affecting facial growth in complete unilateral cleft lip and palate. Part 5: Timing of palate repair" *Cleft Palate J* 42: 54.

85. Ross RB. 1987. "Treatment variables affecting facial growth in complete unilateral cleft lip and palate. Part 6: Techniques of palate repair." *Cleft Palate J* 42: 64.

86. Fudalej P, Obloj B, Miller-Drabikowska D, et al. 2008. "Midfacial growth in a consecutive series of preadolescent children with complete unilateral cleft lip and palate following a one-stage simultaneous repair." *Cleft Palate Craniofac J* 45(6): 667–673.

87. Ozturk Y, and Cura N. 1996. "Examination of craniofacial morphology in children with unilateral cleft lip and palate." *Cleft Palate Craniofac J* 33: 32–36.

88. Savaci N, Hosnuter M, Tosun Z, and Demir A. 2005. "Maxillofacial morphology in children with complete unilateral cleft lip and palate treated by one-stage simultaneous repair." *Plast Reconstr Surg* 115: 1509–1517.

89. Lilja J, Mars M, Elander A, et al. 2006. "Analysis of dental arch relationships in Swedish unilateral cleft lip and palate subjects: 20-year longitudinal consecutive series treated with delayed hard palate closure." *Cleft Palate Craniofac J* 43: 606–611.

90. Molsted K, Brattstrom V, Prahl-Anderson B, et al. 2005. "The Eurocleft Study: intercenter study of treatment outcome in patients with complete cleft lip and palate. Part 3: Dental Arch relationships." *Cleft Palate Craniofac J* 42: 78–82.

91. Friede H, Enemark H, Semb G, et al. 1991. "Craniofacial and occlusal characteristics in unilateral cleft lip and palate patients from four Scandinavian centers." *Scand J Plast Reconstr Surg Hand Surg* 25: 269–276.

92. Kim T, Ishikawa H, Chu S, et al. 2002. "Constriction of the maxillary dental arch by mucoperiosteal denudation of the palate." *Cleft Palate Craniofac J* 39: 425–431.

93. Good PH, Mulliken JB, Padwa BL. 2007. "Frequency of LeFort I osteotomy after repaired cleft lip and palate or cleft palate." *Cleft Palate Craniofac J* 44(4): 396–401.

94. Posnick J. 1991. "Orthognathic surgery in cleft patients treated by early bone grafting (Discussion)." *Plast Reconstr Surg* 87: 840–842.

95. Oberoi S, Chigurupati R, and Vargervik K. 2008. "Morphologic and management characteristics of individuals with unilateral cleft lip and palate who require maxillary advancement." *Cleft Palate Craniofac J* 45(1): 42–49.

96. Costello BJ, Ruiz RL, and Turvey TA. 2002. "Velopharyngeal insufficiency in patients with cleft palate." *Oral Maxillofac Surg Clin* 14: 539.

97. Glaser ER, Skolnick ML, McWilliams BJ, and Shprintzen RJ. 1979. "The dynamics of Passavant's ridge in subjects with and without velopharyngeal insufficiency. A multiview videofluoroscopic study." *Cleft Palate J* 16: 24–33.

98. Passavant G. 1863. "On the closure of the pharynx in speech." *Archiv Heilk* 3: 305.

99. Passavant G. 1869. "On the closure of pharynx in speech." *Virchows Arch* 46: 1.

100. Warren DW. 1986. "Compensatory speech behaviors in cleft palate: a regulation/control phenomenon." *Cleft Palate J* 23: 251–260.

101. Henningsson G, and Isberg A. "Velopharyngeal movements in patients alternating between oral and glottal articulation: A clinical and cineradiographical study." *Cleft Palate J* 23: 1–9.

102. Isberg A, and Henningsson G. 1987. "Influence of palatal fistula on velopharyngeal movements: A cineradiographic study." *Plast Reconstr Surg* 79: 525–530.

103. Lohmander-Agerskov A, Dotevall H, Lith A, and Söderpalm E. "Speech and velopharyngeal function in children with an open residual cleft in the hard palate, and the influence of temporary covering." *Cleft Palate Craniofac J* 33: 324–332.

104. Shprintzen RJ, and Bardach J. 1995. "The use of information obtained from speech and instrumental evaluations in treatment planning for velopharyngeal insufficiency." In: *Cleft Palate Speech Management: A Multidisciplinary Approach.* St Louis: Mosby.

105. Golding-Kushner KJ, Argamaso RV, Cotton RT, et al. 1990. "Standardization for the reporting of nasopharyngoscopy and multi-view videofluoroscopy: A report from an international working group." *Cleft Palate J* 27: 337–347.

106. Warren DW, Dalston RM, and Mayo R. 1994. "Hypernasality and velopharyngeal impairment." *Cleft Palate Craniofac J* 31: 257–262.

107. Turvey TA, Ruiz RL, and Costello BJ. 2002. "Surgical correction of midface deficiency in the cleft lip and palate malformation." *Oral Maxillofac Surg Clin* 14: 491–507.

108. Fonseca RJ, Turvey TA, and Wolford LM. 2000. "Orthognathic surgery in the cleft patient." In: *Oral and Maxillofacial Surgery,* Fonseca RJ, Baker SJ, and Wolford LM, eds. Philadelphia: WB Saunders.

109. Posnick JC, and Tompson B. 1995. "Cleft-orthognathic surgery: complications and long-term results." *Plast Reconstr Surg* 96: 255–266.

110. Posnick JC, and Ruiz RL. 2000. "Discussion of management of secondary orofacial cleft deformities." In: *The Unfavorable Result in Plastic Surgery: Avoidance and Treatment,* 3rd ed., Goldwyn RM, and Cohen MM, eds. Philadelphia: Lippincott Williams & Wilkins.

111. Turvey TA, and Frost D. "Maxillary advancement and velopharyngeal function in the presence of cleft palate." Presented at the 38th Annual Meeting of the American Cleft Palate Association, Lancaster, PA, May 1980.

112. Bernstein L. 1967. "Treatment of velopharyngeal incompetence." *Arch Otolaryngol* 85: 67–74.

113. Rosseli S. 1935–36. "Divisione palatine 3 sua aura chirurgico." *Alu Congr Internaz Stomatal* 391.

114. Schoenborn D. 1876. "Uber eine neue Methode der Staphylorraphies." *Arch Klin Chirurgie* 19: 528.

115. Shprintzen RJ. 1979. "The use of multiview videofluoroscopy and flexible fiberoptic nasopharyngoscopy as a predictor of success with pharyngeal flap surgery." In: *Diagnosis and Treatment of Palatoglossal Malfunction,* Ellis F, and Flack E, eds. London: College of Speech Therapists.

116. Argamaso RV, Levandowski G, Golding-Kushner KJ, and Shprintzen RJ. 1994. "Treatment of asymmetric velopharyngeal insufficiency with skewed pharyngeal flap." *Cleft Palate Craniofac J* 31: 287–294.

117. Shprintzen RJ, Lewin ML, Croft CB, et al. 1979. "A comprehensive study of pharyngeal flap surgery: Tailor-made flaps." *Cleft Palate J* 16: 46–55.

118. Shprintzen RJ, McCall GN, Skolnick ML, and Lencione RM. 1975. "Selective movement of the lateral aspects of the pharyngeal walls during velopharyngeal closure for speech, blowing, and whistling in normals." *Cleft Palate J* 12: 51–58.

119. Hynes W. 1951. "Pharyngoplasty by muscle transplantation." *Br J Plast Surg* 3: 128.

120. Hynes W. 1953. "The results of pharyngoplasty by muscle transplantation in 'failed cleft palate' cases, with special reference to the influence of the pharynx on voice production." *Ann R Coll Surg Engl* 13: 17–35.

121. Orticochea M. 1997. "Physiopathology of the dynamic muscular sphincter of the pharynx." *Plast Reconstr Surg* 100: 1918–1923.

122. Orticochea M. 1968 "Constriction of a dynamic muscle sphincter in cleft palates." *Plast Reconstr Surg* 41: 323–327.

123. Jackson I, and Silverton JS. 1983. "The sphincter pharyngoplasty as a secondary procedure in cleft palates." *Plast Reconstr Surg* 71: 180.

124. Jackson IT. 1985. "Sphincter pharyngoplasty." *Clin Plast Surg* 12: 711.

125. Guilleminault C, and Stoohs R. "Chronic snoring and obstructive sleep apnea syndrome in children." *Lung* 168: 912–919.

126. Sirois M, Caouette-Laberge L, Spier S, et al. 1994. "Sleep apnea following a pharyngeal flap: a feared complication." *Plast Reconstr Surg* 93: 943–947.

127. Ysunza A, Garcia-Velasco M, Garcia-Garcia M, et al. 1993. "Obstructive sleep apnea secondary to surgery for velopharyngeal insufficiency." *Cleft Palate Craniofac J* 30: 387–390.

128. Chen PK, Wu JT, Chen YR, and Noordhoff MS. 1994. "Correction of secondary velopharyngeal insufficiency in cleft palate patients with the Furlow palatoplasty." *Plast Reconstr Surg* 94: 933–941.

129. Poole MD. 1988. "Complications in craniofacial surgery." *Br J Plast Surg* 41: 603–613.

130. Jones BM, Jani P, Bingham RM, et al. 1992. "Complications in paediatric craniofacial surgery: An initial four year experience." *Br J Plast Surg* 45: 225–231.

131. Steig PE, and Mulliken JB. 1991. "Neurosurgical complications in craniofacial surgery." *Neursurg Clin N Am* 2: 703–708.

132. Resnick DK, Pollack IF, and Albright AL. 1995. "Surgical management of the cloverleaf skull deformity." *Pediatr Neurosurg* 22(1): 29–37; discussion 238.

133. Phillips RJ, and Mulliken JB. 1988. "Venous air embolism during a craniofacial procedure." *Plast Reconstr Surg* 82(1):155–159.

134. Greensmith AL, Meara JG, Holmes AD, and Lo P. 2004. "Complications related to cranial vault surgery." *Oral Maxillofac Surg Clin North Am* 16(4): 465–473.

135. Levine JP, Stelnicki E, Weiner HL, et al. 2001. "Hyponatremia in the postoperative craniofacial pediatric patient population: A connection to cerebral salt wasting syndrome and management of the disorder." *Plast Reconstr Surg.* 108(6): 1501–1508.
136. Fearon JA, Ruotolo RA, and Kolar JC. 2009. "Single sutural craniosynostoses: Surgical outcomes and long-term growth." *Plast Reconstr Surg* 123(2): 635–642.
137. Whitaker LA, Munro IR, Salyer KE, et al. 1979. "Combined report of problems and complications in 793 craniofacial operations." *Plast Reconstr Surg* 64: 198–203.
138. Munro IR, and Sabatier RE. 1985. "An analysis of 12 years of craniomaxillofacial surgery in Toronto." *Plast Reconstr Surg* 76: 29.
139. Lo LJ, Hung KF, and Chen YR. 2002. "Blindness as a complication of Le Fort I osteotomy for maxillary distraction." *Plast Reconstr Surg* 109(2): 688–698; discussion 699–700.
140. Rivera-Serrano CM, Oliver CL, Sok J, et al. 2010. "Pedicled facial buccinator (FAB) flap: A new flap for reconstruction of skull base defects." *Laryngoscope* 120(10): 1922–1930.
141. Costello BJ, Shah G, Kumta P, and Sfeir CS. 2010. "Regenerative medicine for craniomaxillofacial surgery." *Oral Maxillofac Surg Clin North Am* 22(1): 33–42.
142. Selber JC, Brooks C, Kurichi JE, et al. 2008. "Long-term results following fronto-orbital reconstruction in nonsyndromic unicoronal synostosis." *Plast Reconstr Surg* 121(5): 251e–260e.

9

Cosmetic Surgery

Jon D. Perenack, DDS, MD
Vernon P. Burke, DMD, MD

INTRODUCTION

Facial cosmetic surgery is a unique area of practice within the scope of oral and maxillofacial surgery in that interventions offered to the patient are typically not required from a medical standpoint but are considered elective procedures. Although some cosmetic procedures offer an adjunctive functional benefit such as the visual field improvement seen with upper blepharoplasty, by and large the goal of the therapy is to achieve a visual appearance that is more aesthetically pleasing to the patient. For this reason, patient tolerance of adverse outcomes is often quite low. The facial cosmetic surgeon must be adept at proper patient selection for cosmetic surgery, as well as prevention of complications and recognition of impending problems with prompt intervention when indicated. Once a complication has been recognized, appropriate intervention is performed in order to correct, or minimize, any adverse sequelae. The surgeon should allocate appropriate additional time to counsel the patient honestly on the nature of the complication, solutions that are available, likely outcomes, and a reasonable timetable until a final result is achievable. This strategy can lead to an acceptable result for the patient, and, often, to one of the more loyal patients to the cosmetic practice.

This chapter aims to outline the more common complications seen with cosmetic procedures of the head and neck. Management strategies will be discussed to minimize or eliminate long-term sequelae of these complications. Common facial cosmetic treatments will be grouped together as either conservative (minimally invasive), or surgical in nature.

CONSERVATIVE COSMETIC PROCEDURE COMPLICATIONS

1. Botulinum toxin
2. Injectable soft tissue volumizers and fillers
3. Nonablative and ablative cosmetic skin therapy
4. Ablative skin resurfacing

Botulinum Toxin

Cosmetic botulinum toxin therapy for the face is typically aimed at reducing mimetic rhytids. Additionally, by adjusting the vector forces of the facial muscles by selective paralysis, nonsurgical brow elevation or lifting of the commissures of the mouth can be achieved. The safety and efficacy of botulinum toxin is well established by the literature and by its extensive use in the population with low reported rate of complications.[1,2] In 2007, there were 4.6 million patients treated with botulinum toxin therapy (BTX) and very few

Management of Complications in Oral and Maxillofacial Surgery, First Edition. Edited by Michael Miloro, Antonia Kolokythas.
© 2012 John Wiley & Sons, Inc. Published 2012 by John Wiley & Sons, Inc.

reports of complications as a result of the medication.[3] Even when evaluating the literature on the use of BTX use for movement disorders such as cervical dystonia where doses reach 300 units, at much higher doses than in the case for cosmetic use (typically much less than 100 units), severe complications are rare.[4] More commonly, there are unsatisfactory results as a result of administration errors or unanticipated effect. Since BTX does not cause permanent paralysis of the musculature, long-term complications are rare. This has contributed greatly to making this treatment the most popular of cosmetic procedures.

Due to its primary use to achieve muscle paralysis, nonselective muscle weakness comprises the most frequent distressing complication encountered following BTX administration. The three most common inadvertent muscle weaknesses seen are lid ptosis, brow droop, and lip droop (from weakness in the marginal mandibular branch of the facial nerve distribution after treatment of the depressor anguli oris muscle) (Fig. 9.1). Rarely, difficulty closing the eye may be seen from excessive BTX administration into the orbicularis oculi muscle.

Upper Lid Ptosis

Ptosis of the upper lid is usually mild and is the result of the inadvertent blocking of Mueller's muscle in the superior orbit. This complication can be avoided by an injection technique that places BTX in an upward direction at least 1 cm above the superior orbital rim. If ptosis is noted following BTX treatment, intervention may be considered if the patient has significant concerns. One therapy commonly recommended for symptomatic ptosis is the ophthalmic administration of apraclonidine (Iodipine), which is an alpha-adrenergic agonist agent (Fig. 9.2). This agent increases sympathetic tone to Mueller's muscle. One

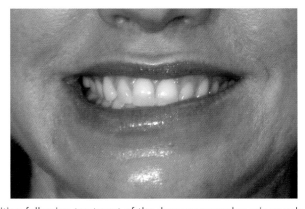

Fig. 9.1. Asymmetric lip position following treatment of the depressor angulae oris muscle with BTX.

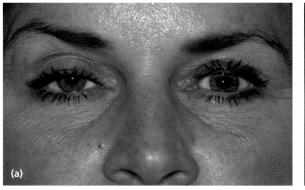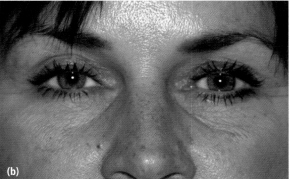

Fig. 9.2. (a) Iatrogenic lid ptosis after BTX treatment of corrugators. (b) Same patient 5 minutes after one drop of ophthalmic iopodine.

to three drops daily of 0.5% ophthalmic solution in the affected eye should limit ptosis for approximately 4 hours.[5]

Brow and Lid Droop

Brow and lip droop result from the overaggressive treatment of the lateral frontalis muscle and depressor anguli oris muscle, respectively. Prevention of this problem is best achieved by undertreating these areas until the practitioner develops a sense of the BTX dose that is best tolerated by an individual patient. Unfortunately, when excessive weakness is noted, there is little option for treatment except to wait for the effects of BTX to diminish. One option is to treat the less weak side of the face with an additional small dose of BTX (1–2 units) in an attempt to achieve symmetry. The patient should be reassured that the undesired weakness typically only lasts 2–3 weeks, far less than the expected duration of usual BTX treatment (3–4 months).

Inability to Close the Eye

A far less frequent complication is the inadvertent block of the orbicularis oculi muscle leading to the inability to close the eye. Typically, a large field dose of BTX encompassing the lateral orbicularis oculi is the culprit initiating this complication. Avoidance of BTX doses in this area of greater than 5–15 units/side, in addition to proper placement technique, should help prevent this problem. If, after treatment with BTX, the patient is unable to close the eye, concern for preventing corneal damage must be considered. The eyelid should be taped shut to protect the globe and prescription of lubricating agents is initiated. It is important to remind the patient that the paralysis will be temporary. The ability to close the eye should return prior to the expected lifespan of the BTX cosmetic effect (3–4 months).

Injection Site Bleeding

Injection site bleeding is usually quite minor and is managed by pressure on the site. The area should not be rubbed or massaged, since this may disseminate the BTX to unintended areas or inactivate the BTX. Bruising with hematoma formation and skin discoloration may be quite distressful for the patient, but this complication has a self-limited course of a few weeks.

Injectable Soft Tissue Volumizers and Fillers

Soft tissue filler materials have been used for years for cosmetic purposes and represent one of the fastest growing areas within facial cosmetic practices. Fillers may be used to smooth folds and wrinkles, replace facial volume, or change actual facial morphology depending on the filler characteristics and placement location (Table 9.1). In the United States there are many choices available based upon patient need, anatomic area, and specific characteristics of the filler material. Although there is great variety in available fillers, many complications are common to all and will be discussed together. Other complications are more specific to individual fillers and will be discussed separately.

Soft tissue fillers are generally considered to have an excellent safety profile, and most complications are not considered life threatening. However, some infrequent complications can lead to exceptional morbidity, and, of course, the patient with a high cosmetic demand can be devastated by an even minor complication. An interesting side effect of the relatively high safety quotient of fillers, and their perceived high profitability, is that an increasing number of medical and dental practitioners with very limited training have introduced filler placement into their practice. In certain communities it has become common for hairdressers and independent aestheticians to integrate the medical placement of fillers into their business practices. Without commenting on the legal or ethical ramifications of this trend, it should be expected that the cosmetic oral and maxillofacial surgeon may see more patients with filler complications from other providers in their region.

The undesirable result in the cosmetic patient can be due to expectations prior to treatment that were not met by the treatment, or by a truly objective unsatisfactory result. Either way, the cosmetic surgeon should have knowledge on treatment of various problems resulting from the injection of fillers and possible techniques for eliminating or decreasing the defect.

Table 9.1. Injectable Fillers Commonly used in the United States

Materials	Type	Placement	Duration of Effect	Disadvantages
Bovine collagen (Zyderm, Zyplast)	Xenograft	Dermal injection or deeper	2–3 months	Allergy testing, short duration
Human collagen (Cosmoderm, Cosmoplast)	Allograft	Dermal injection or deeper	2–3 months	Short duration
Nonanimal, stabilized, hyaluronic acid (Restylane, Juvederm)	Synthetic	Dermal injection or deeper	12–18 months	Moderate duration, increased post-op edema, ecchymosis
Autologous free fat transfer	Autograft	Subcutaneous or deeper	Variable, 30–70% permanent	Prolonged tissue edema, variable efficacy and resorption, uneveness
Poly-L-lactic acid (Sculptra)	Synthetic	Subcutaneous or deeper	2–4 years	Granuloma formation, uneveness
Methylmethacrylate spheres in bovine collagen carrier (Artifil)	Synthetic/ xenograft	Subcutaneous or deeper	Permanent	Granuloma formation, unevenness, surgical removal
Hydroxylapatite (Radiesse)	Synthetic	Subcutaneous or deeper	1–3 years	Granuloma formation, uneveness

Inappropriate Location of Filler Placement

Early post-treatment "lumps," "bumps," and asymmetry are easily recognized problems by patients and surgeons, and are perhaps the most common complications seen with soft tissue fillers. In general, this complication results from injection of the filler material in an inappropriate location, or extension of the material beyond the intended boundaries of the specific site or rhytid, either spontaneously or induced by the patient by manipulating or rubbing the area. The timing of the appearance of the irregularity and the nature of the filler used can provide an important clue as to the source of the problem and the appropriate treatment to resolve it. This may require additional filler material to gently blend the area, or, in some cases, removal of the material surgically. It is best to plan appropriately and isolate the filler material to the specific area of concern to avoid this complication.

Injection Hematoma

Since most fillers are placed using a needle, an injection hematoma at either the site of skin penetration or filler deposition must be considered as a possible cause of early skin irregularities in the area. Typically, injection hematomas will be noticed sometime after filler placement, either at the treatment visit, or within the next 24 hours (Fig. 9.3). The clinician can be fairly certain that if the treated area appears smooth and symmetric initially, but becomes asymmetric or uneven within 24 hours, a small hematoma or uneven edema is the likely cause. In the case of fillers that provide immediate substance (e.g., the hyaluronic acids), one must also consider that the patient may have manipulated the material into a new location if it is first recognized after the treatment visit, as discussed. If a hematoma is suspected, the patient should be reassured that improvement will occur within a few days. Manipulation and massage of the area should be avoided so as not to disturb the location of filler placement. Topically placed cold packs may limit the extent of the hematoma if recognized early. After 24 hours, warm compresses and topical arnica gel placement may help to decrease ecchymosis. Injection hematomas can be best avoided by keeping the number

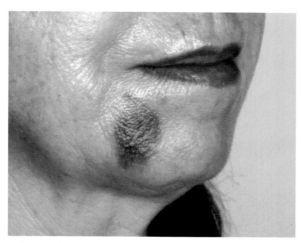

Fig. 9.3. Injection hematoma 24 hours after hyaluronic acid filler placement.

of penetrations of the needle through the dermal plexus to a minimum. If many areas are treated, a fresh needle should be used to prevent tearing of tissue from a dull needle tip. In planning the injection pathway, the surgeon should also consider the anatomical position of major vascular bundles and avoid them when possible.

Inappropriate placement of filler will usually be noticed almost immediately by the astute clinician when using substantive fillers such as the hyaluronic acids, collagens, hydroxyapatite or autologous fat. Poor placement of fillers that rely on the patient's own collagen production to produce volume, such as poly-L-lactic acid, will usually develop late irregularities, after one or more months following placement. Avoidance of this problem is best achieved by considering a number of factors: (1) the recommended tissue depth placement of the filler and its relative viscoelastic properties compared to the regional soft tissues; (2) the relative thickness of the tissue overlying the area to be augmented and the ability to conceal minor irregularities of deep fillers; and (3) avoidance of excessive filler placement to an area in a single visit.

When a clinician recognizes that an irregularity, "lump," " bump," or skin blanching has appeared immediately after placement of a substantive filler, vigorous massage of the area is recommended. This often resolves the undesired result and distributes the filler more evenly. If a large amount of filler has been carelessly injected to form the "lump," consideration must given to either removing the filler via puncture and manual expression, or destruction of the filler agent. Asymmetry that is noticed post-treatment between the right and left side of the face may be caused either by a preexisting, but unrecognized, facial asymmetry, an asymmetric placement of filler, or possible injection hematoma. In the case of asymmetric filler placement, this outcome can be improved by additional injection in the "under-treated" side. A larger problem exists when the patient perceives an asymmetry and believes one side is overcorrected. The only resolution for this complication may be patient management and a tincture of time for the effect of the filler to diminish or consideration of techniques to remove the filler. For this reason it is recommended that in technically demanding areas such as the tear trough deficiency, the use of fillers with a shorter half-life is considered, and underfilling rather than overtreating the location is more prudent (Fig. 9.4). The patient should be made aware that it is always easier to add more filler to achieve a more desirable result than to try to remove filler material. Destruction or removal of fillers depends upon the chemical properties of the agent used. Hyaluronic acid fillers can to some degree be reversed, or their half-life dramatically shortened, by injection of hyaluronidase.[6] Typically, 10–15 units of hyaluronidase is injected directly into the area of excess hyaluronic acid filler. A change is usually noticed by the patient on the following day. Additional hyaluronidase may be injected if needed. Excess collagen injection is often treated by vigorous massage and warm compresses. Older forms of collagen typically have a short half-life and resolve quickly. Newer, cross-linked collagens may be softened by injection of hyaluronidase, or steroid injection (0.1 cc of kenalog-10). Injectable hydroxyapatite (HA) that forms a

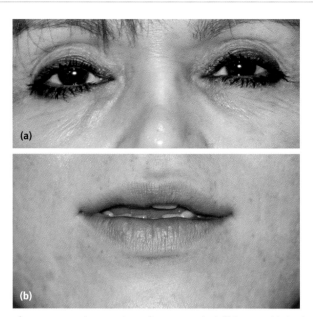

Fig. 9.4. (a) Visible nodularity after attempted correction of tear trough deficiency with hydroxyapatite filler. (b) Lip irregularity after hyaluronic acid filler placement. Both complications were corrected after local injection with hyaluronidase, massage, and placement of camouflaging hyaluronic acid filler.

visible lump can be a very difficult problem to resolve. Massage, warm compresses, and limited steroid injection may be helpful if initiated early. The surgeon may attempt to disrupt a persistent "lump" of hydroxyapatite by passing an 18 g needle transcutaneously and sweeping through the collection of HA particles with multiple passes. If this fails, the final options are either surgical removal or observation with the expectation that the irregularity may remain for several years. Surgical removal often reveals clumped calcium-like deposits spread throughout the underlying soft tissues. Clumping of hydroxyapatite may be minimized by using the recommended technique of the manufacturer to decrease the concentration and viscosity of the material. Occasionally it may be appropriate to add additional filler adjacent to a visible deposit to camouflage the area. It is best to consider using a reversible filler such as hyaluronic acid so that if an increasingly worse result is achieved, it can be returned to the level of the initial complication. Irregular deposits sometimes seen after autologous fat transfer are best avoided by only volumizing areas where thick soft tissue coverage over the augmented area exists. It is not recommended to transfer fat to areas of the face where there is thin soft tissue present over bone, such as over the lateral zygoma or the tear trough region. Irregular fat placement or resorption can create a difficult irregularity to manage. Vigorous massage, steroid injection, and other mesotherapy agent injections may have some success. Liposuction of the localized fat deposit can have an unpredictable result with irregularities. An adjacent camouflage injection with another filler agent is also an option.

Nonsubstantive fillers rely on the patient's natural collagen forming response in reaction to the filler material to create volume. Examples include poly-L-lactic acid and microdroplet silicone injections, and these typically do not form early irregularities; instead, this complication will often appear a month or more after treatment. The degree and dimension of collagen formation can be difficult to predict, making it important to place the material deeply where nodules may not be visible or to use small amounts superficially. Similar to fat transfer, extreme caution should be taken in areas with thin soft tissue covering bone. When visible nodules do appear that are not granulomatous in nature, management is directed at interrupting the collagen formation process. Injection directly into the nodule with low dose steroid is a first line option. Persistent nodules may respond to an intralesional low dose chemotherapy agent (e.g., 5-fluorouracil) or needle disruption. Surgical removal is usually the final option for management of this complication.

Filler Agent Allergic Reaction and Granuloma Formation

Allergic reactions range from minor to life threatening and may be possible with any of the soft tissue filler materials. Minor, local allergic reaction to filler treatment usually presents as an early or late finding of fiery erythema and edema immediately surrounding the area of injection. Infection due to inoculation with skin biofilm must be ruled out. Local allergic reaction often responds well to a tapered dose oral steroid regimen. Local injection with low dose steroid may be useful. If a hyaluronic acid has been used, destruction of the material with hyaluronidase should be considered. Occasionally the affected area may form a sterile abscess that should be drained and irrigated. Systemic anaphylactic reaction is possible, but fortunately is very rare. A systemic reaction should be treated aggressively to stabilize the patient with attention then turned to removing the causative material, if possible. Allergic reaction is most common with the fillers based on bovine collagen, which were more commonly used before the introduction of hyaluronic acid fillers and others. The use of bovine collagen (Zyderm®, Zyplast®) requires allergy testing, which is typically performed 30 days prior to filler placement. A small amount (0.1ml) of the bovine collagen is placed in the forearm; if no reaction is found after 30 days it is assumed filler placement can proceed without risk. This 30-day delay is recommended due to early experience with the material. Many patients were treated after a negative skin reaction evaluated after 6 hours. It was noted that despite negative skin reaction, 1.2–6.3% of patients experienced redness and swelling that lasted for months.[7] This prolonged planning and delay in treatment is in direct contrast to the typical spontaneity of most cosmetic filler procedures used today.[8] The Allergan website (the company that produces Zyderm and Zyplast) states the rate of allergic reaction to be approximately 1–2%.[9]

Granulomatous reactions are more commonly associated with the semi-permanent or permanent fillers such as poly-L-lactic acid, polymethylmethacrylate spheres, and microdroplet silicone injection. Foreign body reaction rarely appears earlier than 1 month after injection and has been reported to occur sometimes years later. Polymethylmethacrylate microspheres (ArteFill®/ArteSense®) are permanent fillers in a bovine collagen transport medium with a low complication profile. Previously, methylmethacrylate microspheres were produced and granulomatous reaction was a more commonly reported incidence. After changes in the production regimen and change of the transport medium from gelatin to bovine collagen, the foreign body granuloma formation rate decreased dramatically.[10] Since ArteFill®/ArteSense® contain bovine collagen, allergy testing similar to Zyderm® and Zyplast® are necessary. A case was reported by Fischer of a patient who developed a sarcoid-like reaction after initiation of antiviral therapy for hepatitis C. The lesions were restricted to the glabellar region, nasolabial area, and lower lips. The patient received an injection of Artecoll® in those areas 10 years prior to initiation of antiviral therapy. The author concluded the low-grade foreign body reaction to the polymethylmethacrylate became exaggerated after treatment for hepatitis C had begun. The foreign body reaction resulted in ulceration of the glabellar region and a quite large nodule in the nasolabial area requiring excision.[11] If foreign body granuloma is noted, an early intralesional steroid is initial treatment as described earlier. Intralesional injection with a chemotherapeutic agent such as 5-FU should also be considered. If the lesion is recalcitrant to intralesional injections then excision may be necessary. If the area allows, a fold or rhytid is used to hide the incision. If the granulomatous reaction extends to the skin, an ellipse should be planned to remove the affected area. If the granuloma is located deeply, a simple linear incision for access is recommended. The granulomatous chain is identified and removed and primary closure is obtained; ablative laser skin resurfacing of the incision may be considered to help blend the resulting scar.

Of all the fillers currently available, the use of silicone injection has been the most fiercely debated and has been the subject of controversy in both the scientific and public literature. Silicone has been used for multiple areas of the body and in different formulations. It continues to be used as facial cosmetic filler because it has excellent flow properties, is thought to have a "natural" feel, and is long lasting. The novice clinician is cautioned about it use because of its permanence. Most cosmetic surgeons who use silicone plan for multiple sessions with injection of small amounts at each visit until the desired effect is achieved. Once the material is placed, massage is prohibited since the material may flow through tissues and diminish its effect, cause asymmetry, or irregular clumping.

Silicone granulomas range from asymptomatic masses to painful erythematous and disfiguring lesions. Occasionally, the silicone masses can ulcerate, cause cellulitis or abscess, or a combination. Like polymethylmethacrylate, the granulomas may be surgically removed. Excision of silicone granulomas is often challenging and many times unsuccessful. Intralesional steroids are often used as the first line of treatment for silicone granulomas, although systemic steroids are another option. Minocycline or imiquinod are treatments used with reportedly good clinical success. Minocycline is prescribed at 100 mg twice daily until resolution of symptoms is observed. A trial decrease in dosage can be attempted after resolution of granulomas but may need to be reinitiated if exacerbation develops.[12] Imiquinod 5% (Aldara®) is available in a cream and is applied twice daily with reportedly good success in the treatment of silicone granulomas.[13] Pasternak has reported on the use of Etanercept, a tumor necrosis factor (TNF) inhibitor, in the treatment of recalcitrant silicone granulomas.[14] Granulomatous reactions are thought to be a T-cell activation by TNF-α. This treatment requires subcutaneous injections biweekly for an extended period of time, and the patient must be tested for tuberculosis prior to initiation of treatment.[15]

Intra-arterial Injection of Filler Materials

Intra-arterial injection of filler material is an extremely rare occurrence but can have severe complications. Intra-arterial injection and its sequelae are theoretically possible with any filler and is the result of inadvertently entering an artery and forcing filler material either anterograde or retrograde along its vascular distribution. For this reason, it is recommended to only inject filler along a defined pathway during retraction of the needle. It is not recommended to inject ahead of the needle as it is advanced into tissue. If blanching of tissue is noticed, then the injection should be immediately discontinued. Case reports of facial skin necrosis and blindness have been reported in the literature;[15–17] De Castro et al.[18,19] described a case of extensive necrosis of the facial artery distribution after injection of polymethylmethacrylate. If occlusion of a vessel is encountered after filler is injected, close observation should be undertaken. Hospital admission with use of heparin and other anticoagulant methods has been employed with unknown benefit. If necrosis occurs then limitation of extension of the area affected is the goal. Judicious debridement and prevention of infection are begun until the time for attempts at secondary reconstruction. Other authors have described blindness after injection of the glabellar region thought to be due to retrograde injection into the ophthalmic artery distribution.[15] If blindness or other ophthalmologic complications are suspected the patient should be referred to an ophthalmologist emergently for assessment in order to salvage sight or eye function.

Nonablative and Ablative Cosmetic Skin Therapy Complications

There are various modalities of therapy available to improve the appearance of the facial and neck skin. Goals of treatment involve the improvement or removal of pigmentations and dyspigmentations, telangectasias and vascular anomalies, tattoo removal, and improvement of age and actinic generated fine lines and rhytids. Therapies can be broadly divided into nonablative and ablative treatments depending upon their effect on the epidermis (Table 9.2).

Nonablative, subsurface therapies include intense pulsed light, Nd-YAG, pulsed dye and the diode (585, 1450 nm) lasers, and radiofrequency delivery systems that are used appropriately to treat dyspigmentations, tattoos, vascular anomalies, very fine rhytids, and loss of skin elasticity. These devices use epidermal surface cooling in combination with deeply penetrating wavelengths and energies that selectively target water-containing tissue, resulting in selective heating and subsequent thermal injury to the dermis. Complications typically relate to exuberant application of energy to the subsurface tissues and may be transitory or long lasting.

Edema is an expected post-treatment finding with most subsurface treatments. It is transitory in nature and usually lasts for 1 to 3 days. Purpura and blistering of the affected area are less common and probably represent an injudicious delivery of energy to the tissue (Fig. 9.5). Patients who normally use topical retin-A homecare should discontinue treatment for several days prior to treatment. If multiple treatments are scheduled for the patient, the clinician should keep an accurate record and change the energy parameters appropriately. Purpura is generally a self-limiting problem. Topical application of an arnica-containing gel may be recommended. Blisters should not be unroofed, but should be maintained as a "biologic dressing" and protected by a moist occlusive dressing and a nonadhering dressing (Telfa) until resolved.

In the treatment of dyspigmentations there is a potential to worsen the initial lesion, or to change the surrounding tissue pigmentation thus creating a new problem. Most modalities for treating pigmentations

Table 9.2. Managing Facelift Complications by Region of Incision

Region	Complication	Solution	Avoidance
Temporal tuft	Elevation or loss of temporal hairline	Follicular hair transplant, local hair-bearing flaps	Trichophyic sideburn incision
Tragus	A) Blunting of tragus with endaural approach B) Visible scar with pretragal approach	A) Advancement flap with cartilage graft B) CO_2 laser resurfacing	A) Generous trimming of skin with 0-tension closure B) Consider endaural approach
Earlobe	Pixie ear	A) V-Y closure with earlobe resuspension B) SMAS advancement with earlobe suspension	A) Incorporate cuff of neck skin around earlobe B) Inferior 2–3 mm of earlobe left unattached with 0-tension
Posterior Hairline	A) Visible scar B) Hairline mismatch	A) Consider hair transplantation B) Reapproximate flap	A) Avoid trichophytic incision B) Careful hairline reapproximation

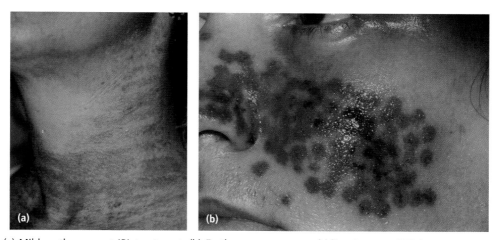

Fig. 9.5. (a) Mild erythema post IPL treatment. (b) Erythema, purpura, and blistering post KTP laser treatment.

require that the patient abstain from tanning or sun exposure for any noticeable extent prior to beginning therapy. Darker skin, and tanned skin, carries a higher risk of generalized damage to melanocytes leading to either temporary or permanent hypopigmentation (Fig. 9.6). Once hypopigmentation occurs, it is notoriously difficult to treat, so avoidance of excessive energy delivery or deferment of treatment in these patients is paramount. Treatment of hypopigmentation is directed at decreasing the general darkness of the skin surrounding the hypopigmented area. High-level sun block, 4% hydroquinone topically twice daily, or topical kojic acid may be helpful. A more limited, low-energy setting using the initial device can be helpful to decrease pigment in the unaffected area surrounding the hypopigmented site, although this has the potential to worsen the problem. Fortunately, most hypopigmentation from subsurface treatments improve with time. Occasionally, in instances of limited permanent hypopigmentation, a medical tattoo artist may be employed to permanently blend the area with surrounding skin. The tattooed skin lacks the ability to tan and thus may be more or less visible as the patient's skin color continues to change with sun exposure. Reactive hyperpigmentation should be treated with topical hydroquinone or kojic acid.

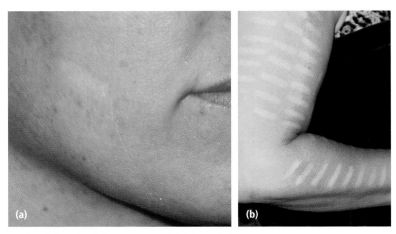

Fig. 9.6. Hypopigmentation following IPL treatment of (a) face; (b) arm.

Subsurface Fat Atrophy and Irregularity

Development of subsurface fat atrophy and irregularity has been reported primarily in conjunction with older modalities of radiofrequency dermal tightening procedures.[20] Utilizing current technologies and recommended energy settings this phenomena is easily avoided but remains as a cautionary reminder of untoward consequences from exuberant treatment. Attempts to correct subsurface irregularity are aimed at adding volume to the affected area. Injectable nonanimal stabilized hyaluronic acid (NASHA), autologous fat transfer, and subcision techniques have been tried with varying levels of success. Areas that exhibit dermal scar tethering to deeper tissues may require scar lysis to allow a potential space to form to accept a filler substance. An easy method of detecting scar adhesions below the dermis is to inject a volume of normal saline subcutaneously into the depressed area. If a "doughnut" of saline forms around the depression, it is prudent to plan on scar lysis prior to filler placement.

Allergic Reaction to Tattoo Removal

Allergic reaction to tattoo ink during the initial placement is well documented, but it also may occur during attempted tattoo removal. Tattoo inks, both temporary and permanent, contain a plethora of substances that can lead to an immediate or delayed reaction. Mercury- and chromium-containing materials are common offenders in permanent tattoo allergic reactions. During the process of tattoo removal by laser, the ink is liberated and is freely exposed to the immune system where it can be labeled as foreign. Though not a common occurrence, with few reports in the literature, the clinician should be aware of this possibility when confronted with a patient who exhibits skin reactions after tattoo removal. In the few case reports, patients have been referred to dermatologists to confirm the diagnosis. During subsequent treatments the patients were treated with prednisone in order to mitigate the immune reaction.[21,22]

Ablative Skin Resurfacing

Ablative skin laser resurfacing and chemexfoliation offer a relatively noninvasive option for patients desiring improvement to actinic changes of the skin, especially fine lines and rhytids. However, unlike the previously discussed subsurface procedures, this spectrum of treatment inherently involves the controlled destruction of the epidermis, in addition to possible injury of the dermis. Complications are more common and can be quite disfiguring if not avoided or managed appropriately in the preoperative and postoperative phases of care. Preoperative evaluation of skin color and type are essential to anticipate potential complications and modify treatment based upon these criteria.

Herpetic Infection

Herpetic infection after laser treatment is a well-known complication. It carries the potential for permanent scarring. Preoperative evaluation of the patient who requests laser surgery should include questions regarding known history of herpes infection or previous symptoms consistent with herpes infection. It is prudent when performing laser therapy to begin antiviral suppressive therapy for herpes prior to surgery. Therapy is continued after treatment until the treated area has re-epithelialized, typically for 10–14 days. Assessment in the early postoperative period may be confounded by the absence of blistering, with pain being the presenting symptom. If herpetic infection is suspected, or confirmed by Tzank smear, than institution of higher dose levels of antiviral medications typical for zoster is provided.

Persistent Erythema

Persistent erythema lasting over 6 months from the time of treatment should trigger investigation since most mild erythema should resolve within 2–3 months (Fig. 9.7). This complication can be vexing for both the patient and clinician due to the multifactorial nature of the possible causes of the problem. Treatable causes include aggressive homecare, allergy to environmental factors, sun exposure, subclinical infection, and early scar formation. A general approach in evaluating erythema is to assess current skin homecare products, environmental factors, and symptoms. Most patients are able to resume homecare products, including retinoids, within 10 days of their ablative procedure. However, as postablative skin is generally more reactive to homecare products and environmental factors, many may require the scaling back of dose or frequency of application of products for a number of months. Aggressive retinoid therapy is a common cause of persistent erythema. It is appropriate in the face of persistent erythema to halt all skin products for a number of weeks in an attempt to limit the number of contributing factors. A tapered dose of oral steroid may be helpful if a contact allergic response is thought to be contributing to the reaction. Topical steroid application is indicated but should be limited in duration, as this can sometimes cause erythema. The patient should be questioned about sun exposure and use of sunblock. Postablative skin is especially sensitive to UV radiation and may present with persistent redness if not adequately protected. Unfortunately, occasionally a contact allergy to sunblock is the root cause of erythema. In this case the blocking agent must be halted. If a subclinical fungal infection is suspected, potassium hydroxide (KOH) prep should be considered to confirm diagnosis and antifungal treatment initiated. Persistent erythema may also represent a precursor to scar formation from overaggressive ablative therapy. Treatment for this will be discussed subsequently.[23]

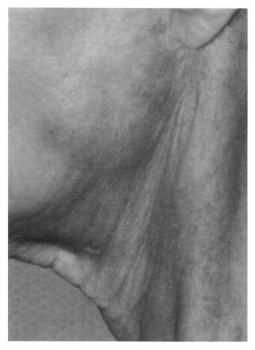

Fig. 9.7. Areas of persistent erythema and hypopigmentation 5 months after CO_2 laser resurfacing of face and neck.

Bacterial and Viral Infections

Bacterial or viral infection after resurfacing therapy, though rare, can range from minor to life threatening. Bacteria or yeast can act as culprit and both should be treated aggressively. Once again, prophylaxis and vigilance in the postoperative period are the keys to prevention of unwanted outcomes. Bacterial infection after laser treatment is most commonly due to *Staphylococcus aureus* and *Pseudomonas aeruginosa*.[16,24] Some surgeons recommend prophylactic administration of cephalosporin antibiotics to cover skin flora while some also recommend quinolone coverage for *Pseudomonas* species. With a postoperative infection rate of 0.4–4.3% this may not be warranted.[16] In a study of 133 patients, Walia and Alster failed to show a benefit of prophylactic administration of antibiotic.[25] If infection is suspected then empirical treatment should begin without delay in order to wait for culture results. Niamtu recommended KOH staining of specimens from the affected area in order to differentiate between bacterial and yeast infection. KOH preparation is timely and can assist with targeting therapy to the offending organism. If yeast infection is diagnosed then treatment with antifungal agents is indicated.[18] Combination therapy with a topical and systemic antifungal should be considered. The most common fungal organism found on culture is *Candida* and empirical treatment should be aimed at this organism.[16]

Milia and Acne Eruption

Milia and acne can also appear in the postoperative period. Milia are common enough that preoperative discussion includes informing the patient that milia are expected and will be treated at their onset. Treatment involves use of topical tretinoin when milia appear. Any recalcitrant lesions can be treated by careful lysis of the lesion. Acne in the postoperative period can range from minor to major and is extremely common.[16] When acne is recognized, systemic antibiotics can begin in the immediate postoperative phase. Topical retinoic acid, acid peels, and topical antibiotics are used once re-epithelialization occurs.

Hyperpigmentation and Hypopigmentation

The practitioner performing ablative laser therapy should be well prepared to treat pigmentation problems after therapy. The patient with darker skin, Fitzpatrick III or greater, is more likely to experience hyperpigmentation although approximately a third of all patients, regardless of Fitzpatrick classification, experience this problem. Many surgeons use preoperative topical medications to reduce the risk of hyperpigmentation. Although this practice is common, studies have yet to support its efficacy. Hyperpigmentation develops approximately 3–4 weeks after treatment. The patient should be instructed to wear high SPF sun-blocking agents. Both skin-bleaching agents and chemical peels are used to treat the hyperpigmented areas.

Hypopigmentation is a later side effect seen in patients six to twelve months after surgery (Fig. 9.7). This complication is seen more often in patients with a history of phenol chemical peels or dermabrasion. It is important to assess whether the hypopigmentation is a true, or relative, hypopigmentation. This phenomenon is exemplified by laser therapy in one cosmetic unit and not another. The lased cosmetic unit will appear lighter than the unit next to it. In true hypopigmentation the skin may contain blotchy lightened areas. The treatment for both is similar. Chemical peels or CO_2 laser blending can be used to smoothen out the transition between areas of hypopigmentation. Minimal sun exposure and the drug oxsoralen can be used to stimulate melanogenesis.[16]

Persistent Erythema and Scarring

Scarring is often a result of poor technique or either contact dermatitis and/or wound infection. Prevention of scarring begins in the preoperative phase. Patients who have used isotretinoin (retin-A) within 2 years prior to laser therapy are at increased risk for scar formation. The practitioner should evaluate the patient for keloid formation due to a high propensity to form scars after treatment. Good technique during laser therapy is the best prevention of scarring. High energy densities and stacking can result in scarring and should be avoided. Periorbital, lower face, and neck skin are more prone to scarring and adjustment in technique and fewer passes at low energies are warranted in these areas. Patients who are undergoing multiple cosmetic procedures along with laser resurfacing may require an adjustment in laser technique.

In areas where skin is undermined subcutaneously, it is generally recommended to limit treatment. Patients who have had prior facelifting surgery require the surgeon to recognize that facial skin present over the area of the mandibular angle may have originally been neck skin, and should be treated less aggressively.

In the postoperative period, scar prevention is best achieved by decreasing the possibility of contact dermatitis, and early recognition of scar formation. Contact dermatitis is recognized as erythematous areas with pruritis frequently reported by the patient. Erythema and induration are indications of early scar formation. For contact dermatitis initial treatment is aimed at removal of the offending agent. Typically these agents are soaps or lotions with fragrance, topical antibiotics, or cosmetics. These substances should be avoided during the period before re-epithelialization, as this is the time of greatest risk for contact dermatitis. Class I topical corticosteroids are recommended when scar formation is suspected. Injection of corticosteroid into the area is also recommended. 585-nm pulsed dye laser can be used on the area and can be very effective in decreasing scarring and accompanying erythema. Alster recommended 4.5 to 5.0 J/cm^2 with a 10-mm spot size, or 6.5 to 7.0 J/cm^2 with a 7-mm spot size. Two to three treatments may be required spaced at 6–8 weeks intervals.[16] Intense pulsed light therapy used with a filter to treat vascular lesions is also effective.

Exuberant Skin Tightening and Ectropion Formation

Skin tightening is usually one of the desirable consequences of ablative skin resurfacing. Unfortunately, when treating the thin lower eyelid skin this may lead to lower lid retraction and inferior scleral display or ectropion. This is a more frequent finding in patients who have been previously treated in the area with ablative laser, had an aggressive skin resection from lower blepharoplasty, or present with a lax lower canthal tendon. Although this complication frequently resolves with time, persistent ectropion is a problem that often takes surgical correction to remedy. Initial evaluation of the patient to assess for risk of this complication involves an assessment of skin laxity and canthal laxity in the lower lid. To assess skin laxity we recommend having the patient look up with the mouth moderately open. This stretches the lower eyelid skin to its maximal extent. If a caliper can pinch the lower eyelid skin without inferiorly displacing the lid margin, a lower risk of ectropion is expected. The vertical and horizontal snap test is used to evaluate laxity in the lower canthal tendon. Increased lower lid laxity increases the risk of ectropion and lid shortening as the forces of inferior tightening overcome the tendon's ability to hold the lid in a superior position. When lid shortening or ectropion are noted, topical and intralesional steroids coupled with lower lid massage are initial therapy recommendations. Typically, therapy is delayed until after re-epithelialization is complete. As both lower lid retraction and ectropion are a result of scarring, they are initially treated similarly. Correction of persistent ectropion and lid shortening will be discussed in the surgical blepharoplasty section to follow.

SURGICAL COSMETIC PROCEDURE COMPLICATIONS

1. Blepharoplasty
2. Forehead and brow procedures
3. Lower facial procedures (Rhytidectomy, Neck Lift, Liposculpture)
4. Facial implants
5. Rhinoplasty

Blepharoplasty

Blepharoplasty is reported to be the most commonly performed facial cosmetic surgical procedure, which, if not performed correctly, can lead to very unsatisfactory results. Many of patients' early complaints are related to ecchymosis, edema, conjunctival irritation, or minor corneal abrasion. The more problematic complications of blepharoplasty may be avoided by a good preoperative evaluation, as most are correlated to the position and function of the lids relative to the globe and their appearance in contrast with the surrounding periorbital area. Rarely complications can lead to visual disturbances or blindness.

Edema, Ecchymosis, Conjunctival Irritation, and Corneal Abrasion

Patients should be instructed to expect periorbital edema and ecchymosis after any eyelid procedure. Edema may be present to some extent often up to 3 months after blepharoplasty and this should be explained to the patient preoperatively. Patients who wear corrective lenses should expect their prescription to be changed slightly during this time and may experience a degree of blurry vision. Limitation of these problems by the surgeon is best accomplished by atraumatic technique and, optimally, to avoid all bleeding during surgery, and to remove any blood from the field prior to closure. Arnica- or bromoline-containing topical solutions may aid in resolution of edema and ecchymosis. Conjunctival irritation or minor corneal abrasion may be noted after surgery. Conjunctival injection, with thin watery discharge, is likely due to mechanical or chemical irritation during surgery and does not represent infection in the early post-op period. Steroid ophthalmic drops four times daily (QID) for 5 days may be started immediately. If infection is suspected or present, an antibiotic–steroid solution may be prescribed. One should check for an adequate lid seal on closure to exclude early progression of keratoconjunctivitis. If the eyelid seal is weak, copious artificial tears should be used during daytime hours with the addition of a viscous lubricant for sleep periods.

Corneal abrasion is diagnosed by inspection of the eye after instillation of fluorescein drops and blue light examination. Occasionally the use of a cycloplegic agent such as homotropine to prevent blepharospasm may aid the examination. Once diagnosed, antibiotic–steroid drops and copious eye lubricants are the initial recommended treatment. For serious corneal abrasions, referral to an ophthalmologist for placement of a soft corneal bandage should be considered. Fortunately, most symptoms resolve within 48 hours, but close follow-up is needed to ensure that bacterial or fungal super-infection does not develop.

Ectropion, Entropion, Lid Shortening, Poor Lid Seal, and Ptosis

Common lower lid malposition complications include ectropion, entropion, lid shortening with scleral display, inability of the lids to form a seal, and ptosis. Patients who are at risk of these problems can often be identified during preoperative evaluation. Ectropion, entropion, and lid shortening are complications related to lower lid blepharoplasty. An inability to form a lid seal with resulting symptoms of dry eyes and keratoconjunctivitis can be seen with overaggressive upper or lower blepharoplasty. Lid ptosis is a complication of upper blepharoplasty. As mentioned previously, a proper assessment of lid skin and canthal laxity (snap test) should be performed prior to lower blepharoplasty. Patients with a deficient infraorbital rim, or proptotic eyes are particularly prone to lower lid position complications. Ectropion is usually the result of over-resection of lower lid skin and/or muscle. Early surgery to correct this problem is not recommended since many cases will respond to simple massage therapy and time. Three months is a typical period to delay further treatment. Another option is to attempt to elevate cheek soft tissue and to remove tension from the lower lid. This has been accomplished with varying degrees of success using larger volumes of soft tissue fillers or suborbicularis oculi fat (SOOF) lift procedures. This can be particularly effective in patients having a deficient infraorbital rim projection. Skin grafting is performed only for persistent ectropion. If available, the skin graft may be obtained from the upper lid, or less optimally from the retroauricular or supraclavicular regions. Excessive inferior scleral display after blepharoplasty (lid shortening) is more commonly seen after subciliary approach blepharoplasty that involves opening the septum to remove orbital fat (Fig. 9.8). The septum heals with scar

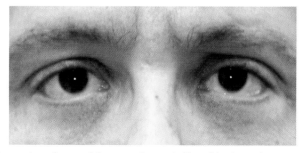

Fig. 9.8. Ectropion and lid shortening observed 5 years after subciliary blepharoplasty.

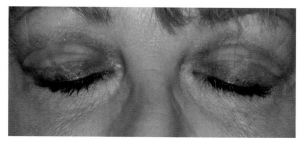

Fig. 9.9. Patient 10 years post skin grafting to upper lids. Grafting was done to create adequate lid seal after previous aggressive upper blepharoplasty led to keratoconjunctivitis.

contracture that pulls the lower lid inferiorly. To avoid this issue some have recommended a transconjunctival approach to the orbital fat. When lid shortening is noted, we recommend massage and superior taping depending on severity. For cases with greater than 2 mm of inferior scleral display, the surgeon may consider placement of a Frost suture, although it is of limited value. Conservative treatment should be continued for at least 3 months postoperatively if tolerated by the patient. It is often necessary to treat symptoms of dry eyes and conjunctival irritation during this period. If the scleral show is recalcitrant to these interventions then scar lysis along the infraorbital rim with lateral canthopexy may be necessary. It is often of value to place a spacer graft along the orbital rim to support the septum in the new position. If the excessive scleral show is long-standing then an interpositional mucosal and cartilage graft is recommended along with canthopexy. Patients may present with a combination of both lid shortening and ectropion. In these cases both problems need to be considered if corrective surgery is necessary. Entropion commonly results from overclosure of a transconjuctival incision or after resolution of a local infection of the same incision. To avoid imbrication of the conjunctiva, most surgeons do not close the incision, or place one or two fine loose sutures. Entropion can be a very painful complication for patients as eyelashes constantly abrade the conjunctiva and can cause corneal abrasion. If noticed early, massage, and/or opening the incision can be helpful. For longer-standing cases, grafting of the conjunctiva below the tarsus with an interpositional palatal mucosal graft is effective. Lack of adequate lid seal after blepharoplasty may be transitory and related to lid edema, or permanent and related to excessive skin removal and/or removal of excessive muscle with resultant movement impairment. Revision blepharoplasty patients are particularly prone to this complication and accurate preoperative marking with use of skin calipers is standard. Massage, eye lubricants, and steroids are useful in cases of inability to close the eyes. If unresolved, skin grafting may be required to allow the upper lid sufficient laxity to close (Fig. 9.9). In cases of excessive orbicularis oculi resection and movement impairment, gold weight placement in the upper lid may be necessary. Ptosis often results from disruption of the levator aponeurosis. Repair of ptosis involves shortening of the levator aponeurosis to its appropriate length. This procedure can be performed through an incision either transconjunctivally or through the blepharoplasty incision as an outpatient procedure.[26]

Dry Eyes (Keratoconjunctivitis Sicca)

Dry eyes (keratoconjunctivitis sicca) after blepharoplasty is a common complication. In a recent study by Hamaway and colleagues, they noted a rate of 11% of patients with complaints of dry eyes 2 weeks after blepharoplasty with 2% persisting after 2 months.[27] This problem can vary from a mild annoyance to a serious problem requiring referral and long-term treatment. Preoperative evaluation should include assessment for patients with dry eyes and those at risk for developing the condition postoperatively (Schirmer's test). In an algorithm proposed by Hamaway, patients with dry eye after blepharoplasty are managed with a topical lubricant, topical steroid, and nighttime taping. If chemosis is present, then systemic corticosteroid and eye patching may be warranted. If the condition persists for over 3 months, consultation should be made to an ophthalmologist.[27]

Acute Angle Glaucoma

Acute angle closure glaucoma after blepharoplasty is an exceedingly rare complication but with potentially devastating result. There have been approximately five cases reported in the literature, with three of those resulting in blindness.[28–31] Early recognition of signs and symptoms of acute angle closure glaucoma and prompt referral is key to limiting long-term sequelae. The eye may show signs of injection and a mid-dilated pupil. Complaints of pain and blurry vision after surgery should be investigated for increased intraocular pressure. It should be remembered that patients with acute angle closure glaucoma often have nausea, vomiting, or headache. These symptoms can blur the diagnosis and cause a delay in appropriate care.

The underlying cause of **retrobulbar hemorrhage** in the postoperative period following blepharoplasty is unknown. Three causes are frequently believed to be responsible: damage to posterior orbital veins, extraocular muscle bleeding, and orbital fat bleeding following fat resection. Retrobulbar hematoma can produce a spectrum of problems, from pain to blindness. It is thought to cause visual disturbance by increased retrobulbar pressure causing compression of the optic nerve.[32] Signs of retrobulbar hematoma include stabbing eye pain, proptosis, loss of visual field, and severe headache. Most retrobulbar hematomas are managed with medical therapy in the way of osmotic agents, steroids, or other agents to decrease intraocular pressure. If necessary, a lateral canthotomy is the surgical treatment of choice. This is performed by scissor release of the lower arm of the lateral canthus and release of the arcus marginalis. Dissection into the posterior orbit is almost never necessary and is not recommended in most cases.

Blindness is a relatively rare complication of blepharoplasty. In a report by McCarthy and colleagues, developed from a questionnaire, they reported a rate of postoperative blindness of 0.04% among 98,514 surgeries.[33] Unfortunately, the questionnaire did not address the cause of blindness. Though blindness is often the permanent result of a complication, disturbances in vision and ocular signs and symptoms should be aggressively investigated to prevent this most feared outcome.

Infection is a quite rare occurrence in blepharoplasty, as well as in other head and neck procedures due to the extensive vascularity in the area. In a study by Lee, 2,227 patients underwent eyelid surgery and only one had a postoperative infection. This infection was reported as mild and was remedied by oral antibiotics without permanent deficit.[34]

Forehead and Brow Procedures

When brow ptosis and/or deep forehead rhytids are not amenable to less invasive treatments, brow lifting procedures can provide excellent results in upper facial rejuvenation. There are many methods of brow lifting, with various advantages and disadvantages. Techniques can be broadly described as short scar (endoscopic) or as long scar using a hairline incision (coronal, pretrichial, trichophytic, or direct brow approaches). Methods for maintaining brow position following the lift are numerous and include suture or screw anchorage. Complications of brow lifting in general will be discussed with a focus on both early and late complications. Early complications of brow surgery include infection, bleeding or hematoma formation, pain, and swelling. Infection after brow lifting is quite rare in published reports.[35–37] and is managed with antibiotic therapy, removal of infection source, and incision and drainage. Folliculitis is a specific type of infection seen after brow lifting procedures, and treatment includes antibiotics targeted toward skin flora, especially *Staphylococcus aureus*.

Bleeding and hematoma formation are more common postoperative complications than infections. Typically, drains are not placed after brow-lifting procedures. Limiting the use of anticoagulants, good surgical technique and hemostasis, and the use of epinephrine-containing tumescent solutions are the keys to limiting the occurrence of this complication. Hematomas are usually evacuated in the office setting. If bleeding or reaccumulation of a hematoma occurs, a return to the operating room may be considered to achieve adequate visualization and hemostatic control. Commonly, branches of the superficial temporal artery or vein that have not been appropriately cauterized at surgery are the contributing vessels to the hematoma.

Postoperative pain after a brow lift typically presents as a tension-like headache. Narcotic medication is usually effective for control of discomfort, and pain is noticeably improved within 24–48 hours as edema and inflammation begins to resolve.

Edema after brow lifting is more common in patients who are smokers. This is usually a mild problem, which resolves with time. Reassurance and recommendations such as head elevation are given to the patient, as well as preoperatively smoking cessation counseling.

Long-term complications of brow lifting include sensory disturbances, incisional alopecia, facial motor nerve weakness, brow asymmetry, and relapse. Fortunately, all of these complications are rare and generally managed with acceptable results.

As most brow-lifting procedures involve manipulating the periosteum near the supraorbital and supratrochlear nerves, **sensory disturbances** are a frequent complaint in the early period. Most sensory disturbances are related to a neuropraxic (nerve stretch or conduction block) type injury and may resolve within a few weeks. Long-lasting sensory loss is often well tolerated by patients but it has a very low occurrence rate.[30,31] Dysesthesia, burning, and itching are often distressing for patients, and attempts at treatment may be required. Conservative pain medication management for this complaint is recommended. Additional medications include low dose amitryptaline, medrol dose pack, or neurontin (gabapentin). The use of lidocaine and triamcinolone injection at the supraorbital nerve has been reported to have good results.[30]

Incisional alopecia is a common complication of both endoscopic or open brow lift surgery. Hair loss is often temporary and reassurance in the early postoperative period is warranted. One may consider using medrol dose packs in the perioperative period to decrease the likelihood of "hair shock" and subsequent exfoliation. The surgical technique is critical during the surgical procedure; a beveled skin incision in the direction of the hair may be used to prevent follicular damage, and skin tension should be avoided at the incision line and suture location. If the alopecia is cosmetically unacceptable, excisional scar revision is performed, or in some cases hair grafting may be warranted.

Facial motor weakness in the frontal branch of the facial nerve is fortunately an uncommon complication, and, is almost always temporary. When encountered, weakness in brow elevation is often only seen on one side. Treatment with botulinum toxin in the functional brow is used to increase symmetry until recovery of the weakened brow has taken place.

Relapse should be expected after brow lifting surgery, and overcorrection is typically performed to account for this phenomenon. Minimizing relapse is dependent upon technique during the surgical procedure including attention to fixation techniques, adequate release of periosteum and muscle attachments. Greater degrees of relapse may be found in patients who present with thick, sebaceous forehead skin, deep horizontal brow rhytids, severe brow ptosis, or high foreheads. The surgeon faced with relapse must consider reoperation to provide the patient with an acceptable final result.

Lower Facial Procedures (Rhytidectomy, Neck Lift, Liposculpture)

Facelift procedures, otherwise known as cervicofacial rhytidectomy, are an effective way to treat facial rhytids not amenable to less invasive forms of therapy. A neck lift procedure may be considered a facelift that lacks a preauricular and temporal component. Submental liposuction, or liposculpture, is a lower facial and neck procedure that is often performed either alone or in conjunction with a facelift to recontour superficial fat deposits. Though many techniques have been described, as a group of lower facial procedures, these technqiues share many of the same complications. The purpose of this section is to describe the treatment of the complications of cervicofacial rhytidectomy, neck lift and submental liposuction, and not to argue the benefit of one technique over another.

Hematoma is a common complication of cervicofacial rhytidectomy, neck lift, and liposculture procedures and can lead to skin necrosis if not identified and treated promptly. It occurs in approximately 3% to 15% of all cases.[38–40] Prevention of hematoma begins in the preoperative period, when patients should be evaluated for use of anticoagulant medications or bleeding disorders. Intraoperatively, patients should be maintained in a normotensive state as intraoperative hypertension has been positively correlated with postoperative hematoma development. In addition, blood pressure control in the perioperative period is also advisable since hypertension has also been associated with increased postoperative hematoma formation.

Most hematomas appear early in the postoperative period, likely in the first 24–48 hours. Two classifications of hematomas exist: major hematoma and microhematoma. The difference between the two is the size of the hematoma, as well as the method required to treat each. If the hematoma is large and/or

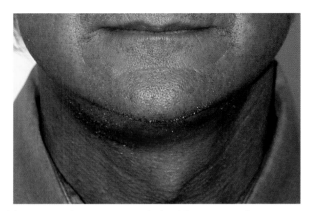

Fig. 9.10. Delayed submental hematoma formation in male facelift patient 7 days post-op.

expanding and requires surgical drainage then it is classified as a major hematoma. If a major hematoma is encountered, the management is partial or complete opening of the surgical wound with evacuation of the hematoma. It is prudent at that time to try to identify and control any active bleeding sources. Microhematoma is managed by needle aspiration and application of external pressure dressings. Occasionally these small hematomas may be observed and needle evacuated 7–10 days after the procedure when the clot has liquefied to some degree. Patients should be encouraged to limit activity for at least 7–10 days since late hematoma formation has been observed, especially in males, as late as 1 week after surgery (Fig. 9.10).

Facial nerve injury is a rare complication of face and neck procedures occurring in only 2–4% of cases, although transient weakness due to edema may occur more commonly.[41,42] The risk of permanent nerve injury is considered greater in deep plane versus superficial rhytidectomy procedures. Most frequently the temporal and marginal mandibular branches are affected. To avoid trauma to the facial nerve it is imperative that the surgeon maintain a plane of dissection that allows for anatomic protection of the nerve. Use of liposuction cannulas and dissecting scissors should be done cautiously when elevating tissue over the prejowl region since the facial nerve is least protected and most vulnerable in this area. When weakness of the muscles of facial expression is noted postoperatively it is important to realize that most cases will resolve spontaneously. It is advisable to monitor any decreased facial animation for a period of 3 weeks to 6 months for likely spontaneous recovery. Minor asymmetries may be unnoticed by the patient but apparent to the skilled observer. Persistent asymmetry may be amenable to botulinum toxin treatment of the unaffected side. Paralysis of the periorbital musculature necessitates protection of the globe. This may include eye drops and/or wearing a patch or the use of a gold weight in the upper lid. In severe cases, one may also consider a temporary tarsorrhaphy suture (Frost stitch) to protect the globe.

Superficial epidermolysis and more problematic full thickness loss of skin after face and neck procedures occurs most often in the post auricular region, but can occur anywhere in an area of undermined skin. Gentle soft tissue handling, proper depth of dissection, and avoiding overly tense closure are methods to avoid ischemia and subsequent skin compromise. Hematoma, if present, should be drained as soon as recognized. If ischemia persists despite preventative measures, areas of skin slough usually are allowed to heal by secondary intention. The wound should be treated with Aquafor or another moist occlusive, and any signs of infection should be treated promptly. As the wound heals, hypertrophic scarring can be addressed with steroid (kenalog) injections and/or laser treatment. If required, formal scar revision should be delayed for 6 months although in unusual instances primary revision may be accomplished immediately (Fig. 9.11).[37] In many cases there is insufficient skin laxity to allow the excision of scar tissue and closure. In these instances scar camouflage therapies are attempted to minimize the deformity. Erythema may be reduced by pulsed dye laser or intense pulse light (IPL) therapy. Skin irregularity may be smoothed with low energy ablative laser treatment and steroid injection. Areas of hypopigmentation are often the most difficult problem to improve and referral to a medical tattoo artist may be helpful.

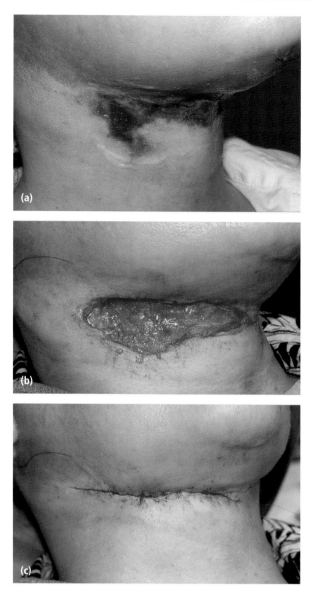

Fig. 9.11. (a) Skin breakdown 1 week after facelift. (b) Debridement of necrotic tissue 2 weeks after facelift. (c) Primary closure of defect.

Neurosensory disturbances after lower face and neck procedures are common, but are for the most part also self-limited. Most commonly the greater auricular nerve is affected from the plane of dissection along the area of the sternocleidomastoid muscle. Sullivan found an incidence of permanent numbness to the ear in 1% of their facelift patients. Besides paresthesia and anesthesia, which are difficult to manage, patients may also suffer from dysesthesia.[42] If dysesthesia develops in the postoperative period investigation into the cause is mandatory. A diagnostic nerve block with local anesthesia injected at the proximal nerve distribution can elucidate the responsible sensory nerve and also provide temporary relief. If a neuroma is suspected, high-resolution magnetic resonance imaging may help to locate the lesion. Neuromas may be amenable to surgical resection to provide permanent relief if done early. A less invasive option is the use of tricyclic antidepressants or gabapentin. Canter et al. describe a case of a female patient who developed intractable pain after rhytidectomy and was successfully treated with neurontin 300 mg three times a day.[43]

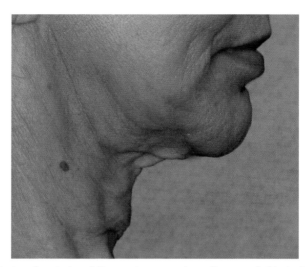

Fig. 9.12. Submental irregularity after isolated liposuction procedure. Degree of skin laxity dictates that correction will require a skin tightening procedure such as facelift.

Contour irregularities are a potential complication that can be seen after liposuction, facelift, and neck lift procedures. Avoidance of this problem begins with maintaining liposuction and lipodissection in a consistent plane. Also, care must be taken not to be overly aggressive in fat removal. Patients requiring large amounts of submental lipoosuction alone may benefit from the subcutaneous release of skin from deeper structures to allow passive redraping of the soft tissue envelope (Fig. 9.12). In cases where there is clearly a postoperative contour irregularity after 3 months, consideration must be given to correction. Fat deficiencies may be corrected with fat transfer or soft tissue fillers. Lateral sweep, or irregularities of skin redraping may benefit from subcutaneous release and resuspension. Hamra has described in several articles the contour abnormalities resulting from lateral vector rhytidectomy. The lateral sweep is a late sequelae and a sign of previous facelifting procedures:

> The unopposed tension of lateral vector face lifts allows the cheek tissues to descend eventually over the tightened jaw line, creating a "lateral sweep" or pulled appearance of the face. A crescent-shaped mound over the malar area is the inferior orbicularis oculi muscle, not repositioned with conventional procedures.[44]

This late sequelae can be prevented by adding a superior vector to the original facelift procedure to reposition the periorbital soft tissue and improve contour of the malar area. Hamra recommends arcus marginalis release to achieve this along with minimal removal of periorbital fat to avoid hollow eyes, which can accentuate facial contour imbalance. Correction of lateral sweep may require revectoring skin tension lines via revision facelift. Additional improvement may be achieved by improving skin tonicity via ablative skin resurfacing, radiofrequency tightening, or by optimizing facial volume with fat grafting or fillers (Fig. 9.13).

A number of cosmetic facelift and neck-lift complications can be related to various regions of the incision. The temporal tuft, tragus, earlobe, retroauricular sulcus, and the posterior hairline are all regions that may require modification of technique to avoid undesired sequelae (Table 9.2).

Pixie ear is a postoperative complication of rhytidectomy in which the normal architecture of the earlobe is changed and becomes pulled inferiorly towards the neck (Fig. 9.14). Normally, the free segment of the ear lobe typically meets the cheek and retromandibular skin in a notched area called the otobasion inferius. After rhytidectomy, the pull of the attached skin in this area is anterior and inferior. Drawing this attachment down and forward eliminates the free lobe and gives it a "stuck on" appearance. Avoidance of this complication is based upon proper incision design. One choice is to include a small amount of "cheek tissue" on the incision at the area of the earlobe (Fig. 9.15). This enables the closure of the otobasion inferius with a loose edge. It is imperative this closure is tension-free to help avoid "pixie ear."[45] Another

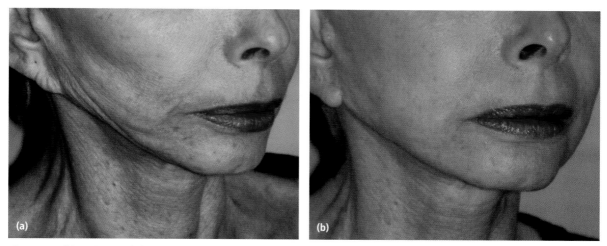

Fig. 9.13. (a) Patient with lateral sweep and pixie ear deformity. (b) Correction with revision facelift, CO_2 laser resurfacing, and free fat grafting.

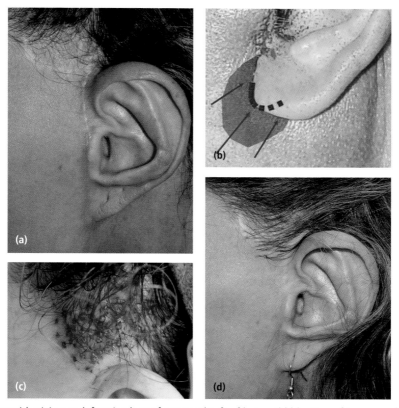

Fig. 9.14. (a) Patient with pixie ear deformity, loss of temporal tuft of hair, mild blunting of tragus and persistent incisional erythema at 5 years. Constellation of deformities suggests original facelift created excessive skin tension superficial undermining across the incision. (b) Original incision is reopened with subcutaneous undermining, and SMAS advancement is performed. Closure with inferior aspect of earlobe left unattached. (c) Temporal tuft is recreated with one and two hair follicular unit transplants. (d) Final result at 1 year post-op. CO_2 laser resurfacing of incisions was performed at 1 month post-op.

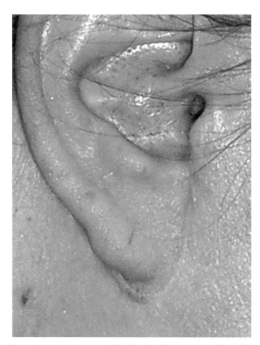

Fig. 9.15. Facelift incision designed to incorporate a cuff of neck tissue around earlobe.

option is to leave the inferior aspect of the earlobe unattached and overlapping the neck skin to heal by secondary intention. If pixie ear develops then surgery is required to correct the deformity. One method described involves removing a triangular amount of tissue on the lobe. The base of the triangle is the junction of lobe and cheek skin. The triangle is excised and the lobe is reattached in a superior and posterior direction.[45] In severe cases it may become necessary to undermine neck skin and tighten the underlying superficial muscular aponeurotic system (SMAS) to relieve tension on the earlobe.

Facial Implants

Facial implants offer a minimally invasive method to augment the patient's face and improve contour to normal or a more aesthetic form. Though implants have the advantage of being a less invasive method compared to orthognathic surgery, they should not be thought of as a complete substitute for correction of skeletal deformities. Facial implants have a low complication rate, yet occasionally cause problems severe enough to warrant their removal or revision.

Infection is the most common reason for implant removal. In their series, Wang et al. showed infection as the cause of removal of 3.7% of all implants placed in the face.[46] Late infection 10–20 years after implant placement is possible as well and has been reported. Meticulous technique should be used when placing implants, especially through the oral cavity. It is recommended that any infective odontogenic process be addressed before placement of implants through an intraoral incision. Preoperative chlorhexidine rinse and tooth brushing should be performed to decrease pathologic oral flora.

Infection may present with pain and swelling of the implant site. Physical examination may reveal erythema or fluctuance in the area of the implant. Sinus tract communication to the skin or fistula formation to the oral cavity is not unusual. Once recognized, infected implants should be removed. Implant therapy may be abandoned, or, a wait period of at least 6 months should pass before attempt at re-implantation.

Bone Resorption and Exposed Implant

Bone erosion deep to an implant is a concern related to the long-term stability of the implant and its safety. Bone remodeling and erosion has been a long-noted problem with implants of the chin.[47,48] Implants of all types have been found to cause changes to adjacent bone. In the case of chin implants it was thought that the pressure exerted on the implant from the mentalis muscle was the cause of the resorption. Many

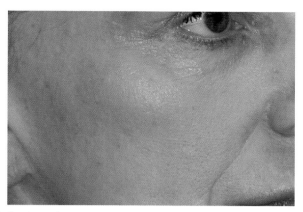

Fig. 9.16. Visible malar shell silastic implant.

others thought the resorption might result from subperiosteal placement of the implant. Contrary evidence in an animal study model challenges these two assumptions. Pearson et al. found that placement related to periosteum did not change resorption. They also found that resorption was greater in implants in which less pressure was exerted upon them.[49] Though not a definitive answer to the question of bone erosion, this study shows there is much to learn about erosion and its causes. Erosion and bone changes under implants are noted often on radiographs in patients who are happy with their surgical result and have no symptoms. It is an ill-advised decision to remove an implant due to this radiographic finding. Implant removal can lead to dimpling and disfigurement of the chin and must be considered prior to implant retrieval. If erosion becomes a problem, removal may be necessary.

Implants that are exposed or readily visible are usually the result of either poor selection of type and size, or inadequate creation of a surgical pocket. Correction of the visible implant typically involves removal and possible replacement with an appropriate implant in an adequate surgical dissection (Fig. 9.16).

Implant mobility is a well-recognized problem with all the implant materials used. Mobility of the implant has prompted many surgeons to use some form of fixation to maintain the implants in place such as titanium screws. A downside of this technique is that it may require a larger dissection in order to place the implant. If the implant has migrated on long-term evaluation a capsule may have formed. Repositioning at this stage may require a larger dissection and may destroy the implant. The surgeon should discuss the options and possibilities prior to removal. These include repositioning with fixation or complete removal of the old implant with a rest period or placement of a new implant. One should remember that contamination of the implant and subsequent infection is always a concern, and exposure of the implant increases this risk.

Neurosensory disturbances related to facial implants may be a result of the surgical access or a result of the implant impinging on the nerve. With chin implants patients should be warned of the possibility of mental nerve distribution paresthesia. With malar implant augmentation the infraorbital, zygomatico-frontal and zygomaticofacial nerve distribution are most likely to be involved. If the implant has become mobile and is causing pressure to any nerve then the implant should be exposed, repositioned, and fixed. If no obvious trauma was noted at the time of surgery, sensation is likely to return.

Rhinoplasty

Rhinoplasty is often referred to as the most demanding of all the facial cosmetic procedures. As the nose is centrally located on the face, any mishaps in nasal repair or cosmetic refinement will be readily apparent. The anatomy is intricate and small intraoperative adjustments produce seemingly large changes in the patient's appearance, for better or worse. These facts cause many surgeons to avoid rhinoplasty and others to specialize in the procedure. Many patients benefit from rhinoplastic surgery whether it be cosmetic, functional, or both. Dealing with the complications of rhinoplasty is as much an art as dealing with the surgery itself. Complications of rhinoplastic surgery may be considered functionally related, such as bleeding, infection, airway compromise, or primarily cosmetic issues. Often a cosmetic deformity will be related to a functional problem.

Hemorrhage to some degree during or after rhinoplasty is a fairly common occurrence. The nose is highly vascular with blood supply from branches of the internal and external carotid arteries. Bleeding can be a minor annoyance or can be serious and require hospital admission and possibly a return trip to the operating room. Most postoperative hemorrhage is minor, and packing along with topical vasoconstrictor application is sufficient to control the bleeding. Other methods include fibrin glue, thrombin, chemical cautery, and electrocautery. If bleeding persists or is pronounced, the improved visibility and access afforded in the operating room may be necessary.

Significant nasal hemorrhage is often from one of two sources, anterior bleeding from Kiesselbach's plexus, or posterior bleeding from a turbinate or septal branch of the sphenopalatine artery. Anterior bleeding is the more common of the two types, and fortunately is generally more amenable to control with conservative measures. Posterior bleeding is typically more profuse and difficult to control outside of the operative setting. In the unlikely event that complete control of bleeding cannot be obtained in the operating room, inflatable posterior nasal packs may be considered. The patient should be admitted for observation in an intensive care unit (ICU) level of care. Removal of nasal packs may be attempted after 24–48 hours. The patient should be observed for an appropriate period thereafter for signs of re-bleeding.

Infection incidence occurring after rhinoplasty can be divided into two categories based on the level of complexity of the procedure performed. Nasal surgery may be considered complex if it involves revision surgery, severe post-traumatic surgery, or the use of complex auto, alloplastic, or synthetic grafting techniques. The use of synthetic grafts has a particularly high rate of infection compared to simple nasal surgery. Routine nasal surgery has a low infection rate at approximately 2.5%, while more complex nasal corrective procedures have a postoperative infection rate up to 27%. Postoperative antibiotics have not been shown to reduce the rate of infection in routine rhinoplasty, but have been shown assist in complex cases.[50] Minor suture abscess and skin wound infections with cellulites can be treated with oral or intravenous antibiotics. Infected grafts typically require removal of the graft and debridement for resolution. Failure to recognize and treat an infected graft may lead to skin compromise and soft tissue loss (Fig. 9.17). Septal abscess in patients following septoplasty is almost always seen after hematoma. Once septal abscess recognized it must be treated aggressively because pronounced loss of nasal septal and lateral cartilage may occur (Fig. 9.18). The septal mucosa must be opened and all foreign or graft material removed; tissue debridement should be undertaken for all involved areas. Systemic antibiotics for *Staphylococcal* species coverage should also be employed. The surgeon must decide whether to reconstruct immediately or delay reconstruction.[51] Often, a waiting period of 6 months is advisable prior to reconstruction.

Airway obstruction may be present prior to rhinoplasty, or may develop postoperatively from the procedure itself. A thorough preoperative functional examination may alert the surgeon to patients who either have a compromised airway, or who may be at risk for an airway obstruction post rhinoplasty. In addition to intranasal speculum exam, nasopharyngoscopy or CT radiographic examination may be warranted. Particular care in these patients must be directed at maintaining the function of the internal and external nasal valves. Narrowing procedures for example may be contraindicated, use of a spreader graft may be required when decreasing a dorsal hump or alar/batten grafting maybe needed to support the external nasal valve (Fig. 9.19). Extreme caution must be exercised in destructive techniques such as cartilage removal or osteotomies. Most patients will observe some nasal stuffiness in the immediate postoperative period. Nasal obstruction present beyond 3 months will typically not resolve and may require surgical intervention. Functional revision rhinoplasty is often a complex procedure that may require the procurement of either ear or rib cartilage and at best may yield compromised functional and cosmetic results. For this reason, all rhinoplasties should be considered "functional" as well as cosmetic during the planning phase.

Intracranial communications are an extremely rare complication of rhinoplasty. The mechanism is typically violation of the cribiform plate by the instruments used during septorhinoplasty. Rhinorrhea should be managed by admission to a hospital and consultation with the neurosurgical service. Head of bed elevation and other efforts to decrease and prevent spikes in intracranial pressure are employed as a first line. Prophylactic antibiotics are an area of controversy. If the cerebral spinal fluid leak is recalcitrant

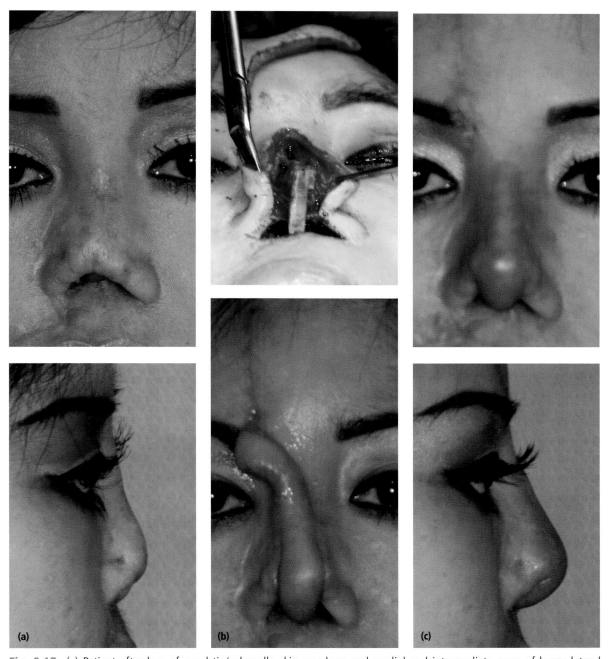

Fig. 9.17. (a) Patient after loss of nasal tip/columella skin envelope and medial and intermediate crura of lower lateral cartilages secondary to infected dorsal silastic implant. (b) Paramedian forehead flap and costochondral graft to recreate lost tissue. (c) Patient at 5 months post-op.

to the more noninvasive methods, then lumbar drain is sometimes employed to lower intracranial pressure in the hope of spontaneous closure. Invasive local methods are used as a last resort, which include transnasal endoscopic repair or even craniotomy.

Cosmetic complications following rhinoplastic surgery are numerous and may have many causes (Fig. 9.20). Following is a general discussion of common cosmetic complications.

Open roof deformity occurs when the dorsum of the nose is reduced with a chisel, and the nasal bones, septum, and upper lateral cartilage are visible through the skin. It results from an error in judgment at the

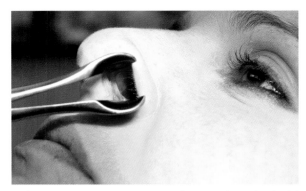

Fig. 9.18. Patient with septal perforation. Patient was unaware of the condition but had history of severe nasal trauma 7 years prior.

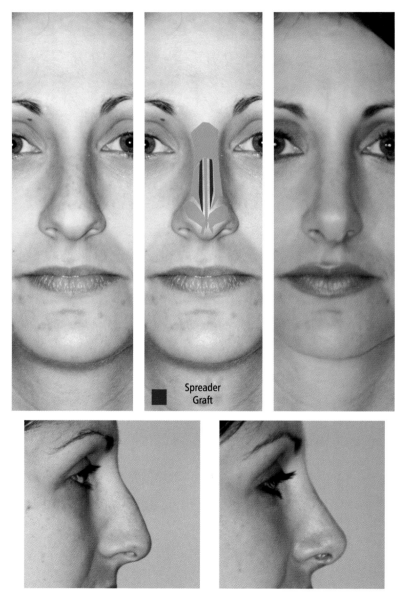

Spreader Graft

Fig. 9.19. Patient with high dorsum and narrow middle nasal vault. Open roof is closed with septal cartilage spreader grafts to preserve nasal function and appearance.

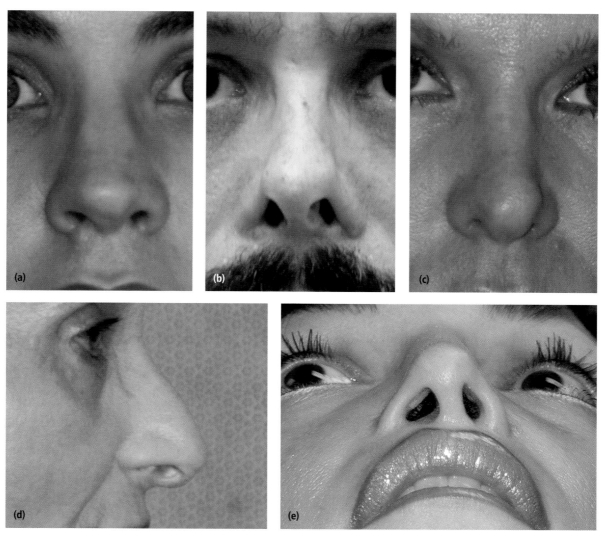

Fig. 9.20. Post-rhinoplasty complications. (a) Open roof deformity—corrected with lateral osteotomies and spreader grafts. (b) Alar rim retraction, tip over-rotation, excessive nasal base resection, and middle nasal vault correction. Corrected with costochondral baton grafts, composite graft to ala, open septorhinoplasty (OSRP). (c) Nasal tip bossae. Corrected with OSRP and onlay auricular cartilage graft. (d) Polly-beak deformity. Corrected with caudal, dorsal septal reduction and OSRP. (e) Unitip deformity, septal deviation, excessive alar base resection, collapse of external nasal valve with nasal stenosis. Corrected with complex OSRP utilizing auricular baton grafts to lower lateral cartilages.

time of original surgery in which osteotomy of the nasal bones is not performed or spreader grafts are not placed. Correction of the deformity requires reoperation. If the internal nasal valve is not too restricted, then osteotomy of nasal bones can be performed; otherwise, spreader grafts should be placed.

Saddle nose deformity denotes a condition in which the dorsum of the nose has been over-reduced. This gives the dorsum a concave profile. It is imperative to evaluate the patient anew when presented with a saddle nose deformity. If the nasal tip is overprojected then revision rhinoplasty may involve reduction of tip projection. If the tip is favorably projected, then a dorsal graft is the treatment of choice. There also exist situations in which tip revision and grafting are done simultaneously. It is important to make an attempt to not create one deformity out of another. Grafts to correct saddle nose deformity are usually placed through an open approach, but many surgeons are doing this through a closed approach and reporting good results. Choice of graft material is varied—from autogenous sources such as cartilage, rib and calvarial bone, among others, to synthetic material such as Gore-Tex or Medpor.

Polly-beak deformity is a frustrating and relatively common complication of rhinoplasty. Three causes are typically identified: (1) failure to reduce the cartilaginous septum, (2) excessive scar formation in the nasal tip, and (3) overzealous cephalic trim or any maneuver leading to unexpected deprojection of the tip relative to the dorsum. With these causes in mind the surgery to correct polly-beak deformity is tailored to the problem. If inadequate reduction of the septal cartilage is the issue, then revision should include reduction of this structure. Polly-beak deformity resulting from excessive scar formation is commonly seen in patients with thick, sebaceous skin. Interception after the primary procedure can help eliminate the need for revision rhinoplasty in some cases. If supratip fullness is noted in the postoperative period, then steroid injections can be attempted to limit scar formation. If revision is necessary it should not be performed until at least 6 months to a year have elapsed from the time of the original surgery. Revision is made by an open technique and excision of fibrous tissue is performed along with redraping of the skin.

Any number of surgical techniques can weaken the support structures that help to maintain tip projection and tip rotation. The act of performing the open rhinoplasty dissection alone can be sufficient to induce undesired tip deprojection and/or superior rotation. Overzealous cephalic trim can result in tip deprojection, tip over-rotation, alar rim retraction, and polly-beak deformity. At the time of the original surgery judicious lateral crural trimming can decrease the incidence of this complication. Placement of a columellar strut graft and alar batten grafts or alar rim grafting may aid to prevent this problem. If the deformity develops after rhinoplasty, then revision surgery is indicated. Revision surgery is often far more complicated and unpredictable than the original operation. The columellar strut and batten grafts are fashioned from septal cartilage or, if unavailable, conchal cartilage can be harvested. An open approach is typically used with suturing of the graft in place to avoid displacement.

Bossae can be congenital or a result of rhinoplasty. This deformity presents as prominences at the nasal tip, usually representing strong cartilage showing through thin skin. A **unitip deformity** is a related deformity where a central singular bossae is present and the ala become retracted, leading to the appearance of a prominent tip that lacks the normal transitional architecture to the cheek. Early bossae are a result of an uncorrected domal irregularity or from splayed medial crura. Late bossae formation result from scar formation and resultant asymmetries. Unitip deformity is often the result of aggressive resection of the lateral crura and excessive narrowing suture/graft techniques of the intermediate/medial crura. Bossae and unitip correction is performed by an open technique and involves modification of the tip cartilage by either suturing, excision of the offending cartilage, or repair with cartilage grafts in an overlapping fashion.[52]

Rocker-deformity, **"inverted-V" deformity, and "keel" deformity** are three complications secondary to a loss of control of lateral nasal osteotomies. A rocker deformity will result after the infracture of a lateral osteotomy that has been carried too far superiorly towards the glabella. An "inverted-V" deformity is the visual result of the inward collapse of the upper lateral cartilages at the junction with the nasal bones and is often accompanied by internal nasal valve dysfunction. This may be seen after aggressive infracturing of a lateral osteotomy when spreader grafts should have been considered to maintain the upper lateral cartilages in a more lateral position. The "keel" deformity is often seen with the "inverted-V" in that as the sidewalls of the nose are collapsed inwards, the dorsum now comes almost to a "keel-like" point. Revision rhinoplasty is indicated to correct these deformities and is directed at reestablishing a more appropriate position of the nasal bones and upper lateral cartilages and often involves complex spreader grafting techniques.

SUGGESTED READINGS

1. Carruthers A, Carruthers J. 2009. "A single-center, dose-comparison, pilot study of the botulinum neurotoxin type A in female patients with upper facial rhytids: Safety and efficacy." *Journal of the American Academy of Dermatology* 60: 972.
2. Carruthers A, Lowe NJ, Menter A, et al.. 2002. "A multicenter, double-blind, randomized, placebo-controlled study of the efficacy and safety of botulinum toxin type A in the treatment of glabellar lines." *Journal of the American Academy of Dermatology* 46: 840.
3. Surgeons ASoP. 2000/2006/2007. "National plastic surgery statistics, cosmetic and reconstructive procedure trends." American Society of Plastic Surgeons, www.plasticsurgery.org.

4. Naumann M, and Jankovic J. 2004. "Safety of botulinum toxin type A: A systemic review and meta-analysis." *Current Medical Research and Opinion* 20: 981.

5. Niamtu JI. 2000. "The use of botulinum toxin in cosmetic facial surgery." In: *Oral and Maxillofacial Surgery Clinics of North America*, Niamtu JI, ed., 595. Philadelphia: W.B. Saunders.

6. Smith KC. 2008. "Reversible vs. nonreversible fillers in facial aesthetics: Concerns and considerations." *Dermatology Online Journal* 14: 3.

7. Klein AW, and Rish DC. 1983. "Bovine injectable collagen." *Western Journal of Medicine* 143: 231.

8. Niamtu JI. 2005. "New lip and wrinkle fillers." In: *Oral and Maxillofacial Surgery Clinics of North America*, Haug RH, ed., 17. Philadelphia: Elsevier.

9. Allergan: ZYDERM® and ZYPLAST® Collagen Implants. 2009. www.allergan.com, accessed June 2011.

10. Fischer J, Metzler G, and Schaller M. 2007. "Cosmetic permanent fillers for soft tissue augmentation: A new contraindication for interferon therapies." *Archives of Dermatology* 143: 507.

11. Wolfram D, Tzankov A, and Piza-Katzer H. "Surgery for foreign body reactions due to injectable fillers." *Dermatology* 213: 300.

12. Senet P, Bachelez H, Ollivaud L, et al. 1999. "Minocycline for the treatment of cutaneous silicone granulomas." *British Journal of Dermatology* 140: 985.

13. Baumann LS, and Halem ML. 2003. "Lip silicone granulomatous foreign body reaction treated with Aldara (imiquimod 5%)." *Dermatologic Surgery* 29: 429.

14. Pasternack FR, Fox LP, and Engler DE. 2005. "Silicone granulomas treated with Etanercept." *Archives of Dermatology* 141: 13.

15. Dreizen NG, and Framm L. 1989. "Sudden unilateral visual loss after autologous fat injection into the glabellar area." *American Journal of Ophthalmology* 107: 85.

16. Egido J, Arroyo R, Marcos A, and Jimenez-Alfaro I. 1993. "Middle cerebral artery embolism and unilateral visual loss after autologous fat injection into the glabellar area." *Stroke* 24: 615.

17. Schanz S, Schippert W, Ulmer A, et al. 2002. "Arterial embolization caused by injection of hyaluronic acid (Restylane)." *British Journal of Dermatology* 148: 379.

18. De Castro ACB, Collares MVM, Portinho CP, et al. 2007. "Extensive facial necrosis after infiltration of polymethylmethacrylate." *Revista Brasileira de Otorrinolaringologia* 73: 850.

19. Cohen SR, and Holmes RE. 2004. "Artecoll: A long-lasting injectable wrinkle filler material: Report of a controlled, randomized, multicenter clinical trial of 251 subjects." *Plastic and Reconstructive Surgery* 114: 964.

20. Bogle MA. 2009. *Non-Surgical Skin Tightening and Lifting: Radiofrequency Energy and Hybrid Devices*. China: Saunders, Elsevier.

21. England RW, Vogel P, and Hagan L. 2002. "Immediate cutaneous hypersensitivity after treatment of tattoo with Nd: YAG laser: A case report and review of the literature." *Annals of Allergy, Asthma & Immunology* 89: 215.

22. Ashinoff R, Levine VJ, and Soter NA. 1995. "Allergic reactions to tattoo pigment after laser treatment." *Dermatologic Surgery* 21: 291.

23. Niamtu JI. 2000. "Common complications of laser resurfacing and their treament." In: *Oral and Maxillofacial Surgery Clinics of North America; Cosmetic Facial Surgery*, Schmidt R, ed., 579. Philadelphia: W.B. Saunders.

24. Alster TS, and Lupton JR. 2002. "Prevention and treatment of side effects and complications of cutaneous laser resurfacing." *Plastic and Reconstructive Surgery* 109: 308.

25. Walia S, and Alster TS. 1999. "Cutaneous CO_2 laser resurfacing infection rate with and without prophylactic antibiotics." *Dermatologic Surgery* 25: 857.

26. Lucarelli MJ, and Lemke BN. 1999. "Small incision external levator repair: Technique and early results." *American Journal of Ophthalmology* 127: 637.

27. Hamaway AH, Farkas JP, Fagien S, and Rohrich RJ. 2009. "Preventing and managing dry eyes after periorbital surgery: A retrospective review." *Plastic and Reconstructive Surgery* 123: 353.

28. Green MF, and Kadri SW. 1974. "Acute closed-angle glaucoma, a complication of blepharoplasty: Report of a case." *British Journal of Plastic Surgery* 27: 25.

29. Gayton JL, and Ledford JK. 1992. "Angle closure glaucoma following a combined blepharoplasty and ectropion repair." *Ophthalmic Plastic & Reconstructive Surgery* 8: 176.

30. Bleyen I, Rademaker R, Wolfs RC, and van Rij G. 2008. "Acute angle closure glaucoma after oculoplastic surgery." *Orbit* 27: 49.

31. Wride NK, and Sanders R. 2004. "Blindness from acute angle-closure glaucoma after blepharoplasty." *Ophthalmic Plastic & Reconstructive Surgery* 20: 476.

32. Wolfort FG, Vaughan TE, Wolfort SF, and Nevarre DR. 1999. "Retrobulbar hematoma and blepharoplasty." *Plastic and Reconstructive Surgery* 104: 2154.

33. McCarthy D, Wood T, and Austin W. 1974. "Eye complications with blepharoplasty or other eyelid surgery." *Plastic and Reconstructive Surgery* 53: 634.

34. Lee EW, Holtebeck AC, and Harrison AR. 2009. "Infection rates in outpatient eyelid surgery." *Ophthalmic Plastic & Reconstructive Surgery* 25: 109.

35. Jones BM, and Grover R. 2004. "Endoscopic brow lift: A personal review of 538 patients and comparison of fixation techniques." *Plastic and Reconstructive Surgery* 113: 1251.

36. De Cordier BC, de la Torre JI, Al-Hakeem MS, et al. 2002. "Endoscopic forehead lift: Review of technique, cases, and complications." *Plastic and Reconstructive Surgery* 110: 1558.

37. Elkwood A, Matarasso A, Rankin M, et al. 2001. "National plastic surgery survey: Brow lifting techniques and complications." *Plastic and Reconstructive Surgery* 108: 2143.

38. Grover R, Jones BM, and Waterhouse N. 2001. "The prevention of haematoma following rhytidectomy: A review of 1078 consecutive facelifts." *British Journal of Plastic Surgery* 54: 481.

39. Niamtu JI. 2005. "Expanding hematoma in face-lift surgery: Literature review, case presentations, and caveats." *Dermatologic Surgery* 32: 1134.

40. Griffin JE, and Jo C. 2007. "Complications after superficial plane cervicofacial rhytidectomy: A retrospective analysis of 178 consecutive facelifts and review of the literature." *Journal of Oral and Maxillofacial Surgery* 65: 2227.

41. Ghali GE, and Lustig JH. 2003. "Complications associated with facial cosmetic surgery." In: *Oral and Maxillofacial Surgery Clinics of North America*, August M, ed., 265. Philadelphia: W.B. Saunders.

42. Sullivan CA, Masin J, Maniglia AJ, and Stepnick DW. 1999. "Complications of rhytidectomy in an otolarygology program." *Laryngoscope* 109: 198.

43. Canter HI, Yilmaz B, Gurunluoglu R, and Algan H. 2006. "Use of gabapentine (neurantin) for relief of intractable pain developed after face-lift surgery." *Aesthetic Plastic Surgery* 30: 709.

44. Hamra ST. 2000. "Prevention and correction of the 'face-lifted' appearance." *Facial Plastic Surgery* 16: 215.

45. Mowlavi A, Meldrum DG, Wilhemi BJ, et al. 2005. "The 'pixie' ear deformity following face lift surgery revisited." *Plastic and Reconstructive Surgery* 115: 1165.

46. Wang TD. 2003. "Multicenter evaluation of subcutaneous augmentation material implants." *Archives of Facial Plastic Surgery* 5: 153.

47. Hasson O, Levi G, and Conley R. 2007. "Late infections associated with alloplastic facial implants." *Journal of Oral and Maxillofacial Surgery* 65: 321.

48. Jobe R, Iverson R, and Vistnes L. 1973. "Bone deformation beneath alloplastic implants." *Plastic and Reconstructive Surgery* 51: 169.

49. Pearson DC, and Sherris DA. 1999. "Resorption beneath silastic mandibular implants: effects of placement and pressure." *Archives of Facial Plastic Surgery* 1: 261.

50. Andrews PJ, East CA, Jayaraj SM, et al. 2006. "Prophylactic vs postoperative antibiotic use in complex septorhinoplasty surgery: A prospective, randomized, single-blind trial comparing efficacy." *Archives of Facial Plastic Surgery* 8: 84.

51. Rettinger G, and Kirsche H. 2006. "Complications in septoplasty." *Facial Plastic Surgery* 22: 289.

52. Kridel RWH, Yoon PJ, and Koch RJ. 2003. "Prevention and correction of nasal tip bossae in rhinoplasty." *Archives of Facial Plastic Surgery* 5: 416.

10

Temporomandibular Joint Surgery

Helen E. Giannakopoulos, DDS, MD
David C. Stanton, DMD, MD

INTRODUCTION

Temporomandibular joint surgery (TMJ) including noninvasive and invasive procedures such as arthrocentesis, arthroscopy, and open joint arthroplasty, like all other types of surgery, can result in complications.[1] While it is not the intent of this chapter, it should be mentioned that nonsurgical therapy, such as bite splint therapy for myofascial pain or internal derangement, may result in complications such as malocclusion. The complications of managing the TMJ patient may be either transient and self-limiting, or long term and irreversible in nature.

For successful TMJ surgery, operative intervention should be reserved for cases where the source of pain and/or dysfunction is the TMJ apparatus itself and, in addition, following a trial of conservative or nonsurgical treatment. Distinction between myofascial and intracapsular pathology is crucial. Concomitant neurologic and psychiatric conditions should be adequately treated beforehand as well.

Appropriate decision making has proven to be difficult with respect to TMJ surgery because of the lack of support from well-designed, randomized, clinical trials. Most of the treatment algorithms are based on the assumption that most TMJ disorders are self-limited or managed with nonsurgical modalities.[2] On the contrary, surgical intervention should not always be considered last resort, as in conditions such as severe ankylosis, tumors, and recurrent dislocation.[2] Progress in our comprehension of molecular, cellular, and biochemical mechanisms has given surgeons the ability to better select the appropriate surgical intervention.[2]

It is also important that the patient's expectations are realistic for a successful outcome. Reasonable expectations from TMJ surgery may include: (1) a postoperative interincisal opening of 30 to 35 mm; (2) pain reductions of 50% to 70%; and (3) 60% to 70% or normal dietary function.[3] The goal of this chapter is to discuss commonly encountered complications associated with TMJ surgery and their management.

VASCULAR INJURY

Vascular injury can occur during arthroscopy or open joint surgery. The blood vessels that are most susceptible to injury during TMJ surgery include the branches of the external carotid artery, most commonly the superficial temporal artery and the internal maxillary artery, and the pterygoid plexus of veins. Rarely, injury to the middle meningeal artery can occur with inadvertent penetration into the middle cranial fossa. Because of the extensive collateralization of the vasculature in the head and neck, adequate tissue perfusion following injury is not compromised.

Punctures or lacerations to these vessels can result in obstruction in visualization of the surgical field and must be controlled to prevent potentially life-threatening hemorrhage. Some degree of bleeding is

Management of Complications in Oral and Maxillofacial Surgery, First Edition. Edited by Michael Miloro, Antonia Kolokythas.
© 2012 John Wiley & Sons, Inc. Published 2012 by John Wiley & Sons, Inc.

existent during most arthroscopic and open joint procedures. Control of hemorrhage includes direct pressure, ligation, electrocautery, laser ablation, local anesthetics with epinephrine, and embolization. Ensuring hemostasis prior to closure in arthrotomy and evacuation of blood clots in arthroscopy is essential to avoid hematoma formation, which can lead to infection and the risk for adhesions formation and potential ankylosis.

Goss and Bosanquet reported three cases of bleeding from branches of the superficial temporal artery in 50 arthroscopies.[4] In a cadaveric study, Westesson et al. demonstrated the close proximity of the superficial temporal vessels to the site of the arthroscopic cannula system insertion.[5] Bleeding from the superficial temporal vessels during arthroscopy can generally be avoided by palpation prior to puncture and with employment of anatomic landmarks for joint entry.[6]

During arthroplasty, branches of the superficial temporal vessels, which are identified during the dissection, can be prophylactically ligated and divided without compromising tissue perfusion because of the vast collateral circulation of the vasculature in the head and neck. On the other hand, injury to the superficial temporal vessels can be avoided by using the flap to retract them anteriorly, during a standard preauricular approach to the TMJ.

Hemorrhage from the internal maxillary artery can arise and be potentially life threatening.[7] Hemostasis following an injury to the internal maxillary artery is challenging due to limited access and visibility of the surgical site. It crosses medial to the condylar neck and sigmoid notch and has been found to be on average 20 mm below the head of the condyle.[8] Blind instrumentation in this area may result in damage to the internal maxillary artery and subsequent hemorrhage. If the injury occurs during condylectomy, the osteotomy should be completed in order to assist in direct visualization of the bleed. Upon discovery of the site of injury, the vessel, depending on its size, can be clamped, then ligated or cauterized. If the bleed cannot be pinpointed or access to it is limited, then the wound should be packed and direct pressure accomplished. Various hemostatic agents can also be used including thrombin-soaked sponges, gelatin sponges (Gelfoam®), microfibrillar collagen (Avitene®), fibrin matrix spray (Tiseel®), and oxidized cellulose (Surgicel®). Flo-Seal Hemostatic Matrix Sealant®, a bovine collagen-derived gelatin matrix consisting of cross-linked granules with topical human-derived thrombin has also been effective.[9] If usual attempts in hemostasis have failed, then more invasive measures should be undertaken.

In total joint replacement surgery, the neck incision should precede the condylectomy so that external carotid artery ligation just distal to common carotid bifurcation can be quickly accomplished, hence halting blood flow to its branches in the event of uncontrollable hemorrhage (Figs. 10.1 and 10.2). However, multiple ligation sites have been found to be more effective since they reduce collateral blood flow.[10] In an animal study, the effectiveness of ligation of the external carotid artery and its major branches, in the control of hemorrhage from the internal maxillary artery, was evaluated.[7] From their findings, the authors concluded that hemorrhage from the internal maxillary artery is most successfully managed with ligation of the external carotid artery in the retromandibular fossa, distal to the origin of the posterior auricular artery, in addition to ligation of the superficial temporal artery at the root of the zygoma.[7]

The ability to access a vessel closer to the area of injury decreases the risk of the collateral blood supply that would otherwise contribute to perfusion. Angiography and selective embolization via percutaneous femoral artery cannulation following hemorrhage in TMJ surgery has been reported.[11] The Seldinger technique under fluoroscopic guidance is used to access the offending branch. A thrombus-inducing material is then introduced into the lumen of the vessel so that it is occluded and blood flow ceases. A variety of agents have been used including methylmethacrylate spheres, balloon catheters, cyanoacrylate tissue adhesives, gelatin sponges, polyvinyl alcohol sponges, silicone spheres, cotton, wool, stainless steel coils, and autologous blood and muscle.[12]

Potential complications, even though rare, can occur with arterial embolization, and include vasospasm, hemorrhage, dissecting aneurysm formation, infection, skin necrosis, cranial nerve injury, and inadvertent internal carotid artery cannulation or reflux with subsequent cerebrovascular accident (CVA) or death.[12] The risk of permanent neurological complications with embolization is generally 1%.[11]

Pseudoaneurysm of the superficial temporal artery following arthroscopy has been reported.[13] A pseudoaneurysm, also known as a false aneurysm, is a leakage of blood from a disrupted artery into the surrounding tissue, forming a hematoma. The hematoma is contained by the surrounding tissues and continues to communicate with the artery. On physical examination, a thrill or a bruit is appreciated.

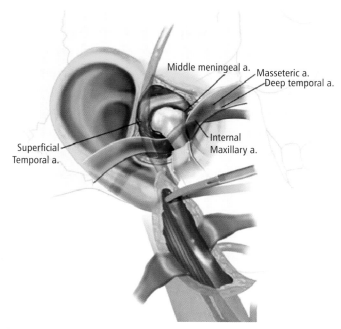

Fig. 10.1. External carotid artery ligation above the posterior auricular branch and below the transverse facial is used to control hemorrhage following injury to the maxillary artery and its branches.

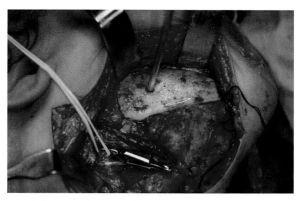

Fig. 10.2. Retromandibular approach for vascular control.

Definitive diagnosis can be made with angiography or magnetic resonance angiography (MRA). Surgical exploration, with vessel isolation, ligation and excision or arterial embolization can be used to treat pseudoaneurysms.

Moses and Topper reported an arterio–venous (A–V) fistula between the right superficial temporal artery and vein following arthroscopy. At a subsequent operation, the A–V fistula was isolated and ligated with 3-0 silk sutures. At the 6-month follow-up, there was no evidence of vascular malformation.[14]

NERVE INJURY

Injury to the branches of cranial nerves V and VII can take place in TMJ surgery. Arthroscopy is less likely than arthrotomy to cause permanent malfunction manifesting as an interference with facial expression and cosmetic deformity. The reported incidence of facial nerve injury following TMJ surgery ranges from 1%

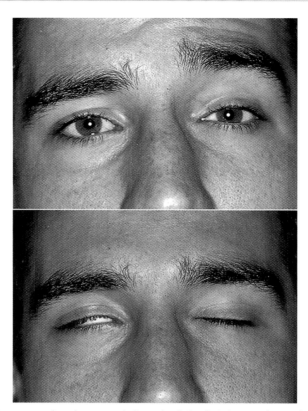

Fig. 10.3. Paresis of the right temporal and zygomatic branch of the facial nerve (CN VII). Inability to wrinkle forehead and raise eyebrow (top) and close eye (bottom) following injury to the temporal and zygomatic branches of the facial nerve (CN VII).

to 25% and is typically transient in nature, resolving within 3 to 6 months.[1] Causes of neuropraxia include edema, excessive flap retraction forces, electrocautery, inadvertent suture ligation, or clamping of tissues.

Surgical approaches to the TMJ have been designed to afford the most protection to the facial nerve. Regardless of the surgical approach that is utilized, facial nerve injury is always a risk. To prevent disruption of the branches of the facial nerve requires a comprehensive knowledge of the anatomy and meticulous surgical dissection. Factors that can increase the risk of nerve damage include use of improper surgical technique or abnormal joint anatomy as a result of a congenital abnormality, trauma, tumor or multiple previous surgeries.

The four basic incisions in TMJ surgery include the preauricular, the endaural, the postauricular, and the submandibular.[15] The incidence of nerve injury has been found to increase when a separate skin flap is raised.[16] During arthroscopy, a rotational versus a straight motion with insertion of the trocar and cannula is more likely to divert any nerves.[6]

The temporal and then the zygomatic branches of the facial nerve are most prone to injury, presenting, respectively, as a loss of ability to raise one's eyebrows, wrinkle one's forehead, or close one's eyes completely (Fig. 10.3). These branches cross the zygomatic arch in their course within the dense, inseparable fusion of the periosteum, temporalis fascia, and the temporoparietal fascia. From their classic cadaveric study, Al-Kayat and Bramley discovered that this dangerous area of fusion was on an average of 2.0 cm (range: 0.8–3.5 cm) from the anterior concavity of the external auditory meatus (Fig. 10.4).[17] Therefore, a vertical incision made over the zygomatic arch that is less than 0.8 cm from the anterior concavity of the external auditory meatus allows safe entry into the joint. Furthermore, the inadequacy of the superficial muscular aponeurotic system (SMAS) at the lateral border of the frontalis muscle leaves the temporal branches susceptible to injury.

Rudolph illustrated in his cadaveric facelift dissections that the facial nerve branches are deepest, or absent, behind the ear, inferior to the zygoma, and near the earlobe, and that the precarious area, where

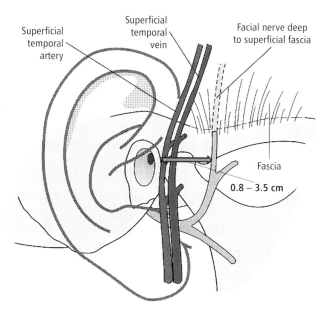

Fig. 10.4. The danger zone of fusion where the facial nerve (CN VII) is most prone to injury is where the upper division of the facial nerve crosses the zygomatic arch 0.8 to 3.5 cm from the anterior concavity of the external auditory meatus.[17]

the temporal branches become superficial, is 5 cm from the parotid border and 2.3 cm ± 0.6 mm deep.[18] Conversely, the zygomatic branch was found to be well protected in the facial fat upon exiting from the parotid gland, and it also has many anastomoses between its branches.[18]

Fortunately, in the majority of the proposed branching patterns of the facial nerve, there is distal branching that allows for multiple points of innervation of the frontalis muscle. Therefore, Hall et al. hypothesized that the most distal branch of the facial nerve that crosses the zygomatic arch could be transected 63% of the time without frontalis dysfunction.[19]

In the patient who has been operated on multiple times, definable surgical planes that make for safe dissection may not be present secondary to scarring. In these cases, the dissection should be carried out to the level of the temporalis muscle.[20]

In patients with facial nerve injury following TMJ surgery, it is necessary to assess the affected area and the degree of the deficit. In patients who have brow or forehead weakness, no immediate intervention is typically necessary. Postoperative measures for management of inadequate eyelid closure include use of artificial tears and ocular lubricant with taping of the eye at bedtime in order to prevent corneal desiccation and keratitis. Conservative treatment with exercises or electrical stimulation may be helpful. Should nerve function fail to return, depending on the affected branches, microneurosurgical repair can be considered. Botulinum toxin A injections to the corresponding muscles of facial expression on the opposite side can be used to mask the deficit. A gold weight implanted into the upper eyelid can also be used to manage permanent insufficient eyelid closure.

Injury to the trigeminal nerve branches (the infraorbital nerve, the inferior alveolar nerve, the lingual nerve, and the auriculotemporal nerve) is less common in TMJ surgery. Extravasation of irrigation fluid can cause paresthesia in the affected branch. In these cases, resolution is rapid without sequelae. More serious injury to the inferior alveolar nerve can occur from instruments used to clamp the mandible in order to distract the condyle inferiorly. It can also be damaged during condylectomy, or screw placement used to fixate mandibular implants, in TMJ replacement surgery. The prognosis for recovery from these injuries is less predictable.

The auriculotemporal nerve travels alongside the superficial temporal vessels commonly encountered with a standard preauricular approach to the TMJ. It is a mixed nerve and carries both sympathetic and parasympathetic nerve fibers. Auriculotemporal nerve injuries were found to represent 59% of all neurologic injuries during TMJ arthroscopy.[21] Dolwick et al. found that in 56 patients who had undergone TMJ arthrotomy via a preauricular approach, all had subsequent paresthesia associated with the auriculotemporal nerve.[22] However, its occurrence is most often temporary.

Auriculotemporal nerve syndrome, otherwise known as Frey's syndrome, is a gustatory sweating, flushing, and warmth over the distribution of the auriculotemporal nerve and/or the greater auricular nerve during mastication of foods that are potent stimulants of saliva. It is believed to result from the misdirected regeneration of injured parasympathetic fibers to the eccrine sweat glands in the skin. Frey's syndrome is an unlikely complication of TMJ surgery, and a small incision without an oblique superior extension may further decrease the risk.[23] Kryshtalsky and Weinberg reported that 3 of 20 patients (15%) developed Frey's syndrome following open TMJ surgery in which a preauricular approach was utilized.[24]

A Minor's starch-iodine test can be used to diagnose Frey's syndrome.[24] A solution of 3 g of iodine, 20 g of castor oil, and 200 ml of absolute alcohol is applied. The region is then lightly dusted with starch powder. The patient is instructed to chew on a lemon drop for 4 minutes. A positive result occurs when sweat dissolves the starch powder and reacts with the iodine to produce a dark blue discoloration. A negative result occurs when there is no color change.

Treatment of Frey's syndrome includes topical application of anticholinergic compounds, such as glycopyrolate, transection of the auriculotemporal nerve, or implantation of freeze-dried dura or fascia lata under the skin of the involved area.[25]

INFECTION

Postsurgical infections in TMJ surgeries when an implant is not placed occur infrequently. There are few case reports of postarthroscopic infections, including otitis media,[26] joint infection,[27,28] and infratemporal space infection.[29]

Forty-four out of 2,106 (2.09%) patients and 44 of 3,285(1.34%) implants had an infection following TMJ reconstruction with the TMJ Concepts® system. With total TMJ replacement, immediate infection of the components is atypical. Late infection can occur and is associated with biofilm formation.[30] These are matrix-enclosed, surface-associated communities that are protected from host defenses and antibiotics.[2] Biomaterial–associated infections of orthopedic joint replacements are the second most common cause of implant failure.[31]

Mercuri described a protocol to treat biofilm infected TMJ alloplastic prostheses: (1) removal of the biofilm infected medical device; (2) application of an antibiotic-impregnated orthopedic bone cement spacer; (3) long-term systemic antibiotic therapy; (4) replacement of the device; and (5) another course of systemic antibiotic therapy.[32] Fossa components made of high molecular weight polyethylene are replaced, and undistorted, all-metal components are sterilized and reused with new screws.[30]

The bacteria that are most commonly isolated from biofilm infected medical devices are *Staphylococcus epidermidis*,[32] *Staphylococcus aureus*, *Pseudomonas aerugenosa*, and the *Enterococcus* species. Infrequently, the *Candida* species are also encountered.[32] Broad-spectrum antibiotics should be used empirically, followed by culture and microanalysis of the explanted prosthesis.[32]

Future research aimed at decreasing device-related biofilms and enhancing the success of treatment is based on the following objectives: (1) creating implant surfaces that are less likely to attract planktonic cells and thus accrete biofilms; (2) fabricating coatings that release conventional antibiotics into the surrounding tissues and fluids to kill planktonic cells; (3) using chemical inhibitors to block the cell–cell signaling necessary for biofilm production; (4) delivering an ultrasonic pulse to increase transport of antibiotics across biofilms; (5) employing low electric current, combined with antibiotics, to enhance the killing of biofilm-associated bacteria.[33] Basically, the utilization of aseptic technique, perioperative antibiotics, and meticulous surgery can minimize the occurrence of device-related biofilm.

OTOLOGIC COMPLICATIONS

The close proximity of the ear to the TMJ makes it susceptible to injury during surgery. In 1986, Sanders reported the first otologic complication, a case of otitis media from TMJ arthroscopy.[26] In 1987, Van Sickels et al., reported a middle ear injury resulting in hearing loss and tinnitus.[34] Several other large series of arthroscopies reported low otologic complication rates of 0–1%.[35–38]

Otologic complications developed in 26 of 202 patients (8.6%) who underwent arthroscopic lysis and lavage. These consisted of blood clots in the external auditory canal (9), laceration of the external auditory canal (7), partial hearing loss (5), ear fullness (2), vertigo (1), and perforation of the tympanic membrane with laceration of the external auditory canal (1).[39] Ear lacerations were frequently identified intraoperatively when there was sudden extravasation of irrigation fluid from the external auditory canal.[39] External auditory canal lacerations and tympanic membrane perforations were treated with placement of antibiotic-coated gauze packing in the external auditory canal, which was removed on postoperative day 4.[39] An otorhinolaryngology consultation was subsequently obtained and patients were prescribed antibiotics or hydrocortisone suspension ear drops. There was complete resolution of all of the cases within a few weeks. The five cases of partial hearing loss were diagnosed as postoperative edema of the external auditory canal or middle ear. Three cases resolved spontaneously and two cases were treated with oral or otic steroids. After 1 month, hearing loss completely resolved in all of the cases.[39]

Puncture of the tragal cartilage and tympanic membrane laceration with middle ear damage during TMJ arthroscopy can be avoided with careful surgical technique and planning. Superior joint space entry can be facilitated by using anatomic landmarks like the canthal–tragal line.[40] McCain advised review of preoperative radiographic studies with attention to anatomic structures. He also cautioned awareness of the average puncture depths, with the approximate distance from the skin to middle of the joint and to the medial capsule being 25 and 50 ± 5 mm, respectively.[6]

With open joint surgery, the postauricular approach to the TMJ, when compared to the standard preauricular approach, is associated with a higher risk of otologic complications, particularly external auditory canal (EAC) stenosis. Cerumen can accumulate and can lead to external otitis.[41] The patient can also experience a conductive hearing loss from the iatrogenic obliteration of the EAC.[40] Kreutziger described stenting the EAC open and avoiding this complication by utilizing subcuticular interrupted mattress sutures around the canal and placing an antibiotic-impregnated sponge dressing within it.[41]

INTRACRANIAL INJURY

Intracranial perforation through the glenoid fossa during arthroscopic cannula insertion is an unlikely, but a reported injury. Patel et al. reported a case of skull base entry during TMJ arthroscopy resulting in vertigo and palsies of the right oculomotor and trochlear nerves, which they attributed to a fluid collection in the region of the ipsilateral temporal lobe and cavernous sinus.[42]

The average thickness of the fossa is 0.9 mm.[43] Entrance into the middle cranial fossa may result in a dural tear and a subsequent cerebrospinal fluid (CSF) leak. Inadvertent intracranial puncture can cause permanent neurologic deficits. Penetration into the middle cranial fossa can also transpire during eminectomy or eminoplasty. Additionally, foreign body reaction from alloplastic implants, a late complication of TMJ surgery, can lead to fossa destruction and a communication into the middle cranial fossa.

If such an injury is suspected, a CT scan and/or MRI, and a neurosurgery consultation should be obtained. Dural tears that are recognized intraoperatively and are of significant size can be repaired immediately. Most small dural tears and ensuing CSF leaks, though, resolve spontaneously with appropriate measurements. Persistent CSF leaks that do not respond to nonsurgical management may require surgical innervation. Vigilant preoperative preparation using imaging to identify individuals who may have an increased risk, knowledge of anatomic landmarks, and avoidance of excessive force during cannula insertion should be utilized in order to prevent this injury from arising.

ALLERGIC REACTIONS

After encountering patients with foreign body giant cell reactions to a chrome–cobalt–molybdenum alloy following joint reconstruction with the Christensen system, Sidebottom et al. introduced routine preoperative skin testing.[44] For patients with a positive test, a titanium condylar prosthesis should be used instead.[45]

COMPLICATIONS LIMITED TO ARTHROSCOPY

TMJ arthroscopy has been considered generally safe. In a study consisting of 500 consecutive patients (670 joints) with internal derangement of the TMJ who were treated with arthroscopy between 1995 and 2004, an overall complication rate of 1.34% was observed. Bleeding within the joint space was the most common complication, occurring in 57 cases (8.5%).[46] In another study of 373 patients (451 joints) followed over a 10-year period, a 1.77% complication rate was reported.[38] In both studies, most problems were self-limited.

Instrument Breakage

The fine, delicate instruments used in TMJ arthroscopy are subject to breakage. Retrieval of small broken pieces can be accomplished with a hemostat-like instrument passed through the cannula system of the scope.[6]

However, certain measures can be made to minimize instrumentation breakage. Verifying that the selected armamentarium is specifically intended for TMJ arthroscopy and that the individual instruments are intact prior to introduction to the joint is essential. Placement of instruments through cannulas and the avoidance of excessive force will also prevent instrument breakage. Retrieval of a broken instrument should be accomplished with a systematic approach. If the instrument cannot be visualized, radiography can be used to localize it. Conversion to open joint surgery may be necessary should arthroscopic attempts fail. Accordingly, patients who have arthroscopy should be counseled and consent obtained for this possibility.

Extravasation of Irrigating Fluid

Irrigation using normal saline or lactated Ringer's solution during arthrocentesis or arthroscopy is administered intermittently or continuously. Extravasation of fluid beyond the joint space and into the neighboring tissues has been reported. This fluid will result in edema that can clinically present as paresthesia, paresis, airway obstruction, and infection. In a study of 43 joints, extravasation of fluid through the articular capsule occurred in nine joints (20.9%) and was attributed to a thin capsule anteromedially.[47] Indresano reported extravasation of fluid in 3 of 100 (3%) arthroscopies. Two of three cases were not associated with any functional deficits and resolved within 24 hours, and one case resulted in a CN VII paralysis of the temporal and zygomatic branches, lasting for 6 months.[35] The authors believe that all complications may have been related to operator skill, as they coincided with the first 20 arthroscopies performed.[35]

Extravasation of fluid medially can result in lateral pharyngeal space edema and potential airway obstruction (Fig. 10.5). The incidence of lateral pharyngeal space edema has been reported to be between 0.45% and 2.0%.[36,43]

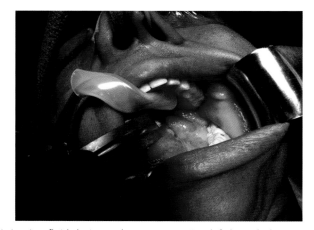

Fig. 10.5. Extravasation of irrigating fluid during arthroscopy, causing left lateral pharyngeal edema.

In a case report, extensive facial, cervical, and laryngeal edema required prolonged intubation following arthroscopy. Direct laryngoscopy confirmed resolution prior to extubation 8 hours later.[48] Airway obstruction was also reported by Hendler and Levin and resulted in pulmonary edema. In both of these cases, there was increased technical difficulty due to fibrous ankylosis in the joint.[49] Troublesome and extensive procedures, utilizing large amounts of irrigation fluid, can lead to serious sequelae secondary to the extravasation of fluids beyond the confines of the joint space.

Attention to trocar insertion depths, continuous confirmation of unobstructed outflow, and close monitoring of inflow and outflow volumes are essential in preventing extravasation of irrigating fluids into the surrounding tissues. After completion of the surgery and prior to extubation, careful inspection of the airway should be performed.

Scuffing of the Fibrocartilage

Scuffing of the articular fibrocartilage of the glenoid fossa, condyle, and disk can occur during arthroscopy. These injuries can be prevented, with use of careful joint entry, switching to a blunt trocar to advance further into the joint space, and continuous visualization of instruments.

LONG-STANDING COMPLICATIONS

Malocclusion

Malocclusions following arthrocentesis and lysis and lavage arthroscopy are a consequence of edema that can produce a posterior open bite on the operated side. This open bite is of brief duration and self-resolving. More invasive TMJ surgery, with significant alteration in joint anatomy, as in arthroplasty with meniscectomy, removal of failed implants, or in gap arthroplasty for treatment of ankylosis can cause more of a dysfunction. There could be a substantial loss in vertical height resulting in occlusal changes, such as an ipsilateral premature contact and a contralateral open bite of the posterior teeth, as well as, bilateral crossbites. An anterior open bite can occur following bilateral TMJ surgery. Similar occlusal changes have been observed with the modified condylotomy.[50]

Managing the malocclusion and facial asymmetry entails a multidisciplinary approach. Consultation with an orthodontist and a prosthodontist should be done. Treatment may consist of dental occlusal equilibration, prosthodontic rehabilitation, orthodontics, orthognathic surgery, alloplastic temporomandibular joint reconstruction, or combinations of these options.

Ankylosis

Ankylosis is clinically demonstrated as an inability to achieve adequate mouth opening, with subsequent difficulties in oral hygiene, mastication, and speech (Fig. 10.6). The functional problems and associated facial deformity could be expressed as psychosocial distress.[51,52]

Radiographic imaging with CT scans is necessary for evaluation of the status of the joint and appropriate surgical planning (Figs. 10.7 and 10.8). A combination of CT imaging with angiography has been employed to further delineate vascular structures. Recently, several authors have been reporting on the use CT navigation systems for preoperative planning and precise surgical guidance in real time.[53]

Treatment goals of joint reconstruction for correction of ankylosis should include sufficient mouth opening for mastication and speech, restoration of facial symmetry, and reduction of pain to at least more manageable levels.[54] In 1990, Kaban et al. proposed a protocol for the management of temporomandibular joint ankylosis.[55] Since this time, most authors have reported cases that have followed the basic tenets of the principles suggested in that series.[56,57]

The concept of critical size defect has been identified as being paramount in playing a role in reankylosis. A critical size defect is a bone-to-bone gap that cannot be bridged by callus formation in secondary healing. An accepted standard for the critical surgical defect has not been fully elicited with respect to TMJ ankylosis. Recommended resection to prevent reankylosis has ranged anywhere from 0.5 to 4.0 cm.[58] A larger defect, theoretically, decreases the likelihood of reankylosis, but at the expense of ramus height and associated facial deformities.[59]

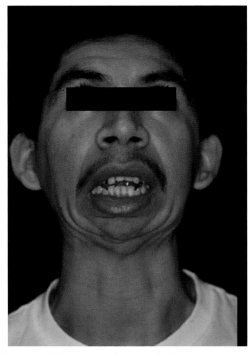

Fig. 10.6. Limited maximal incisal opening of patient with TMJ ankylosis.

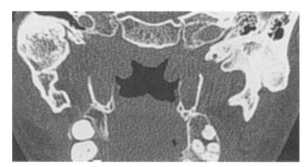

Fig. 10.7. CT scan depicting bilateral TMJ ankylosis.

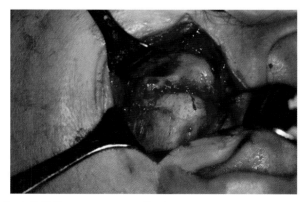

Fig. 10.8. Ankylotic mass of the left TMJ seen on open arthrotomy.

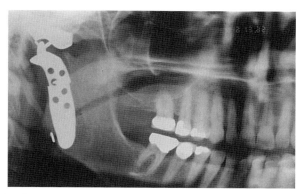

Fig. 10.9. Fractured condylar implant.

The preferred method of reconstruction has varied in the literature.[54,57,59,60] Current treatment approaches encompass gap athroplasty with alloplastic or autogenous grafting, costrochondral grafting, distraction osteogenesis, and total joint replacement.[51,56,61]

Despite the technique chosen for joint reconstruction, avoidance of reankylosis is imperative. Early joint mobilization must take place. A variety of other medical therapies have also been applied. Postsurgical radiation therapy has been supported as a treatment option for reankylosis. The use of 10 Gy (1,000 rads) in five fractionated daily doses following surgical re-excision has been found to be beneficial.[62] Evidence has also suggested that nonsteroidal anti-inflammatory drugs may inhibit reankylosis.[63] In a study by Wolford and Karras, autologous abdominal fat grafts were placed around custom total joint replacements. Of the grafted group, 100% had no evidence of ankylosis, whereas, while 35% of the nongrafted (control) group required reoperation for ankylosis.[64]

Materials Failure

Quinn states:

> Unfortunately, the history of alloplastic TMJ reconstruction has been characterized by multiple highly publicized failures based on inappropriate design, lack of attention to biomechanical principles, and ignorance of what already had been documented in the orthopaedic literature.[65]

Mercuri and Anspach published a comprehensive review of the various types of materials failure, including: (1) foreign body reaction with implant loosening; (2) component fracture; and (3) fixation failure (Fig. 10.9).[66]

Fricton and colleagues demonstrated more favorable outcomes for nonsurgical management and arthroplasty, in which, neither a temporary or permanent alloplastic implant was placed.[67] Several authors have published treatment sequences for patients with failed alloplastic implants. Kearns and colleagues had good results with pedicled temporalis muscle/fascial flaps after aggressive debridement.[68] Mercuri and Giobbie-Hurder established the efficacy of total joint reconstruction for patients with Proplast, Teflon, and Silastic implants.[69] Henry and Wolford compared 62 patients who underwent TMJ reconstruction with autogenous or alloplastic means, subsequent to proplast/Teflon implant removal, and found higher success rates (88%) with prosthetic replacement.[70]

Chronic Pain in the Multiply-Operated Patient

It is important to recognize that some multiply-operated TM joints are "iatrogenic" failures that should not have had surgery to begin with. Israel and colleagues found that "misdiagnosis and multiple failed treatments were common in those patients with chronic orofacial pain."[71] Milam postulated that TMJ pain could be perpetuated by neuroplastic changes, even in the absence of peripheral pathology.[72]

Previous medical records should be obtained. A team approach including pain management, neurology, physical therapy, and psychology is recommended. Alloplastic joint reconstruction may be necessary to improve mechanical function. Surgical intervention, however, may not improve pain and may even exacerbate it.[73]

CONCLUSIONS

Surgical intervention is appropriate for a small percentage of patients with TMJ disorders. The decision to proceed should be based on a specific diagnosis of intracapsular pathology not responsive or amenable to nonsurgical treatment modalities. When TMJ surgery is considered, the potential complications and their management should be discussed with the patient.

SUGGESTED READINGS

1. Keith DA. 2003. "Complications of temporomandibular joint surgery." *Oral and Maxillofacial Surgery Clinics of North America* 15: 187–194.
2. Quinn PD, Giannakopoulos H, and Carrasco L. 2006. "Management of surgical failures." *Oral and Maxillofacial Surgery Clinics of North America* 18: 411–417.
3. Quinn PD. 2000. "Pain management in the multiply-operated temporomandibular joint patient." *Journal of Oral and Maxillofacial Surgery* 58(Suppl 2): 12–14.
4. Goss AN, and Bosanquet AG. 1986. "Temporomandibular joint arthroscopy." *Journal of Oral and Maxillofacial Surgery* 44: 614–617.
5. Westesson PL, Ericksson L, and Leidberg J 1986. "The risk of damage to facial nerve, superficial temporal vessels, disk and articular surfaces during arthroscopic examination of the temporomandibular joint." *Oral Surgery, Oral Medicine, Oral Pathology, Oral Radiology, and Endodontology* 62: 124–127.
6. McCain JP. 1988. "Complications of TMJ arthroscopy." *Journal of Oral and Maxillofacial Surgery* 46: 256.
7. Rosenberg I, Austin JC, Wright PG, et al. 1982. "The effect of experimental ligation of the external carotid artery and its major branches on haemorrhage from the maxillary artery." *International Journal of Oral Surgery* 11: 251–259.
8. Greene MW, Hackney FL, and VanSickels JE. 1989. "Arthoscopy of the tempormandibular joint: An anatomic perspective." *Journal of Oral and Maxillofacial Surgery* 47: 386–389.
9. Cillo JE, Jr., Sinn D, and Truelson JM. 2005. "Management of middle meningeal and superficial temporal artery hemorrhage from total temporomandibular joint replacement surgery with a gelatin-based hemostatic agent." *The Journal of Craniofacial Surgery* 16: 309–312.
10. Yin NT. 1994. "Hemorrhage of the initial part of the internal maxillary artery treated by multiple ligations: Report of four cases." *Journal of Oral and Maxillofacial Surgery* 52: 1066–1071.
11. Peoples JR, III, Herbosa EG, and Dion J. 1988. "Management of internal maxillary artery hemorrhage from temporomandibular joint surgery via selective embolization." *Journal of Oral and Maxillofacial Surgery* 46: 1005–1007.
12. Frame JW, Putnam G, Wake MJ, et al. 1987. "Therapeutic arterial embolisation of vascular lesions in the maxillofacial region." *British Journal of Oral and Maxillofacial Surgery* 25: 181–194.
13. Kornbrot A, Shaw AS, and Toohey MR. 1991. "Pseudoaneurysm as a complication of arthroscopy: A case report." *Journal of Oral and Maxillofacial Surgery* 49: 1226–1228.
14. Moses JJ, and Topper DC. 1990. "Arteriovenous fistula: An unusual complication associated with arthroscopic temporomandibular joint surgery." *Journal of Oral and Maxillofacial Surgery* 48: 1220–1222.
15. Kreutziger KL. 1984. "Surgery of the temporomandibular joint. I. Surgical anatomy and surgical incisions." *Oral Surgery, Oral Medicine, Oral Pathology, Oral Radiology, and Endodontology* 58: 637.
16. Brown WA. 1980. "Internal derangement of the temporomandibular joint: Review of 214 patients following meniscectomy." *Canadian Journal of Surgery* 23: 30–32.
17. Al-Kayat A, and Bramley P. 1979. "A modified pre-auricular approach to the temporomandibular joint and malar arch." *British Journal of Oral and Maxillofacial Surgery* 17: 91–103.
18. Rudolph R. 1990. "Depth of the facial nerve in face lift dissections." *Plastic and Reconstructive Surgery* 85: 537–544.
19. Hall MB, Brown RW, and Lebowitz MS. 1985. "Facial nerve injury during surgery of the temporomandibular joint: A comparison of two dissection techniques." *Journal of Oral and Maxillofacial Surgery* 43: 20–23.
20. Weinberg S, and Kryshtalskyj B. 1992. "Facial nerve function following temporomandibular joint surgery using the preauricular approach." *Journal of Oral and Maxillofacial Surgery* 50: 1048–1051.
21. Carter J, and Testa L. 1988. "Complications of TMJ arthroscopy: A review of 2,225 cases: Review of the 1988 Annual Scientific Sessions abstracts." *Journal of Oral and Maxillofacial Surgery* 46: M14.
22. Dolwick MF, and Kretzschmar DP. 1982. "Morbidity associated with the preauricular and perimeatal approaches to the temporomandibular joint." *Journal of Oral and Maxillofacial Surgery* 40: 699–700.
23. Swanson KS, Laskin DM, and Campbell RL. 1991. "Auriculotemporal syndrome following the preauricular approach to temporomandibular joint surgery." *Journal of Oral and Maxillofacial Surgery* 49: 680–682.

24. Kryshtalskyj B, and Weinberg S. 1989. "An assessment for auriculotemporal syndrome following temporomandibular joint surgery through the preauricular approach." *Journal of Oral and Maxillofacial Surgery* 47: 3–6.

25. Berrios RJ, and Quinn PD. 1986. "Frey's syndrome: Complication after orthognathic surgery." *The International Journal of Adult Orthodontics and Orthognathic Surgery* 1: 219–224.

26. Sanders B. 1986. "Arthroscopic surgery of the temporomandibular joint: Treatment of internal derangement with persistent closed lock." *Oral Surgery, Oral Medicine, Oral Pathology, Oral Radiology, and Endodontology* 62: 361–372.

27. Tarro AW. 1989. "Arthroscopic treatment of anterior disc displacement: A preliminary report." *Journal of Oral and Maxillofacial Surgery* 47: 353–358.

28. McCain JP, Zabiegalski NA, and Levine RL. 1993. "Joint infection as a complication of temporomandibular joint arthroscopy: A case report." *Journal of Oral and Maxillofacial Surgery* 51: 1389–1392.

29. Chossegros C, Cheynet F, Conrath J. 1995. "Infratemporal space infection after temporomandibular arthroscopy: An unusual complication." *Journal of Oral and Maxillofacial Surgery* 53: 949–951.

30. Speculand B. 2009. "Current status of replacement of the temporomandibular joint in the United Kingdom." *British Journal of Oral & Maxillofacial Surgery* 47: 37–41.

31. Neut D, vanHorn JR, vanKooten TG, et al. 2003. "Detection of biomaterial-associated infections in orthopaedic joint implants." *Clinical Orthopaedics and Related Research* 413: 261–268.

32. Mercuri LG. 2006. "Microbial biofilms: A potential source of alloplastic device failure." *Journal of Oral and Maxillofacial Surgery* 64: 1303–1309.

33. Costerton JW. 2005. "Biofilm theory can guide the treatment of device-related orthopaedic infections." *Clinical Orthopaedics and Related Research* 437: 7–11.

34. Van Sickels JE, Nishioka GJ, Hegewald MD, et al. 1987. "Middle ear injury resulting from temporomandibular joint arthroscopy." *Journal of Oral Maxillofacial Surgery* 45: 92–965.

35. Indresano AT. 1989. "Arthroscopic surgery of the temporomandibular joint: Report of 64 patients with long-term follow-up." *Journal of Oral and Maxillofacial Surgery* 47: 439–441.

36. White RD. 1989. "Retrospective analysis of 100 consecutive surgical arthroscopics of the temporomandibular joint." *Journal of Oral and Maxillofacial Surgery* 47: 1014–1021.

37. McCain JP, Sanders B, Koslin MG, et al. 1992. "Temporomandibular joint arthroscopy: A 6-year multicenter retrospective study of 4831 joints." *Journal of Oral and Maxillofacial Surgery* 50: 926–930.

38. Carls FR, Engelke W, Locher MC, et al. 1996. "Complications following arthroscopy of the temporomandibular joint: Analysis covering a 10-year period (451 arthroscopies)." *Journal of Cranio-Maxillo-Facial Surgery* 24: 12–17.

39. Tsuyama M, Kondob T, Seto K, et al. 2000. "Complications of temporomandibular joint arthroscopy: A retrospective analysis of 301 lysis and lavage procedures performed using the triangulation technique." *Journal of Oral and Maxillofacial Surgery* 58: 500–505.

40. Holmund A, and Hellsing G. 1985. "Arthroscopy of the TMJ. An autopsy study." *International Journal of Oral Surgery* 14: 169–175.

41. Kreutziger KL. 1987. "Extended modified postauricular incision of the temporomandibular joint." *Oral Surgery, Oral Medicine, Oral Pathology, Oral Radiology, and Endodontology* 63: 2–8.

42. Patel S, Jerjes W, Upile T, et al. 2010. "TMJ arthroscopy: Rare neurological complications associated with breach of the skull base." *British Journal of Oral & Maxillofacial Surgery* 48: 18–20.

43. Greene MW, and Van Sickels JE. 1989. "Survey of TMJ arthroscopy in oral and maxillofacial surgery programs." *Journal of Oral and Maxillofacial Surgery* 47: 574–576.

44. Sidebottom AJ, Speculand B, and Hensher R. 2008. "Foreign body response around total prosthetic metal-on-metal replacements of the temporomandibular joint in the UK." *British Journal of Oral & Maxillofacial Surgery* 46: 288–292.

45. Speculand B, Hensher R, and Powell D. 2000. "Total prosthetic replacement of the TMJ: Experience with two systems 1988–1997." *British Journal of Oral & Maxillofacial Surgery* 38: 360–369.

46. González-García R, Rodríguez-Campo FJ, Escorial-Hernández V, et al. 2006. "Complications of temporomandibular joint arthroscopy: A retrospective analytic study of 670 arthroscopic procedures." *Journal of Oral and Maxillofacial Surgery* 64: 1587–1591.

47. Sasaki K, Watahiki R, Tamura H, et al. 2002. "Fluid extravasation of the articular capsule as a complication of temporomandibular joint pumping and perfusion." *The Bulletin of Tokyo Dental College* 43: 237–242.

48. Goudot P, Jaquinet AR, and Richter M. 1999. "Upper airway compression after arthroscopy of the temporomandibular joint." *International Journal of Oral and Maxillofacial Surgery* 28: 419–420.

49. Hendler BH, and Levin LM. 1993. "Postobstructive pulmonary edema as a sequela of temporomandibular joint arthroscopy: A case report." *Journal of Oral and Maxillofacial Surgery* 51: 315–317.

50. Hall DH, Nickerson JW, Jr., and McKenna SJ. 1993. "Modified condylotomy for treatment of the painful temporomandibular joint with a reducing disc." *Journal of Oral and Maxillofacial Surgery* 51: 133–142.

51. Rowe NL. 1982. "Ankylosis of the temporomandibular joint." *Journal of the Royal College of Surgeons of Edinburgh* 27: 67–79.

52. Chidzonga MM. 1999. "Temporomandibular joint ankylosis: Review of thirty-two cases." *British Journal of Oral & Maxillofacial Surgery* 37: 123–126.

53. Malis DD, Xia JJ, Gateno J, et al. 2007. "New protocol for 1-stage treatment of temporomandibular joint ankylosis using surgical navigation." *Journal of Oral and Maxillofacial Surgery* 65: 1843–1848.

54. Rowe NL. 1982. "Ankylosis of the temporomandibular joint. Part 2." *Journal of the Royal College of Surgeons of Edinburgh* 28: 167–173.

55. Kaban LB, Perrott DH, and Fisher K. 1990. "A protocol for management of temporomandibular joint ankylosis." *Journal of Oral and Maxillofacial Surgery* 48: 1145–1151.

56. Chossegros C, Guyot L, Cheynet F, et al. 1999. "Full-thickness skin graft interposition after temporomandibular joint ankylosis surgery. A study of 31 patients." *International Journal of Oral and Maxillofacial Surgery* 28: 330–334.

57. Su-Gwan K. 2001. "Treatment of temporomandibular joint ankylosis with temporalis muscle and fascia flap." *International Journal of Oral and Maxillofacial Surgery* 30: 189–193.

58. Topazian RG. 1966. "Comparison of gap and interposition arthroplasty in the treatment of temporomandibular joint ankylosis." *Journal of Oral Surgery* 24: 405–409.

59. Salins PC. 2000. "New perspectives in the management of craniomandibular ankylosis." *International Journal of Oral Maxillofacial Surgery* 29: 337–340.

60. Saeed NR, and Kent JN. 2003. "A retrospective study of the costochondral graft in TMJ reconstruction." *International Journal of Oral Maxillofacial Surgery* 32: 606–609.

61. Ortak T, Ulusoy MG, Sungur N, et al. 2001. "Silicon in temporomandibular joint ankylosis surgery." *Journal of Craniofacial Surgery* 12: 232–236.

62. Reid R, and Cooke H. 1999. "Postoperative ionizing radiation in the management of heterotopic bone formation in the temporomandibular joint." *Journal of Oral and Maxillofacial Surgery* 57: 900–905.

63. Vuolteenaho K, Moilanen T, and Moilanen E. 2007. "Non-steroidal anti-inflammatory drugs, cyclooxygenase-2 and the bone healing process." *Basic & Clinical Pharmacology & Toxicology* 102: 10–14.

64. Wolford LM, and Karras SC. 1997. "Autologous fat transplantation around temporomandibular joint total joint prostheses: Preliminary treatment outcomes." *Journal of Oral and Maxillofacial Surgery* 55: 245–251.

65. Quinn PD. 1999. "Alloplastic reconstruction of the temporomandibular joint." *Selected Readings in Oral and Maxillofacial Surgery* 7(5): 1–23.

66. Mercuri LG, and Anspach WE. 2003. "Principles for the revision of total alloplastic TMJ prostheses." *International Journal of Oral and Maxillofacial Surgery* 32: 353–359.

67. Fricton JR, Look JO, Schiffman E, et al. 2002. "Long-term study of temporomandibular joint surgery with alloplastic implants compared with nonimplant surgery and nonsurgical rehabilitation for painful temporomandibular joint disc displacement." *Journal of Oral and Maxillofacial Surgery* 60: 1400–1411.

68. Kearns GJ, Perrott DH, and Kaban LB. 1995. "A protocol for the management of failed alloplastic temporomandibular joint disc implants." *Journal of Oral and Maxillofacial Surgery* 53: 1240–1247.

69. Mercuri LG, and Giobbie-Hurder A. 2004. "Long-term outcomes after total alloplastic temporomandibular joint reconstruction following exposure to failed materials." *Journal of Oral and Maxillofacial Surgery* 62: 1088–1096.

70. Henry CH, and Wolford LM. 1993. "Treatment outcomes for temporomandibular joint reconstruction after proplast-teflon implant failure." *Journal of Oral and Maxillofacial Surgery* 51: 352–358.

71. Israel HA, Ward JD, Horrell B, et al. 2003. "Oral and maxillofacial surgery in patients with chronic orofacial pain." *Journal of Oral and Maxillofacial Surgery* 61: 662–667.

72. Milam SB. 2000. "Chronic temporomandibular joint arthralgia." *Oral and Maxillofacial Surgery Clinics of North America* 12(1): 5–26.

73. Quinn PD. 2000. "Lorenz prosthesis." *Oral and Maxillofacial Surgery Clinics of North America* 12: 93–104.

11

Ablative Oral/Head and Neck Surgery

Eric R. Carlson, DMD, MD, FACS
Daniel Oreadi, DMD

INTRODUCTION

Patients undergoing benign and malignant ablative surgery of the oral cavity and head and neck region may experience a variety of medical and surgical complications perioperatively and postoperatively. These complications may be related to the surgery itself or to the patient's preexisting physiologic compromise. Patients with a diagnosis of oral/head and neck cancer, for example, are occasionally elderly and should be considered to exhibit an immunocompromised state. Many of these patients are also malnourished. Patients with benign and malignant tumors with social habits such as smoking and medical comorbidities such as diabetes mellitus, anemia, and other diagnoses are prone to postoperative wound healing complications. As such, efforts should be made to optimize health status preoperatively and minimize perioperative and postoperative complications so as to permit patients to resume normal quality lives post ablative surgery. It is the purpose of this chapter to categorize complications associated with ablative surgery into those that occur in patients with malignant and benign tumors.

COMPLICATIONS RELATED TO ABLATIVE SURGERY FOR MALIGNANT TUMORS

Predictive Factors

Patients with malignant disease of the head and neck region are at high risk for the development of perioperative complications.[1] Avoiding surgical complications in this patient cohort requires identification of those individuals with unfavorable prognostic indices such as advanced age, compromised nutritional status, and the presence of medical conditions predisposing them to higher complication rates.

Advanced Age

The effect of advanced age on surgical morbidity is a highly contested issue in the management of patients with malignant disease. One time-honored discussion showed an operative mortality of nearly 20% for patients older than 80 years of age compared to less than 5% for younger patients.[2] Another study examined more than 4,300 patients undergoing orthopedic, intrathoracic, abdominal, and other surgical procedures.[3] Complications were segregated according to patient decade and categorized as cardiac, such as cardiogenic pulmonary edema, myocardial infarction, unstable angina, and cardiac arrest; or as noncardiac events such as bacterial pneumonia, respiratory failure, renal failure, or pulmonary embolism. It was determined that in-hospital mortality was significantly higher in patients 80 years of age or older (2.6%) versus those patients younger than 80 years of age (0.7%). Major perioperative complications occurred in 4.3% of patients 59 years of age or younger, 5.7% of patients 60–69 years of age, 9.6% of patients 70–79 years of

Management of Complications in Oral and Maxillofacial Surgery, First Edition. Edited by Michael Miloro, Antonia Kolokythas.
© 2012 John Wiley & Sons, Inc. Published 2012 by John Wiley & Sons, Inc.

age, and 12.5% of patients 80 years of age or older. The authors concluded that age significantly affects the risk for perioperative cardiac and noncardiac complications after noncardiac surgery. Surgery was not prohibitive, however, in patients older than 80 years of age. In the final analysis, postoperative surgical complications such as wound infection and postoperative bleeding with hematoma formation seem to be no more common overall compared to younger patients. Medical complications, however, do seem to occur with greater frequency in older patients, including those related to a preoperative diagnosis of cardiac and pulmonary compromise.

Compromised Nutritional Status

Patients with oral cancer are often malnourished. The negative nitrogen balance noted in these patients is a reflection of poor nutrition as may exist in those with chronic alcohol abuse, inadequate oral intake due to the presence of a bulky oral tumor that may be painful, or in the case of tumor-induced weight loss.[4] Surgeons have appreciated the unfavorable effects of nutritional compromise on postoperative surgical wound healing for decades, as well as the understanding that malnutrition translates to immune compromise. The observation that improved T- and B-lymphocyte mediated immune responses develop after correction of malnutrition lends credence that malnourished patients are immunocompromised.[5] The prognostic nutritional index is one means to quantitatively assess the potential for cancer treatment complications. The prognostic nutritional index, as originally developed by Buzby et al.,[6] uses the variables of serum albumin and transferrin values, triceps skinfold measurement, and cutaneous delayed hypersensitivity to develop a percentage value. The authors indicated that a prognostic nutritional index greater than 40% placed patients at high risk for developing treatment complications, those between 20% and 39% were at intermediate risk, and those patients with a prognostic nutritional index below 20% were at low risk of developing treatment complications. The high-risk group experienced an 89% major complication rate compared to a 12.5% major complication rate in the low-risk group. Preoperative nutritional support for longer than 7 days has been shown to decrease operative complications in patients in the high-risk group.[7] While these studies were not directed at patients with oral/head and neck cancer, addressing malnutrition in this patient population preoperatively and providing chemical support of its efficacy (increased prealbumin) prior to surgery will provide a reduction in the risk of perioperative complications.

Medical Comorbidity

The traditional staging system for oral cavity and head and neck cancer is the tumor, node, metastasis (TNM) classification. This system stages cancer according to the size of the primary tumor, and the presence or absence of lymph node and distant metastatic disease. While staging systems attempt to prognosticate patients with cancers, unfortunately, their shortcoming is that they only consider the patient's cancer and not comorbid medical conditions that may accompany the cancer and negatively affect the prognosis.[8] Many patients with oral cavity and head and neck cancer have multiple medical comorbidities that can influence treatment recommendations as well as the prognosis related to ablative surgery. These comorbidities involve nearly every organ system, including the cardiac, pulmonary, endocrine, and hepatic systems. The risk of myocardial infarction or death, for example, exceeded 4% in patients with nonrevascularized coronary artery disease undergoing head and neck surgery in one study.[9] Interestingly, this study identified vascular, thoracic, abdominal, and major head and neck surgery procedures as being associated with the highest risk of cardiac complications in the face of nonrevascularized coronary artery disease. The ideal method of quantifying comorbidity has not been established although several indices have been discussed in the literature including the Kaplan–Feinstein index (KFI) and the Charlson comorbidity index (CCI).[10] The CCI assigns weights for diseases (Table 11.1) that are thought to alter the risk of mortality and is based on a cohort of 604 medical patients admitted to a medical service of one hospital during a 1-month period in 1984. Complete 1-year follow-up information was obtained for 559 of the 604 patients. The intention of this original report was to develop a prognostic taxonomy for comorbid conditions that singly or in combination might alter the risk of short-term mortality for patients enrolled in longitudinal studies. Results of this study indicated that the weighted index of comorbidity was a significant predictor of 1-year survival. Kim et al.[1] briefly discussed unpublished data from their medical center that correlated the CCI score with survival in 117 oral cancer

Table 11.1. Weighted Index of Comorbidity

Assigned weights for diseases	Conditions
1	Myocardial infarction
	Congestive heart failure
	Peripheral vascular disease
	Cerebrovascular disease
	Dementia
	Chronic pulmonary disease
	Connective tissue disease
	Ulcer disease
	Mild liver disease
	Diabetes
2	Hemiplegia
	Moderate or severe renal disease
	Diabetes with end organ damage
	Any tumor
	Leukemia
	Lymphoma
3	Moderate or severe liver disease
6	Metastatic solid tumor
	AIDS

patients. For example, a CCI score of 2–4 showed a 5-year survival of 64% while a CCI score of 8–10 showed a 5-year survival of 14%.

The American Society of Anesthesiologists' classification (ASA) of physical status has been developed for preoperative risk assessment of perioperative adverse events. This classification is not used, however, as a predictor of complications beyond the perioperative period. In addition, the main concern with the use of the ASA classification is the subjectivity involved in its assignment. Reid et al.[11] assessed the ASA classification as a measure of prognosis of a cohort of head and neck surgical patients with a comparison to the Charlson index. Their study concluded that the ASA classification was slightly superior to the Charlson index for prognostic value. Clearly, the presence of comorbid medical disease impacts the prognosis of patients with oral/head and neck cancer.[12]

Complications

Failure to Cure

Failure to cure the disease remains the most significant and devastating negative outcome for the cancer patient and the treating team. Persistent disease, local or regional recurrence, distant metastasis, or presence of second primary cancer are among the commonest reasons for failure. The vast majority of recurrences occur within the first 2 to 3 years following completion of treatment. As it turns out, "recurrence" is a catchall term for the development of disease at the local site, the regional lymph nodes, or at distant sites. Although survival rates from treatment of squamous cell carcinoma of the oral cavity have not improved significantly over the past 30 years, the patterns of failure have changed.[1] Specifically, progressive improvement in local and regional disease has been coupled with increased mortality from second primary cancers and distant metastatic disease. Local, regional, and distant failures seem to occur early following treatment

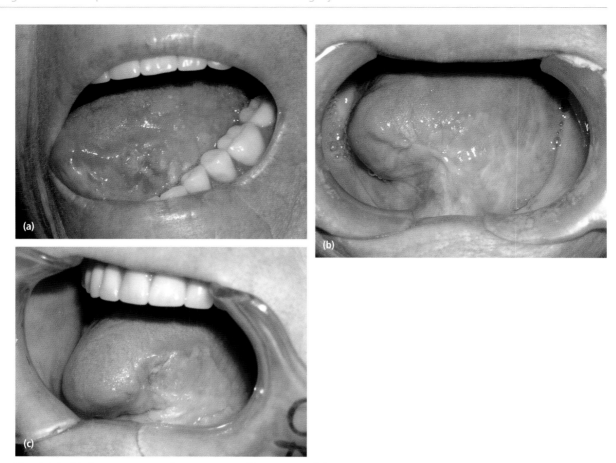

Fig. 11.1. (a) The appearance of a squamous cell carcinoma of the tongue in a 74-year-old woman who did not use alcohol or tobacco. (b) She underwent left partial glossectomy and neck dissection following diagnosis. She healed well as noted at 3 years postoperatively. (c) She displayed recurrent disease at 4 years postoperatively. A repeat partial glossectomy was performed that identified infection with human papilloma virus.

for oral squamous cell carcinoma. In addition, failure is a function of stage of the cancer, particularly related to the histologic status of the cervical lymph nodes.[13]

Local Recurrence

Recurrence of cancer at its primary site usually represents failure to eliminate the entire cancer and achieve negative margins. In this sense, reappearance of cancer at its local site is either indicative of persistence of disease at that primary site or persistence of carcinogenic exposure to that site (Fig. 11.1). Histologically negative margins have been defined as the absence of invasive carcinoma, carcinoma *in situ*, and dysplasia within 5 mm of the resection margins. As such, the oncologic surgeon plans surgical ablation of oral cancers with a 1- to 1.5-cm linear margin of normal appearing tissue. The use of frozen sections of soft tissue margins in the specimen may be of assistance to this end, with a reported accuracy rate of 99%.[14] Ord and Aisner[14] reported a 100% recurrence rate when margins were microscopically involved by infiltrating carcinoma although Slootweg et al. reported local recurrence in 21.9% of their patients with positive margins.[15] Kovacs retrospectively analyzed three subsets of patients with free or positive margins related to surgery for squamous cell carcinoma of the oral cavity and oropharynx.[16] This analysis included 143 patients treated only surgically, 122 patients treated with surgery and adjuvant systemic chemotherapy, and 94 patients treated with surgery and adjuvant chemoradiation therapy. The author concluded that patients treated with adjuvant therapy following surgery with healthy margins had a survival advantage compared to those patients who underwent surgery only. Overall, disease-free survival was better in the groups with adjuvant therapy irrespective of free or positive margins. Survival rates following positive surgical margins were worse in all three groups as compared to the respective subgroups with healthy margins. A second resection in patients with positive margins who subsequently underwent chemoradiation therapy did not result in improvement in survival. The combination of healthy margins and adjuvant treatment is clearly the most favorable scenario for patient survival.

When local recurrence is noted, the time between identification of the recurrence and subsequent treatment is of prognostic significance. Schwartz et al. noted recurrent disease in 28% of their 350 patients with oral squamous cell carcinoma.[17] Recurrent disease that occurred within 6 months of treatment of the primary tumor showed a mean survival time of 20 months, and no patients were cured. Recurrences occurring after 6 months resulted in a mean survival time of 58 months, and 21% of patients were salvaged with further surgery.

Regional Recurrence

Proper execution of the prophylactic neck dissection in the absence of clinically and radiographically nodal involvement (N0 cases) is one oncologically sound method to decrease the chances of regional recurrence following surgical treatment of the primary oral cancer. This concept requires an appreciation for the presence of occult neck disease that in cancers of certain subsites (i.e., oral tongue, floor of mouth) has been reported to range between 36% and 42%.[18,19] The supraomohyoid neck dissection that involves an en bloc excision of lymph nodes in levels I, II, and III represents a scientifically sound approach to the management of the N0 neck in cases of oral tongue cancers with depth of invasion greater than 3–4 mm, as well as floor of mouth lesions (Fig 11.2). In general, when the risk of occult nodal involvement is greater than 20%, the regional lymphatics require treatment. This can be in the form of surgery, selective neck dissection, or radiotherapy to the "at risk" neck. Given the low overall morbidity and complication rates of the selective neck dissection, it is the preferred approach. This is further supported by the reported poor survival (less than 50%) in cases of regional failure, especially post radiotherapy. The international literature supports the performance of this elective neck dissection for T1N0 and T2N0 squamous cell carcinomas of the oral cavity, with the identification of occult neck disease in these specimens ranging from 36% to 42%.[20–22] As such, numerous authors have recommended the routine performance of the supraomohyoid neck dissection in the management of early squamous cell carcinoma of the oral cavity.[23–25] Locoregional control has been reported to increase from 50% to 91% when supraomohyoid neck dissection is performed.[26] A study examining 501 patients undergoing radical neck dissection showed that only 9% of patients had metastatic disease in cervical lymph nodes in level IV when the neck dissection was elective in nature and the incidence of positive lymph nodes in level V was only 2%.[27] These data point to the unnecessary dissection of lymph node levels IV and V when managing the N0 neck. The only exception to this rule occurs when managing tongue cancer in which case extending the elective neck dissection into level IV is probably warranted.[28]

Proper execution of a neck dissection for the N+ neck also represents a method of reducing the likelihood of regional recurrences. The modified radical neck dissection and its variants are preferable in the management of the N+ neck due to the opportunity to preserve the spinal accessory nerve that otherwise would lead to a shoulder syndrome of pain and limited mobility of the upper extremity.[29] The surgical principle of the modified radical neck dissection (MRND) is based on the knowledge that the aponeurotic system of the neck encases the internal structures that are routinely removed in radical neck dissection. The MRND works within these planes of dissection yet removes an en bloc specimen of metastatic and nonmetastatic lymph nodes and surrounding structures. The MRND intentionally preserves anatomic structures, most commonly the spinal accessory nerve (Fig. 11.3). For example, the type I MRND involves preservation of the spinal accessory nerve, a type II MRND involves preservation of the spinal accessory nerve and the internal jugular vein, and a type III MRND involves preservation of the spinal accessory nerve, internal jugular vein, and the sternocleidomastoid muscle. The international literature indicates that the type I MRND is the preferred neck dissection for the N+ neck in oral cavity cancers.[30] This neck dissection effectively manages metastatic cervical lymph nodes, does not compromise oncologic safety, maintains function when properly performed, and should provide patients with a reduced incidence of regional recurrence depending on the final histopathology of the neck dissection specimen.[13] This approach is advocated due to the observation that palpable lymph nodes even smaller than 3 cm in diameter have a substantial incidence of extracapsular spread of disease.[31] The presence of extracapsular extension of cervical lymph node metastases might breech the aponeurotic planes relied upon when the sternocleidomastoid

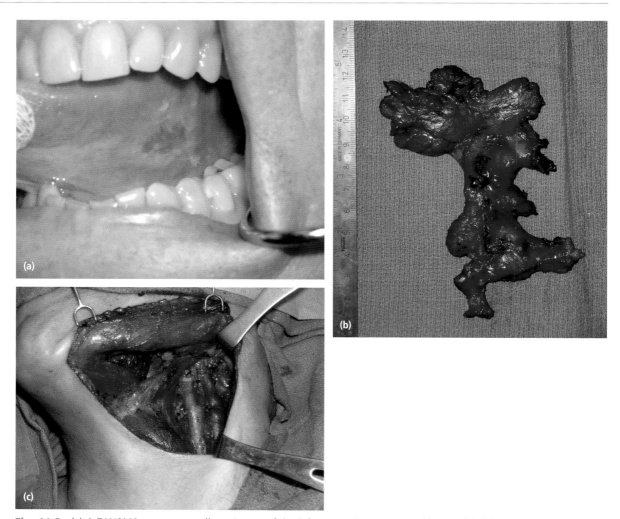

Fig. 11.2. (a) A T1N0M0 squamous cell carcinoma of the left tongue in a 60-year-old man. (b), (c) The patient underwent a left partial glossectomy and selective neck dissection (I–IV). The final histopathology of the neck specimen identified three lymph nodes with metastatic squamous cell carcinoma. The patient underwent postoperative radiation therapy and showed no evidence of disease in the neck at 3 years postoperatively.

muscle and internal jugular vein are otherwise preserved. Such a surgical maneuver would likely result in recurrence in the neck postoperatively.

The functional neck dissection was originally described by Bocca and Pignataro in 1967.[32] In 1984, these authors described their findings of 1,500 functional neck dissections performed in 843 patients operated on between 1961 and 1982.[33] Cancer of the larynx made up 87% of the patients in this report where only lymphatic tissue of the neck was sacrificed, and the sternocleidomastoid muscle, internal jugular vein, and spinal accessory nerve were preserved. Out of these 1,500 neck dissections, 1,200 were elective in nature (N0) while 300 were therapeutic in their execution (N+). Regional recurrences were noted in 68 cases (8.1%). Sixteen cases of regional recurrence occurred in patients with N0 necks (1.33%), while 52 cases of recurrence occurred in N+ necks noted in 171 patients (30.4%). Of interest to the oral cancer surgeon is the absence of dissection of lymph nodes in level I in the functional neck dissection.[34] Since level I lymph nodes are sentinel nodes related to oral cancer, failure to dissect this important oncologic level may result in cervical lymph node recurrence when managing the N0 or N+ neck. As such, it would seem that the functional neck dissection has no role in the management of cervical lymph nodes in patients with oral squamous cell carcinoma.

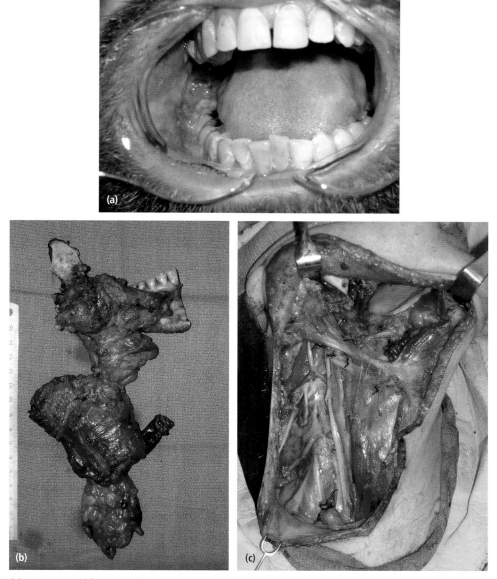

Fig. 11.3. (a) A 39-year-old man with a T4N1M0 squamous cell carcinoma of the right mandibular gingiva, mandible, and neck. (b), (c) He underwent a composite resection of the right mandible, gingiva, and type I modified radical neck dissection.

Distant Metastatic Disease

The development of distant metastatic disease related to oral cavity squamous cell carcinoma has historically been believed to represent a rare phenomenon, seen only in 2–9% of patients.[35] The presence of distant metastatic disease may be disclosed by abnormal findings on a routinely ordered plain film of the chest, a PET/CT scan or a CT scan (Fig. 11.4), the presence of pain in the case of bone metastases, or the incidental discovery of metastatic foci during autopsy as may occur in a previously asymptomatic patient. Since autopsies are performed relatively infrequently following death of a patient with oral cancer, it is likely that the incidence of distant metastatic disease is underestimated.[36] The most common site of distant metastatic spread has been noted as the lungs, with a mean survival time of approximately 9 months.[35] The second most common distant metastatic site is bone with a mean survival time of approximately 2 months.[37]

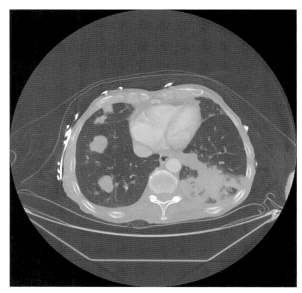

Fig. 11.4. A CT of the chest in a patient treated for stage IV squamous cell carcinoma of the oral cavity 2 years earlier. The CT demonstrates evidence of metastatic disease in the right lung.

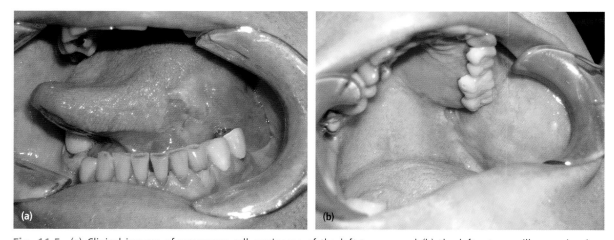

Fig. 11.5. (a) Clinical images of squamous cell carcinoma of the left tongue and (b) the left retromaxillary region in a 66-year-old man with metachronous primary cancers. Eighteen months separated the diagnosis of these cancers.

Second Primary Disease

Second primary cancers are those tumors that develop either synchronously or metachronously in patients with a diagnosed squamous cell carcinoma of the oral/head and neck region (Fig. 11.5). They are believed to exist at a rate of 5% to 7% annually in these patients.[38] Some controversy exists regarding the most appropriate definition of second primary tumors, but most authors use the criteria from Warren and Gates[39]: (1) each of the tumors must present a definite picture of malignancy, (2) each must be distinct, and (3) the probability of one being a metastasis of the other must be excluded. In general, if an individual continues to smoke after a first squamous cell carcinoma of the oral cavity, that patient has a 33% rate of developing a second primary cancer in the upper aerodigestive tract within 5 years compared to a 3–5% rate of developing a second primary cancer if smoking cessation occurs.[4]

Chemoprevention has historically represented one means to prevent the development of second primary cancers. Because retinoids are required for normal developmental differentiation, and since they reverse cellular characteristics associated with malignant disease, they have been studied for their efficacy in reversing premalignant changes in the oral cavity, as well as in the prevention of second primary cancers of the upper aerodigestive region.[40] Encouraging results were once realized with the use of retinoids; however, drug toxicity and the rapid reversal of beneficial effects once the drug was discontinued limited the utility of these agents. Second line agents included cyclooxygenase-2 inhibitors. Many human malignancies, including oral squamous cell carcinoma, are known to produce higher levels of prostaglandins than the normal tissues from which they arise. Increased synthesis of prostaglandins in transformed cells and neoplasms is thought to be a consequence of enhanced expression of cyclooxygenase-2 (COX-2).[41] Prostaglandins are also believed to be important in the pathogenesis of cancer due to their effects on cell proliferation, angiogenesis, immune surveillance, and apoptosis. Nonsteroidal anti-inflammatory drugs and aspirin are known to prevent colon cancer in patients with arthritis.[42] Moreover, it has been determined that COX-2 is overexpressed in the oral mucosa of active smokers versus those who never smoked.[43] Increased levels of COX-2 are commonly found in premalignant and malignant conditions such as oral leukoplakia and invasive cancer.[42] Several lines of medical evidence indicate that COX-2 is a promising molecular target for the prevention or treatment of cancer. In October 2004, Merck pulled rofecoxib (Vioxx) off the market after research showed that the drug could increase the risk of heart attacks and strokes. On December 17, 2004, Pfizer announced a long-term study on celecoxib (Celebrex) that also suggested an increased risk of heart attack, although doses up to twice as high as those that had been recommended for the treatment of arthritis patients were being investigated.[44]

Neurologic Dysfunction

Sensory and motor nerve dysfunction related to ablative surgery for malignant disease may represent inadvertent nerve injury or intentional sacrifice. Although many of the cranial and cervical nerves are at risk related to extirpation of oral/head and neck malignancies, the incidence of injury to each nerve is a function of the site and stage of the primary cancer.

Spinal Accessory Nerve

The dissection and preservation of the spinal accessory nerve is paramount to the performance of a type I MRND. As previously discussed, this surgical maneuver reduces or eliminates the morbidity associated with the radical neck dissection that intentionally sacrifices the spinal accessory nerve, most notably shoulder syndrome. Transection of the spinal accessory nerve does not uniformly cause total loss of trapezius muscle function,[45] and preservation of this nerve has been found to be associated with a permanent shoulder droop in 25% of patients.[46] This finding may be explained by traction injury, devascularization of the nerve, or unrecognized transection of the nerve. When spinal accessory nerve dysfunction is observed, patients exhibit limitation of arm abduction at the shoulder, loss of the rhythm of abduction due to abnormal rotation of the scapula, winging of the scapula, and loss of the normal sloping contour of the shoulder (Fig. 11.6). Patients typically also complain of pain. Shoulder function following neck dissection is a multifactorial issue. Although the spinal accessory nerve is usually regarded as the sole innervation of the trapezius muscle, anatomists have described variable motor innervations that form a plexus with the spinal accessory nerve and account for the variability in motor innervation and function of the muscle.[47] Contributions to innervation of this muscle include fibers from the greater auricular nerve, phrenic nerve, and branches of the brachial plexus.

Facial Nerve

Dissection and preservation of the main trunk of the facial nerve and its peripheral branches typically occurs related to the surgical management of neoplasms of the parotid gland. Under such circumstances, the incidence of temporary facial nerve palsy after superficial parotidectomy can be as high as 40–58% but permanent palsy is 0–3%.[1] The incidence of temporary and permanent facial nerve palsy increases with recurrent superficial lobe tumors and deep tumors. The most commonly affected branch during parotidectomy is the marginal mandibular branch due to the infrequent incidence of crossover innervation from other branches (Fig. 11.7). The marginal mandibular branch of the facial nerve is routinely encountered during a neck dissection. Identification and superior transposition is warranted during the dissection of the N0 neck and may also be performed during surgical management of the N+ neck provided that its

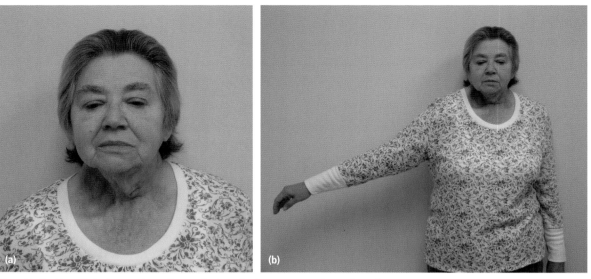

Fig. 11.6. The clinical sequelae of a radical neck dissection performed in this 64-year-old woman. (a) She displays a shoulder droop and (b) the inability to fully elevate the ipsilateral upper extremity.

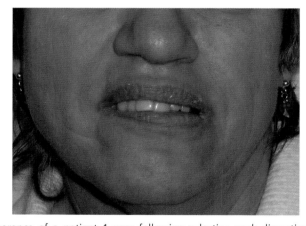

Fig. 11.7. The clinical appearance of a patient 1 year following selective neck dissection in which the right marginal mandibular nerve was inadvertently sacrificed. The patient displays abnormal posturing of the ipsilateral lower lip.

preservation does not compromise oncologic safety, particularly when level I lymph nodes are clinically positive. Under such circumstances, separation of the neck dissection specimen from the inferior border of the mandible without dissection of the marginal mandibular nerve within the investing fascia may be prudent. Sacrifice of this nerve certainly has cosmetic implications and may also have functional consequences. Lack of lower lip competence as may occur when the marginal mandibular nerve has been sacrificed, for example, may result in difficulty eating.

Phrenic Nerve

Phrenic nerve injury during neck dissection usually represents a complication of surgery rather than direct tumor infiltration of the nerve. An overall 8% incidence of phrenic nerve injury has been reported with resultant diaphragmatic paralysis following neck dissection.[47] The diagnosis is most commonly made postoperatively by chest radiograph. Ipsilateral elevation of the diaphragm at least one intercostal space

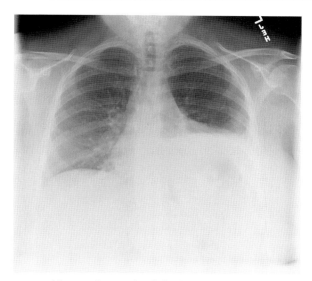

Fig. 11.8. A left hemidiaphragm noted in a patient with a left phrenic nerve injury.

above the unaffected side is the radiologic parameter that must be met to make a diagnosis of a hemidiaphragm due to phrenic nerve injury (Fig. 11.8). Signs of phrenic nerve injury include diminished, absent, or paradoxical movement of the diaphragm on inspiration; mediastinal shifting toward the contralateral side with inspiration; and paradoxical movement of the diaphragm during cough. These abnormal diaphragmatic movements may be seen with fluoroscopy. Patient symptoms include those related to respiratory compromise and include dyspnea, as well as cardiac irritation by the displaced diaphragm, which can result in palpitations, tachycardia, and premature ventricular contractions. In addition, gastrointestinal complaints include abdominal pain, and nausea and vomiting, also likely due to the superior displacement of the abdominal contents secondary to the change in position of the diaphragm. A review of 176 patients undergoing neck dissection revealed 11 patients who experienced permanent paralysis of the diaphragm postoperatively and three patients who demonstrated paralysis that resolved within 3 weeks of surgery.[48] Evaluation of the operative reports of these patients revealed that tumor infiltration near the nerve, bleeding with ligation of vessels near the nerve and electrocoagulation near the nerve occurred during these neck dissections.

Miscellaneous Nerve Injuries

Other nerves that are intentionally isolated during neck dissection include the hypoglossal nerve (cranial nerve XII) and the vagus nerve (cranial nerve X). The hypoglossal nerve predictably crosses the carotid artery approximately 2 cm superior to its bifurcation. It is surrounded by branches of the internal jugular vein that must be anticipated so as to prevent bleeding while attempting to identify and preserve the hypoglossal nerve. Hypoglossal nerve dysfunction results in difficulties with speech and swallowing postoperatively.

Sacrifice of the hypoglossal nerve will result in ipsilateral deviation when asking the patient to protrude the tongue (Fig. 11.9). The vagus nerve is located posterior to the carotid artery. Its location must be visualized prior to ligating the internal jugular vein in the supraclavicular fossa when performing MRND. As such, a thorough dissection of the inferior aspect of the internal jugular vein as well as level IV lymph nodes must be performed so as to visualize the vagus nerve. Injury to the vagus nerve results in a hoarse voice and severe swallowing difficulties with predisposition to aspiration.

Wound Infection

Ablative surgical procedures in head and neck and oral cavity are prone to infection by virtue of representing clean-contaminated cases. Prophylactic antibiotics should be routinely administered and have limited

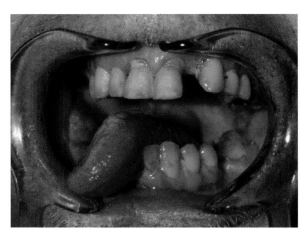

Fig. 11.9. Abnormal movement of the tongue on protrusion in a patient who underwent sacrifice of the right hypoglossal nerve during neck dissection.

the incidence of postoperative infection to approximately 10%.[1] Even so, wound infections are particularly problematic to surgeons who care for these patients due to the potential for delay of adjuvant therapy, as well as due to the concern for patient morbidity and length of stay in the hospital. Identification of risk factors for wound infection include tumor stage, duration of surgery, previous radiation or chemotherapy, the concurrent placement of a soft tissue flap, unfavorable nutritional status, and comorbid medical conditions such as diabetes that place a patient at risk for wound infection.

A bacterial inoculum of 10^5 bacteria per gram of tissue is required for a wound infection to develop. Salivary contamination in surgical wounds allows for the introduction of 10^{8-9} bacteria per milliliter of saliva, and these organisms are most commonly cultured in wound sepsis after head and neck surgery. The purpose of perioperative antibiotics is to decrease the bacterial count at the time of surgery. Antibiotic selection should be directed at the organisms indigenous to the oral cavity including *Streptococcus*, *Staphylococcus*, and *Enterobacter* species, as well as *Eikenella corrodens*, *Fusobacterium*, *Escherichia coli*, and others.

Chylous Fistula

Thoracic duct injury during neck dissection with the subsequent development of a chylous fistula occurs in about 1.0–2.5% of cases and is reported to occur primarily in the left neck.[49] The risk of this complication is increased with reoperations for persistent or recurrent disease.[50] Anatomically, the thoracic duct originates in the cisterna chyli and passes through the aortic hiatus in the diaphragm. In the posterior mediastinum, the duct crosses from right to left and then traverses the superior mediastinum to the left of the esophagus and behind the aortic arch and proximal left subclavian artery. Multiple branching of the intrathoracic portion of the duct has been noted.[51] The duct arches superiorly and laterally as it exits the thoracic inlet, passing anteriorly to the vertebral artery and thyrocervical trunk and posterior to the carotid sheath structures. Finally, it empties into the great veins at the root of the neck, with a valve near its terminus preventing backflow. Many anatomic variations in the course of the duct exist, including approximately 5% of main thoracic ducts terminating on the right side of the neck, thereby explaining the occurrence of a major chyle leakage following right neck surgery. The superior extent of the duct is also variable. It may extend as high as 5 cm superior to the clavicle, making it vulnerable to injury higher in the neck than might be typically expected. Furthermore, multiple terminations of the duct are common, with two or more branches occurring in 11–45% of cases.[51] These branches may empty into the same vein or different veins. Identification and ligation of the thoracic duct, therefore, does not eliminate injury to another branch such that a chyle fistula could occur even in association with meticulous surgical technique.

Chyle contains a major portion of the ingested fat intake, as well as electrolytes, protein, and white blood cells in a concentration similar to serum. Chronic loss of chyle, therefore, can result in serious metabolic

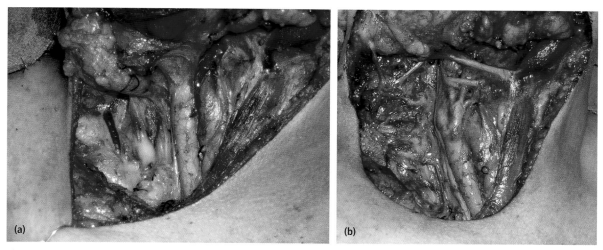

Fig. 11.10. (a) The presence of chyle in the wound of a patient undergoing right modified radical neck dissection following a valsalva maneuver. (b) Successful suturing of the right thoracic duct resulted in no further leakage of chyle in the wound upon a repeat valsalva maneuver.

derangements secondary to depletion of fluid, electrolytes, protein, and lymphocytes. Loss of lymphocytes in a chylous fistula will result in reduced immune competence due to the development of a peripheral lymphocytopenia.

The management of a chyle fistula is controversial. Both operative and nonoperative techniques for its management have been suggested. Clearly, identification of a chyle leak during neck dissection is desirable. This is accomplished by the observation of a chyle leak in the supraclavicular fossa during or following delivery of the specimen. Due to the *non per os* (NPO) status of the patient undergoing surgery, chyle appears as cloudy fluid and should be readily identified if a breach of integrity of the thoracic duct occurs during neck dissection (Fig. 11.10). Even if not identified, the anesthesia team should deliver a valsalva maneuver so as to increase intrathoracic pressure and permit egress of chyle through the injured duct if this complication has occurred. If so, primary operative control of a lacerated thoracic duct should remedy the problem. The treatment of iatrogenic chyle leak after neck dissection is divided into an early conservative management and a delayed surgical intervention. Early treatment consists of diet modification, specifically a fat-free diet, the use of a pressure dressing, maintaining a closed vacuum suction drainage of the neck wound, and the institution of prophylactic broad-spectrum antibiotics.[52] Other diet modifications can include the use of total parenteral nutrition (TPN) and the use of medium chain fatty acids in enteral feeds. Somatostatin analogs such as octreotide have also been used successfully to permit seal of a thoracic duct fistula.[50] Octreotide reduces gastrointestinal chyle production by decreasing splanchnic blood flow and decreasing gastric, biliary, pancreatic, and intestinal secretions.

Surgical management of thoracic duct injuries is indicated in patients with persistent high-output fistulas (>500 ml/d) with severe metabolic and nutritional complications or coexisting chylothorax with respiratory compromise. Surgery should also be considered in low-output fistulas (<500 ml/d) of duration longer than 14 days where conservative measures have been unsuccessful.

Wound Dehiscence, Reconstruction Plate Exposure

Intraoral wound breakdown is not an uncommon complication following composite resection for oral squamous cell carcinoma. Nutritional compromise, unfavorable medical comorbidity, tension on mucosal closures, and oral infections can lead to mucosal breakdown with bone or bone plate exposure. The use of axial pattern myocutaneous flaps and free flaps with generous skin paddles can reduce the chance for mucosal dehiscence due to the provision of tension-free closures in the oral cavity. Nonetheless, soft tissue flaps may have a compromised blood supply that could also result in wound breakdown. The end result of wound dehiscence is the need to provide enteral nutritional feeds so as to bypass the oral cavity, frequent wound care with oral irrigations, and often the delay of postoperative adjuvant therapy (radiation and chemotherapy). The delay in the delivery of radiation therapy may be to the detriment of the patient's long-term survival. Studies have identified a significant survival advantage when radiotherapy is initiated no later than 6–8 weeks after surgical resection and completion of treatment is achieved within 100 days, ideally with no interruptions. Surgical care must be performed so as to reduce the incidence of postoperative wound dehiscence.

The use of reconstruction bone plates for the stabilization of segmental defects of the mandible was first reported by Spiessl et al.[53] in 1976. Advantages of the use of reconstruction bone plates includes proper maintenance of occlusion, support of the facial soft tissues, and stabilization of the mandible in concert with a free microvascular reconstruction of a mandibular segmental defect. Initially bone plates were made of stainless steel and vitallium followed by the development of first-generation titanium bone plates. Such first-generation titanium bone plates were typically of higher profile than second-generation titanium reconstruction bone plates. Lavertu et al. examined early and late complications associated with the placement of 27 reconstruction bone plates.[54] Early complications were noted in 44% of patients that included wound dehiscence and plate exposure. Ten of 12 patients who experienced early complications had received radiation therapy. Late complications were mainly related to tumor recurrence, but also included pain, plate exposure, infection, screw loosening, and plate fracture that were reported as being unrelated to tumor recurrence. At least one late complication was experienced by 63% of patients. Boyd et al.[55] examined plate failure and concluded that reconstruction bone plates placed across the symphysis are particularly prone to exposure.

Second-generation titanium bone plates utilize locking screws and are lower profile than first-generation reconstruction bone plates. The complication rate associated with the use of second-generation reconstruction bone plates has been reported as 36%.[56] Specific complications included plate fracture, screw loosening, plate exposure, wound infection, and malocclusion. The average time for hardware failure was 14 months following placement. The authors recommended the use of a primary vascularized bone reconstruction in conjunction with plate placement. Such a reconstruction was reported to permit additional soft tissue support around the bone plate so as to minimize the risk of plate exposure. Osseous support of the plate is also provided thereby minimizing the risk of plate fracture.

Wound dehiscence may occasionally result in exposure of reconstruction bone plates (Fig. 11.11). When this occurs, it is our experience that attempts at coverage of the exposed plate with soft tissue flaps is unsuccessful, such that the surgeon must resort to plate removal.

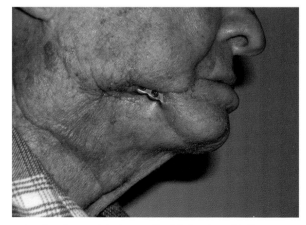

Fig. 11.11. Exposure of a reconstruction bone plate in a patient following ablative surgery of the right mandible and the subsequent delivery of radiation therapy.

COMPLICATIONS RELATED TO ABLATIVE SURGERY FOR BENIGN TUMORS

Predictive Factors

Patients undergoing ablative surgery for benign tumors of the oral/head and neck region are generally not as likely to experience perioperative complications as patients undergoing ablative surgery for malignant tumors. In general terms, patients who undergo ablative surgery for benign neoplasms have relatively more favorable prognostic indices such as younger age, acceptable nutritional status, and often times the relative lack of medical comorbidity compared to patients who undergo surgery for malignant neoplasms. This latter issue may reflect the younger age of patients with benign tumors. Unless known to be immunocompromised, patients who undergo benign tumor surgery need not be routinely classified or treated as such. Due to all of this information, complications seen in patients undergoing benign tumor surgery are generally related to the surgery itself rather than to the patient's preexisting physiologic compromise. This being the case, benign tumor surgery must be executed with preoperative and intraoperative precision as technique sensitivity is of utmost importance to reduce complications. The two most common types of benign head and neck tumors are odontogenic and salivary.

Recurrence

Odontogenic Tumors

From a surgical standpoint, odontogenic tumors are classified as those that require resection for cure and those that may be cured with enucleation and curettage (Table 11.2). The prototypical benign odontogenic tumor is the solid or multicystic ameloblastoma that requires resection with 1 cm linear bone margins in order to predict cure.[57] The management of this tumor by more conservative measures including enucleation and curettage, surgical excision and peripheral ostectomy, and enucleation with liquid nitrogen cryotherapy has a lower rate of cure than resection with adequate margins (Fig. 11.12). When these tumors reappear after treatment, they have been incorrectly referred to as "recurrences" when in fact they represent persistent disease.[58] Persistent disease represents the most common complication associated with the solid or multicystic ameloblastoma. Persistent ameloblastomas may result in death.[59] A

Table 11.2. Surgical Treatment of Odontogenic Tumors With Curative Intent

Odontogenic tumors requiring resection
Solid or multicystic ameloblastoma

Unicystic ameloblastoma
   Mural subtype

Odontoameloblastoma

Odontogenic myxoma

Pindborg tumor

Odontogenic tumors treated properly by enucleation and curettage
Odontoma

Adenomatoid odontogenic tumor

Unicystic ameloblastoma
   Luminal subtype
   Intraluminal subtype

Ameloblastic fibroma

Ameloblastic fibro-odontoma

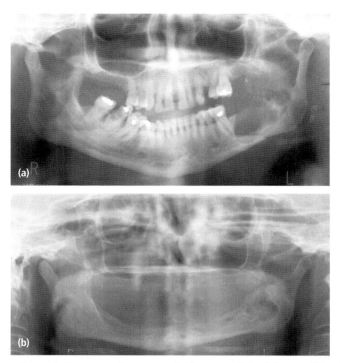

Fig. 11.12. (a) Panoramic radiograph demonstrating an ameloblastoma of the left mandible. (b) The patient underwent enucleation and curettage of her tumor and was noted to have persistent disease on a panoramic radiograph obtained 5 years later.

scientific approach to the linear and anatomic barriers as part of a marginal or segmental resection of the mandible or a maxillectomy where negative soft and hard tissue histopathologic sections are realized is likely to result in cure of the patient. Anything short of this approach is likely to not result in cure of the patient.

One additional and enigmatic issue related to recurrence of odontogenic tumors is the development of metastatic disease. This issue has been exclusively noted in relationship to the diagnosis of a solid or multicystic ameloblastoma. Numerous sites of metastatic disease have been identified related to the solid or multicystic ameloblastoma, although the lung is the most common site.[60-65] This being the case, aspiration of the ameloblastoma has been purported as being the cause of distant disease in the lungs, likely related to enucleation and curettage procedures. This premise has been debated widely, with one author indicating that the aspiration hypothesis leaves unanswered the questions as to why other odontogenic tumors have not undergone metastatic spread to the lungs.[66] In addition, if aspiration of an ameloblastoma were to occur, it would most likely result in middle and lower lobe metastases, and this has not been noted in the literature. With this and other issues in mind related to this tumor, other authors have indicated that the only way to explain the observation of metastatic spread of the ameloblastoma is that this tumor is a low-grade malignancy.[67]

Parotid Tumors

The pleomorphic adenoma is the most common benign salivary gland tumor, the most common salivary gland tumor overall, and the most common tumor of the parotid gland. As such, significant data exist regarding the recurrence of this tumor as a function of various forms of surgical treatment. Although pleomorphic adenomas have a pseudocapsule of compressed fibrous tissue, buds and pseudopodia from the tumor involve the pseudocapsule such that simple enucleation of the tumor will leave remnants of tumor in the surrounding parotid gland that was not extirpated, thereby leading to multifocal recurrence (Fig. 11.13). Due to this observed dilemma, surgeons have performed a superficial parotidectomy or partial

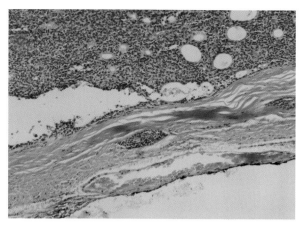

Fig. 11.13. Invasion of the pseudocapsule of a pleomorphic adenoma of the parotid gland.

superficial parotidectomy (limited superficial parotidectomy) for treatment of this diagnosis. This not-withstanding, the tumor pseudocapsule's proximity to the facial nerve that is preserved during the surgery translates to the dissection leaving no tissue at some points surrounding the pseudocapsule. Nonetheless, the recurrence rate of the pleomorphic adenoma of the parotid treated with partial or complete superficial parotidectomy is extremely low.[68] Ghosh et al. indicated that microscopic invasion of the capsule had no influence on recurrence, suggesting that a fraction of a millimeter of normal tissue was an adequate margin and that only tumors that actually involved the margin were at risk for recurrence.[69] These authors recommended that preservation of vital structures, such as the facial nerve, is a more important consideration than preserving a cuff of normal tissue at the periphery of the pseudocapsule.[69]

Nerve Injury

Sensory Nerve Injury

The inferior alveolar nerve is commonly intentionally sacrificed during segmental resection of the mandible for benign odontogenic tumors, such as the ameloblastoma. While this tumor is still considered to be benign without nerve invasion, most surgeons sacrifice this nerve with the tumor specimen so as not to spill tumor that might occur during a nerve pull-through procedure.[70]

Motor Nerve Injury

As pointed out earlier in this chapter, the facial nerve is the motor nerve most likely to be injured during ablative surgery for benign neoplasms of the parotid gland. Witt reported a zero incidence of permanent facial nerve paralysis in a series of 59 partial parotidectomies with facial nerve dissection for benign and low-grade malignant tumors.[71] Klintworth et al.[72] evaluated 377 patients undergoing extracapsular dissection of benign parotid gland tumors. Postoperative facial nerve function was normal in 346 patients (92%) in the immediate postoperative period, whereas 23 patients (6%) showed temporary facial nerve paresis, and 8 patients (2%) developed permanent facial nerve paresis. Interestingly, Ellingson et al.[73] compared the facial nerve function following parotidectomy in 67 patients with benign disease versus 52 patients with malignant disease. Of patients with benign disease, 94% had normal postoperative facial nerve function (House-Brackmann grade I) or only slight weakness (House-Brackmann grade II) compared to 76.9% of patients with malignant disease exhibiting the same. The final facial nerve function was the same for both groups. It is unclear if a greater degree of medical comorbidity existed with resultant compromised wound healing or if a dissection of greater magnitude occurred in the patients with malignant disease versus patients with benign disease in this series.

SUGGESTED READINGS

1. Kim DD, and Ord RA. 2003. "Complications in the treatment of head and neck cancer." *Oral Maxillofacial Surg Clin N Am* 15: 213–227.
2. McGuirt WF, Loevy S, McCabe BF, et al. 1977. "The risks of major head and neck surgery in the aged population." *Laryngoscope* 87: 1378–1382.
3. Polanczyk CA, Marcantonio E, and Goldman L. 2001. "Impact of age on perioperative complications and length of stay in patients undergoing noncardiac surgery." *Ann Intern Med* 134: 637–643.
4. Marx RE. 1990. "Complications of head and neck cancer." *Oral Maxillofacial Surg Clin N Am* 2: 567–591.
5. Law DK, Dudrick DJ, and Abdou NI. 1973. "Immunocompetence of patients with protein-calorie malnutrition." *Ann Int Med* 79: 545–550.
6. Buzby GP, Mullen JL, Matthews DC, et al. 1980. "Prognostic nutritional index in gastrointestinal surgery." *Am J Surg* 139: 160–167.
7. Mullen JL, Buzby GP, Matthews DC, et al. 1980. "Reduction of operative morbidity and mortality by combined preoperative and postoperative nutritional support." *Ann Surg* 192: 604–613.
8. Piccirillo JF. 1995. "Purposes, problems, and proposals for progress in cancer staging." *Arch Otolaryngol Head Neck Surg* 121: 145–149.
9. Eagle KA, Rihal CS, Mickel MC, et al. 1997. "Cardiac risk of noncardiac surgery. Influence of coronary disease and type of surgery in 3368 operations." *Circulation* 96: 1882–1887.
10. Charlson ME, Pompei P, Ales KL, and MacKenzie CR. 1987. "A new method of classifying prognostic comorbidity in longitudinal studies: Development and validation." *J Chron Dis* 40: 373–383.
11. Reid BC, Alberg AJ, Klassen AC, et al. 2001. "The American Society of Anesthesiologists' class as a comorbidity index in a cohort of head and neck cancer surgical patients." *Head Neck* 23: 985–994.
12. Piccirillo JF. 2000. "Importance of comorbidity in head and neck cancer." *Laryngoscope* 110: 593–602.
13. Kalmins IK, Leonard AG, Sako K, et al. 1977. "Correlation between prognosis and degree of lymph node involvement in carcinoma of the oral cavity." *Am J Surg* 134(4): 450–454.
14. Ord RA, and Aisner S. 1997. "Accuracy of frozen sections in assessing margins in oral cancer resection." *J Oral Maxillofac Surg* 55: 663–669.
15. Slootweg PJ, Hordijk GL, Schade Y, et al. 2002. "Treatment failure and margin status in head and neck cancer. A critical view on the potential value of molecular pathology." *Oral Oncol* 38: 500–503.
16. Kovacs AF. 2004. "Relevance of positive margins in case of adjuvant therapy of oral cancer." *Int J Oral Maxillofac Surg* 33: 447–453.
17. Schwartz GJ, Mehra RM, Wening BL, et al. 2000. "Salvage treatment for recurrent squamous cell carcinoma of the oral cavity." *Head Neck* 22: 34–41.
18. Carlson ER, Cheung A, Smith BC, and Pfohl C. 2006. "Neck dissections for oral/head and neck cancer 1906–2006." *J Oral Maxillofac Surg* 64: 4–11.
19. Carlson ER, and Miller I. 2006. "Management of the neck in oral cancer." *Oral Maxillofac Surg Clin N Am* 18: 533–546.
20. Yen APW, Lam KY, Chan CL, et al. 1999. "Clinicopathological analysis of elective neck dissection for N0 neck of early oral tongue carcinoma." *Am J Surg* 177: 90–92.
21. Ho CM, Lam KH, and Wei WI. 1992. "Occult lymph node metastasis in small oral tongue cancers." *Head Neck* 14: 359–363.
22. Beenken SW, Krontiras H, and Maddox WA. 1999. "T1 and T2 squamous cell carcinoma of the oral tongue: Prognostic factors and the role of elective lymph node dissection." *Head Neck* 21: 124–130.
23. Medina JE, and Byers RM. 1989. "Supraomohyoid neck dissection: Rationale, indications, and surgical technique." *Head Neck* 11: 111–122.
24. Kligerman J, Lima RA, and Soares JR. 1994. "Supraomohyoid neck dissection in the treatment of T1/T2 squamous cell carcinoma of oral cavity." *Am J Surg* 168: 391–394.
25. Kowalski LP, Magrin J, Waksman G, et al. 1993. "Supraomohyoid neck dissection in the treatment of head and neck tumors." *Arch Otolaryngol Head Neck Surg* 119: 958–963.
26. Jalisi S. 2005. "Management of the clinically negative neck in early squamous cell carcinoma of the oral cavity." *Otolaryng Clin North Am* 38: 37–46.
27. Shah JP, Candela FC, and Podar AK. 1990. "The patterns of cervical lymph node metastasis from squamous cell carcinoma of the oral cavity." *Cancer* 66: 109–113.
28. Byers RM, Weber RS, Andrews T, et al. 1997. "Frequency and therapeutic implications of 'skip metastases' in the neck from squamous carcinoma of the oral tongue." *Head Neck* 19: 14–19.
29. Nahum AM, Mullally W, and Marmor I. 1961. "A syndrome resulting from radical neck dissection." *Arch Otolaryngol* 74: 424–428.
30. Myers EN, and Fagan JJ. 1998. "Treatment of the N+ neck in squamous cell carcinoma of the upper aerodigestive tract." *Otolaryngol Clin North Am* 31: 671–686.
31. Snow GB, Annyas AA, Van Slooten EA, et al. 1982. "Prognostic factors of neck node metastasis." *Clin Otolaryngol* 7: 185–192.
32. Bocca E, and Pignataro O. 1967. "A conservation technique in radical neck dissection." *Ann Otol Rhinol Laryngol* 76: 975–987.
33. Bocca E, Pignataro O, Oldini C, et al. 1984. "Functional neck dissection: An evaluation and review of 843 cases." *Laryngoscope* 94: 942–945.

34. Ferlito A, Rinaldo A, Robbins KT, et al. 2003. "Changing concepts in the surgical management of the cervical node metastasis." *Oral Oncol* 39: 429–435.
35. Kademani D, and Dierks E. 2006. "Management of locoregional recurrence in squamous cell carcinoma." *Oral Maxillofac Surg Clin N Am* 18: 615–625.
36. Carlson ER, and Ord RA. 2002. "Vertebral metastases from oral squamous cell carcinoma." *J Oral Maxillofac Surg* 60: 858–862.
37. Kowalski LP, Carvalho AL, Prinate AVM, et al. 2005. "Predictive factors for distant metastasis from oral and oropharyngeal squamous cell carcinoma." *Oral Oncol* 41: 534–541.
38. Gonzalez-Garcia R, Naval-Gias L, Roman-Romero L, et al. 2009. "Local recurrences and second primary tumors from squamous cell carcinoma of the oral cavity: A retrospective analytic study of 500 patients." *Head Neck* 31: 1168–1180.
39. Warren S, and Gates O. 1932. "Multiple primary malignant tumors. A survey of the literature and statistical study." *Am J Cancer* 16: 1358–1414.
40. Conley BA, and Ord RA. 1996. "Current status of retinoids in chemoprevention of oral squamous cell carcinoma: An overview." *J Craniomaxillofac Surg* 24: 339–345.
41. Lin DT, Subbaramaiah K, Shah JP, et al. 2002. "Cyclooxygenase-2: A novel molecular target for the prevention and treatment of head and neck cancer." *Head Neck* 24: 792–799.
42. Boyle JO. 2004. "Cyclooxygenase inhibition as a target for prevention of tobacco-related cancers." *Clinical Cancer Research* 10: 1557–1558.
43. Moraitis D, Du B, DeLorenzo MS, et al. 2005. "Levels of cyclooxygenase-2 are increased in the oral mucosa of smokers: Evidence for the role of epidermal growth factor receptor and its ligands." *Cancer Res* 65: 664–670.
44. http://www.cbc.ca/news/background/drugs/cox-2.html
45. Stell PM, and Jones TA. 1983. "Radical neck dissection: Preservation of function of the shoulder." *J Laryngol Otol* 8 (Suppl): 106–107.
46. Leipzig G, Suen JY, et al. 1983. "Functional evaluation of the spinal accessory nerve after neck dissection." *Am J Surg* 146: 526–530.
47. August M. 1997. "Complications associated with treatment of head and neck cancer." In: *Complications in Oral and Maxillofacial Surgery*, Pogrel MA, Perrott DH, and Kaban LB, eds., 179–192. Philadelphia: WB Saunders Co.
48. De Jong AA, and Manni JJ. 1991. "Phrenic nerve paralysis following neck dissection." *Eur Arch Otorhinolaryngol* 248: 132–134.
49. Belloso A, Saravanan K, de Carpentier J. 2006. "The community management of chylous fistula using a pancreatic lipase inhibitor (orlistat)." *Laryngoscope* 116: 1934–1935.
50. Valentine CN, Barresi RB, and Prinz RA. 2002. "Somatostatin analog treatment of a cervical thoracic duct fistula." *Head Neck* 24: 810–813.
51. Spiro JD, Spiro RH, and Strong EW. 1990. "The management of chyle fistula." *Laryngoscope* 100: 771–774.
52. De Gier HH, Balm AJ, Bruning PF, et al. 1996. "Systematic approach to the treatment of chylous leakage after neck dissection." *Head Neck* 18: 347–351.
53. Spiessl B, Prein J, and Schmoker R. 1976. "Anatomic reconstruction and functional rehabilitation of mandibular defects after ablative surgery." In: *New Concepts in Maxillofacial Bone Surgery*, Spiessl B, ed., 160–166. Berlin: Springer-Verlag.
54. Lavertu P, Wanamaker JR, Bold EL, et al. 1994. "The AO system for primary mandibular reconstruction." *Am J Surg* 168: 503–507.
55. Boyd JB, Morris S, Rosen IB, et al. 1994. "The through-and-through oromandibular defect: Rationale for aggressive reconstruction." *Plast Reconstr Surg* 93: 44–53.
56. Colletti DP, Ord R, and Liu X. 2009. "Mandibular reconstruction and second generation locking reconstruction plates: Outcome of 110 patients." *Int J Oral Maxillofac Surg* 38: 960–963.
57. Carlson ER, and Marx RE. 2006. "The ameloblastoma: Primary, curative surgical management." *J Oral Maxillofac Surg* 64: 484–494.
58. Carlson ER, August M, and Ruggiero S. 2004. "Locally aggressive benign processes of the oral and maxillofacial region." *Selected Readings in Oral and Maxillofacial Surgery* 12: 1–52.
59. Ramon Y, Mozes M, and Buchner A. 1964. "A fatal case of ameloblastoma (Adamantinoma)." *Br J Plast Surg* 17: 320–324.
60. Sugimura M, Yamauchi T, Yashikawa K, et al. 1969. "Malignant ameloblastoma with metastasis to the lumbar vertebra: Report of case." *J Oral Surg* 27: 350–357.
61. Clay RP, Weiland LH, and Jackson IT. 1989. "Ameloblastoma metastatic to the lung." *Ann Plast Surg* 22: 160–162.
62. Oka K, Fukui M, Yamashita M, et al. 1986. "Mandibular ameloblastoma with intracranial extension and distant metastasis." *Clin Neurol Neurosurg* 88: 303–309.
63. Newman L, Howells GL, Coghlan KM. 1995. "Malignant ameloblastoma revisited." *Br J Oral Maxillofac Surg* 33: 47–50.
64. Byrne MP, Kosmala RL, Cunningham MP. 1974. "Ameloblastoma with regional and distant metastases." *Am J Surg* 128: 91–94.
65. Laughlin EH. 1989. "Metastasizing ameloblastoma." *Cancer* 64: 776–780.
66. MacIntosh RB. 1991. "Aggressive management of ameloblastoma." *Oral Maxillofac Surg Clin N Am* 3: 73–97.
67. Gold L, and Williams TP. 2009. "Odontogenic tumors: Surgical pathology and management." In: *Oral and Maxillofacial Surgery*, 2nd ed., Fonseca R, Turvey T, and Marciani R, eds., 466–508. St. Louis: Elsevier.
68. Carlson ER, and Ord RA. 2008. *Textbook and Color Atlas of Salivary Gland Pathology. Diagnosis and Management*, 171–198. Ames, IA: Wiley-Blackwell.

69. Ghosh S, Panarese A, Bull PD, and Lee JA. 2003. "Marginally excised parotid pleomorphic adenomas: Risk factors for recurrence and management. A 12.5 year mean follow-up study of histologically marginal excisions." *Clin Otolaryngol* 28: 262–266.

70. Ishikawa T, Nomura M, Nagahata H, et al. 1986. "A new method of conserving the inferior alveolar nerve during resection of the mandible." *Br J Oral Maxillofac Surg* 24: 107–113.

71. Witt RL. 1999. "Facial nerve function after partial superficial parotidectomy: An 11 year review 1987–1997." *Otolaryngol Head Neck Surg* 121: 210–213.

72. Klintworth N, Zenk J, Koch M, and Iro H. 2010. "Postoperative complications after extracapsular dissection of benign parotid lesions with particular reference to facial nerve function." *Laryngoscope* 120(3): 484–490.

73. Ellingson TW, Cohen JI, and Andersen P. 2003. "The impact of malignant disease on facial nerve function after parotidectomy." *Laryngoscope* 113: 1299–1303.

12

Lip Cancer

Cole Anderson, DMD
Jonathan S. Bailey, DMD, MD, FACS

INTRODUCTION

Lip cancer comprises 30% of all head and neck malignancies and is second only to cutaneous malignancies.[1,2] The oral and maxillofacial surgeon (OMS) has a unique opportunity to participate in the diagnoses and management of these patients. General dental practitioners often identify premalignant and malignant lesions and have traditional referral pattern to their surgical colleagues and traditionally the OMS is greatly involved in the management of lip cancer.[3,4,5] While the prognosis for early stage lip cancer is generally good,[1] up to 20% of the patients can develop nodal metastasis. Those cancers with nodal metastasis are noted to be of larger size (greater than 2 cm) or higher histologic grade. Elective cervical lymphadenectomy can be justified for lip cancers that are very poorly differentiated or undifferentiated and for locally recurrent lip cancers when the initial tumor size is greater than 2 cm. High grade histologic tumors have been found to present with regional metastasis more frequently regardless of T stage.[6]

The incidence of lip cancer is approximately 10–12 cases per 100,000 persons in the United States,[2] and sun exposure is one of the most common risk factors. The Sun Belt region in the south and southwest of the United States has been identified as having a greater prevalence of lip cancer. Other risk factors include smoking, particularly cigar and pipe smoking.[7] Men represent 95% of all diagnosed cases[8] and this is presumed to be due to traditional gender roles such as labor activities in the sun. Additionally, women may decrease their risk due to the use of lipstick or lip coverage.[9] Generally, most patients are 53–66 years of age, likely due to a cumulative effect of chronic sun exposure. Squamous cell carcinoma is the most common histological variant reported at 90%,[10] melanoma, basal cell carcinoma, and minor salivary malignancies represent the minority of lesions.[8]

DIAGNOSIS/STAGING

Lip cancer lesions are typically diagnosed early given the fact that the lesion is in a conspicuous area, which prompts individuals to seek treatment. These lesions may present with a variety of clinical features. A persistent ulcerative wound on the vermilion, and endophytic or exophytic variants are typical (Figs. 12.1, 12.2, and 12.3). Early lesions can present as a limited leukoplakia to advanced lesions being obviously malignant, invading the adjacent anatomic structures. The lower lip is most often affected and accounts for 89% of lesions. The upper lip and oral commissure represent 7% and 4% of lesions, respectively (Figs. 12.4, 12.5, 12.6).

The American Joint Committee on Cancer has established the tumor, node, metastasis (TNM) classification for staging lip cancer, which is also used in staging of oral cancer[11,12] (Table 12.1). Seventy percent of

Management of Complications in Oral and Maxillofacial Surgery, First Edition. Edited by Michael Miloro, Antonia Kolokythas.
© 2012 John Wiley & Sons, Inc. Published 2012 by John Wiley & Sons, Inc.

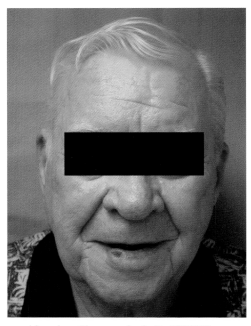

Fig. 12.1. Frontal view of an 84-year-old male with an endophytic T2N0M0 squamous cell carcinoma of the lower lip. (Miloro M. 2004. *Peterson's Principles in Oral and Maxillofacial Surgery*, 2nd ed., BC Decker Inc., Hamilton, Ontario, Canada.)

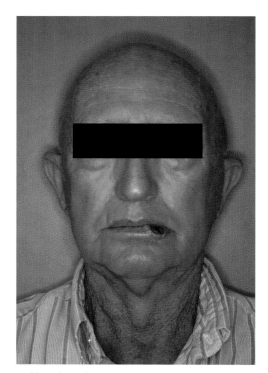

Fig. 12.2. Frontal view of a 76-year-old male with an exophytic T2N0M0 squamous cell carcinoma of the left lower lip. (Miloro M. 2004. *Peterson's Principles in Oral and Maxillofacial Surgery*, 2nd ed., BC Decker Inc., Hamilton, Ontario, Canada.)

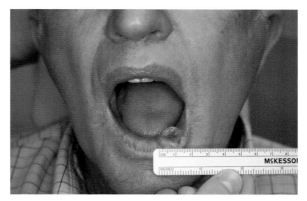

Fig. 12.3. Close-up view of the umbilicated exophytic T2 lesion. (Miloro M. 2004. *Peterson's Principles in Oral and Maxillofacial Surgery*, 2nd ed., BC Decker Inc., Hamilton, Ontario, Canada.)

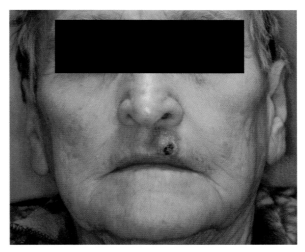

Fig. 12.4. Frontal view of a 73-year-old female with a T1N0M0 squamous cell carcinoma of the upper lip.

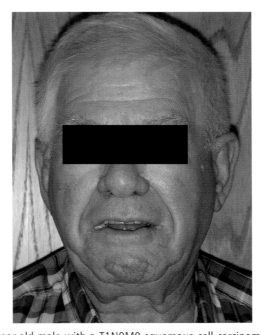

Fig. 12.5. Frontal view of a 78-year-old male with a T1N0M0 squamous cell carcinoma of the right oral commissure.

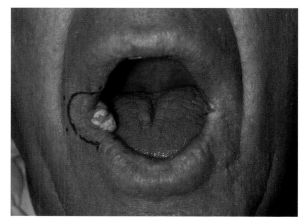

Fig. 12.6. Intraoral view of the right oral commissure squamous cell carcinoma.

Table 12.1. American Joint Committee on Cancer TNM (Tumor, Node, Metastasis) Classification

Primary Tumor (T)	
TX	Primary tumor cannot be assessed
T0	No evidence of primary tumor
Tis	Carcinoma *in situ*
T1	Tumor 2 cm or less in greatest dimension
T2	Tumor more than 2 cm but not more than 4 cm in greatest dimension
T3	Tumor more than 4 cm in greatest dimension
T4a	Moderately advanced local disease; superficial erosion alone of bone/tooth socket by gingival primary is not sufficient to classify a tumor as T4
	(Lip) Tumor invades through cortical bone, inferior alveolar nerve, floor of mouth, or skin of face, that is chin or nose
	(Oral cavity) Tumor invades adjacent structures only [e.g.. through cortical bone (mandible or maxilla) into deep extrinsic muscle of tongue (genioglossus, hyoglossus, palatoglossus, and styloglossus), maxillary sinus, skin of face]
T4b	Very advanced local disease
	Tumor invades masticator space, pterygoid plates, or skull base and/or encases internal carotid artery

Regional Lymph Nodes (N)	
NX	Regional lymph nodes cannot be assessed
N0	No regional lymph node metastasis
N1	Metastasis in a single ipsilateral lymph node, 3 cm or less in greatest dimension
N2	Metastasis in a single ipsilateral lymph node, more than 3 cm but not more than 6 cm in greatest dimension; or in multiple ipsilateral lymph nodes, none more than 6 cm in greatest dimension; or in bilateral or contralateral lymph nodes, none more than 6 cm in greatest dimension
N2a	Metastasis in single ipsilateral lymph node more than 3 cm but not more than 6 cm in greatest dimension
N2b	Metastasis in multiple ipsilateral lymph nodes, none more than 6 cm in greatest dimension
N2c	Metastasis in bilateral or contralateral lymph nodes, none more than 6 cm in greatest dimension
N3	Metastasis in a lymph node more than 6 cm in greatest dimension

Distant Metastasis (M)	
M0	No distant metastasis
M1	Distant metastasis

Table 12.1. *Continued*

Anatomic Stage/Prognostic Groups for Lip and Oral Cavity			
Stage 0	Tis	N0	M0
Stage I	T1	N0	M0
Stage II	T2	N0	M0
Stage III	T3	N0	M0
	T1	N1	M0
	T2	N1	M0
	T3	N1	M0
Stage IVA	T4a	N0	M0
	T4a	N1	M0
	T1	N2	M0
	T2	N2	M0
	T3	N2	M0
	T4a	N2	M0
Stage IVB	Any T	N3	M0
	T4b	Any N	M0
Stage IVC	Any T	Any N	M1

all lip cancers present as stage I while stages II, III, and IV comprise 16%, 10%, and 4%, respectively.[8] Diagnostic tools include a incisional biopsy, thorough history and clinical evaluation for cervical lymphadenopathy, and imaging of the neck most commonly via computed tomography (CT) with contrast or magnetic resonance imaging (MRI) when indicated.

The mainstay in treatment modalities for lip cancer is surgical excision[7,13] or radiation therapy. The surgical defect and the undesirable side effects of radiation contribute to the morbidity of treating lip cancer. Surgical margins for resection may vary with a 5-mm margin in lesions smaller than 10 mm in diameter and up to a 20-mm margin for larger lesions.[14,15,16] Preoperative planning of the anticipated surgical defect is paramount. Maintaining the facial aesthetics, speech, and oral competence are the pivotal reconstructive goals.

Many proposed techniques have been utilized for lip reconstruction following ablative surgery. Options include primary closure, local tissue rearrangement and microvascular free tissue transfer. A simple approach when considering reconstruction is to estimate the size of the defect. T1 lesions may be managed with a wedge resection and primary closure due to elasticity of the perioral tissue. Vermilionectomy should be included with the wedge resection when indicated. For larger defects that are one-third to two-thirds of the lip, horizontal advancement flaps may be employed. For defects greater than two-thirds of the lip, a number of differing local tissue rearrangement techniques have been proposed (e.g., nasolabial flaps and fan flaps),[17,18] (Figs. 12.7–12.12). Free flaps can also be employed for large defects [Figs. 12.13(a)–(e); Table 12.2). No matter which reconstructive option is utilized, many of the complications associated with the treatment of lip cancer revolve around the challenges to restore the premorbid function, anatomy, and aesthetics.

COMPLICATIONS ASSOCIATED WITH LIP RECONSTRUCTION

Wound Dehiscence

Wound dehiscence is a common complication related to lip cancer surgery. Compromised wound healing and dehiscence of the reconstruction are the cause of these complications. This can be attributed to two main issues: limitations of the chosen reconstructive option and comorbid health conditions.

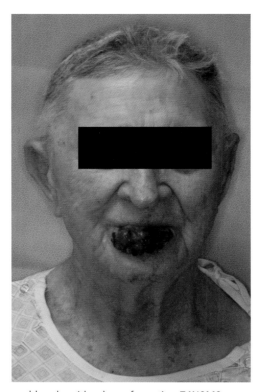

Fig. 12.7. Frontal view of an 86-year-old male with a large fungating T4N0M0 squamous cell carcinoma of the lower lip.

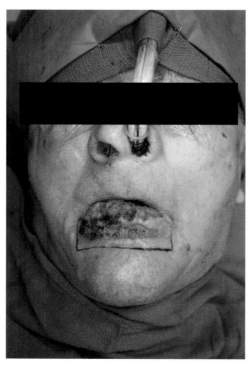

Fig. 12.8. Intraoperative view demonstrating planned excision margins.

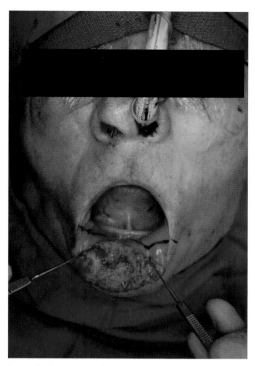

Fig. 12.9. Intraoperative intraoral view of planned excision margins.

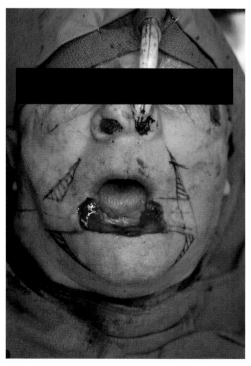

Fig. 12.10. Intraoperative view of defect and planned reconstruction with Bernard flaps.

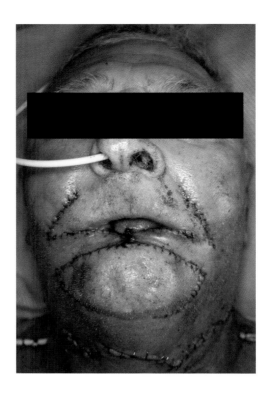

Fig. 12.11. Immediate postoperative view of the lower lip reconstruction using the Bernard's flaps technique. Note the wound tension and venous congestion.

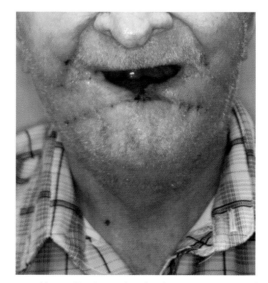

Fig. 12.12. Dehiscence of a reconstructed lower lip. Secondary healing is occurring at the midline where the wound margins have broken down.

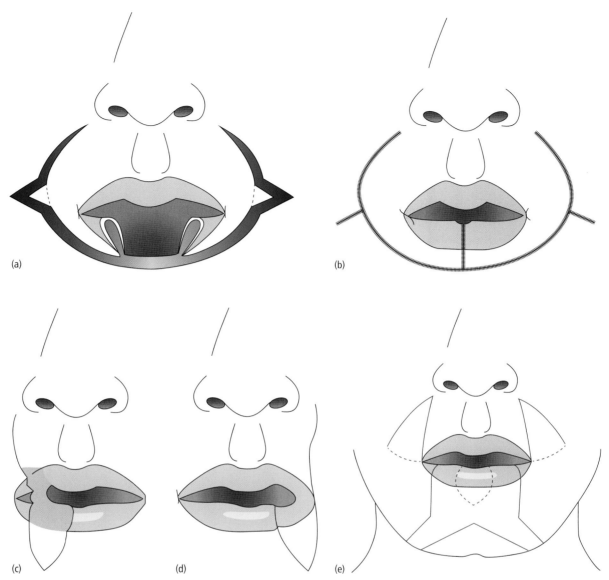

Fig. 12.13. Intraoperative view of planned resection and reconstruction with the Karapandzic Flaps. (a), (b). The figure presents the Karapandzic flap reconstruction technique for excision of a lower lip lesion that comprises greater than one-third of the lower lip. (c) The two-staged Abbé flap. The opposing vermillion is interpolated to the opposing lip. Approximately 3 weeks following the initial procedure, the pedicle is divided and primary closure of the harvest site and reconstruction site occurs. (d) The Estlander flap with advancement of the upper lip to the defect of the lower lip. Note the rounding of the commissure. (e) The Bernard flap is useful for reconstruction of defects that comprise nearly the entirety of the lip. (Edge SE, Byrd DR, Compton CC, eds. 2010. *AJCC Cancer Staging Manual*, 7th ed. New York, NY: Springer.)

Table 12.2. Lip Reconstruction Techniques

V Excision
Vermilionectomy with mucosal advancement
V-Y mucosal advancement flaps
Tongue flap
Transpositional flaps
Abbé–Estlander flap
Karapandzic flap
Bernard flap
Stair step flap
Circumoral advancement flaps
Cheek advancement flap
Gillies fan flaps
McGregor flaps
Microvascular free flap

Table 12.3. Wound Care

Debridement of necrotic tissue
Keep wound moist
Wet to wet dressings
Pack dead space
Control oral secretions
Treat infections
Protect from mechanical injury
Optimize nutritional and medical status

A common contributor of wound break down is marginal ischemia as a result of tension (Fig. 12.11). Reconstructing the perioral anatomy is influenced by functional limits, such as the desired dimensions of the stoma and available tissue. If the flap design does not provide for a tension-free closure or if the pedicled flap is not passive, tissue ischemia and wound dehiscence may occur. The microenvironment of the acute surgical wound inherently has reduced oxygenation of the tissues from a direct surgical disruption of the blood supply. Tension created by rearrangement of local tissue can further compromise the vascular supply. Initial signs of tissue ischemia include venous congestion with tissue edema, suggestive of venous insufficiency (Fig. 12.12). Other signs include poor capillary refill and pale color of the tissue that indicate arterial compromise.

Many patients who suffer from lip cancer have comorbidities that may compromise the success of the reconstruction. Common conditions include metabolic conditions (diabetes and renal failure), respiratory [chronic obstructive pulmonary disease (COPD)] or cardiovascular [congestive heart failure (CHF)] disease, immunosuppression, and/or malnutrition. Optimization of these medical conditions can increase success of treatment and reduce the risk of poor wound healing and breakdown of the reconstructed wounds. Preoperative consultation with the primary care physician to optimize these conditions may be indicated.

Due to the robust vascularity of the head and neck, most wound problems are somewhat limited. Management usually includes simple wound care and minimal debridement. Other interventions include identification and treatment of infection, dressings to absorb excessive exudates and maintain open and clean wound margins (Table 12.3).[19]

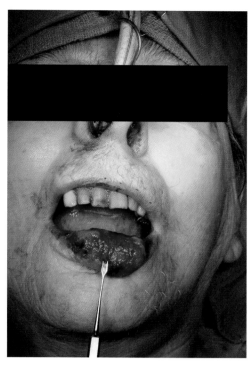

Fig. 12.14. Intraoperative view of an 82-year-old female with a rapidly growing T3N0M0 squamous cell carcinoma of the lower lip.

Hyperbaric oxygen (HBO) therapy has been utilized to improve wound healing. Many studies have demonstrated that HBO therapy has been very successful in the salvage of flaps in situations of hypoxia and decreased perfusion. HBO maximizes tissue viability reducing the need for repeat procedures.[20,21] This is due to the physiologic effects of HBO that include control of infection by the potentiation of neutrophils' ability to kill bacteria, angiogenesis to improve oxygenation of ischemic tissue, and epithelial migration of the wound edge.[22]

Microstomia

Large T3 and T4 lip cancers that require surgical excision present a difficult reconstructive challenge to avoid microstomia. Microstomia may result in speech articulation errors, loss of oral competence, difficulties with oral intake, and for patients with removable dental prosthesis, the inability to use their prosthesis (Figs. 12.14–12.17).[23]

For example, following the Karapandzic flap technique for lip reconstruction, up to 24% of patients require surgical revision for microstomia.[24] Several revision techniques, variations of commissuroplasty, to increase the size of the oral stoma can be employed. Regardless of the technique used, reconstruction of the oral sphincter is essential. Oral competence and control of secretions depend on the restoration of this anatomic feature.[25]

A nonsurgical option for managing microstomia is the use of a graduated lip expander or semidynamic acrylic splints. Consultation with a maxillofacial prosthodontist would be essential in designing the expander appropriately. The device is designed with two opposing arms that are placed at each of the oral commissures and an expanding mechanism is at midline to incrementally increase the oral stoma over a number of weeks to achieve a greater opening. A combination of commissuroplasty and tissue-expanding therapy can optimize the correction of microstomia and reduce relapse.[26]

Consultation with a speech pathology therapist directed toward swallowing, speech articulation, and intelligibility may also be helpful.[27]

Poor tolerance for use of removable dental prosthesis is another associated complication related to microstomia, as mentioned earlier. The patient with microstomia can find it very challenging to insert and

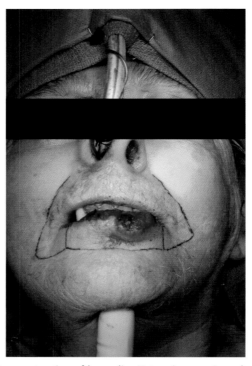

Fig. 12.15. Intraoperative view of reconstruction of lower lip. Note microstomia and potential trauma to lower lip due to the presence of the remaining dentition.

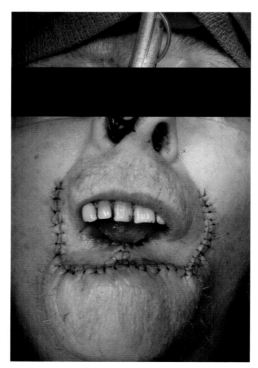

Fig. 12.16. Contracture and thinning of the lower lip status post (s/p) resection and reconstruction of advanced lower lip cancer.

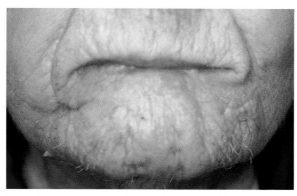

Fig. 12.17. Profile view of patient with contracture and inward rotation of lower lip.

remove the prosthesis through a small oral stoma. Furthermore, loss of the normal oral vestibule, in cases of vermilionectomy when mucosa advancement is used for reconstruction, retention of a complete denture may be compromised. This is more problematic for patients with significant mandibular alveolar ridge resorption and shallow vestibules. A possible alternative to labial mucosa advancement for reconstruction of the vermilion in these cases is a tongue flap, as it allows for preservation of the labial vestibule depth.

Prosthetic dental rehabilitation of the lip cancer patient may require the assistance of a maxillofacial prosthodontic specialist. Sectional impression techniques may be required and have been utilized in patients with microstomia for denture fabrication. Flexible dentures have also been used for delivery into and out of the small stoma. These methods use a number of segments of impressions that can be passed through the stoma and later assembled to create the prosthesis.[28,29]

Patients with advanced stage lip cancer often require postoperative radiation therapy. Xerostomia in conjunction with microstomia creates a difficult problem in providing dental care. The development of chronic periodontal disease, dental caries, and dental abscesses are real and significant problems for these patients.[30] Lip cancer patients at stages T3 and T4 may require dental extractions at the time of the ablative surgery to limit radiation caries, the need for future extractions, and the potential risk for osteoradionecrosis. Additionally, the presence of the anterior mandibular teeth needs to be considered when planning the reconstruction of the lower lip since some flaps (such as tongue flaps) may not be possible to utilize without modifications.

Neurologic Injury

Ablative surgery for lip cancer can result in altered sensation to the lower lip and chin. The mental nerve branch of the inferior alveolar nerve supplies sensation of the lower lip and chin. Injury to this nerve can result in paresthesia, which is abnormal sensation often characterized as decreased sensation, or dysesthesia, which is abnormal painful sensation. Patients with decreased sensation often accommodate well without a significant impact on their quality of life. However, patients with neuropathic pain have a significant impact on their quality of life and may require medical treatment with a neurologist. There are a number of pharmacological agents to treat nerve pain that include carbamezepine, oxcarbazepine, baclofen, lamotrigine, pimozide, gabapentin, and phenytoin. Neurology consultation is also useful in long-term management.[31]

Scarring and Poor Cosmetic Outcome

There are a number of notable unfavorable outcomes related to the aesthetic aspect of reconstruction. Scarring, asymmetry, unbalanced facial proportions, inconsistent tissue color and texture, and discontinuity of the defined anatomy of the lips are some of the related complications.

Contracture of the lower or upper lip can result in thinning of the lips (Fig. 12.17). Vermilion reconstruction is most often reconstructed with mucosal advancement flaps. The vermilion is a

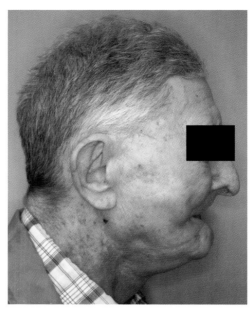

Fig. 12.18. Patient with lip inversion and shaving irritation.

modified mucosal tissue and thus oral mucosa presents as a good alternative for reconstruction. Mucosal advancement may result in thinning of the visible vermilion and inward rotation of the lip. The latter in male patients can cause irritation of the upper lip from the facial hair of the lower lip. Shaving may also be more troublesome for these patients (Fig. 12.18). Although this may represent a minor complication, patients will often note this change. At the time of reconstruction, generous dissection of the mucosal flap to the depth of the vestibule to allow for adequate advancement may improve the outcome.[31,32]

Appropriate preoperative planning for flap reconstruction is also imperative to maximize the cosmetic outcome. Placing incisions in the relaxed skin tension lines and natural skin creases such as nasolabial, labiomandibular, submental, melolabial, and rhytids of the lips will aid in hiding incisions for improved aesthetic outcomes.[33,34]

COMPLICATIONS RELATED TO RADIATION THERAPY

Radiotherapy is used either as an adjunct to surgery for advanced lip cancers or as a primary modality for treatment of small lesions. The common problems encountered with use of radiotherapy in the head and neck, such as dermatitis, mucositis, poor wound healing, and poor saliva production, will occur when treating for lip cancer. Symptomatic management of mucositis during treatments, and fundamental principles of wound care post surgery should be used as indicated. Long-term management of the fragile radiated facial skin in the chin, lip area (or neck if included in fields of radiation) is based on prevention of further injury. Skin protection from environmental elements includes relief from cold, wind, and sunlight that along with meticulous hygiene may minimize problems.[35]

The complications related to mucositis are based on the ability to eat and swallow. For minor symptoms, sialogogues, oral hydration, and palliative oral rinses (i.e., viscous lidocaine and sedative medicaments) can be beneficial. If symptoms become so severe that the patient is unable obtain adequate oral intake, consideration should be given to provide nutritional support via feeding tubes that bypass the oral cavity. Encouragement to return to oral intake and swallowing, though, is paramount to preventing long-term swallowing difficulties from the radiation. Poor nutrition compounds the healing ability related to radiation therapy and may result in wound breakdown and associated sequelae.

CONCLUSIONS

In summary, the surgical treatment of lip cancer can be a challenging and rewarding aspect in the practice of oral and maxillofacial surgery. The treating surgeon and patient can often be hopeful of an optimistic outcome. However, potential complications may result in a significant alteration on the patient's quality of life. It is incumbent upon the surgeon to proactively identify and navigate the potential complications that can arise with treating lip cancer. Adherence to the fundamental principles of surgery is essential in minimizing complications. Accurate diagnosis, planning, appropriate medical management, and meticulous surgical technique are at the center of successful management of the lip cancer patient.

SUGGESTED READINGS

1. Hoffman HT, Karnel LH, Funk GF, et al. 1998. "The national cancer data base report on cancer of the head and neck." *Archives of Otolaryngology Head and Neck Surgery* 124: 951–962.
2. Moore S, Johnson N, Pierce A, et al. 1999. "The epidemiology of lip cancer: A review of global incidence and aetiology." *Oral Diseases* 5(3): 185–195.
3. Kaugars GE, Aggey LM, Page DG, et al. 1999. "Prevention and detection of lip cancer—the dentist's role. *Journal of the California Dental Association* 27(4): 318–323.
4. Awde JD, Kogon SL, and Morin RJ. 1996. "Lip cancer: A review." *Journal of the Canadian Dental Association* 62(8): 634–636.
5. Kademani D, Bell B, Schmidt B, et al. 2008. "Oral and maxillofacial surgeons treating oral cancer: A preliminary report from the American Association of Oral and Maxillofacial Surgeons Task Force on Oral Cancer." *Journal of Oral and Maxillofacial Surgery* 66: 2151–2157.
6. Zitsch RP, Lee BW, Smith RB. 1999. "Cervical lymph node metastases and squamous cell carcinoma of the lip." *Head Neck: Journal for the Sciences & Specialties of the Head and Neck* 21(5): 447–453.
7. De Vissher JGAM, van den Elsaker K, Grond AJK, et al. 1998. "Surgical treatment of squamous cell carcinoma of the lower lip: Evaluation of long-term results and prognostic factors—A retrospective analysis of 184 patients." *Journal of Oral and Maxillofacial Surgery* 56: 814.
8. Shah J. 2003. "The lips." In: *Head and Neck, Surgery and Oncology*, 3rd ed., 149–172. Edinburgh: Mosby.
9. Pogoda J, and Preston-Martin S. 1996. "Solar radiation, lip protection, and lip cancer in Los Angeles County women (California, United States)." *Cancer Causes and Control* 7: 458–463.
10. Chen J, Katz RV, Krutchkoff DJ, et al. 1992. "Lip cancer, incidence trends in Connecticut, 1935–1985. *Cancer* 70: 2025.
11. Lipincott JB. 1992. *American Joint Committee on Cancer: Manual for Staging of Cancer*, 4th ed. Philadelphia: Saunders Elsevier.
12. Larson D. 2006. "Tumors of the lips, oral cavity, and oropharynx." In: *Plastic Surgery*, Vol. V, 2nd ed., Mathes S, ed., 159–167. Philadlephia: Saunders Elsevier.
13. Hasson O. 2008. "Squamous cell carcionma of the lower lip." *Journal of Oral and Maxillofacial Surgery* 66: 1259–1262.
14. Cruse CW, and Radocha RF. 1987. "Squamous cell carcinoma of the lip." *Plastic and Reconstructive Surgery* 80: 787–791.
15. Brodland DG, and Zitelli JA. 1992. "Surgical margins for excision of primary cutaneous squamous cell carcinoma." *Journal of the American Academy of Dermatology* 27: 241–248.
16. Sikes JW, and Ghali GE. 2004. "Lip cancer." In: *Peterson's Principles of Oral and Maxillofacial Surgery*, Vol. 1, 2nd ed., Miloro M, ed., 559–570. Hamilton: BC Decker Inc.
17. Ord RA, and Pazoki AE. 2003. "Flap designs for lower lip reconstruction." *Oral Maxillofacial Surgery Clinics of North America* 15: 497–511.
18. Calhoun KH. 1992. "Reconstruction of small-medium sized defects of the lower lip." *American Journal of Otolaryngology* 13(1): 16–22.
19. Hom DB, and Dresner H. 2009. "General approach to a poorly healing problem wound: Practical and clinical overview." In: *Essential Tissue Healing of the Face and Neck*, Hom DB, et al., eds., 293–305. Shelton, CT: PMPH USA.
20. Zamboni WA, and Shah HR. 2003. "Skin grafts and flaps (compromised)." In: *Hyperbaric Oxygen 2003, Indications and Results: The Hyperbaric Oxygen Therapy Committee Report*," 101–107. Kensington, MD: Undersea and Hyperbaric Medical Society.
21. Tibbles PM, and Edelsberg JS. 1996. "Hyperbaric oxygen therapy." *New England Journal of Medicine* 334: 1642–1648.
22. Feldmeier JJ. 2009. "Hyperbaric oxygen and wound healing in the head and neck." In: *Essential Tissue Healing of the Face and Neck*, Hom DB, et al., eds., 367–378. Shelton, CT: PMPH USA.
23. Neligan PC. 2009. "Strategies in lip reconstruction." *Clinical Plastic Surgery*, 36(3): 477–485.
24. Karapandzic M. 1974. "Reconstruction of lip defects by local arterial flaps." *British Journal of Plastic Surgery* 27: 93.
25. Luce EA. 1995. "Reconstruction of the lower lip." *Clinical Plastic Surgery* 22(1): 109–121.
26. Koymen R, Gulses A, Karacayli U, et al. 2009. "Treatment of microstomia with commissuroplasties and semidynamic acrylic splints." *Oral Surgery, Oral Medicine, Oral Pathology, Oral Radiology, Endodontology* 107(4): 503–507.
27. Clayton NA, Ledgard JP, Haertsch PA, et al. 2009. "Rehabilitation of speech and swallowing after burns reconstructive surgery of the lips and nose." *Journal of Burn Care and Research* 30(6): 1039–1045.

28. Prithviraj DR, Ramaswamy S, and Romesh S. 2009. "Prosthetic rehabilitation of patients with microstomia." *Indian Journal of Dental Research* 20(4): 483–486.

29. Givan DA, Auclair WA, Seidenfaden JC, et al. 2010. "Sectional impressions and simplified folding complete denture for sever microstomia." *J Prosthodont* 19(4): 299–302.

30. Nussbaum BL. 2009. "Dental care for patients who are unable to open their mouths." *Dental Clinics of North America* 53(2): 323–328.

31. Gronseth G, Cruccu G, Alksne J, et al. 2008. "Practice parameter: The diagnostic evaluation and treatment of trigeminal neuralgia (an evidence-based review): Report of the Quality Standards Subcommittee of the American Academy of Neurology and the European Federation of Neurological Societies." *Neurology* 71(15): 1183–1190.

32. Sanchez-Conejo-Mir J, Perez Bernal AM, Moreno-Giminez JC, et al. 1986. "Follow-up of vermilionectomies: Evaluation of the technique." *Journal of Dermatologic Surgery and Oncology* 12(2): 180–184.

33. Renner GJ. 2007. "Reconstruction of the lip." In: *Local Flaps in Facial Reconstruction*, 2nd ed., Baker SR, ed., 475–524. St. Louis: Mosby.

34. Dupin C, Metzinger S, and Rizzuto R. 2004. "Lip reconstruction after ablation for skin malignancies." *Clinical Plastic Surgery* 31(1): 69–85.

35. Hom DB, Ho V, and Lee C. 2009. "Irradiated skin and its postsurgical management." In: *Essential Tissue Healing of the Face and Neck*, Hom DB, et al., eds., 224–238. Shelton, CT: PMPH USA.

13

Hard Tissue Reconstruction

Miller Smith, DDS, MD
Fayette Williams, DDS, MD
Brent B. Ward, DDS, MD, FACS

INTRODUCTION

Successful bone continuity restoration is the basis for the success of the majority of reconstructive surgery procedures in the oral maxillofacial skeleton. There are a number of preoperative, intraoperative and postoperative considerations the surgeon must be aware of with the use of bone grafts (transfer of free cancellous, cortical, or corticocancellous bone without a blood supply), bone flaps (bone pedicled or transferred free with its own vascular system), or bone substitutes (growth factors, allogeneic, alloplastic, and xenogenic materials). Knowing the potential risks and complications with each method can provide effective informed consent and allow measures for quality control. Ultimately surgeons must provide the best possible care to the patients by minimizing known risks and complications, and having a clear understanding of their effective management.

CONTRIBUTORY PATIENT FACTORS IN COMPLICATIONS

Preoperative Comorbidity

Primary reconstruction with nonvascularized bone graft at the time of pathological resection or during trauma reconstruction, although ideal, is not always undertaken for several reasons. Occasionally the added time or blood loss from harvesting the graft may be limiting factors in certain patients. Bone graft harvesting may be associated with increased risk of surgical site blood loss perioperatively and in the postoperative period that can cause adverse patient outcomes. Risks from significant blood loss especially in older or medically compromised patients include perioperative or postoperative cardiopulmonary complications such as myocardial infarction or cardiac arrhythmias, or even neurologic sequelae, such as stroke. In addition, blood transfusions harbor the risk of several adverse reactions that may even be life threatening, while aggressive crystalloid or colloid resuscitation may add to cardiopulmonary system's stress. Intraoperative hemostasis is essential for minimizing these risks. A complete medical history including cardiopulmonary history and functional status in the preoperative period can provide accurate risk assessment and determine if any additional evaluation is necessary.[1–5] While most grafting procedures are low risk in their overall morbidity and mortality, the frail, the elderly, and the medically unfit should all be carefully evaluated and optimized preoperatively to ensure a safe treatment can be performed with minimal adverse effects. This is especially true in cases of elective reconstructive procedures that can be delayed for a period of time to maximize patient health. In cases of more urgent surgery, preoperative evaluation and discussion of risks

Management of Complications in Oral and Maxillofacial Surgery, First Edition. Edited by Michael Miloro, Antonia Kolokythas.
© 2012 John Wiley & Sons, Inc. Published 2012 by John Wiley & Sons, Inc.

with both the patient and anesthesiologist can allow for appropriate care and avoidance of adverse outcomes.

Risks of Blood Transfusion

With many maxillofacial surgical procedures, and especially those requiring bone reconstruction, there may be need for blood transfusion in the perioperative period. In the past, patients were transfused more liberally in an attempt to minimize major cardiopulmonary complications; however, good supportive evidence for this practice did not exist. It is well known that numerous risks exist with the transfusion of blood products including: disease transmission, systemic inflammatory response syndrome (SIRS), wound infection, sepsis, pneumonia, acute lung injury (TRALI), acute respiratory distress syndrome (ARDS), extended length of hospitalization, and increased post-transfusion complications.[6–10] Some additionally have cited that there may exist an immunomodulation effect on the host that may increase the risk of cancer recurrence, though it is impossible to define the precise risk involved.[11–27] Currently it is accepted that transfusions do offer some beneficial actions with improved oxygen delivery; however, this should be limited to use primarily in symptomatic patients with hemoglobin levels below 7 gm/dl. There is significant controversy on acceptable transfusion guidelines for cardiovascular and cerebrovascular compromised patients based on overall risk. While some suggest hemoglobin levels between 8 and 10 gm/dl can be tolerated by these patients, others believe transfusions at these levels are acceptable to prevent adverse outcomes.[6,7] Excess blood loss and/or the need for transfusions prolong postoperative recovery with risks associated with increased hospitalization (pneumonia, hematoma, wound infection and breakdown, thromboembolism) among others.[28]

Meticulous hemostasis to the soft tissues from the donor site, along with use of adjunctive agents can effectively minimize procedural and postoperative blood loss. Medullary bleeding has often been minimized with the use of bone wax applied directly on the exposed cancellous marrow. There have been reports of granulomas at the site of bone wax use as well as possible delayed infections[29–37] The use of other hemostatics such as oxidized cellulose (Surgicel® Ethicon, www.ethicon.com) can prove beneficial, but are also known to cause nerve paresthesias when applied directly on or in immediate vicinity to nerves.[38–41] Newer resorbable wax substitutes are also available for use (Ostene®, Ceremed, www.ostene.com).

There has been interest in utilizing perioperative erythropoietin in cases where patients are anemic preoperatively or significant blood loss is anticipated to minimize the risk of blood transfusions.[25,42] This is especially true for patients whose religious beliefs prevent them from receiving autologous blood transfusions.[43,44] Further trials are necessary to demonstrate a reliable cost-benefit for erythropoietin use in elective surgery with minimal to moderate risk. Most recently, the use of hemoglobin-based oxygen-carrying substitutes is being explored. Their benefits include a prolonged shelf life, decreased immunogenic potential, lack of risk for disease transmission, and a potential for greater oxygen carrying capacity.[45] Continued investigation will be necessary to delineate the benefit of these products.

Nutritional Status Issues

Nutritional status is becoming an important determinant of overall success during bone reconstruction procedures. Patients presenting with malnutrition must be identified preoperatively through clinical assessment and appropriate serum laboratory testing. Some studies have noted that 20% to 67% of head and neck cancer patients (many of whom may require bone reconstruction procedures with the use of free tissue transfers) are malnourished based on a number of variables at the time of surgical intervention.[46] Patients with a recent weight loss of greater than 10% prior to surgery are prone to major postoperative complications including wound infection, fistula, respiratory complications, myocardial injury, and even progression to sepsis.[46,47] Albumin, prealbumin, preoperative CRP levels, and BMI have all been described as useful determinants of outcome.[48–52] Those patients with low albumin and prealbumin are more likely to proceed with slower postoperative recovery and delayed soft and hard tissue healing; however, these markers can be affected by renal and hepatic dysfunction as well as acute inflammation and should be used in the context of the patients overall status.[53–56] Conversely, providing patients with protein nutrition preoperatively can decrease hospital stay and improve bone healing as evidenced in the general surgery and orthopedic populations.[57,58] In the postoperative setting, many bone graft and bone flap procedures require intraoral incisions. There is substantial debate and no consensus regarding the use of oral rest postoperatively. Patients do require adequate nutrition for wound healing. It is well documented that early nutrition in the postoperative period equates to better patient outcomes, which is especially true of larger flap reconstructions in a critical care setting.[59,60] In any circumstance, four options are available. First, a period of oral rest for up to a week is sometimes advocated for gastrointestinal procedures but has never openly been advocated for maxillofacial surgery wound healing. It is generally felt that particulate food can harbor bacteria and predispose to infection and wound breakdown if it is not being cleared adequately. For large reconstructions or difficult wounds, enteral feeding tubes may offer the benefit of nutrition by bypassing the oral wound. While the oral tissues are rested, the patient can still achieve appropriate nutritional support. Complications from nasogastric tube placement have been reported, including intracranial placement in trauma patients, intrapulmonary feeding, tracheoesophageal fistula, sinusitis, diarrhea from dumping syndrome, and gastric ulcerations among other problems. For certain cancer reconstructions, a prolonged oral rehabilitation may be encountered and selected patients may benefit from a percutaneous or open gastrostomy tube. Major complications may include peritoneal placement, colon or intestinal perforation, peristomal infection and granulation, and other feed-related problems.[61–64] Some have felt that parenteral nutrition has its advantages in specific populations, but it is associated with a higher rate of sepsis and intestinal atrophy, most notably in a critical care setting.[59,62,65]

Effects of Diabetes Mellitus and the Use of Corticosteroids

Poorly controlled diabetes mellitus as well as perioperative corticosteroid use are shown to decrease bone and tissue healing. High glucose concentrations, as well as prolonged corticosteroid use, inhibit collagen cross-linking, which is necessary for proper bone and soft tissue healing.[66] Additional inhibitive properties on angiogenesis, macrophage and neutrophil chemotaxis, migration, and phagocytosis are also exhibited.[67–69] Bone healing is impaired with alterations in osteoblastic and osteoclastic function as well as vascular ingrowth and remodeling.[69–75] Poor glucose control is a known risk factor for bone graft site dehiscence and subsequent failure.[76] Glucocorticoid therapy is commonly used in the perioperative period with minimal effect on wound healing and infection rates when given over short courses, and without excess dosing. Prolonged corticosteroid use, though, inhibits collagen synthesis and cross-linking, decreases osteoblast and osteoclast differentiation and function, and thus impacts healing.[77–80]

Nicotine Effects

Nicotine has been shown to have substantial effects on the vascularity of all tissues. By eliciting microvascular vasoconstriction, promoting hypercoagulation with increased fibrinogen levels and platelet aggregation, and creating volatile agents and free radicals, an inflammatory environment is produced that limits healing. Even in low doses, nicotine has been shown to have deleterious effects on bone healing with suppression of pro-osteogenic bone morphogenetic proteins.[81–83] Smoking should optimally be stopped well in advance of elective bone reconstructive procedures to maximize bone regenerative capacity. Smoking during the postoperative healing phase has been shown to be detrimental to bone graft survival,[84–86] and smokers may have twice the rate of complications as nonsmokers in monocortical onlay grafts.[87]

The Influence of Active Infections

In rare circumstances, patients may have an underlying infection or severe inflammation to the recipient bed or at the donor site. It is imperative that formal infections be properly evaluated clinically prior to proceeding with any grafting procedure as risks for potential failure or adverse outcomes increase.[88] A vascularized flap does offer some protection to mild inflammation at the recipient site; however, prudence is imperative to minimize graft loss and failure. Appropriate patient selection is essential and use of reconstructive procedures in infected sites is best avoided when possible.

DONOR BONE SELECTION CONSIDERATIONS

Autogenous Bone Grafts

Autogenous bone is the current gold standard of hard tissue transfer, and both bone grafts and bone flaps can be utilized to reconstruct ablative, traumatic, infective, and congenital defects. Autogenous grafts carry some viable cells but require ingrowth of adjacent vascular supply (primarily from periosteum and adjacent marrow) to promote successful healing and integration to the native bone. Data suggest that defect shape and size will determine appropriate reconstructive options, as volume and quality of necessary bone can determine the appropriate donor site. Segmental defects of the mandible are among the largest and most difficult grafting procedures performed in the maxillofacial region due to geometry, chin projection, and curved shape. Complications are commonly related to infection, dehiscence, or nonunion. Postoperative wound dehiscence is the most common complication that can result in loss of a portion or all of the graft.[89–92] While infection among both vascularized and nonvascularized groups range between 8% and 10%, overall complication rates for nonvascularized bone grafts may be as high as 69%. In a retrospective review of 47 maxillary reconstructions, Smolka and Lizuka[93] compared the outcomes and complications of nonvascularized bone grafts, microvascular soft tissue flaps combined with free bone grafts, and composite osteocutaneous microvascular flaps. Postoperative infection occurred in over half the cases of free bone grafts wrapped in vascularized soft tissue, while only 8% of osteocutaneous free flaps developed infection. Complete graft loss was noted in 25% and 16% of free bone grafts and osteocutaneous free flaps, respectively, mainly due to infection. Other complications included wound dehiscence and oroantral/oronasal fistula. One of the largest series of nonvascularized iliac crest bone grafts for segmental mandibular defects in 74 patients was reviewed by van Gemert et al.[94] While 76% of patients ultimately had a successful outcome, 43% of patients had postoperative complications. These complications were significantly associated with the site of the defect and the presence of intraoral communication. The authors concluded that nonvascularized iliac bone grafts for the mandible are best used for lateral defects and only with an extraoral approach. Pogrel has published that segmental mandibular defects less than 6 cm portray only a 20–25% complication rate with use of nonvascularized cortical grafts. When grafts greater than 6 cm are used the risk of failure increases significantly. Although a successful bony union rate of 40% was demonstrated for defects up to 14 cm, vascularized bone offers a more predictable and viable option and should be considered when possible.[95,96] A determination of morbidity based on defect characteristics (including presence of soft tissue coverage), donor site risk, and procedural length must be weighed for defects between 4 and 7 cm. Use of vascularized bone should be limited for defects under 4 cm due to established success with nonvascularized bone, unless a substantial amount of soft tissue is necessary.

For maxillary sinus grafts, postoperative complications are generally related to infection. When a sinus graft is jeopardized by infection, complete removal and healing for 6 weeks may be required to eliminate infection before regrafting.[97] Hematomas in the sinus cavity can occur due to the difficulty in controlling bone bleeding.[98] Patients with a preoperative history of sinusitis have a higher incidence of postoperative complications after sinus augmentation procedures including infections, dehiscence, and development of oralantral fistulas.[99,100] Soft tissue coverage for bone grafting is occasionally necessary and an assessment of appropriate coverage must be made prior to undertaking surgery. While locoregional flaps may be used for soft tissue coverage, they must be accounted for during the initial plan to allow for proper consent for the patient, given the known risks of each soft tissue coverage flap [random pattern mucosal finger flap, facial artery myomucosal (FAMM) flap, palatal rotation flap, anterior- and posterior-based tongue flap, buccal fat pad, temporoparietal galeal flap, superiorly based platysma flap, submental island flap, pectoralis major pedicled flap]. Microvascular soft tissue flaps can be used for coverage with known risks and complications of each flap.

Risks of Allografts and Xenografts

Allografts and xenografts have increasing use given their availability, low cost, lack of donor site morbidity, and sterile shelf-life. Many options are available for use with particulate cancellous, particulate cortical, and corticocancellous sheets being available. There have been some concerns with the risk of disease transmission, but with proper screening procedures and appropriate sterility assurance levels (below 10^{-6}), the chance of organism transmission overall is 1:1 million. Estimations for specific transmission such as HIV range between 1:1.6 million and 1:8 million and substantially lower when using demineralized formulations.[101–104] There are a multitude of techniques used to disinfect and sterilize off-the-shelf graft materials. These include physical debridement, ultrasonic washes, antimicrobial therapy, ethanol soaking, ethylene oxide, electron beam irradiation, and gamma irradiation. Based on the type of bone graft and the techniques employed by the distributer, a combination of these are used while trying to maintain beneficial properties of the graft.[102–104] Xenografts have their own concerns due to recent media concern over prion transmission and bovine spongiform encephalopathy. While no reports for transmission have occurred in the maxillofacial literature, a theoretical estimated risk has been calculated by groups, based on purification techniques. A worst-case scenario has listed the risk on the order of 1 in $10^{10.3}$ correlating to a virtually nonexistent transmission risk based on preparation and animal selection processes.[105,106]

Bone Morphogenetic Proteins

Recombinant bone morphogenetic protein-2 (rhBMP-2) has shown some promise for bony reconstruction, although the indications are still not completely defined at present. Perhaps the most concerning postoperative sequela associated with this treatment relates to the impressive swelling, which ensues after placement of the graft. The use of rhBMP-2 in cervical spine reconstruction has been associated with significant neck swelling and dysphagia in up to 27% of patients, sometimes resulting in prolonged hospital stay or readmission.[107,108] While the relevance for maxillofacial reconstruction is difficult to ascertain, similar concerns have been raised in the use of rhBMP-2 for segmental mandibular defects.[109] Another phenomenon unique to rhBMP-2 is ectopic bone formation.[110,111] This is likely due to intraoperative spilling of the reconstituted solution onto the surgical field around the defect being treated. The most serious consequence of ectopic bone would be ankylosis of the temoporomandibular joint if used around the condyle but to date this problem has not been reported.

Reconstruction of mandibular continuity defects using rhBMP-2 is currently being explored, although only small case series exist at this time. In 2008, Herford and Boyne reported their technique in 14 patients, which resulted in successful outcomes in all 14 patients.[112] Herford later reported on two cases of using rhBMP-2 with demineralized bone in the successful reconstruction of lateral segmental defects.[113] These articles both discuss the need for a technique that maintains space for the graft since the sponge carrier is soft and easily compressed under the soft tissue envelope. A separate series demonstrated successful outcomes using BMP-7 for segmental defects of the mandible in seven patients and a large peripheral ostectomy in three others with no reported complications. Others have not been as successful, as evidenced by Carter et al. in their series of five patients described in 2008. While three patients achieved union, two suffered from nonunion due to chronic infection and collapse of the soft tissue envelope resulting in graft loss.[114,115] Other complications of rhBMP-2 include hematoma, seroma, and bone resorption at the graft site.[111,116]

Specific Donor Site Morbidity and Complications

Autogenous bone reconstruction must take into account the possible complications and morbidity of the donor site. Each donor site has inherent advantages, limitations, and potential complications. For very small defects, intraoral sources are ideal. Extraoral donor sites by contrast imply higher morbidity and risk, but do offer greater amounts of reconstructive material.

Intraoral Donor Sites

Common intraoral sources of bone grafts include the mandibular ramus, symphysis, tuberosity, and coronoid process. A comparison of two sites in 50 patients by Misch suggested that the symphysis donor site is associated with more problems in postoperative healing compared to ramus grafts.[117] Wound dehiscence occurred in 3 of 28 patients who underwent grafting from the symphysis, while all ramus donor sites healed without wound breakdown. The author noted that only the vestibular incisions suffered from healing problems in the symphysis, while sulcular incisions healed with fewer problems. Postoperative neurosensory changes from intraoral donor sites are related to proximity of the long buccal nerve, inferior alveolar nerve, and mental nerve. Patients seem less likely to notice sensory changes in the buccal nerve distribution as compared to the lower lip.[117] Misch reported a 10% incidence of temporary mental nerve paresthesia after symphysis grafts, but all patients eventually recovered. In the same series, 29% of patients with symphysis grafts reported altered sensation to the lower incisors, which lasted up to 6 months. No patients who underwent ramus grafts demonstrated permanent postoperative changes along the inferior alveolar or long buccal nerve distribution, although other authors have reported low rates of temporary neurosensory changes.[118] Postoperative infection seems to be uncommon with intraoral donor sites. A 2009 review of 32 patients who underwent ramus grafts found only one site with a localized postoperative infection, which responded well to incision and drainage.[118] While not directly reported, coronoid bone grafts have inherent risks of trismus related to injury of the temporalis muscle, injury to the inferior alveolar and lingual nerves, and injury to the masseteric branch of the internal maxillary artery, which can cause profound acute blood loss. This latter risk is minimized by performing the osteotomy from medial to lateral. The tuberosity harvest site yields poor quality and limited quantity of bone that lead to early resorption of the graft. In addition, sinus exposure and associated sequelae or oral antral fistulas or sinus infections may occur. For these reasons the tuberosity is rarely used as a donor site.

Iliac Crest Harvest Site

The iliac crest is one of the most commonly used donor sites to reconstruct moderate to large bony defects. Both the anterior and posterior iliac crests are available for harvest. Gait disturbance and pain in the early postoperative period is considered normal sequelae of surgery that should resolve with time.[119–121] Gait disturbance has been attributed to muscle dissection of the gluteus, iliacas, and tensor fascia lata, particularly when block grafts are required. In contrast, when only cancellous bone is harvested this complication may be limited with careful technique. Although repositioning the patient intraoperatively is required to access the posterior crest, this location has gained the reputation of having less morbidity from gait disturbance, less pain, and fewer hematomas.[120,122] The need for repositioning the patient perioperatively carries its own risks of endotracheal tube displacement or occlusion, eyes or nose injury, and requires special attention to taping and padding. In a prospective study of 50 patients that compared the morbidity between the anterior and posterior approaches for iliac crest bone harvest, the authors preferred the posterior ilium due to the lower severity of pain and gait disturbance.[123]

Infection at this donor site is uncommon and usually minor. Resolution can often be obtained simply with local measures that may require removal of sutures and drainage through the incision site.[121,124,125] Postoperative hematomas may occur in up to 6% of cases and are generally minor as well.[121,122,126] Most are the result of blood oozing from the marrow, although the deep circumflex iliac artery and muscular perforators may also contribute to bleeding.[119] While some surgeons recommend the placement of drains,[119,127] this can usually be avoided with use of bone wax, oxidized cellulose, activated thrombin–gelatin matrix (Floseal®, Baxter, www.baxter.com; Surgiflo®, Ethicon, www.ethicon360.com), and meticulous hemostasis of the soft tissues. An exceedingly rare complication of retroperitoneal bleeding with patient death has been reported.[128] Hematoma formation in the posterior ilium may be minimized by postoperative bed rest in the supine position the first night after surgery. Seromas have been reported commonly as a complication and may be treated with aspiration and pressure dressing. If these conservative measures fail, seromas and hematomas may require a return to the operating room for formal evacuation.[129] Fractures of the iliac crest may occur after harvest of the anterior or posterior ilium. While this fracture may occur intraoperatively, postoperative fractures have been described secondary to sudden contraction of the lateral musculature along a weakened iliac crest.[130] Pelvic instability may also occur after posterior iliac crest harvest and is due to weakening of the sacroiliac crest ligaments.[131] Removal of a full thickness segment of anterior ilium has been associated with postoperative contour deformities of the hip.[126,132,133] This may be prevented by leaving the crest intact while harvesting bone only from the medial table when possible. Alternatively, trephination allows removal of deep cores of bone while maintaining the overall integrity of the ilium.

Postoperative paresthesia has been reported most commonly in the distribution of the lateral femoral cutaneous nerve (0–17%).[121,125,134,135] Injury to this nerve may be minimized by avoiding excessive traction and preserving 1 cm of bone at the anterior superior iliac spine. Other nerves at risk include the ilioinguinal, iliohypogastric, cluneal, sciatic, and subcostal nerves. A postoperative hernia may develop (0–0.8%) with poor reapproximation of muscular and fascial landmarks.[135–137] Postoperative ileus is considered extremely rare and has been described in a case report of two patients.[138] Careful dissection with protection of the periosteum along with detailed knowledge of the local anatomy should assist in avoidance of severe complications that usually are due to loss of orientation and aggressiveness.

Calvarial Bone Grafts

The calvarium is commonly used as a corticocancellous bone source for maxillofacial reconstruction. The donor site is easily included in the surgical field, and minimal dissection is required to reach bone. Grafts can be easily and quickly harvested from the calvarium for a wide range of purposes including nasal recon-struction, orbital reconstruction, and mandibular onlays, to name a few. While a fullthickness graft is possible, harvesting only the outer table of bone is generally the safest approach. Postoperative hematoma and seroma are the most common complications associated with calverial bone graft harvest and minimal pain has been reported.[139] Avoidance of hematoma may be minimized by ensuring hemostasis with bone wax or a scalp head wrap dressing. A review of 586 calvarial bone grafts observed five seromas and two intracranial hematomas for a 1% overall complication rate.[140] This report also highlights the potentially serious complication from calvarial bone harvesting in which inadvertent perforation of the inner cortical plate with dural tear or direct cerebral cortex injury can ensue. Neurologic complications, including post-operative hemiparesis, were reported although these were ultimately found to be temporary. Overall, inner table violation has been reported in the range of 0 to 13% resulting variably in subdural hematoma, cere-brospinal fluid leak, central nervous system infection, and sagittal sinus penetration. A number of surgical considerations are important to avoid this complication. First, the surgeon should consider the location of the graft carefully. Some have advocated grafting from the nondominant hemisphere to limit the extent of injury should complications occur. In addition, regardless of side, the overall thickness of calverial bone, which is variably based on the location of harvest, needs to be considered. The thickest and most desirable for grafting in the adult is generally located high on the parietal bone but at least 2 cm lateral to the midline to avoid the region of the sagittal sinus. Preoperative imaging with computed tomography (CT) scanning has been advocated by some surgeons but would generally not be required in the adult population. In children, cranial bone split procedures are generally not undertaken prior to 3 years of age, and at that point a CT scan to assure a diploic space may be warranted. At around 9 years of age, the parietal bone reaches a thickness of approximately 6 mm. Surgical techniques have been variably reported. For outer cortex grafts, carefully outlining the donor site to diploic bone followed by judicious beveling of a least one edge will allow for appropriate angulation of the osteotome for cortical separation. Surgeon preference regarding osteotomy size, shape, and thickness is likely secondary to meticulous technique.[139–143] Dural exposure without a tear is generally not a serious event, but dural coverage with pericranium or off-the-shelf dural substitutes is warranted as well as extended spectrum antibiotic coverage. Consideration for neurosurgical input is warranted, particularly when the complication results in dural tear requiring repair or frank injury to the intracranial contents.[140]

Postoperative donor site infections tend to be superficial and may resolve with drainage.[144] Progression to central nervous system infection is rare but may have devastating results. Delayed wound healing of the scalp is uncommon and was reported in only two cases of a series of 247 cranial bone harvests over a 6-year period.[142] Postoperative contour deformities of the skull tend to be minimal, although patients may be bothered when the defect is palpable.[142,145] These defects may be minimized by generous beveling of the defect edges after graft harvest.[140,146] Alternatively, the surgeon may place cranial bone shavings in the defect to augment the contour.[142]

Alopecia, scarring, or keloid formation along the incision line can occur, and there may be significant cosmetic complications associated with cranial bone graft harvest especially when these sequelae are visible. Care not to transect hair follicles, avoiding the use of hemostatic clips and electrocautery on the scalp flap, and placement of the incision with consideration to the hair receding along hair line, coupled with meticu-lous wound closure, will assist in minimizing occurrence of these potential complications.

Costochondral Grafts

Costochondral grafts are frequently employed for bony reconstruction of the face particularly when both bone and cartilage are needed. Postoperative complications include atelectasis, pneumonia, pneumothorax, and wound infection. Normal postoperative pain leads to splinting of the chest wall by the patient to decrease movement and further pain. An additional consideration for this pain occurs when the graft is harvested is from the left chest where pain can mimic the findings of acute chest pain from myocardial infarction. Surgeons should consider this carefully particularly in patients with higher risk for cardiac complications. This reduced inspiratory effort can promote atelectasis and pneumonia. A series of 300 patients who underwent rib harvesting noted pneumonia was the most common complication (eight patients) while persistent atelectasis occurred in two patients.[147] Postoperative respiratory difficulty is increased as the number of harvested ribs increases.[148] Since pain control plays a vital role in the

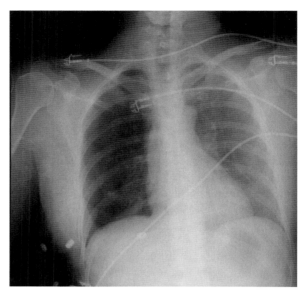

Fig. 13.1. Right pneumothorax following rib harvest.

postoperative respiratory recovery of these patients, the surgeon may consider an intercostal nerve block with a long-acting local anesthetic at the termination of the procedure.[149] Aggressive use of incentive spirometry and chest physiotherapy should be employed to minimize risk of postoperative respiratory sequelae that could progress to pneumonia.

Intraoperative pneumothorax is generally avoided with wide access and precise surgical technique. The complication is increased when multiple ribs are harvested in a single setting or when large portions of cartilage are removed. As an average, this complication occurs in approximately 5% of patients (Fig. 13.1). Care should be taken particularly when unwrapping the periosteum from the deep portions of the rib and when working in the area of the cartilage to avoid damage to the underlying tissues. Careful inspection of the surgical site should be undertaken after harvest is completed with underwater examination of the wound while the anesthesiologist applies positive pressure. Notation of any clinical tear or bubbles on positive pressure is indicative of pleural tear. Treatment of pleural tear depends on the size and extent of injury. Repair may be attempted over a small Foley or red Robinson catheter with evacuation of pleural air underwater prior to final closure. Muscle patches for larger tears may be helpful, and ultimately a decision for chest tube placement may need to be made. In addition, it should be recognized that a delayed pneumothorax may occur if sharp edges of the remaining cut ribs lacerates the pleura during respiration.[149] These remaining ends of cut ribs should be inspected and smoothed if necessary prior to closure. Regardless of intraoperative perception, a postoperative radiograph for evaluation of pneumothorax is indicated given that pneumothorax can be present despite the lack of corroborating intraoperative findings. Treatment of pneumothorax is dependent on size, symptoms, and patient-related factors.

Wound infections following rib harvest are fortunately rare and occur in fewer than 3% of cases.[132,150–152] Long-term pleuritic pain has been described[132] and may be attributed to scar formation that tethers the pleura to the chest wall. Chest scars occasionally become widened[133] and often heal with suture tracks.[132] These deformities may be minimized by placing adequate deep dermal sutures,[149] removing skin sutures early, and by placing incisions in lines of minimal tension such as the inframammary crease.

Intraoperative and postoperative complications at the recipient site with costochondral grafts deserve consideration. The current role of costochondral grafts tends to be in condylar reconstruction where rib and cartilage are used. Placement of the appropriate amount of cartilage has been debated, particularly in the growing child where some have suggested that the resulting mandibular growth potential, including the risk for excessive growth, is determined by the cartilaginous component. Though not studied prospectively, a 3-mm cartilaginous cap has generally been accepted to be adequate for reconstruction without risking the potential for excess growth or its accidental severance from the rib perioperatively. To avoid this latter complication, some have advocated maintaining a cuff of periosteum and pericondrium at the junction of these tissues. This technique may add to the durability of the costochondral junction but does increase the risk of pneumothorax.

Additional complications arise in the placement of the rib into the glenoid fossa and its ability to remain in place during the postoperative period. Intermaxillary fixation is employed to assist in joint stability during the healing process. In addition, some have described the use of wires or nonresorbable sutures suspended from the glenoid fossa or temporal region to the rib providing additional support. Immediate and long-term malocclusion is a complication attributed to intraoperative failure and the innate growth potential or lack thereof of the graft. Overall, patients should be prepared for the potential need of a period of occlusal elastic therapy to assist in train the musculature to the new joint characteristics.

Tibial Bone Grafts

Tibial bone has gained popularity due to the ability to harvest distant bone in an in-office setting with relatively low morbidity. Postoperative complications include delayed wound healing, infection, gait disturbance, fracture, and persistent pain or paresthesia. A review of 230 tibial bone grafts from the orthopedic literature revealed an overall complication rate of 1.3%.[153] Delayed wound healing may occur in the range of 0 to 4.5% of cases.[153–155] One review noted delayed wound healing in an obese patient who developed a seroma requiring surgical debridement and closure over a suction drain.[154] Ecchymosis is commonly reported although it resolves with time.[154,156] Pathologic fractures may occur at the donor site in up to 2.7% of cases.[153,157] Gait disturbance is usually short-lived and resolves within 10 days,[158] although ambulatory difficulty as long as 3 weeks after surgery has been reported.[155] Persistent pain at the donor site occurs in up to 5% of cases.[153,155] A series of 44 tibial bone grafts noted one patient with persistent postoperative joint pain due to surgical entry into the joint space during harvest, which can be prevented by avoiding bone excavation in the region of the tibial plateau.[154] Neurosensory disturbance may occur in up to 7.5% of cases, although the paresthesia tends to resolve within a few weeks.[156]

Pedicled Bone Flaps

A number of harvest sites are available for bone transfer with a pedicled blood supply. Calvarial bone as described above can be transferred with the blood supply from a temporoparietal fascia pedicled flap into the lateral maxilla, orbit, or lateral mandible region. Transfer of the fascia can allow for a larger bone graft to be harvested from the outer cranium;[159] however, the resultant bony and soft tissue defect can be more prominent following the reconstruction. In addition, there are additional risks associated with temporoparietal galeal harvest, such as alopecia, facial nerve injury, and trismus.[159–163]

A variety of other pedicled bone flaps have been described with similar risks and complications as their free bone graft counterparts. While they may provide a larger volume of bone due to the pedicled periosteal blood supply, their applications can be limited due to the amount of soft tissue bulk provided and the limitations in orientation. Such examples are costochondral rib grafts pedicled on pectoralis major muscle or latissimus dorsi muscle, scapula tip pedicled on latissimus dorsi, and clavicle pedicled on sternocleidomastoid.[164,165]

ADJUNCTS TO MICROVASCULAR BONE FLAPS

Fibula Myoossesous (Cutaneous) Flap

Vascularized fibula bone grafts are often required for reconstruction of larger composite or segmental defects. Preoperative considerations focus on the suitability of harvesting the peroneal vessels while maintaining adequate leg perfusion via the anterior and posterior tibial vessels. Although palpable dorsalis pedis and posterior tibial pulses have been recommended as reliable guides,[166] this is no guarantee that sacrifice of the peroneal artery is safe given the possibility of peripheral vascular disease and normal anatomic variants. Kim et al. reviewed 495 lower extremity angiograms and noted hypoplasia or the absence of anterior

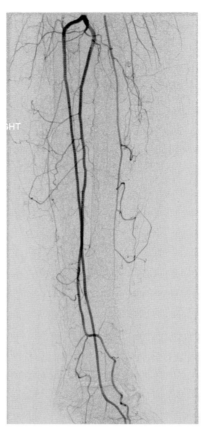

Fig. 13.2. Right dominant peroneal artery.

tibial arteries in 4% of patients.[167] Hypoplasia or absence of posterior tibial arteries was noted in 2%. Peroneal arteria magna may occur when both the anterior and posterior tibial arteries are inadequate, resulting in only the peroneal artery supplying blood to the foot. Peroneal arteria magna is estimated to be present in up to 7% of the population (Fig. 13.2).[168,169] An absent peroneal artery occurs in 0.1 to 4.0% of the population. Importantly, normal pedal pulses are present in both peroneal arteria magna and with absent peroneal arteries.[170] Choice of preoperative lower extremity imaging is often based on surgeon preference and available services in the surgeon's practice environment. While arteriography is considered by many to be the gold standard, this is an invasive study that carries a 3–5% complication rate. Such problems include contrast allergy, renal failure, hematoma, aortic dissection, and arterial occlusion.[168] While the least invasive modality is color flow Doppler imaging, this study is highly technique-sensitive and requires an experienced technician.[171] Computed tomography angiography (CTA) and magnetic resonance angiography (MRA) have become standard preoperative modalities in many institutions. MRA has been suggested to be nearly equal to conventional angiography in the preoperative assessment of fibula harvest.[170] High sensitivity and positive predictive value have led some authors to utilize this modality routinely in all patients.[172] An additional advantage of MRA over conventional angiography is the ability to view the lower extremity vasculature in three dimensions.

Intraoperative complications in fibula free flap harvest are often related to maintaining the vascular integrity of the skin paddle. While septocutaneous perforators are more easily incorporated into the flap, musculocutaneous perforators are commonly encountered and require inclusion of a muscle cuff around the perforators. Schusterman et al. reported only 33% of skin paddles survived based on a septocutaneous supply, while survival rose to 93% with the inclusion of a muscle cuff.[173] Additional complications may occur if the vascular pedicle to the bone is injured. Extreme care should be taken when proximal dissection of the pedicle is undertaken, for injury to the pedicle at this level may render the flap unusable. Distally,

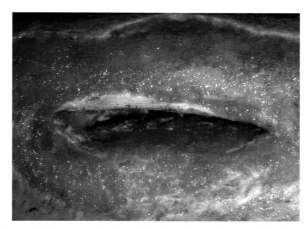

Fig. 13.3. Fibula flap with skin paddle harvest site in a diabetic patient that was closed primarily with wound breakdown and infection treated with debridement and wound dressings.

aggressive retraction of the osteotomized bone prior to pedicle division may cause separation of the blood supply to the distal bone. To avoid this scenario, some authors recommend removing a small segment of bone at the distal osteotomy.[174] This maneuver provides a window through which the pedicle may be accessed and divided prior to lateral mobilization of the fibula.

The fibula donor site occasionally suffers from delayed wound healing, orthopedic complications, contour or cosmetic deformities, and weak or diminished great toe function. Donor site wound healing difficulty is mainly related to the soft tissue component of a composite flap (Fig. 13.3). Incomplete skin graft healing can lead to tendon exposure requiring local wound care for several weeks as healing progresses. A suprafascial dissection under the skin paddle may provide a wound bed more amenable to skin grafting by minimizing the exposure of peroneus longus tendons. Similar wound healing problems may occur if primary closure is attempted after harvesting a skin paddle greater than 3 cm in width. The increased tension along the closure often leads to dehiscence and requires prolonged wound care. The temptation to close the soft tissue defect primarily to avoid a skin graft should be weighed carefully against the possibility of wound breakdown that results in the same cosmetic outcome as a skin graft. Compartment syndrome is fortunately a rare postoperative phenomenon that occurs in less than 1% of cases.[175] Orthopedic problems are related to the detachment of muscles from the fibula, injury to the peroneal nerve, or joint instability. The fibula serves to stabilize the ankle joint during function, which requires a 6- to 8-cm distal segment to remain in place. A 10-year follow-up study by Hidalgo[176] studied donor site morbidity of 20 patients who underwent fibula free flap harvest. Three of the 20 patients reported intermittent leg weakness or pain and only one was unable to perform rigorous activities such as jogging. One patient in the group was able to run a marathon without difficulty. Postoperative physical therapy should be routinely instituted to minimize functional disturbances.[177]

Deep Circumflex Iliac Artery Myoosseous (Cutaneous) Flap

The iliac crest free flap based on the deep circumflex iliac artery is an excellent source of bone for maxillofacial reconstruction. However, significant donor site morbidity precludes the use of this donor site as a first choice in many institutions. In contrast to nonvascularized corticocancellous grafts, the extent of dissection required for free tissue harvest significantly increases morbidity. Common postoperative problems include ambulatory difficulty, abdominal wall hernia, and chronic pain.[178] Hernias may form in up to 12% of patients.[179–181] Long-term abdominal wall weakness is most likely to develop into a hernia when a portion of the abdominal wall musculature is harvested. In these cases, a mesh repair of the defect is recommended at the time of harvest.[182] Two cases have been reported in the literature describing bowel obstruction due to herniation at the donor site requiring emergent surgery.[183] A 2008 review of 24 iliac crest flaps revealed only one donor site hematoma that upon exploration was found to be caused by oozing bone marrow.[184] A similar small study found two seromas in 12 patients, which resolved spontaneously.[185] No other early postoperative complications were noted in either study. A small number of patients report chronic pain or long-term neurosensory changes. Chronic pain may be related to the use of synthetic mesh for repair of the abdominal wall defect.[186] Rare complications reported in the literature include ureteral injury, pelvic instability, and tumor seeding.[179]

Radial Forearm Osteofasciocutaneous Flap

Preoperative evaluation of the radial forearm donor site must assess the ability of the ulnar circulation to maintain hand viability after sacrifice of the radial artery. Communication between the superficial and deep palmar arches must be present for safe harvest of the flap. This assessment is traditionally performed using the Allen test. The donor radial and ulnar arteries are occluded by the examiner's thumbs while the hand is exsanguinated by repeated fist clinching. The ulnar artery is released to reveal the extent of hand perfusion while the radial artery remains occluded. Although this test is easily performed at bedside, the assessment is subjective and variable amounts of pressure may be required to reliably occlude the radial artery. Additional error can be introduced if the donor hand is hyperextended. The reliability of the Allen test is well accepted, although some others recommend an objective Allen test using Doppler imaging and photoplethysmography. Nuckols et al. compared the traditional Allen test with an objective Doppler-assisted Allen test in 65 patients and noted an improved ability to detect vascular variations using the Doppler.[187] Notably, of the 25 patients found to have equivocal or poor subjective Allen tests, the Doppler exam revealed that 18 of these could safely undergo radial forearm harvest.

The radial forearm free flap is occasionally harvested as an osteocutaneous flap incorporating a segment of the radius. Fracture of the remaining radius is the most feared postoperative complication, occurring in up to 40% of cases.[188] Some authors recommend routine prophylactic plating across the radius defect to minimize the chance of fracture.[188–190] Others employ postoperative casting of the arm for 6–8 weeks or bone grafting the donor site, although these techniques seem to be utilized infrequently.[189] More common donor site problems include decreased pinch and grip strength, reduced sensation over the dorsum of the hand, delayed wound healing, and cosmetic deformities.[191–194] A retrospective review of 52 patients who underwent osteocutaneous radial forearm free flap harvest revealed a 7.7% rate of donor site complications.[190] These included one radius fracture and three cases of delayed wound healing with exposed tendons. The fracture occurred on postoperative day 3 despite prophylactic plating and was felt to be due to a loose screw. Reoperation and cast immobilization for 4 weeks was required.

Scapula Myoosseous (Cutaneous) Flap

The scapula is a versatile source of vascularized bone that can be tailored to complex defects. Postoperative donor site complications include hematoma, seroma, infection, wound breakdown, shoulder weakness, and chronic pain. While hematoma formation is likely minimized by the normal postoperative bed rest and sleeping supine, seroma formation is common after such extensive dissection of the back. Donor site problems in 36 patients were reviewed that revealed a 25% rate of persistent seroma.[195] Little long-term data exist regarding the functional compromise after harvesting the scapula. A 2009 publication reviewed 20 patients who underwent scapula harvest to assess shoulder function 1 and 6 months after surgery.[196] Compared with the nondonor arm, the study demonstrated limited mobility in the operated shoulder at 1 month with improvement at 6 months.

BONY RECONSTRUCTION

Distraction Osteogenesis

Distraction osteogenesis has become increasingly common in bony reconstruction as an alternative to standard grafting techniques, with the advantage to generate bone from adjacent sites. Transport disc distraction for segmental defects and alveolar distraction for atrophic ridges are specific examples. Difficulties and complications with distraction have tempered much of the initial enthusiasm with these techniques. While limitations do exist, many of the common complications can be avoided with careful presurgical planning and surgical precision.

The majority of complications relate to the distraction hardware, and the need for exposure through the skin or mucosa. While infection is uncommon, pin-track infections may occur secondary to the open wound, which must be maintained through mucosa or skin during the distraction phase. Because these openings allow drainage, local wound care and irrigation are usually all that are required. Mechanical device failure, instability, or breakage occurs uncommonly and is described as less than 6% for all types of distraction in two large case series.[197,198] In two retrospective case series of 37 and 45 patients who underwent alveolar distraction, only one case of a broken distractor was noted.[199,200] Other complications were reported as minor (up to 75% of cases), including soft tissue dehiscence (14% to 38%) with infections in 6% to 7%. Major complications included fracture of the basal bone and/or transport segment (8% to 17%).[199,200] Another review of 20 patients undergoing alveolar distraction revealed a 55% overall complication rate including fracture of the transport segment in one patient.[201] Other reported complications include paresthesia (14% to 28%), hematomas (4%), and postoperative bone defects at the site of the distractor.[199,200] Transport distraction is not as widely used with free flap techniques being at the forefront of treatment protocols; however, one series presented 28 patients of maxillary, mandibular, and skull defects with a failure rate of 21% through a variety of causes, including three patients (10%) who died of disease prior to completion of distraction: one patient had device failure with screw loosening on two occasions in an irradiated site, one patient developed early consolidation, and one patient with fulminant infection. Defects up to 80 mm were reported as being successfully distracted.[202] Other authors report small case series with custom fabricated distraction devices.[203] Additional complications arise when distraction does not result in a bony matrix adequate for healing. This is of particular importance in patients following radiation treatment, where some believe distraction may be of limited use and bone quality is poor; however, a small case series of six patients has shown beneficial results with only one failure (17%). There was soft tissue dehiscence over the distractor that was successfully treated conservatively in two patients.[204] Further evaluation of larger case series with both transport and alveolar distraction methods is needed as there is substantial variability of success comparing maxilla to mandible and anterior to posterior with supraperiosteal and subperiosteal methods used.

The most frequent complication for larger defects results from the inability to position the final bone matrix in the desired location. This complication may result from hardware failure itself or more commonly from the surgeon's inability to appropriately place the distraction device consistent with the desired vectors.[197,198,202,205–207] In order to overcome this limitation surgeons have employed computer modeling for accuracy[208] and devices that can be adjusted mid-distraction.[209] Computer-assisted surgery with surgical planning and modeling allows for the creation of templates, which will guide distractor placement in the operating room.[208,210,211] Still, care must be taken to assure that the templates accurately reflect the anatomy since many do not "lock in" to a single position. In addition, the bulky nature of the templates often requires additional surgical exposure, which should be weighed when considering their use.

Hyperbaric Oxygen

Hyperbaric oxygen therapy (HBO) has been recommended by some authors[212–217] in the treatment of osteoradionecrosis (ORN) in conjunction with surgical reconstruction. While the initial data seemed promising, the utility of HBO has been challenged by recent more strenuous scientific investigations.[218] Conceptually, it seems plausible that HBO therapy would promote angiogenesis and revascularization; however, Annane's randomized controlled trial evaluating the effectiveness of HBO compared to a control without HBO was halted prematurely due to a demonstration of worse outcomes in using HBO therapy.[218] Microvascular reconstruction with free tissue transfer makes possible the reconstruction of bone and soft tissue that is reliable even in the vascularly compromised wound setting and avoids the costs, potential complications, and current uncertainty of the utility of HBO therapy.[219–226] Complications from HBO include barotrauma to the middle ear and sinuses, myopia, and oxygen toxicity to the lungs or central nervous system.[227,228] An additional consideration is that one study has demonstrated trends toward increased complications with free tissue transfer after HBO therapy compared to patients who have never been exposed to this modality.[222] There continues to be substantial debate over the application of HBO for maxillofacial practitioners as highlighted by two recent articles.[229,230] Further randomized controlled trials are currently being undertaken.

Fixation Schemes

There is substantial variability in usage of reconstructive plates in bone reconstruction. Many have debated size and rigidity of plate with supporters of both miniplates and rigid reconstruction plates. Plating technology in North America and Europe has advanced substantially over the past 30 years with the advent of more biocompatible and rigid titanium alloys with improving success rates.[231] While it is known that the plate must offer rigidity for stabilizing the bone segments to allow for healing, fracture healing concepts and the identification of stress shielding have evolved significant changes in treatment philosophy.[232–234] If a plate is used and torque from muscle pull provides detrimental forces on the plate, it may proceed to weakening screws and result in failure of the graft with malunion or nonunion. Similarly, bending plates puts undue stress into the metal and with repetitive use in cases of malunion/nonunion, the plate can run the risk of fracture (Fig. 13.4). There are additional debates regarding the use of standard nonlocking screws versus threadlock screws for plate-to-bone adaptation, with many studies evaluating the advantages and disadvantages of each technique the fracture literature.[235–245]

When reconstructing continuity with grafts and flaps, both rigid and nonrigid/semirigid fixation has been employed and advocated in the literature. Despite the beneficial characteristics of locking plate systems through stabilization of the screw to the plate for spatial maintenance of the segments, the screw may not be fully engaging the bone. The locking mechanism, though, of the screw to the plate prevents identification of this problem intraoperatively, with subsequent risk of graft failure due to inadequate stabilization. In addition, absorption of all masticatory forces by the plate and stress shielding of the graft may prevent healing and union with the native mandible. Overall, complications from plates result from screw loosening (0.8% of locking screws), plate exposure (10–15% intraorally and extraorally), plate fracture (0–8%) with resultant acute and chronic infections (up to 30%), orocutaneous fistulas, and malunion/nonunion (0.7–8%) (Fig. 13.5).[238,246–259]

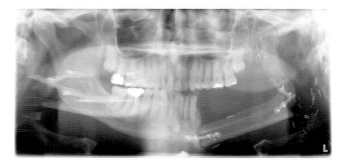

Fig. 13.4. Postoperative fibula flap with plate fracture and condylar dislocation.

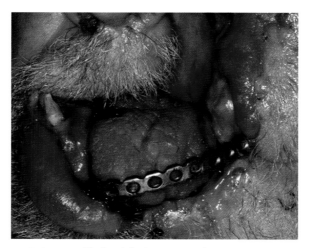

Fig. 13.5. Plate exposure in an anterior mandibular defect reconstruction.

Newer resorbable techniques have been shown to be of use with certain clinical applications, especially in the pediatric population, where less rigidity is required for fixation.[260] Some authors have demonstrated success with resorbable screws used to fixate small bone grafts for preprosthetic applications, so as to obviate the need to retrieve screws when implant placement occurs.[261–265] Further evaluation is necessary to determine the overall success and indications for resorbable systems in bone reconstruction.

SPECIAL CONSIDERATIONS

Bone Necrosis and Infection

One of the most difficult situations to reconstruct is the exposure of bone without soft tissue coverage intraorally and/or extraorally. Chronic nonhealing wounds can be related to various factors resulting in nonviable bone. This could be from tissue loss from ballistic wounds or avulsive traumatic defects, infected segments from osteomyelitis or hardware failure, necrotic bone from failed bone reconstruction (vascularized and nonvascularized osseous tissues), osteoradionecrosis (ORN), osteonecrosis of the jaws (ONJ), etc. (Figs. 13.6 and 13.7). In any situation, the soft tissues are often chronically inflamed or infected and fibrotic.[220,225,226,266–274] The soft tissue envelope retracts to expose more bone and often a composite defect may result. Managing this complicated situation is onerous and must be dealt with in a strategic manner that considers both the hard tissue and soft tissue needs as well as the reality that native bone involvement may be more extensive than what is appreciated clinically or radiographically. Determining an intraoperative margin of normal bone is an important and often difficult task. In these cases, strong consideration should be given for the use of vascularized tissue transfer.

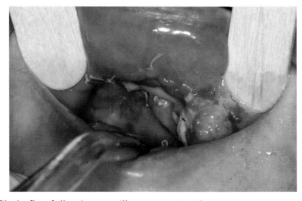

Fig. 13.6. Exposed necrotic fibula flap following maxillary reconstruction.

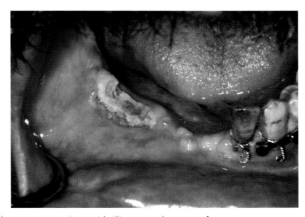

Fig. 13.7. Necrotic mandibular reconstruction with iliac crest bone graft.

Debridement Issues

While specific management for necrotic infected bone may vary based on etiology it is universally accepted that broad spectrum antibiotics are initiated and accordingly changed based on cultures and sensitivity results. Management with antibiotics and drainage of fluid collections as necessary will often settle the inflammatory process, and on occasion soft tissue healing and coverage may result. If persistent exposure of nonviable bone is evident, debridement may be necessary. Bone may be curetted and debrided to viable bleeding bone when possible with an attempt at preserving nerve function. If necessary, a load-bearing rigid reconstruction plate with locking screws can be applied to support segmental defects or weakened areas of the mandible.[89,275-277] In addition, maxillomandibular fixation can assist with segment positioning intraoperatively.[89]

Hardware Removal

Hardware can elicit a foreign body reaction when stability is not achieved and gross mobility of the segments with function occurs. Hardware failure can result from various causes: poor engagement of screws at the time of placement (locking and nonlocking), overheating of bone (drill hole preparation or osteotomy sites), lack of stability at time of placement, small thickness plates that cannot appropriately share or bear the functional load, poorly adapted plates with nonlocking screws, and use of nonbiocompatible materials.[238,258,259] The latter is less common due to rigorous standards imposed by FDA for product approval. It is routinely recommended that chronically exposed or failed hardware be removed once it is identified to allow for soft tissue healing and possible coverage. Assessment of healing and consolidation at the time of hardware removal is essential. Grafts that have consolidated and been replaced by an adequate quantity and quality of viable noninfected bone can tolerate hardware removal without difficulty. In contrast, early hardware removal may result in long-term failure if osseous healing has not occurred. Consideration should be given to replacement of hardware, external fixation, or intermaxillary fixation to stabilize bony segments when necessary. If infection is noted at the time of removal, appropriate cultures and antibiotic coverage are warranted.

RECIPIENT SITE CONSIDERATIONS IN RECONSTRUCTION

Based on numerous individual patient factors and the reconstructive needs, different strategies can be implemented. As mentioned earlier, the preoperative status of the patient and availability of donor sites is one level that will determine the reconstructive options. Poor functional status, nonoptimized cardiopulmonary disease and poor health may preclude the patient from being able to undergo a microvascular free tissue transfer due to the length of general anesthetic needed. Case selection is often dependent on operator and anesthesiologist skill and comfort level as well as facility capabilities for intraoperative and postoperative care; however, good surgical results can be achieved in elderly patients and those with comorbidities.[278-282] A poor nutritional status with hypoalbuminemia, poor glucose control, or high-dose steroid use may need to be optimized prior to considering an operation. Patients may require extensive preoperative nutrition using nasogastric tube feedings for both protein nutrition and to avoid further contamination of the wound. Though previously reviewed to some extent in our review of donor sites, several clinical scenarios deserve specific mention and/or reiteration.

Anterior Mandibular Defects

The anatomic complexity coupled with the multidirectional muscle pull on the anterior mandible make defects in this region difficult to manage. Reconstruction should establish bony continuity in order to prevent hardware failure and/or exposure. If mandibular continuity is not established, the lack of lip and tongue support will result in the characteristic "Andy Gump" deformity and associated catastrophic functional outcomes.[252,253,283,284] Mandibular continuity with the use of a reconstruction plate alone should be avoided or used as temporary measure for stability until final reconstruction is undertaken; nonvascularized block bone grafts are well documented to offer very good results when placed in noninflamed defects ideally measuring less than 6 cm. Defects greater than 6 cm are fraught with a greater number of complications and have a lower success rate. As tissues can be quite tense anteriorly, an extraoral approach will avoid oral contamination and can offer a more reliable result due to ease in achieving water tight closure of the tissues intraoperatively.[94] Particulate bone grafts in the anterior region[285–288] should be avoided for larger defects as the particulate matter does not offer any resistance to compression caused by the soft tissue envelope in this area.

Vascularized osseous, myoosseous, and osteocutaneous options provide very good results for reconstruction of larger osseous defects and composite defects of all sizes. It may remain difficult to achieve complete bony union in ORN or ONJ cases, but successful wound closure and restoration of function can be achieved. Various free flap options are available, and reconstruction is tailored to each patient based on operator skill and preference and site selection. While some may advocate vascularized bone transfer for all defect sizes, the morbidity related to donor site harvest and prolonged anesthetic time must be taken into account. For larger defects in the anterior mandible, vascularized bone has a significant advantage with capabilities of providing soft tissue coverage with a single flap.

Lateral Mandibular Defects

A greater number of reconstructive options exist for lateral mandibular defects. Nonvascularized block and particulate bone grafts or vascularized bone flaps can be employed, and the choice depends on the defect size to be reconstructed.[289–294]

Condylar Defects

The condyle should be preserved if at all possible. Even a small condylar stump can be maintained if at least two screws can be passed and secured to the reconstructed bone.[295] When the condyle must be removed, costochondral grafts have proven to be quite effective in maintaining articular function of the mandible.[296] Additionally, they can be attached to vascularized bone flaps to offer function, though many believe they are unnecessary, and direct placement of bone into the fossa can be effective, with or without the presence of an articular disk.[295,297–303] Both custom and stock condylar–fossa replacements are available and can reestablish the hinge function of the mandible.[296,304–307] Custom implants can be manufactured to reconstruct larger defects even to the angle of the mandible. While they can be quite effective and successful for 10 years and more, they can have their own complications and should never be placed into an inflamed tissue bed as they will invariably fail and require removal.[305–307] Long-term placement of stock condyle replacements without an imposing fossa implant must be avoided as they can erode and migrate into the cranial fossa over time.[308] If the condyle can be maintained with resection without compromising postoperative outcome,[303] then this should be the reconstructive option of choice.

Maxillary Defects

Patients can do well with maxillary defects even without reconstruction. Many tolerate obturation of anterior and posterior defects using a properly fitting prosthesis fabricated by a maxillofacial prosthodontist.[309–312] Speech and swallowing can be optimized with this technique if stability of the prosthesis is ensured. This can be difficult with large defects, anterior defects, and minimal remaining palatal support. Occasionally zygomatic implants can offer additional stability.[313] Soft tissue closure of oroantral and oronasal fistulas can be accomplished with locoregional soft tissue transfer (one or a combination of buccal advancement, buccal fat pad, palatal rotation or facial artery myomucosal soft tissue flaps)[314,315] or with soft tissue free flaps (radial forearm, rectus abdominis, parascapular).[316,317] For definitive fixed prosthetic rehabilitation, bone is necessary, and nonvascularized grafts can only be utilized if soft tissue coverage can be achieved. Larger defects warrant soft tissue transfer including myoosseous or osteocutaneous flaps.[272,317–320]

COMPUTER-ASSISTED SURGERY

In the process of planning and executing the surgical plans, emerging technology has given the surgeon of the 21st century the ability to preoperatively plan major bony reconstruction as well as the ability for intraoperative guidance that can assist the surgeon. It is our impression that the authors' adoption of this technology has significantly limited complications and optimized outcomes by simulating the surgical plan, including prefabrication of plates and surgical templates, which adds to the operative efficiency with a resulting decrease in operative times (thereby decreasing the risk of bleeding that might require transfusion, and the need for long-acting anesthetics), augmenting the surgical accuracy of bone placement for future implant reconstruction. With that in mind, consideration of computer-assisted surgery (CAS) is appropriate for discussion in this chapter, which has the ultimate goal of assisting surgeons in limiting the complications of major bony reconstruction.

Thanks to advances in CAS, such surgery will have an expanding role to play with bony maxillofacial reconstruction. The use of in-office cone beam computed tomography and the decreased intraoperative time achieved with rapid prototyping techniques such as stereolithography are very marketable to the head and neck surgeon, and they certainly have the potential to decrease complications.[321,322] There is an increasing use of cutting guides as well to optimize osteotomies for bone reconstruction that use free tissue transfer.[210,323–327]

With bone reconstruction, the goals are to recapitulate preoperative form so that function can follow. While perfect bone replacement does not guarantee complete restoration of function, every effort is made to support the soft tissues for rehabilitative purposes. It has recently become apparent that CAS has numerous advantages to the surgeon. While these highlight decreased operative time, preoperative planning and intraoperative use of prefabricated templates and navigation has aided the operator to foresee difficulties in advance and avoid them in a coordinated fashion.[210,322–336] This ultimately allows for improved predictable outcomes.

Software programs for preoperative planning are becoming ever more powerful; among these are Brain-suite®, Brainlab, www.brainlab.com; Mimics® and Surgicase®, Materialise, www.materialise.com; Voxim®, IVS technology GmbH, www.ivs-technology.de/en; InVivo, Anatomage, www.anatomage.com; Nobelguide, NobelBiocare, www.nobelbiocare.com; and 3dMDVultus, 3dMD, www.3dmd.com. The surgeon now has many options to reduce operating time and attempt more predictable results (Figs. 13.8–13.10).

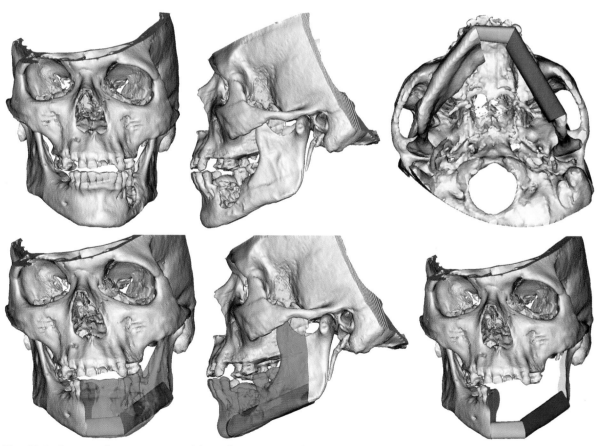

Fig. 13.8. Preoperative computer modeling of surgical plan for mandibular resection and reconstruction.

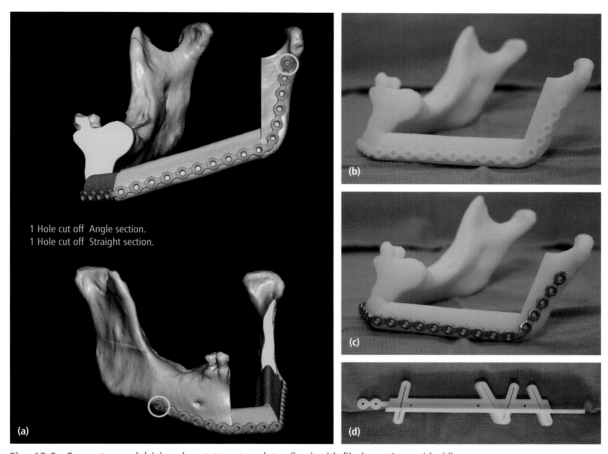

1 Hole cut off Angle section.
1 Hole cut off Straight section.

Fig. 13.9. Computer model (a) and prototype templates (b, c) with fibula cutting guide (d).

Unfortunately there is no single unified program for all modalities, but each has its own application. We can therefore separate CAS modalities into imaging, tactile models, preoperative planning, and intraoperative navigation.

Digital Imaging and Communications in Medicine

The ever-improving accuracy of imaging and a standardized image format [digital imaging and communications in medicine (DICOM)] has allowed computed tomography (CT) and magnetic resonance imaging (MRI) scans to be readily accessed and easily visualized by multiple viewers for interactive purposes. Technological advances afford improved clarity of images at decreased slice intervals for CT and MRI studies with ever-decreasing radiation doses due to improvement in scanner and sensor sensitivities.[337,338] Image scatter caused by radiodense objects in the visualized field (dental restorations, piercings, implants, and hardware), continues to be problematic for seamless image viewing. Software programs now offer image processing to clean up the data loss caused by artifact.[210,339] These programs offer advanced imaging strategies to allow the surgeon to identify key structures and landmarks. Not only can linear measurements and angles be identified as with cephalometry, but areas and volumes can also be appreciated.[339] Surgeons can appreciate anticipated defect size and plan appropriately in advance.[340] Three-dimensional (3D) image reconstruction can afford an appreciation of fracture displacement for trauma victims and extent of bone involvement for pathological cysts and tumors requiring resection. Key structures (nerves, vessels) can be identified along their entire course and margin involvement predicted for anatomical resection. Current studies are ongoing to predict area and volume airway measurements pre- and postoperatively for successful outcomes with surgery.

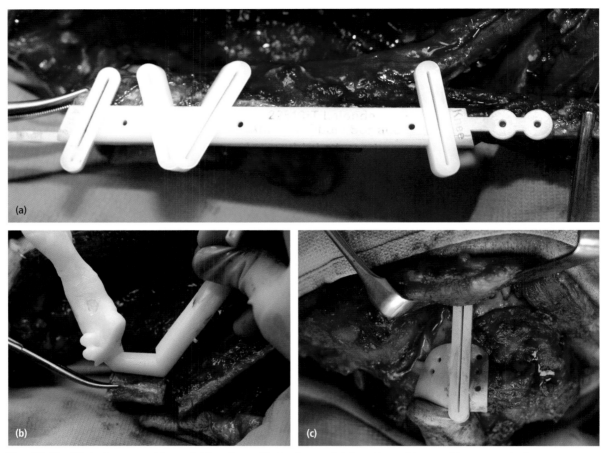

Fig. 13.10. Fibula (upper and lower left) and mandibular (lower right) cutting guides used intraoperatively.

Orbital Reconstruction

There is a large amount of supportive literature on the use of volumetric data records for orbital reconstruction. While it had been previously felt that orbital floor reconstruction could be undertaken with titanium mesh, porous polyethylene, resorbable polydioxanone (PDS) or calvarial bone, suboptimal results became evident for several reasons. These included improper access procedures causing difficult scarring of the lids (entropion and ectropion), but more importantly errors in repositioning the globe in the anteroposterior and superoinferior planes. This becomes an important factor in reconstructing an orbital floor or orbital rim that was lost due to trauma or pathological resection.[341–346] Metzger and Schmelzeisen have demonstrated through orbital volume analysis, that while humans are individually unique, the image data mapped and noted average values of specific orbital contours. This afforded the fabrication of two sizes (small and large) of precontoured titanium plates to three-dimensionally recreate orbital volume of males and females. These plates can be extremely useful in the vast majority of patients and greatly reduce operating time while minimizing volumetric problems after primary orbital reconstruction.[347–349] Synthes (www.synthes.com) is currently the only company that offers precontoured plates for this application.

Tactile Rapid-Prototyped Models

Conversion of DICOM files to a universal format (.stl) results in a loss-less reconstruction of surface anatomy to allow for fabrication of a representative tactile model. A model can be made to replicate, in a 1:1 fashion, the areas of interest. This then allows an operator several advantages preoperatively and intraoperatively. Anatomical definition of the model is limited by accuracy of the scan and can be lost if

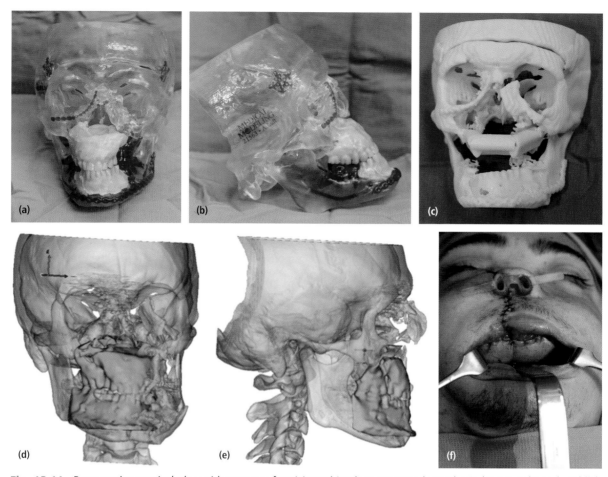

Fig. 13.11. Preoperative surgical plan with wax-up of anticipated implant supported prosthesis (upper right and middle); image fusion (lower right and middle). Preoperative computer-generated fibula placement (upper right); intraoperative placement (lower right).

image processing does not reduce the artifact prior to fabrication. In addition, regions of thin bone may appear as defects on the models due to the inherent limitations of prototyping technology unless the image is manipulated in advance. There are numerous prototyping techniques available including stereolithography, selective laser sintering, 3D printing, fused deposition modeling, and multijet printing. Each has its own advantages and can be readily accessible, but stereolithography and selective laser sintering can be more expensive. Stereolithography has the unique capability of being able to produce clear models with a second color to highlight predetermined areas of interest (teeth, nerves, vessels, tumors, or other unique structures) (Fig. 13.11). There is increasing familiarity of commercial stereolithographic models and services produced by companies such as Medical Modeling® (www.medicalmodeling.com); however, access to local prototyping facilities is becoming more widespread. The costs for rapid prototyping printers and materials are decreasing, and they are becoming more readily available to the mass market for both sterile and nonsterile use. Using the model, a surgeon can make preoperative measurements to determine bony osteotomies for pathological resection and similarly know the approximate dimensions for osseous reconstruction. Some surgeons even carry out the surgery on the models preoperatively. Titanium plates can be prebent to closely adapt to the underlying bone with free exposure and less work hardening the metal. This greatly reduces intraoperative time and can improve patient outcomes with reduction of further complications.[321,322,335,350,351] Custom temporomandibular joint (TMJ) implants are fabricated directly on the model as a wax-up prior to being cast in metal.[306] One can hypothesize that reconstruction plates in the future can be manufactured to the specific requirements of each individual patient; unfortunately their properties cannot be reliably reproduced for customized applications at this time.

Preoperative Software Planning

Some programs offer the capabilities of virtual surgery to allow a surgeon to have a better understanding of what will occur intraoperatively. Reconstructive procedures requiring manipulation of bone structures (orthognathic surgery, distraction osteogenesis, craniomaxillofacial surgery, trauma reconstruction and pathological resection) can all be planned to offer an avenue toward more predictable outcomes. This strategy is most commonly applied in both 2D and 3D for patient education and postoperative prediction with orthognathic surgery, although many more avenues are evolving. While soft tissues can be manipulated individually, normative algorithms have been established to offer the closest estimation of results.[352] It is impossible to accurately predict each individual patient and this must be relayed appropriately so they do not have unreasonable expectations. Contour deformity caused by pathological or developmental processes can undergo virtual planning to mimic the nonaffected side or create a normal template. A sterilizable tactile model can be created to prebend plates or shape bone grafts/flaps intraoperatively. Orthognathic surgery splints/wafers can be manufactured based on preoperative virtual plans that use rapid prototyping strategies and avoid the pitfalls of laboratory planning with articulators and their inherent inaccuracies. For various reconstructive procedures, preoperative planning can allow the surgeon to perform the osteotomies virtually and develop cutting guide templates through rapid prototyping strategies to be used on the maxilla or mandible. This can minimize damage to vital structures caused by wayward osteotomy cuts. In addition, bone grafts and osseous flaps can be shaped, contoured and positioned virtually to allow for an individually tailored reconstruction. Cutting guide templates with known predetermined measurements can also be prepared for predictable osteotomies, thereby decreasing operative time.[210,322–336] Lastly, distraction devices can be virtually planned to ensure proper orientation in all three planes of space. Rapid prototyping can create positioning templates for reliable placement, thereby avoiding early consolidation or premature binding of the devices.[210]

In all surgical fields there is an aim for functional reconstruction, and this is always imperative with maxillofacial surgery. As reconstruction of underlying bone has an impact with the surrounding teeth, comprehensive oral rehabilitation requires recapitulation of not only bone in an anatomical position but also placement of implants in a functional position to allow proper restoration of functional dentition. Using surgical planning and guidance, the underlying bone can be placed in a proper location and implants can be positioned where they will be in stable bone and properly oriented to accept functional loads. Using preoperative planning, multiple surgeries can be planned at once to offer optimal results and minimize future complications with other necessary procedures.

Navigation and Intraoperative Imaging

Computer-assisted surgery has drastically improved the outcomes related to neurosurgical procedures by offering identification of instrument positioning in 3D in real time (also known as 4D when performed real time). Thin-cut preoperative imaging is necessary to be able to register the patient accurately. Registration on hard tissues such as teeth and bone offers improved accuracy, although laser scanners and electromagnetic sensors are improving the accuracy of soft tissue measurements. Maxillofacial surgery has evolving applications for its use particularly in the fields of pathological resection and post-traumatic reconstruction. Many tumors can be accessed and resected with avoidance of critical vital structures by being able to identify their proximity and safe tissue planes. This is especially true for tumors that involve the skull base or the posterior naso- or oropharynx.[210,323,328,329,332,334] Osteotomy cuts can be performed with precision, and vessels and nerves can be avoided by using locating devices on the handpiece.[210,323] Orbital reconstruction procedures are optimized with navigation through identification of instruments and their proximity to the orbital nerve, as well as proper positioning of implants posteriorly. Preoperative planning software can also be used for reconstructive procedures to allow for accurate positioning of bone in complex cases and when other stable landmarks are lost. Intraoperative navigation using virtual plans can help with confirmation on bone placement minimizing critical errors.[323,336]

Intraoperative imaging has become standard of care for many orthopedic and vascular procedures while its use for maxillofacial procedures is in its infancy. The literature supports the use of intraoperative CT as a quality assurance measure to identify correct bone positioning in post-traumatic reconstruction.[353,354] More predictable outcomes are noted for orbital floor reconstruction and zygoma repositioning, while further procedure applications are continuing to evolve.

Computer-Assisted Surgery Complications

It should be recognized that while assisting to avoid complications, the technology described in this section does innately have its own potential set of complications that the surgeon should recognize. Templates can provide the surgeon with some difficulties intraoperatively despite their increasing use. In an ideal situation, guides can be used to reposition bone reconstructive segments, but on occasion there may be bony interferences that may limit the perfect adaptation of the graft/flap. An astute surgeon must be cognizant that they be used only as guides and if intraoperative judgment involves any concerns, appropriate measures must be taken to ensure an optimal result (whether it relates to following the template/guide or surgical judgment). For instance, there are guides for osteotomizing fibula flap segments but these may not allow for perfect adaptation of the flap or create unwarranted gaps when positioned into the donor site with a prebent plate. Prebending a plate to a rapid prototyped model is dependent on the accuracy of the scan, the similarity in tumor size as compared to when the scan was first obtained, and the bone graft shape to be able to closely adapt to the plate.[355] In the end, computer guidance can significantly augment surgical technique but should never completely replace clinical judgment.

CONCLUSIONS

It has been said that the best way to manage complications is to avoid them. Considerations that have to be addressed, and which are among those that need be taken into account for each patient, include patient comorbidities, availability of donor sites, body habitus, defect size and location, defect type (bone vs. composite), and recipient site condition. In addition, frank discussion with patients is important as a part of informed consent with the realization that a number of approaches may be feasible, each with specific risks and benefits particular to the patient. Allowing patients to be involved in the decision process is important when a number of options may ultimately lead to similar results. Computer technologies offer one new avenue to attempt to limit a number of the potential complications of bony reconstruction.

There are ample data from the literature in other surgical specialties to support the fact that complications arise from a number of avoidable and unavoidable sources. In addition, the complication rate of each surgeon, surgery, and patient will be unique. Surgeons should utilize procedures they can perform competently in order to optimize the outcome for each patient and monitor their complications in a way that allows for optimization of their techniques.

SUGGESTED READINGS

1. Mukherjee D, and Eagle KA. 2003. "Perioperative cardiac assessment for noncardiac surgery: Eight steps to the best possible outcome." *Circulation* 107: 2771–2774.
2. Fleisher LA, Beckman JA, Brown KA, et al. 2009. "2009 ACCF/AHA focused update on perioperative beta blockade incorporated into the ACC/AHA 2007 guidelines on perioperative cardiovascular evaluation and care for noncardiac surgery." *J Am Coll Cardiol* 54: e13–e118.
3. Schroeder BM. 2002. "Updated guidelines for perioperative cardiovascular evaluation for noncardiac surgery. American College of Cardiology. American Heart Association." *Am Fam Physician* 66: 1096; 1099–1100; 1103–1094 passim.
4. ACC/AHA Task Force Report. 1996. "Special report: Guidelines for perioperative cardiovascular evaluation for noncardiac surgery. Report of the American College of Cardiology/American Heart Association Task Force on practice guidelines (Committee on Perioperative Cardiovascular Evaluation for Noncardiac Surgery)." *J Cardiothorac Vasc Anesth* 10: 540–552.
5. Eagle KA, Brundage BH, Chaitman BR, et al. 1996. "Guidelines for perioperative cardiovascular evaluation for noncardiac surgery. Report of the American College of Cardiology/American Heart Association Task Force on Practice Guidelines (Committee on Perioperative Cardiovascular Evaluation for Noncardiac Surgery)." *J Am Coll Cardiol* 27: 910–948.
6. Napolitano LM, Kurek S, Luchette FA, et al. 2009. "Clinical practice guideline: Red blood cell transfusion in adult trauma and critical care." *J Trauma* 67: 1439–1442.
7. Napolitano LM, Kurek S, Luchette FA, et al. 2009. "Clinical practice guideline: Red blood cell transfusion in adult trauma and critical care." *Crit Care Med* 37: 3124–3157.

8. Taniguchi Y, and Okura M. 2003. "Prognostic significance of perioperative blood transfusion in oral cavity squamous cell carcinoma." *Head Neck* 25: 931–936.

9. Bove JR. 1987. "Transfusion-associated hepatitis and AIDS. What is the risk?" *N Engl J Med* 317: 242–245.

10. Ward JW, Holmberg SD, Allen JR, et al. 1988. "Transmission of human immunodeficiency virus (HIV) by blood transfusions screened as negative for HIV antibody." *N Engl J Med* 318: 473–478.

11. Vamvakas EC, and Blajchman MA. 2007. "Transfusion-related immunomodulation (TRIM): An update." *Blood Rev* 21: 327–348.

12. Blajchman MA. 2005. "Transfusion immunomodulation or TRIM: What does it mean clinically?" *Hematology* 10(Suppl 1): 208–214.

13. Blajchman MA. 2002. "Immunomodulation and blood transfusion." *Am J Ther* 9: 389–395.

14. Bock M, Grevers G, Koblitz M, et al. 1990. "Influence of blood transfusion on recurrence, survival and postoperative infections of laryngeal cancer." *Acta Otolaryngol* 110: 155–160.

15. Von Doersten P, Cruz RM, Selby JV, et al. 1992. "Transfusion, recurrence, and infection in head and neck cancer surgery." *Otolaryngol Head Neck Surg* 106: 60–67.

16. Schuller DE, Scott C, Wilson KM, et al. 1994. "The effect of perioperative blood transfusion on survival in head and neck cancer." *Arch Otolaryngol Head Neck Surg* 120: 711–716.

17. Johnson JT, Taylor FH, and Thearle PB. 1987. "Blood transfusion and outcome in stage III head and neck carcinoma." *Arch Otolaryngol Head Neck Surg* 113: 307–310.

18. Jackson RM, and Rice DH. 1989. "Blood transfusions and recurrence in head and neck cancer." *Ann Otol Rhinol Laryngol* 98: 171–173.

19. Jones KR, and Weissler MC. 1990. "Blood transfusion and other risk factors for recurrence of cancer of the head and neck." *Arch Otolaryngol Head Neck Surg* 116: 304–309.

20. Woolley AL, Hogikyan ND, Gates GA, et al. 1992. "Effect of blood transfusion on recurrence of head and neck carcinoma. Retrospective review and meta-analysis." *Ann Otol Rhinol Laryngol* 101: 724–730.

21. Ell SR, and Stell PM. 1991. "Blood transfusion and survival after laryngectomy for laryngeal carcinoma." *J Laryngol Otol* 105: 293–294.

22. Alun-Jones T, Clarke PJ, Morrissey S, et al. 1991. "Blood transfusion and laryngeal cancer." *Clin Otolaryngol Allied Sci* 16: 240–244.

23. Barra S, Barzan L, Maione A, et al. 1994. "Blood transfusion and other prognostic variables in the survival of patients with cancer of the head and neck." *Laryngoscope* 104: 95–98.

24. McCulloch TM, VanDaele DJ, Hillel A. 1995. "Blood transfusion as a risk factor for death in stage III and IV operative laryngeal cancer. The Department of Veterans Affairs Laryngeal Cancer Study Group." *Arch Otolaryngol Head Neck Surg* 121: 1227–1235.

25. Sturgis EM, Congdon DJ, Mather FJ, et al. 1997. "Perioperative transfusion, postoperative infection, and recurrence of head and neck cancer." *South Med J* 90: 1217–1224.

26. Waymack JP, Fernandes G, Yurt RW, et al. 1990. "Effect of blood transfusions on immune function. Part VI. Effect on immunologic response to tumor." *Surgery* 108: 172–177; discussion 177–178.

27. Waymack JP, and Chance WT. 1988. "Effect of blood transfusions on immune function: IV. Effect on tumor growth." *J Surg Oncol* 39: 159–164.

28. Patel RS, McCluskey SA, Goldstein DP, et al. 2010. "Clinicopathologic and therapeutic risk factors for perioperative complications and prolonged hospital stay in free flap reconstruction of the head and neck." *Head Neck* 32: 1345–1353.

29. De Riu G, Meloni SM, Raho MT, et al. 2008. "Delayed iliac abscess as an unusual complication of an iliac bone graft in an orthognathic case." *Int J Oral Maxillofac Surg* 37: 1156–1158.

30. Sudmann B, Bang G, and Sudmann E. 2006. "Histologically verified bone wax (beeswax) granuloma after median sternotomy in 17 of 18 autopsy cases." *Pathology* 38: 138–141.

31. Anfinsen OG, Sudmann B, Rait M, et al. 1993. "Complications secondary to the use of standard bone wax in seven patients." *J Foot Ankle Surg* 32: 505–508.

32. Sudmann B, Anfinsen OG, Bang G, et al. 1993. "Assessment in rats of a new bioerodible bone-wax-like polymer." *Acta Orthop Scand* 64: 336–339.

33. Solheim E, Pinholt EM, Bang G, et al. 1992. "Effect of local hemostatics on bone induction in rats: A comparative study of bone wax, fibrin-collagen paste, and bioerodible polyorthoester with and without gentamicin." *J Biomed Mater Res* 26: 791–800.

34. Low WK, and Sim CS. 2002. "Bone wax foreign body granuloma in the mastoid." *ORL J Otorhinolaryngol Relat Spec* 64: 38–40.

35. Wolvius EB, van der Wal KG. 2003. "Bone wax as a cause of a foreign body granuloma in a cranial defect: A case report." *Int J Oral Maxillofac Surg* 32: 656–658.

36. Aurelio J, Chenail B, and Gerstein H. 1984. "Foreign-body reaction to bone wax. Report of a case." *Oral Surg Oral Med Oral Pathol* 58: 98–100.

37. Mattsson T, Anderssen K, Koendell PA, et al. 1990. "A longitudinal comparative histometric study of the biocompatibility of three local hemostatic agents." *Int J Oral Maxillofac Surg* 19: 47–50.

38. Loescher AR, and Robinson PP. 1998. "The effect of surgical medicaments on peripheral nerve function." *Br J Oral Maxillofac Surg* 36: 327–332.

39. Alkan A, Inal S, Yildirim M, et al. 2007. "The effects of hemostatic agents on peripheral nerve function: An experimental study." *J Oral Maxillofac Surg* 65: 630–634.

40. Nagamatsu M, Podratz J, Windebank AJ, et al. 1997. "Acidity is involved in the development of neuropathy caused by oxidized cellulose." *J Neurol Sci* 46: 97–102.

41. Nagamatsu M, Low PA. 1995. "Oxidized cellulose causes focal neuropathy, possibly by a diffusible chemical mechanism." *Acta Neuropathol* 90: 282–286.

42. Helfaer MA, Carson BS, James CS, et al. 1998. "Increased hematocrit and decreased transfusion requirements in children given erythropoietin before undergoing craniofacial surgery." *J Neurosurg* 88: 704–708.

43. Pogrel MA, and McDonald A. 1995. "The use of erythropoietin in a patient having major oral and maxillofacial surgery and refusing blood transfusion." *J Oral Maxillofac Surg* 53: 943–945.

44. Genden EM, and Haughey BH. 1996. "Head and neck surgery in the Jehovah's Witness patient." *Otolaryngol Head Neck Surg* 114: 669–672.

45. Natanson C, Kern SJ, Lurie P, et al. 2008. "Cell-free hemoglobin-based blood substitutes and risk of myocardial infarction and death: A meta-analysis." *JAMA* 299: 2304–2312.

46. Van Bokhorst-de van der Schueren MA, van Leeuwen PA, Sauerwein HP, et al. 1997. "Assessment of malnutrition parameters in head and neck cancer and their relation to postoperative complications." *Head Neck* 19: 419–425.

47. Sepehr A, Santos BJ, Chou C, et al. 2009. "Antibiotics in head and neck surgery in the setting of malnutrition, tracheotomy, and diabetes." *Laryngoscope* 119: 549–553.

48. Tang YJ, Sheu WH, Liu PH, et al. 2007. "Positive associations of bone mineral density with body mass index, physical activity, and blood triglyceride level in men over 70 years old: A TCVGHAGE study." *J Bone Miner Metab* 25: 54–59.

49. Wang CS, and Sun CF. 2009. "C-reactive protein and malignancy: Clinico-pathological association and therapeutic implication." *Chang Gung Med J* 32: 471–482.

50. Heikkila K, Ebrahim S, and Lawlor DA. 2007. "A systematic review of the association between circulating concentrations of C reactive protein and cancer." *J Epidemiol Community Health* 61: 824–833.

51. Iizuka T, and Lindqvist C. 1991. "Changes in C-reactive protein associated with surgical treatment of mandibular fractures." *J Oral Maxillofac Surg* 49: 464–467.

52. Khandavilli SD, Ceallaigh PO, Lloyd CJ, et al. 2009. "Serum C-reactive protein as a prognostic indicator in patients with oral squamous cell carcinoma." *Oral Oncol* 45: 912–914.

53. Kudsk KA, Tolley EA, DeWitt RC, et al. 2003. "Preoperative albumin and surgical site identify surgical risk for major postoperative complications." *JPEN J Parenter Enteral Nutr* 27: 1–9.

54. Fang JC, Chirag DN, and Dym H. 2006. "Nutritional aspects of care." *Oral Maxillofac Surg Clin North Am* 18: 115–130; vii.

55. Gibbs J, Cull W, Henderson W, et al. 1999. "Preoperative serum albumin level as a predictor of operative mortality and morbidity: Results from the National VA Surgical Risk Study." *Arch Surg* 134: 36–42.

56. Beck FK, and Rosenthal TC. 2002. "Prealbumin: A marker for nutritional evaluation." *Am Fam Physician* 65: 1575–1578.

57. Schurch MA, Rizzoli R, Slosman D, et al. 1998. "Protein supplements increase serum insulin-like growth factor-I levels and attenuate proximal femur bone loss in patients with recent hip fracture. A randomized, double-blind, placebo-controlled trial." *Ann Intern Med* 128: 801–809.

58. Ruberg RL. 1984. "Role of nutrition in wound healing." *Surg Clin North Am* 64: 705–714.

59. Hernandez G, Velasco N, Wainstein C, et al. 1999. "Gut mucosal atrophy after a short enteral fasting period in critically ill patients." *J Crit Care* 14: 73–77.

60. Kubrak C, Olson K, Jha N, et al. 2010. "Nutrition impact symptoms: Key determinants of reduced dietary intake, weight loss, and reduced functional capacity of patients with head and neck cancer before treatment." *Head Neck* 32: 290–300.

61. Ziccardi VB, Ochs MW, and Braun TW. 1993. "Indications for enteric tube feedings in oral and maxillofacial surgery." *J Oral Maxillofac Surg* 51: 1250–1254.

62. Falender LG, Leban SG, and Williams FA. 1987. "Postoperative nutritional support in oral and maxillofacial surgery." *J Oral Maxillofac Surg* 45: 324–330.

63. Urban KG, and Terris DJ. 1997. "Percutaneous endoscopic gastrostomy by head and neck surgeons." *Otolaryngol Head Neck Surg* 116: 489–492.

64. Koretz RL. 2007. "Do data support nutrition support? Part II. Enteral artificial nutrition." *J Am Diet Assoc* 107: 1374–1380.

65. Koretz RL. 2007. "Do data support nutrition support? Part I: Intravenous nutrition." *J Am Diet Assoc* 107: 988–996; quiz 998.

66. Goodson WH, 3rd, and Hunt TK. 1979. "Wound healing and the diabetic patient." *Surg Gynecol Obstet* 149: 600–608.

67. Devlin H, Garland H, and Sloan P. 1996. "Healing of tooth extraction sockets in experimental diabetes mellitus." *J Oral Maxillofac Surg* 54: 1087–1091.

68. Yoo HK, and Serafin BL. 2006. "Perioperative management of the diabetic patient." *Oral Maxillofac Surg Clin North Am* 18: 255–260; vii.

69. Loder RT. 1988. "The influence of diabetes mellitus on the healing of closed fractures." *Clin Orthop Relat Res* 232: 210–216.

70. Goodman WG, and Hori MT. 1984. "Diminished bone formation in experimental diabetes. Relationship to osteoid maturation and mineralization." *Diabetes* 33: 825–831.

71. Frost HM, and Villanueva AR. 1961. "Human osteoblastic activity. III. The effect of cortisone on lamellar osteoblastic activity." *Henry Ford Hosp Med Bull* 9: 97–99.

72. Hahn TJ, Halstead LR, Teitelbaum SL, et al. 1979. "Altered mineral metabolism in glucocorticoid-induced osteopenia. Effect of 25-hydroxyvitamin D administration." *J Clin Invest* 64: 655–665.

73. Hough S, Avioli LV, Bergfeld MA, et al. 1981. "Correction of abnormal bone and mineral metabolism in chronic streptozotocin-induced diabetes mellitus in the rat by insulin therapy." *Endocrinology* 108: 2228–2234.

74. Levin ME, Boisseau VC, and Avioli LV. 1976. "Effects of diabetes mellitus on bone mass in juvenile and adult-onset diabetes." *N Engl J Med* 294: 241–245.

75. Yano H, Ohya K, and Amagasa T. 1996. "Insulin enhancement of in vitro wound healing in fetal rat parietal bones." *J Oral Maxillofac Surg* 54: 182–186.

76. Schwartz-Arad D, Levin L, and Sigal L. 2005. "Surgical success of intraoral autogenous block onlay bone grafting for alveolar ridge augmentation." *Implant Dent* 14: 131–138.

77. Dan AE, Thygesen TH, and Pinholt EM. 2010. "Corticosteroid administration in oral and orthognathic surgery: A systematic review of the literature and meta-analysis." *J Oral Maxillofac Surg* 68: 2207–2220.

78. Tiwana PS, Foy SP, Shugars DA, et al. 2005. "The impact of intravenous corticosteroids with third molar surgery in patients at high risk for delayed health-related quality of life and clinical recovery." *J Oral Maxillofac Surg* 63: 55–62.

79. Thoren H, Snall J, Kormi E, et al. 2009. "Does perioperative glucocorticosteroid treatment correlate with disturbance in surgical wound healing after treatment of facial fractures? A retrospective study." *J Oral Maxillofac Surg* 67: 1884–1888.

80. Canalis E, Mazziotti G, Giustina A, et al. 2007. "Glucocorticoid-induced osteoporosis: Pathophysiology and therapy." *Osteoporos Int* 18: 1319–1328.

81. Ma L, Zheng LW, Sham MH, et al. 2010. "Effect of nicotine on gene expression of angiogenic and osteogenic factors in a rabbit model of bone regeneration." *J Oral Maxillofac Surg* 68: 777–781.

82. Ma L, Sham MH, Zheng LW, et al. 2011. "Influence of low-dose nicotine on bone healing." *J Trauma* 70: E117–121.

83. Zheng LW, Ma L, and Cheung LK. 2008. "Changes in blood perfusion and bone healing induced by nicotine during distraction osteogenesis." *Bone* 43: 355–361.

84. Haber J, and Kent RL. 1992. "Cigarette smoking in a periodontal practice." *J Periodontol* 63: 100–106.

85. Riebel GD, Boden SD, Whitesides TE, et al. 1995. "The effect of nicotine on incorporation of cancellous bone graft in an animal model." *Spine (Phila Pa 1976)* 20: 2198–2202.

86. Kan JY, Rungcharassaeng K, Lozada JL, et al. 1999. "Effects of smoking on implant success in grafted maxillary sinuses." *J Prosthet Dent* 82: 307–311.

87. Lambert PM, Morris HF, and Ochi S. 2000. "The influence of smoking on 3-year clinical success of osseointegrated dental implants." *Ann Periodontol* 5: 79–89.

88. Lewis VL, Jr., Cook JQ, and Bailey MH. 1990. "Infection following cranial bone grafting—A need for caution?" *Ann Plast Surg* 24: 276–278.

89. Benson PD, Marshall MK, Engelstad ME, et al. 2006. "The use of immediate bone grafting in reconstruction of clinically infected mandibular fractures: Bone grafts in the presence of pus." *J Oral Maxillofac Surg* 64: 122–126.

90. Tolman DE. 1995. "Reconstructive procedures with endosseous implants in grafted bone: A review of the literature." *Int J Oral Maxillofac Implants* 10: 275–294.

91. Misch CM, and Misch CE. 1995. "The repair of localized severe ridge defects for implant placement using mandibular bone grafts." *Implant Dent* 4: 261–267.

92. Adamo AK, and Szal RL. 1979. "Timing, results, and complications of mandibular reconstructive surgery: Report of 32 cases." *J Oral Surg* 37: 755–763.

93. Smolka W, and Iizuka T. 2005. "Surgical reconstruction of maxilla and midface: Clinical outcome and factors relating to postoperative complications." *J Craniomaxillofac Surg* 33: 1–7.

94. van Gemert JT, van Es RJ, Van Cann EM, et al. 2009. "Nonvascularized bone grafts for segmental reconstruction of the mandible—A reappraisal." *J Oral Maxillofac Surg* 67: 1446–1452.

95. Foster RD, Anthony JP, Sharma A, et al. 1999. "Vascularized bone flaps versus nonvascularized bone grafts for mandibular reconstruction: An outcome analysis of primary bony union and endosseous implant success." *Head Neck* 21: 66–71.

96. Pogrel MA, Podlesh S, Anthony JP, et al. 1997. "A comparison of vascularized and nonvascularized bone grafts for reconstruction of mandibular continuity defects." *J Oral Maxillofac Surg* 55: 1200–1206.

97. Garg AK. 1999. "Augmentation grafting of the maxillary sinus for placement of dental implants: Anatomy, physiology, and procedures." *Implant Dent* 8: 36–46.

98. Levin L, Herzberg R, Dolev E, et al. 2004. "Smoking and complications of onlay bone grafts and sinus lift operations." *Int J Oral Maxillofac Implants* 19: 369–373.

99. Raghoebar GM, Batenburg RH, Timmenga NM, et al. 1999. "Morbidity and complications of bone grafting of the floor of the maxillary sinus for the placement of endosseous implants." *Mund Kiefer Gesichtschir* 3(Suppl 1): S65–69.

100. Timmenga NM, Raghoebar GM, Boering G, et al. 1997. "Maxillary sinus function after sinus lifts for the insertion of dental implants." *J Oral Maxillofac Surg* 55: 936–939; discussion 940.

101. Eneroth CM, and Martensson G. 1961. "Closure of antro-alveolar fistulae." *Acta Otolaryngol* 53: 477–485.

102. Holtzclaw D, Toscano N, Eisenlohr L, et al. 2008. "The safety of bone allografts used in dentistry: A review." *J Am Dent Assoc* 139: 1192–1199.

103. Buck BE, Malinin TI, and Brown MD. 1989. "Bone transplantation and human immunodeficiency virus. An estimate of risk of acquired immunodeficiency syndrome (AIDS)." *Clin Orthop Relat Res* 240: 129–136.

104. Khan SN, Cammisa FP, Jr., Sandhu HS, et al. 2005. "The biology of bone grafting." *J Am Acad Orthop Surg* 13: 77–86.

105. Wenz B, Oesch B, and Horst M. 2001. "Analysis of the risk of transmitting bovine spongiform encephalopathy through bone grafts derived from bovine bone." *Biomaterials* 22: 1599–1606.

106. Sogal A, and Tofe AJ. 1999. "Risk assessment of bovine spongiform encephalopathy transmission through bone graft material derived from bovine bone used for dental applications." *J Periodontol* 70: 1053–1063.

107. Shields LB, Raque GH, Glassman SD, et al. 2006. "Adverse effects associated with high-dose recombinant human bone morphogenetic protein-2 use in anterior cervical spine fusion." *Spine (Phila Pa 1976)* 31: 542–547.

108. Smucker JD, Rhee JM, Singh K, et al. 2006. "Increased swelling complications associated with off-label usage of rhBMP-2 in the anterior cervical spine." *Spine (Phila Pa 1976)* 31: 2813–2819.

109. Bell RB, and Gregoire C. 2009. "Reconstruction of mandibular continuity defects using recombinant human bone morphogenetic protein 2: A note of caution in an atmosphere of exuberance." *J Oral Maxillofac Surg* 67: 2673–2678.

110. Bennett M, Reynolds AS, and Dickerman RD. 2006. "Recent article by Shields et al. titled 'Adverse effects associated with high-dose recombinant human bone morphogenetic protein-2 use in anterior cervical spine fusion.'" *Spine (Phila Pa 1976)* 31: 2029–2030.

111. Benglis D, Wang MY, and Levi AD. 2008. "A comprehensive review of the safety profile of bone morphogenetic protein in spine surgery." *Neurosurgery* 62: ONS423–431; discussion ONS431.

112. Herford AS, and Boyne PJ. 2008. "Reconstruction of mandibular continuity defects with bone morphogenetic protein-2 (rhBMP-2)." *J Oral Maxillofac Surg* 66: 616–624.

113. Herford AS. 2009. "rhBMP-2 as an option for reconstructing mandibular continuity defects." *J Oral Maxillofac Surg* 67: 2679–2684.

114. Carter TG, Brar PS, Tolas A, et al. 2008. "Off-label use of recombinant human bone morphogenetic protein-2 (rhBMP-2) for reconstruction of mandibular bone defects in humans." *J Oral Maxillofac Surg* 66: 1417–1425.

115. Clokie CM, and Sandor GK. 2008. "Reconstruction of 10 major mandibular defects using bioimplants containing BMP-7." *J Can Dent Assoc* 74: 67–72.

116. Tumialan LM, Pan J, Rodts GE, et al. 2008. "The safety and efficacy of anterior cervical discectomy and fusion with poly-etheretherketone spacer and recombinant human bone morphogenetic protein-2: A review of 200 patients." *J Neurosurg Spine* 8: 529–535.

117. Misch CM. 1997. "Comparison of intraoral donor sites for onlay grafting prior to implant placement." *Int J Oral Maxillofac Implants* 12: 767–776.

118. Soehardi A, Meijer GJ, Strooband VF, et al. 2009. "The potential of the horizontal ramus of the mandible as a donor site for block and particular grafts in pre-implant surgery." *Int J Oral Maxillofac Surg* 38: 1173–1178.

119. Marx R. 2005. "Bone harvest from the posterior ilium." *Atlas of the Oral and Maxillofacial Surgery Clinics of North America* 13: 109–118.

120. Kessler P, Thorwarth M, Bloch-Birkholz A, et al. 2005. "Harvesting of bone from the iliac crest—Comparison of the anterior and posterior sites." *Br J Oral Maxillofac Surg* 43: 51–56.

121. Tayapongsak P, Wimsatt JA, LaBanc JP, et al. 1994. "Morbidity from anterior ilium bone harvest. A comparative study of lateral versus medial surgical approach." *Oral Surg Oral Med Oral Pathol* 78: 296–300.

122. Marx RE, and Morales MJ. 1988. "Morbidity from bone harvest in major jaw reconstruction: A randomized trial comparing the lateral anterior and posterior approaches to the ilium." *J Oral Maxillofac Surg* 46: 196–203.

123. Nkenke E, Weisbach V, Winckler E, et al. 2004. "Morbidity of harvesting of bone grafts from the iliac crest for preprosthetic augmentation procedures: A prospective study." *Int J Oral Maxillofac Surg* 33: 157–163.

124. Keller EE, and Triplett WW. 1987. "Iliac bone grafting: Review of 160 consecutive cases." *J Oral Maxillofac Surg* 45: 11–14.

125. Canady JW, Zeitler DP, Thompson SA, et al. 1993. "Suitability of the iliac crest as a site for harvest of autogenous bone grafts." *Cleft Palate Craniofac J* 30: 579–581.

126. Wolfe SA, and Kawamoto HK. 1978. "Taking the iliac-bone graft." *J Bone Joint Surg Am* 60: 411.

127. David R, Folman Y, Pikarsky I, et al. 2003. "Harvesting bone graft from the posterior iliac crest by less traumatic, midline approach." *J Spinal Disord Tech* 16: 27–30.

128. Brazaitis MP, Mirvis SE, Greenberg J, et al. 1994. "Severe retroperitoneal hemorrhage complicating anterior iliac bone graft acquisition." *J Oral Maxillofac Surg* 52: 314–316.

129. Mazock JB, Schow SR, and Triplett RG. 2003. "Posterior iliac crest bone harvest: Review of technique, complications, and use of an epidural catheter for postoperative pain control." *J Oral Maxillofac Surg* 61: 1497–1503.

130. Zijderveld S, ten Bruggenkate CM, van Den Bergh JPA, et al. 2004. "Fractures of the iliac crest after split-thickness bone grafting for preprosthetic surgery: Report of 3 cases and review of the literature." *Journal of Oral and Maxillofacial Surgery* 62: 781–786.

131. Coventry MB, and Tapper EM. 1972. "Pelvic instability: A consequence of removing iliac bone for grafting." *J Bone Joint Surg Am* 54: 83–101.

132. Laurie SW, Kaban LB, Mulliken JB, et al. 1984. "Donor-site morbidity after harvesting rib and iliac bone." *Plast Reconstr Surg* 73: 933–938.

133. Korlof B, Nylen B, and Rietz KA. 1973. "Bone grafting of skull defects. A report on 55 cases." *Plast Reconstr Surg* 52: 378–383.

134. Grillon GL, Gunther SF, and Connole PW. 1984. "A new technique for obtaining iliac bone grafts." *J Oral Maxillofac Surg* 42: 172–176.

135. Beirne OR. 1986. "Comparison of complications after bone removal from lateral and medial plates of the anterior ilium for mandibular augmentation." *Int J Oral Maxillofac Surg* 15: 269–272.

136. Cockin J. 1971. "Autologous bone grafting: Complications at the donor site." *J Bone Joint Surg Br* 53: 153.

137. Kinninmonth AW, and Patel P. 1987. "Herniation through a donor site for iliac bone graft." *J R Coll Surg Edinb* 32: 246.

138. James JD, Geist ET, and Gross BD. 1981. "Adynamic ileus as a complication of iliac bone removal: Report of two cases." *J Oral Surg* 39: 289–291.

139. Jackson IT, Helden G, and Marx R. 1986. "Skull bone grafts in maxillofacial and craniofacial surgery." *J Oral Maxillofac Surg* 44: 949–955.

140. Kline RM, Jr., and Wolfe SA. 1995. "Complications associated with the harvesting of cranial bone grafts." *Plast Reconstr Surg* 95: 5–13; discussion 14–20.

141. Pensler J, and McCarthy JG. 1985. "The calvarial donor site: An anatomic study in cadavers." *Plast Reconstr Surg* 75: 648–651.

142. Jackson IT, Adham M, Bite U, et al. Update on cranial bone grafts in craniofacial surgery. *Ann Plast Surg* 1987;18: 37–40.

143. Whitaker LA, Munro IR, Salyer KE, et al. 1979. "Combined report of problems and complications in 793 craniofacial operations." *Plast Reconstr Surg* 64: 198–203.

144. Jackson IT, Smith J, and Mixter RC. 1983. "Nasal bone grafting using split skull grafts." *Ann Plast Surg* 11: 533–540.

145. Petroff MA, Burgess LP, Anonsen CK, et al. 1987. "Cranial bone grafts for post–traumatic facial defects." *Laryngoscope* 97: 1249–1253.

146. Frodel JL, Jr., Marentette LJ, Quatela VC, et al. 1993. "Calvarial bone graft harvest. Techniques, considerations, and morbidity." *Arch Otolaryngol Head Neck Surg* 119: 17–23.

147. Sawin PD, Traynelis VC, and Menezes AH. 1998. "A comparative analysis of fusion rates and donor-site morbidity for autogeneic rib and iliac crest bone grafts in posterior cervical fusions." *J Neurosurg* 88: 255–265.

148. Munro IR, and Guyuron B. 1981. "Split-rib cranioplasty." *Ann Plast Surg* 7: 341–346.

149. Caccamese JF, Jr., Ruiz RL, and Costello BJ. 2005. "Costochondral rib grafting." *Atlas Oral Maxillofac Surg Clin North Am* 13: 139–149.

150. Skouteris CA, and Sotereanos GC. 1989. "Donor site morbidity following harvesting of autogenous rib grafts." *J Oral Maxillofac Surg* 47: 808–812.

151. James DR, and Irvine GH. 1983. "Autogenous rib grafts in maxillofacial surgery." *J Maxillofac Surg* 11: 201–203.

152. Woods WR, Hiatt WR, and Brooks RL. 1979. "A technique for simultaneous fracture repair and augmentation of the atrophic edentulous mandible." *J Oral Surg* 37: 131–135.

153. O'Keeffe RM, Jr., Riemer BL, and Butterfield SL. 1991. "Harvesting of autogenous cancellous bone graft from the proximal tibial metaphysis. A review of 230 cases." *J Orthop Trauma* 5: 469–474.

154. Mazock JB, Schow SR, and Triplett RG. 2004. "Proximal tibia bone harvest: Review of technique, complications, and use in maxillofacial surgery." *Int J Oral Maxillofac Implants* 19: 586–593.

155. Catone GA, Reimer BL, McNeir D, et al. 1991. "Tibial autogenous cancellous bone as an alternative donor site in maxillofacial surgery: A preliminary report." *J Oral Maxillofac Surg* 50: 1258–1263.

156. Chen YC, Chen CH, Chen PL, et al. 2006. "Donor site morbidity after harvesting of proximal tibia bone." *Head Neck* 28: 496–500.

157. Hughes CW, and Revington PJ. 2002. "The proximal tibia donor site in cleft alveolar bone grafting: Experience of 75 consecutive cases." *J Craniomaxillofac Surg* 30: 12–16; discussion 17.

158. Marchena JM, Block MS, and Stover JD. 2002. "Tibial bone harvesting under intravenous sedation: Morbidity and patient experiences." *J Oral Maxillofac Surg* 60: 1151–1154.

159. McCarthy JG, and Zide BM. 1984. "The spectrum of calvarial bone grafting: Introduction of the vascularized calvarial bone flap." *Plast Reconstr Surg* 74: 10–18.

160. Lai A, and Cheney ML. 2000. "Temporoparietal fascial flap in orbital reconstruction." *Arch Facial Plast Surg* 2: 196–201.

161. Parhiscar A, Har-El G, Turk JB, et al. 2002. "Temporoparietal osteofascial flap for head and neck reconstruction." *J Oral Maxillofac Surg* 60: 619–622.

162. Cesteleyn L. 2003. "The temporoparietal galea flap." *Oral Maxillofac Surg Clin North Am* 15: 537–550; vi.

163. Cesteleyn L, Helman J, King S, et al. 2002. "Temporoparietal fascia flaps and superficial musculoaponeurotic system plication in parotid surgery reduces Frey's syndrome." *J Oral Maxillofac Surg* 60: 1284–1297; discussion 1297–1288.

164. Cuono CB, and Ariyan S. 1980. "Immediate reconstruction of a composite mandibular defect with a regional osteomusculocutaneous flap." *Plast Reconstr Surg* 65: 477–484.

165. Kowalik S. 1980. "Reconstruction of mandible with pedicle bone grafts." *Int J Oral Surg* 9: 45–48.

166. Wood MB. 2007. "Free vascularized fibular grafting—25 years' experience: Tips, techniques, and pearls." *Orthop Clin North Am* 38: 1–12; v.

167. Kim D, Orron DE, and Skillman JJ. 1989. "Surgical significance of popliteal arterial variants. A unified angiographic classification." *Ann Surg* 210: 776–781.

168. Ahmad N, Kordestani R, Panchal J, et al. 2007. "The role of donor site angiography before mandibular reconstruction utilizing free flap." *J Reconstr Microsurg* 23: 199–204.

169. Young DM, Trabulsy PP, and Anthony JP. 1994. "The need for preoperative leg angiography in fibula free flaps." *J Reconstr Microsurg* 10: 283–287; discussion 287–289.

170. Fukaya E, Grossman RF, Saloner D, et al. 2007. "Magnetic resonance angiography for free fibula flap transfer." *J Reconstr Microsurg* 23: 205–211.

171. Futran ND, Stack BC, Jr., and Zaccardi MJ. 1998. "Preoperative color flow Doppler imaging for fibula free tissue transfers." *Ann Vasc Surg* 12: 445–450.

172. Kelly AM, Cronin P, Hussain HK, et al. 2007. "Preoperative MR angiography in free fibula flap transfer for head and neck cancer: Clinical application and influence on surgical decision making." *AJR Am J Roentgenol* 188: 268–274.

173. Schusterman MA, Reece GP, Miller MJ, et al. 1992. "The osteocutaneous free fibula flap: Is the skin paddle reliable?" *Plast Reconstr Surg* 90: 787–793; discussion 794–788.

174. Cascarini L, Coombes DM, and Brown AE. 2007. "Minimizing risk to the vascularity of the osteotomized fibula: A technical note." *Int J Oral Maxillofac Surg* 36: 751.

175. Han CS, Wood MB, Bishop AT, et al. 1992. "Vascularized bone transfer. *J Bone Joint Surg Am* 74: 1441–1449.

176. Hidalgo DA, and Pusic AL. 2002. "Free-flap mandibular reconstruction: A 10-year follow-up study." *Plast Reconstr Surg* 110: 438–449; discussion 450–431.

177. Anderson AF, and Green NE. 1991. "Residual functional deficit after partial fibulectomy for bone graft." *Clin Orthop Relat Res* 267: 137–140.

178. Boyd JB, Rosen I, Rotstein L, et al. 1990. "The iliac crest and the radial forearm flap in vascularized oromandibular reconstruction." *Am J Surg* 159: 301–308.

179. Seiler JG, 3rd, and Johnson J. 2000. "Iliac crest autogenous bone grafting: Donor site complications." *J South Orthop Assoc* 9: 91–97.

180. Rogers SN, Lakshmiah SR, Narayan B, et al. 2003. "A comparison of the long-term morbidity following deep circumflex iliac and fibula free flaps for reconstruction following head and neck cancer." *Plast Reconstr Surg* 112: 1517–1525; discussion 1526–1517.

181. Lyons AJ, James R, and Collyer J. 2005. "Free vascularised iliac crest graft: An audit of 26 consecutive cases." *Br J Oral Maxillofac Surg* 43: 210–214.

182. Iqbal M, Lloyd CJ, Paley MD, et al. 2007. "Repair of the deep circumflex iliac artery free flap donor site with Protack (titanium spiral tacks) and Prolene (polypropylene) mesh." *Br J Oral Maxillofac Surg* 45: 596–597.

183. Tan NC, Brennan PA, Senapati A, et al. 2009. "Bowel obstruction following deep circumflex iliac artery free flap harvesting." *Br J Oral Maxillofac Surg* 47: 645–647.

184. Yilmaz M, Vayvada H, Menderes A, et al. 2008. "A comparison of vascularized fibular flap and iliac crest flap for mandibular reconstruction." *J Craniofac Surg* 19: 227–234.

185. Puxeddu R, Ledda GP, Siotto P, et al. 2004. "Free-flap iliac crest in mandibular reconstruction following segmental mandibulectomy for squamous cell carcinoma of the oral cavity." *Eur Arch Otorhinolaryngol* 261: 202–207.

186. Flum DR, Horvath K, and Koepsell T. 2003. "Have outcomes of incisional hernia repair improved with time? A population-based analysis." *Ann Surg* 237: 129–135.

187. Nuckols DA, Tsue TT, Toby EB, et al. 2000. "Preoperative evaluation of the radial forearm free flap patient with the objective Allen's test." *Otolaryngol Head Neck Surg* 123: 553–557.

188. Nunez VA, Pike J, Avery C, et al. 1999. "Prophylactic plating of the donor site of osteocutaneous radial forearm flaps." *Br J Oral Maxillofac Surg* 37: 210–212.

189. Villaret DB, and Futran NA. 2003. "The indications and outcomes in the use of osteocutaneous radial forearm free flap." *Head Neck* 25: 475–481.

190. Kim JH, Rosenthal EL, Ellis T, et al. 2005. "Radial forearm osteocutaneous free flap in maxillofacial and oromandibular reconstructions." *Laryngoscope* 115: 1697–1701.

191. Bardsley AF, Soutar DS, Elliot D, et al. 1990. "Reducing morbidity in the radial forearm flap donor site." *Plast Reconstr Surg* 86: 287–292; discussion 293–284.

192. Smith AA, Bowen CV, Rabczak T, et al. 1994. "Donor site deficit of the osteocutaneous radial forearm flap." *Ann Plast Surg* 32: 372–376.

193. Swanson E, Boyd JB, and Manktelow RT. 1990. "The radial forearm flap: Reconstructive applications and donor-site defects in 35 consecutive patients." *Plast Reconstr Surg* 85: 258–266.

194. Inglefield CJ, and Kolhe PS. 1994. "Fracture of the radial forearm osteocutaneous donor site." *Ann Plast Surg* 33: 638–642; discussion 643.

195. Germann G, Bickert B, Steinau HU, et al. 1999. "Versatility and reliability of combined flaps of the subscapular system." *Plast Reconstr Surg* 103: 1386–1399.

196. Nkenke E, Vairaktaris E, Stelzle F, et al. 2009. "Osteocutaneous free flap including medial and lateral scapular crests: Technical aspects, viability, and donor site morbidity." *J Reconstr Microsurg* 25: 545–553.

197. Norholt SE, Jensen J, Schou S, et al. 2011. "Complications after mandibular distraction osteogenesis: A retrospective study of 131 patients." *Oral Surg Oral Med Oral Pathol Oral Radiol Endod* 111: 420–427.

198. Shetye PR, Warren SM, Brown D, et al. 2009. "Documentation of the incidents associated with mandibular distraction: Introduction of a new stratification system." *Plast Reconstr Surg* 123: 627–634.

199. Enislidis G, Fock N, Millesi-Schobel G, et al. 2005. "Analysis of complications following alveolar distraction osteogenesis and implant placement in the partially edentulous mandible." *Oral Surg Oral Med Oral Pathol Oral Radiol Endod* 100: 25–30.

200. Perdijk FB, Meijer GJ, Strijen PJ, et al. 2007. "Complications in alveolar distraction osteogenesis of the atrophic mandible." *Int J Oral Maxillofac Surg* 36: 916–921.

201. Wolvius EB, Scholtemeijer M, Weijland M, et al. 2007. "Complications and relapse in alveolar distraction osteogenesis in partially dentulous patients." *Int J Oral Maxillofac Surg* 36: 700–705.

202. Gonzalez-Garcia R, and Naval-Gias L. 2010. "Transport osteogenesis in the maxillofacial skeleton: Outcomes of a versatile reconstruction method following tumor ablation." *Arch Otolaryngol Head Neck Surg* 136: 243–250.

203. Hibi H, and Ueda M. 2011. "Supraperiosteal transport distraction osteogenesis for reconstructing a segmental defect of the mandible." *J Oral Maxillofac Surg* 69: 742–746.

204. Gonzalez-Garcia R, Rodriguez-Campo FJ, Naval-Gias L, et al. 2007. "The effect of radiation in distraction osteogenesis for reconstruction of mandibular segmental defects." *Br J Oral Maxillofac Surg* 45: 314–316.

205. Ettl T, Gerlach T, Schusselbauer T, et al. 2010. "Bone resorption and complications in alveolar distraction osteogenesis." *Clin Oral Investig* 14: 481–489.

206. Shetye PR, Giannoutsos E, Grayson BH, et al. 2009. "Le Fort III distraction: Part I. Controlling position and vectors of the midface segment." *Plast Reconstr Surg* 124: 871–878.

207. McCarthy JG, Stelnicki EJ, and Grayson BH. 1999. "Distraction osteogenesis of the mandible: A ten-year experience." *Semin Orthod* 5: 3–8.

208. Poukens J, Haex J, and Riediger D. 2003. "The use of rapid prototyping in the preoperative planning of distraction osteogenesis of the cranio-maxillofacial skeleton." *Comput Aided Surg* 8: 146–154.

209. Hurmerinta K, and Hukki J. 2001. "Vector control in lower jaw distraction osteogenesis using an extra-oral multidirectional device." *J Craniomaxillofac Surg* 29: 263–270.

210. Edwards SP. 2010. "Computer-assisted craniomaxillofacial surgery." *Oral Maxillofac Surg Clin North Am* 22: 117–134.

211. Gateno J, Teichgraeber JF, and Aguilar E. 2000. "Distraction osteogenesis: A new surgical technique for use with the multiplanar mandibular distractor." *Plast Reconstr Surg* 105: 883–888.

212. Marx RE, Johnson RP, Kline SN. 1985. "Prevention of osteoradionecrosis: A randomized prospective clinical trial of hyperbaric oxygen versus penicillin." *J Am Dent Assoc* 111: 49–54.

213. Myers RA, and Marx RE. 1990. "Use of hyperbaric oxygen in postradiation head and neck surgery." *NCI Monogr* 9: 151–157.

214. Aitasalo K, Niinikoski J, Grenman R, et al. 1998. "A modified protocol for early treatment of osteomyelitis and osteoradionecrosis of the mandible." *Head Neck* 20: 411–417.

215. Hart GB, and Mainous EG. 1976. "The treatment of radiation necrosis with hyperbaric oxygen (OHP)." *Cancer* 37: 2580–2585.

216. Hao SP, Chen HC, Wei FC, et al. 1999. "Systematic management of osteoradionecrosis in the head and neck." *Laryngoscope* 109: 1324–1327; discussion 1327–1328.

217. Mounsey RA, Brown DH, O'Dwyer TP, et al. 1993. "Role of hyperbaric oxygen therapy in the management of mandibular osteoradionecrosis." *Laryngoscope* 103: 605–608.

218. Annane D, Depondt J, Aubert P, et al. 2004. "Hyperbaric oxygen therapy for radionecrosis of the jaw: A randomized, placebo-controlled, double-blind trial from the ORN96 study group." *J Clin Oncol* 22: 4893–4900.

219. Chang DW, Oh HK, Robb GL, et al. 2001. "Management of advanced mandibular osteoradionecrosis with free flap reconstruction." *Head Neck* 23: 830–835.

220. Hirsch DL, Bell RB, Dierks EJ, et al. 2008. "Analysis of microvascular free flaps for reconstruction of advanced mandibular osteoradionecrosis: A retrospective cohort study." *J Oral Maxillofac Surg* 66: 2545–2556.

221. Curi MM, Oliveira dos Santos M, Feher O, et al. 2007. "Management of extensive osteoradionecrosis of the mandible with radical resection and immediate microvascular reconstruction." *J Oral Maxillofac Surg* 65: 434–438.

222. Gal TJ, Yueh B, and Futran ND. 2003. "Influence of prior hyperbaric oxygen therapy in complications following microvascular reconstruction for advanced osteoradionecrosis." *Arch Otolaryngol Head Neck Surg* 129: 72–76.

223. Coskunfirat OK, Wei FC, Huang WC, et al. 2005. "Microvascular free tissue transfer for treatment of osteoradionecrosis of the maxilla." *Plast Reconstr Surg* 115: 54–60.

224. Sandel HDt, and Davison SP. 2007. "Microsurgical reconstruction for radiation necrosis: An evolving disease." *J Reconstr Microsurg* 23: 225–230.

225. Suh JD, Blackwell KE, Sercarz JA, et al. 2010. "Disease relapse after segmental resection and free flap reconstruction for mandibular osteoradionecrosis." *Otolaryngol Head Neck Surg* 142: 586–591.

226. Cannady SB, Dean N, Kroeker A, et al. 2011. "Free flap reconstruction for osteoradionecrosis of the jaws—Outcomes and predictive factors for success." *Head Neck* 33: 424–428.

227. Tibbles PM, and Edelsberg JS. 1996. "Hyperbaric–oxygen therapy." *N Engl J Med* 334: 1642–1648.

228. Ambiru S, Furuyama N, Aono M, et al. 2008. "Analysis of risk factors associated with complications of hyperbaric oxygen therapy." *J Crit Care* 23: 295–300.

229. Freiberger JJ, and Feldmeier JJ. 2010. "Evidence supporting the use of hyperbaric oxygen in the treatment of osteoradionecrosis of the jaw." *J Oral Maxillofac Surg* 68: 1903–1906.

230. Bessereau J, and Annane D. 2010. "Treatment of osteoradionecrosis of the jaw: The case against the use of hyperbaric oxygen." *J Oral Maxillofac Surg* 68: 1907–1910.

231. Klotch DW, Gal TJ, and Gal RL. 1999. "Assessment of plate use for mandibular reconstruction: Has changing technology made a difference?" *Otolaryngol Head Neck Surg* 121: 388–392.

232. Dechow PC, Ellis E, 3rd, and Throckmorton GS. 1995. "Structural properties of mandibular bone following application of a bone plate." *J Oral Maxillofac Surg* 53: 1044–1051.

233. Throckmorton GS, Ellis E, 3rd, Winkler AJ, et al. 1992. "Bone strain following application of a rigid bone plate: An in vitro study in human mandibles." *J Oral Maxillofac Surg* 50: 1066–1073; discussion 1073–1064.

234. Zoumalan RA, Hirsch DL, Levine JP, et al. 2009. "Plating in microvascular reconstruction of the mandible: Can fixation be too rigid?" *J Craniofac Surg* 20: 1451–1454.

235. Chiodo TA, Ziccardi VB, Janal M, et al. 2006. "Failure strength of 2.0 locking versus 2.0 conventional Synthes mandibular plates: A laboratory model." *J Oral Maxillofac Surg* 64: 1475–1479.

236. Collins CP, Pirinjian-Leonard G, Tolas A, et al. 2004. "A prospective randomized clinical trial comparing 2.0-mm locking plates to 2.0-mm standard plates in treatment of mandible fractures." *J Oral Maxillofac Surg* 62: 1392–1395.

237. Doty JM, Pienkowski D, Goltz M, et al. 2004. "Biomechanical evaluation of fixation techniques for bridging segmental mandibular defects." *Arch Otolaryngol Head Neck Surg* 130: 1388–1392.
238. Gellrich NC, Suarez-Cunqueiro MM, Otero-Cepeda XL, et al. 2004. "Comparative study of locking plates in mandibular reconstruction after ablative tumor surgery: THORP versus UniLOCK system." *J Oral Maxillofac Surg* 62: 186–193.
239. Haug RH, Fattahi TT, and Goltz M. 2001. "A biomechanical evaluation of mandibular angle fracture plating techniques." *J Oral Maxillofac Surg* 59: 1199–1210.
240. Haug RH, Peterson GP, and Goltz M. 2002. "A biomechanical evaluation of mandibular condyle fracture plating techniques." *J Oral Maxillofac Surg* 60: 73–80; discussion 80–71.
241. Haug RH, Street CC, and Goltz M. 2002. "Does plate adaptation affect stability? A biomechanical comparison of locking and nonlocking plates." *J Oral Maxillofac Surg* 60: 1319–1326.
242. Madsen MJ, and Haug RH. 2006. "A biomechanical comparison of 2 techniques for reconstructing atrophic edentulous mandible fractures." *J Oral Maxillofac Surg* 64: 457–465.
243. Madsen MJ, McDaniel CA, and Haug RH. 2008. "A biomechanical evaluation of plating techniques used for reconstructing mandibular symphysis/parasymphysis fractures." *J Oral Maxillofac Surg* 66: 2012–2019.
244. Schupp W, Arzdorf M, Linke B, et al. 2007. "Biomechanical testing of different osteosynthesis systems for segmental resection of the mandible." *J Oral Maxillofac Surg* 65: 924–930.
245. Soderholm AL, Rahn BA, Skutnabb K, et al. 1996. "Fixation with reconstruction plates under critical conditions: The role of screw characteristics." *Int J Oral Maxillofac Surg* 25: 469–473.
246. Blackwell KE, and Lacombe V. 1999. "The bridging lateral mandibular reconstruction plate revisited." *Arch Otolaryngol Head Neck Surg* 125: 988–993.
247. Boyd JB. 1994. "Use of reconstruction plates in conjunction with soft-tissue free flaps for oromandibular reconstruction." *Clin Plast Surg* 21: 69–77.
248. Boyd JB, Mulholland RS, Davidson J, et al. 1995. "The free flap and plate in oromandibular reconstruction: Long-term review and indications." *Plast Reconstr Surg* 95: 1018–1028.
249. Davidson J, Boyd B, Gullane P, et al. 1991. "A comparison of the results following oromandibular reconstruction using a radial forearm flap with either radial bone or a reconstruction plate." *Plast Reconstr Surg* 88: 201–208.
250. Head C, Alam D, Sercarz JA, et al. 2003. "Microvascular flap reconstruction of the mandible: A comparison of bone grafts and bridging plates for restoration of mandibular continuity." *Otolaryngol Head Neck Surg* 129: 48–54.
251. Alonso del Hoyo J, Fernandez Sanroman J, Rubio Bueno P, et al. 1994. "Primary mandibular reconstruction with bridging plates." *J Craniomaxillofac Surg* 22: 43–48.
252. Pogrel MA. 2010. "Who was Andy Gump?" *J Oral Maxillofac Surg* 68: 654–657.
253. Steckler RM, Edgerton MT, and Gogel W. 1974. "Andy Gump." *Am J Surg* 128: 545–547.
254. Hannam AG, Stavness IK, Lloyd JE, et al. 2010. "A comparison of simulated jaw dynamics in models of segmental mandibular resection versus resection with alloplastic reconstruction." *J Prosthet Dent* 104: 191–198.
255. Hidalgo DA. 1989. "Titanium miniplate fixation in free flap mandible reconstruction." *Ann Plast Surg* 23: 498–507.
256. Robey AB, Spann ML, McAuliff TM, et al. 2008. "Comparison of miniplates and reconstruction plates in fibular flap reconstruction of the mandible." *Plast Reconstr Surg* 122: 1733–1738.
257. Futran ND, Urken ML, Buchbinder D, et al. 1995. "Rigid fixation of vascularized bone grafts in mandibular reconstruction." *Arch Otolaryngol Head Neck Surg* 121: 70–76.
258. Knott PD, Suh JD, Nabili V, et al. 2007. "Evaluation of hardware-related complications in vascularized bone grafts with locking mandibular reconstruction plate fixation." *Arch Otolaryngol Head Neck Surg* 133: 1302–1306.
259. Farwell DG, Kezirian EJ, Heydt JL, et al. 2006. "Efficacy of small reconstruction plates in vascularized bone graft mandibular reconstruction." *Head Neck* 28: 573–579.
260. Eppley BL. 2005. "Use of resorbable plates and screws in pediatric facial fractures." *J Oral Maxillofac Surg* 63: 385–391.
261. Burger BW. 2010. "Use of ultrasound-activated resorbable poly-D-L-lactide pins (SonicPins) and foil panels (Resorb-X) for horizontal bone augmentation of the maxillary and mandibular alveolar ridges." *J Oral Maxillofac Surg* 68: 1656–1661.
262. Quereshy FA, Dhaliwal HS, El SA, et al. 2010. "Resorbable screw fixation for cortical onlay bone grafting: A pilot study with preliminary results." *J Oral Maxillofac Surg* 68: 2497–2502.
263. Chacon GE, Ellis JP, Kalmar JR, et al. 2004. "Using resorbable screws for fixation of cortical onlay bone grafts: An in vivo study in rabbits." *J Oral Maxillofac Surg* 62: 1396–1402.
264. Ricalde P, Caccamese J, Norby C, et al. 2008. "Strength analysis of 6 resorbable implant systems: Does heating affect the stress-strain curve?" *J Oral Maxillofac Surg* 66: 2493–2497.
265. Reichwein A, Schicho K, Moser D, et al. 2009. "Clinical experiences with resorbable ultrasonic-guided, angle-stable osteosynthesis in the panfacial region." *J Oral Maxillofac Surg* 67: 1211–1217.
266. Nocini PF, Saia G, Bettini G, et al. 2009. "Vascularized fibula flap reconstruction of the mandible in bisphosphonate-related osteonecrosis." *Eur J Surg Oncol* 35: 373–379.
267. Futran ND. 2009. "Maxillofacial trauma reconstruction." *Facial Plast Surg Clin North Am* 17: 239–251.
268. Engroff SL, and Kim DD. 2007. "Treating bisphosphonate osteonecrosis of the jaws: Is there a role for resection and vascularized reconstruction?" *J Oral Maxillofac Surg* 65: 2374–2385.
269. Patel V, McLeod NM, Rogers SN, et al. 2011. "Bisphosphonate osteonecrosis of the jaw—A literature review of UK policies versus international policies on bisphosphonates, risk factors and prevention." *Br J Oral Maxillofac Surg* 49: 251–257.
270. Khan AA, Sandor GK, Dore E, et al. 2008. "Canadian consensus practice guidelines for bisphosphonate associated osteonecrosis of the jaw." *J Rheumatol* 35: 1391–1397.

271. Slough CM, Woo BM, Ueeck BA, et al. 2008. "Fibular free flaps in the management of osteomyelitis of the mandible." *Head Neck* 30: 1531–1534.

272. Chepeha DB, Khariwala SS, Chanowski EJ, et al. 2010. "Thoracodorsal artery scapular tip autogenous transplant: vascularized bone with a long pedicle and flexible soft tissue." *Arch Otolaryngol Head Neck Surg* 136: 958–964.

273. Iseli TA, Yelverton JC, Iseli CE, et al. 2009. "Functional outcomes following secondary free flap reconstruction of the head and neck." *Laryngoscope* 119: 856–860.

274. Buchbinder D, and St Hilaire H. 2006. "The use of free tissue transfer in advanced osteoradionecrosis of the mandible." *J Oral Maxillofac Surg* 64: 961–964.

275. Mehra P, Van Heukelom E, and Cottrell DA. 2009. "Rigid internal fixation of infected mandibular fractures." *J Oral Maxillofac Surg* 67: 1046–1051.

276. Koury ME, Perrott DH, and Kaban LB. 1994. "The use of rigid internal fixation in mandibular fractures complicated by osteomyelitis." *J Oral Maxillofac Surg* 52: 1114–1119.

277. Koury M, and Ellis E, 3rd. 1992. "Rigid internal fixation for the treatment of infected mandibular fractures." *J Oral Maxillofac Surg* 50: 434–443; discussion 443–434.

278. Otto S, Abu-Id MH, Fedele S, et al. 2010. "Osteoporosis and bisphosphonates-related osteonecrosis of the jaw: Not just a sporadic coincidence—A multi-centre study." *J Craniomaxillofac Surg* 39: 272–277.

279. Ruggiero SL, Dodson TB, Assael LA, et al. 2009. "American Association of Oral and Maxillofacial Surgeons position paper on bisphosphonate-related osteonecrosis of the jaw—2009 update." *Aust Endod J* 35: 119–130.

280. Pautke C, Bauer F, Tischer T, et al. 2009. "Fluorescence-guided bone resection in bisphosphonate-associated osteonecrosis of the jaws." *J Oral Maxillofac Surg* 67: 471–476.

281. Patel RS, McCluskey SA, Goldstein DP, et al. 2010. "Clinicopathologic and therapeutic risk factors for perioperative complications and prolonged hospital stay in free flap reconstruction of the head and neck." *Head Neck* 32: 1345–1353.

282. Shaari CM, Buchbinder D, Costantino PD, et al. 1998. "Complications of microvascular head and neck surgery in the elderly." *Arch Otolaryngol Head Neck Surg* 124: 407–411.

283. Bak M, Jacobson AS, Buchbinder D, et al. 2010. "Contemporary reconstruction of the mandible." *Oral Oncol* 46: 71–76.

284. Wolff KD, Holzle F, and Eufinger H. 2003. "The radial forearm flap as a carrier for the osteocutaneous fibula graft in mandibular reconstruction." *Int J Oral Maxillofac Surg* 32: 614–618.

285. Morrison A, and Brady J. 2010. "Mandibular reconstruction using nonvascularized autogenous bone grafting." *Curr Opin Otolaryngol Head Neck Surg* 18: 227–231.

286. Lawson W, and Biller HF. 1982. "Mandibular reconstruction: Bone graft techniques." *Otolaryngol Head Neck Surg* 90: 589–594.

287. Carlson ER, Marx RE. 1996. "Part II. Mandibular reconstruction using cancellous cellular bone grafts." *J Oral Maxillofac Surg* 54: 889–897.

288. Marx RE, Snyder RM, and Kline SN. 1979. "Cellular survival of human marrow during placement of marrow-cancellous bone grafts." *J Oral Surg* 37: 712–718.

289. Zenn MR, Hidalgo DA, Cordeiro PG, et al. 1997. "Current role of the radial forearm free flap in mandibular reconstruction." *Plast Reconstr Surg* 99: 1012–1017.

290. Takushima A, Harii K, Asato H, et al. 2001. "Mandibular reconstruction using microvascular free flaps: A statistical analysis of 178 cases." *Plast Reconstr Surg* 108: 1555–1563.

291. Kroll SS, Robb GL, Miller MJ, et al. 1998. "Reconstruction of posterior mandibular defects with soft tissue using the rectus abdominis free flap." *Br J Plast Surg* 51: 503–507.

292. Hanasono MM, Zevallos JP, Skoracki RJ, et al. 2010. "A prospective analysis of bony versus soft-tissue reconstruction for posterior mandibular defects." *Plast Reconstr Surg* 125: 1413–1421.

293. Alvi A, and Myers EN. 1996. "Skin graft reconstruction of the composite resection defect." *Head Neck* 18: 538–543; discussion 543–534.

294. Iino M, Fukuda M, Nagai H, et al. 2009. "Evaluation of 15 mandibular reconstructions with Dumbach Titan Mesh-System and particulate cancellous bone and marrow harvested from bilateral posterior ilia." *Oral Surg Oral Med Oral Pathol Oral Radiol Endod* 107: e1–8.

295. Potter JK, and Dierks EJ. 2008. "Vascularized options for reconstruction of the mandibular condyle." *Semin Plast Surg* 22: 156–160.

296. Tang W, Long J, Feng F, et al. 2009. "Condyle replacement after tumor resection: Comparison of individual prefabricated titanium implants and costochondral grafts." *Oral Surg Oral Med Oral Pathol Oral Radiol Endod* 108: 147–152.

297. Nahabedian MY, Tufaro A, and Manson PN. 2001. "Improved mandible function after hemimandibulectomy, condylar head preservation, and vascularized fibular reconstruction." *Ann Plast Surg* 46: 506–510.

298. Guyot L, Richard O, Layoun W, et al. 2004. "Long–term radiological findings following reconstruction of the condyle with fibular free flaps." *J Craniomaxillofac Surg* 32: 98–102.

299. Engroff SL. 2005. "Fibula flap reconstruction of the condyle in disarticulation resections of the mandible: A case report and review of the technique." *Oral Surg Oral Med Oral Pathol Oral Radiol Endod* 100: 661–665.

300. Khariwala SS, Chan J, Blackwell KE, et al. 2007. "Temporomandibular joint reconstruction using a vascularized bone graft with Alloderm." *J Reconstr Microsurg* 23: 25–30.

301. Gonzalez-Garcia R, Naval-Gias L, Rodriguez-Campo FJ, et al. 2008. "Vascularized fibular flap for reconstruction of the condyle after mandibular ablation." *J Oral Maxillofac Surg* 66: 1133–1137.

302. Gonzalez-Garcia R, Naval-Gias L, Rodriguez-Campo FJ, et al. 2007. "Predictability of the fibular flap for the reconstruction of the condyle following mandibular ablation." *Br J Oral Maxillofac Surg* 45: 253.

303. Petruzzelli GJ, Cunningham K, and Vandevender D. 2007. "Impact of mandibular condyle preservation on patterns of failure in head and neck cancer." *Otolaryngol Head Neck Surg* 137: 717–721.

304. Infante-Cossio P, Torres-Lagares D, Martinez-de-Fuentes R, et al. 2006. "Dental restoration with endosseous implants after mandibular reconstruction using a fibula free flap and TMJ prosthesis: A patient report." *Int J Oral Maxillofac Implants* 21: 481–485.

305. Mercuri LG, and Swift JQ. 2009. "Considerations for the use of alloplastic temporomandibular joint replacement in the growing patient." *J Oral Maxillofac Surg* 67: 1979–1990.

306. Wolford LM, Dingwerth DJ, Talwar RM, et al. 2003. "Comparison of 2 temporomandibular joint total joint prosthesis systems. *J Oral Maxillofac Surg* 61: 685–690; discussion 690.

307. Mercuri LG, Edibam NR, and Giobbie-Hurder A. 2007. "Fourteen-year follow-up of a patient-fitted total temporomandibular joint reconstruction system." *J Oral Maxillofac Surg* 65: 1140–1148.

308. Westermark A, Koppel D, and Leiggener C. 2006. "Condylar replacement alone is not sufficient for prosthetic reconstruction of the temporomandibular joint." *Int J Oral Maxillofac Surg* 35: 488–492.

309. Moreno MA, Skoracki RJ, Hanna EY, et al. 2010. "Microvascular free flap reconstruction versus palatal obturation for maxillectomy defects." *Head Neck* 32: 860–868.

310. Irish J, Sandhu N, Simpson C, et al. 2009. "Quality of life in patients with maxillectomy prostheses." *Head Neck* 31: 813–821.

311. Kermer C, Poeschl PW, Wutzl A, et al. 2008. "Surgical treatment of squamous cell carcinoma of the maxilla and nasal sinuses." *J Oral Maxillofac Surg* 66: 2449–2453.

312. Eckardt A, Teltzrow T, Schulze A, et al. 2007. "Nasalance in patients with maxillary defects—Reconstruction versus obturation." *J Craniomaxillofac Surg* 35: 241–245.

313. Schmidt BL, Pogrel MA, Young CW, et al. 2004. "Reconstruction of extensive maxillary defects using zygomaticus implants." *J Oral Maxillofac Surg* 62: 82–89.

314. Arce K. 2007. "Buccal fat pad in maxillary reconstruction." *Atlas Oral Maxillofac Surg Clin North Am* 15: 23–32.

315. Cheung LK, Samman N, and Tideman H. 1994. "Reconstructive options for maxillary defects." *Ann R Australas Coll Dent Surg* 12: 244–251.

316. Fernandes R. 2007. "Reconstruction of maxillary defects with the radial forearm free flap." *Atlas Oral Maxillofac Surg Clin North Am* 15: 7–12.

317. Triana RJ, Jr., Uglesic V, Virag M, et al. 2000. "Microvascular free flap reconstructive options in patients with partial and total maxillectomy defects." *Arch Facial Plast Surg* 2: 91–101.

318. Brown JS, and Shaw RJ. 2010. "Reconstruction of the maxilla and midface: Introducing a new classification." *Lancet Oncol* 11: 1001–1008.

319. Valentini V, Gennaro P, Torroni A, et al. 2009. "Scapula free flap for complex maxillofacial reconstruction." *J Craniofac Surg* 20: 1125–1131.

320. Clark JR, Vesely M, and Gilbert R. 2008. "Scapular angle osteomyogenous flap in postmaxillectomy reconstruction: Defect, reconstruction, shoulder function, and harvest technique." *Head Neck* 30: 10–20.

321. Cohen A, Laviv A, Berman P, et al. 2009. "Mandibular reconstruction using stereolithographic 3-dimensional printing modeling technology." *Oral Surg Oral Med Oral Pathol Oral Radiol Endod* 108: 661–666.

322. Chow LK, and Cheung LK. 2007. "The usefulness of stereomodels in maxillofacial surgical management." *J Oral Maxillofac Surg* 65: 2260–2268.

323. Bell RB, Weimer KA, Dierks EJ, et al. 2011. "Computer planning and intraoperative navigation for palatomaxillary and mandibular reconstruction with fibular free flaps." *J Oral Maxillofac Surg* 69: 724–732.

324. Xia JJ, Phillips CV, Gateno J, et al. 2006. "Cost–effectiveness analysis for computer–aided surgical simulation in complex cranio–maxillofacial surgery." *J Oral Maxillofac Surg* 64: 1780–1784.

325. Juergens P, Krol Z, Zeilhofer HF, et al. 2009. "Computer simulation and rapid prototyping for the reconstruction of the mandible." *J Oral Maxillofac Surg* 67: 2167–2170.

326. Hirsch DL, Garfein ES, Christensen AM, et al. 2009. "Use of computer-aided design and computer-aided manufacturing to produce orthognathically ideal surgical outcomes: A paradigm shift in head and neck reconstruction." *J Oral Maxillofac Surg* 67: 2115–2122.

327. Leiggener C, Messo E, Thor A, et al. 2009. "A selective laser sintering guide for transferring a virtual plan to real time surgery in composite mandibular reconstruction with free fibula osseous flaps." *Int J Oral Maxillofac Surg* 38: 187–192.

328. Bell RB, and Markiewicz MR. 2009. "Computer-assisted planning, stereolithographic modeling, and intraoperative navigation for complex orbital reconstruction: A descriptive study in a preliminary cohort." *J Oral Maxillofac Surg* 67: 2559–2570.

329. Bell RB. 2010. "Computer planning and intraoperative navigation in cranio-maxillofacial surgery." *Oral Maxillofac Surg Clin North Am* 22: 135–156.

330. Varol A, and Basa S. 2009. "The role of computer-aided 3D surgery and stereolithographic modelling for vector orientation in premaxillary and trans-sinusoidal maxillary distraction osteogenesis." *Int J Med Robot* 5: 198–206.

331. Gateno J, Xia JJ, Teichgraeber JF, et al. 2007. "Clinical feasibility of computer-aided surgical simulation (CASS) in the treatment of complex cranio-maxillofacial deformities." *J Oral Maxillofac Surg* 65: 728–734.

332. Jayaratne YS, Zwahlen RA, Lo J, et al. 2010. "Computer-aided maxillofacial surgery: An update." *Surg Innov* 17: 217–225.

333. Orentlicher G, Goldsmith D, and Horowitz A. 2010. "Applications of 3-dimensional virtual computerized tomography technology in oral and maxillofacial surgery: Current therapy." *J Oral Maxillofac Surg* 68: 1933–1959.

334. Lubbers HT, Obwegeser JA, Matthews F, et al. 2011. "A simple and flexible concept for computer-navigated surgery of the mandible." *J Oral Maxillofac Surg* 69: 924–930.

335. Farina R, Plaza C, and Martinovic G. 2009. "New transference technique of position of mandibular reconstructing plates using stereolithographic models." *J Oral Maxillofac Surg* 67: 2544–2548.

336. Xia JJ, Gateno J, and Teichgraeber JF. 2009. "A new paradigm for complex midface reconstruction: A reversed approach." *J Oral Maxillofac Surg* 67: 693–703.

337. Ludlow JB, and Ivanovic M. 2008. "Comparative dosimetry of dental CBCT devices and 64–slice CT for oral and maxillofacial radiology." *Oral Surg Oral Med Oral Pathol Oral Radiol Endod* 106: 106–114.

338. Suomalainen A, Kiljunen T, Kaser Y, et al. 2009. "Dosimetry and image quality of four dental cone beam computed tomography scanners compared with multislice computed tomography scanners." *Dentomaxillofac Radiol* 38: 367–378.

339. Schutyser F, and van Cleynenbreugel J. 2009. "From 3-D volumetric computer tomography to 3-D cephalometry." In: *Three-Dimensional Cephalometry: A Color Atlas and Manual*, Swennen GRJ, Schutyser F, and Hausamen J-E, eds., 2–11. Berlin: Springer.

340. Cavalcanti MG, Santos DT, Perrella A, et al. 2004. "CT-based analysis of malignant tumor volume and localization. A preliminary study." *Braz Oral Res* 18: 338–344.

341. Schon R, Metzger MC, Weyer N, et al. 2007. "Microplate osteosynthesis of orbital floor fractures." *Br J Oral Maxillofac Surg* 45: 165.

342. Jaquiery C, Aeppli C, Cornelius P, et al. 2007. "Reconstruction of orbital wall defects: Critical review of 72 patients." *Int J Oral Maxillofac Surg* 36: 193–199.

343. Rohner D, Hutmacher DW, Cheng TK, et al. 2003. "In vivo efficacy of bone-marrow-coated polycaprolactone scaffolds for the reconstruction of orbital defects in the pig." *J Biomed Mater Res B Appl Biomater* 66: 574–580.

344. Gellrich NC, Schramm A, Hammer B, et al. 2002. "Computer-assisted secondary reconstruction of unilateral posttraumatic orbital deformity." *Plast Reconstr Surg* 110: 1417–1429.

345. Hammer B, Kunz C, Schramm A, et al. 1999. "Repair of complex orbital fractures: Technical problems, state-of-the-art solutions and future perspectives." *Ann Acad Med Singapore* 28: 687–691.

346. Hammer B, and Prein J. 1995. "Correction of post-traumatic orbital deformities: Operative techniques and review of 26 patients." *J Craniomaxillofac Surg* 23: 81–90.

347. Metzger MC, Schon R, Tetzlaf R, et al. 2007. "Topographical CT-data analysis of the human orbital floor." *Int J Oral Maxillofac Surg* 36: 45–53.

348. Metzger MC, Schon R, Schulze D, et al. 2006. "Individual preformed titanium meshes for orbital fractures." *Oral Surg Oral Med Oral Pathol Oral Radiol Endod* 102: 442–447.

349. Metzger MC, Schon R, Weyer N, et al. 2006. "Anatomical 3-dimensional pre-bent titanium implant for orbital floor fractures." *Ophthalmology* 113: 1863–1868.

350. Christensen AM. 2007. "Tactile surgical planning using patient-specific anatomic models." In: *Distraction Osteogenesis of the Facial Skeleton*, Bell WH, and Guerrero CA, eds. Hamilton: BC Decker.

351. Derand P, and Hirsch JM. 2009. "Virtual bending of mandibular reconstruction plates using a computer-aided design." *J Oral Maxillofac Surg* 67: 1640–1643.

352. Marchetti C, Bianchi A, Muyldermans L, et al. 2011. "Validation of new soft tissue software in orthognathic surgery planning." *Int J Oral Maxillofac Surg* 40: 26–32.

353. Pohlenz P, Blake F, Blessmann M, et al. 2009. "Intraoperative cone–beam computed tomography in oral and maxillofacial surgery using a C-arm prototype: First clinical experiences after treatment of zygomaticomaxillary complex fractures." *J Oral Maxillofac Surg* 67: 515–521.

354. Heiland M, Schulze D, Blake F, et al. 2005. "Intraoperative imaging of zygomaticomaxillary complex fractures using a 3D C-arm system." *Int J Oral Maxillofac Surg* 34: 369–375.

355. Santler G, Karcher H, and Ruda C. 1998. "Indications and limitations of three-dimensional models in cranio-maxillofacial surgery." *J Craniomaxillofac Surg* 26: 11–16.

14

Soft Tissue Reconstruction

Dongsoo David Kim, DMD, MD, FACS
Daniel Petrisor, DMD, MD

INTRODUCTION

It is critical to understand the potential complications associated with soft tissue reconstruction of the head and neck. This allows the surgeon to anticipate untoward events and take proper action to manage them or help prevent their occurrence. Complications in soft tissue reconstruction can be divided in two general categories: those involving the recipient site and those involving the donor site. Recipient site complications include total or partial flap necrosis, infection, fistula formation, suture line dehiscence, and hematoma or seroma formation. Donor site complications are similar and can include hematoma or seroma formation, infection, poor healing as well as other specific complications based upon the particular donor site. This chapter will discuss complications associated with commonly used myocutaneous flaps and several specific free flaps, and general prevention and management of these complications.

COMPLICATIONS IN PEDICLED SOFT TISSUE FLAPS

Pectoralis Major Myocutaneous Flap

The pectoralis major myocutaneuous flap (PMMF) has traditionally been one of the primary reconstructive options for the oral cavity, oropharynx, and cutaneous head and neck defects. It can be used with a cutaneous skin island or as a myofascial flap by itself. While its popularity has diminished over the past two decades with the widespread use and reliability of microvascular free flaps, the PMMF still plays an important role in head and neck reconstruction. The utilization of this flap is now important for salvage procedures after free flap failure, as muscle bulk for coverage of the great vessels of the neck, and in circumstances where microsurgical reconstruction is contraindicated or expertise is not available.

The overall complication rate for the PMMF has been reported to be as high as 44% to 63%.[1–5] The majority of complications are considered minor, and conservative local wound care is often sufficient to resolve most of these minor complications.[1] Wound dehiscence, flap edge necrosis, local infection, seromas, hematomas, donor site complications, and fistula formation are all possible minor complications. These complications are not unique to the PMMF and can be experienced with any method of reconstruction, particularly in the medically compromised, malnourished, and generally less than ideal surgical head and neck cancer patient.[1]

Although overall complication rates are high, most studies show a relatively low major complication rate with the PMMF ranging from 2.4% to 4%.[1,6,7] Complete necrosis or greater than 25% partial necrosis of the flap are two possible major complications [Figs. 14.1(a), (b)]. Improved cutaneous paddle survival can be achieved by designing the skin paddle to remain over the pectoralis major muscle and minimizing its

Management of Complications in Oral and Maxillofacial Surgery, First Edition. Edited by Michael Miloro, Antonia Kolokythas.
© 2012 John Wiley & Sons, Inc. Published 2012 by John Wiley & Sons, Inc.

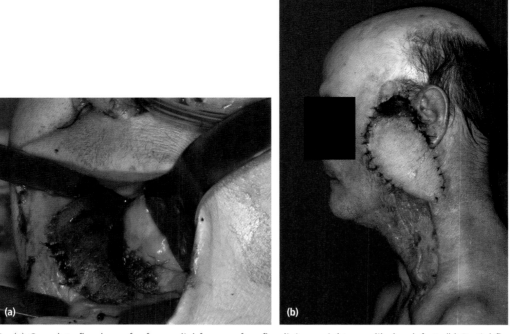

Fig. 14.1. (a) Complete flap loss of a free radial forearm free flap lining a right mandibular defect. (b) Partial flap loss of a pectoralis major myocutaneous flap lining the left preauricular region.

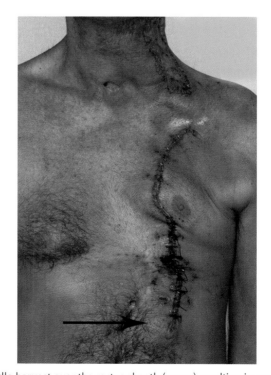

Fig. 14.2. Extension of skin paddle harvest over the rectus sheath (arrow) resulting in partial flap loss [refer to Fig. 14.1(b)].

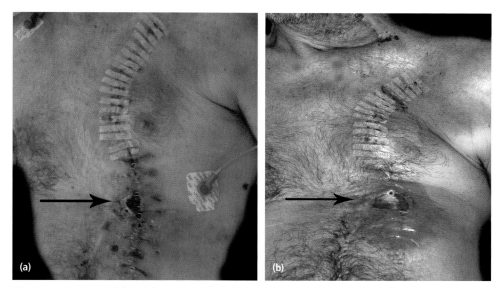

Fig. 14.3. (a) Donor site wound breakdown (arrow) owing to primary closure with tension. (b) Donor site wound after staple removal and debridement of necrotic tissue.

extension over the anterior rectus sheath (Fig. 14.2), careful dissection around the skin paddle without the use of monopolar cautery, and securing the skin paddle to the underlying muscle and fascia with temporary sutures.[7]

Depending on the size of the skin paddle that is required for the defect, primary closure of the pectoralis major flap may not be possible. This can be a more likely issue in very thin, male patients. A split-thickness skin graft may be necessary for closure of these donor sites. This is preferred over having wound breakdown later owing to primary closure with excessive tension [(Figs. 14.3(a), (b)].[8]

Submental Island Flap

The submental island flap is a viable reconstructive option for head and neck defects. Its cervical location assures good color and texture match for facial reconstruction. This flap is based on the submental artery, a consistent branch of the facial artery; venous drainage is through the submandibular vein into the facial vein.[9,10] Dissection of the pedicle allows for good mobility of the flap. This flap can also be harvested as a reverse-flow flap with dependence on the angular artery for its blood flow.[11] One study comparing the two patterns of submental flaps showed a success rate of 95% and 94.4% for the submental artery island flap and the reverse submental artery island flap, respectively.

Complications reported with this flap include venous drainage disruptions, partial or complete flap loss, hematoma formation under the flap, and marginal mandibular nerve injury.[12] In one series, six of the nine cases experienced venous drainage disruption after raising the flap, but this did not cause flap loss.[9] This was overcome in 4 to 5 days without any interventions.

Sterne et al. described the use of the submental island flap in 12 patients for intraoral reconstruction.[12] One patient experienced partial flap loss, one a complete flap loss, one formed a hematoma under the flap, and two patients experienced a marginal mandibular nerve injury. To address the issue of nerve injury, Sterne et al. recommend that identification of the marginal mandibular nerve and preserving it before raising the flap may help prevent inadvertent damage to the nerve. Others advocate staying close to the posterior aspect of the platysma from the angle of the mandible to the midbody area when incising the ipsilateral upper limit of the flap. This will adequately protect the nerve and make it unnecessary to identify the nerve.[13]

Paramedian Forehead Flap

The forehead skin is acknowledged as an ideal donor site with which to resurface the nose due to its good color and texture match, as well as its favorable anatomic location. The paramedian forehead flap is thus a commonly used flap for nasal reconstruction. Complications associated with the paramedian forehead flap are rare, as the superficial axial blood supply provides for robust vascularity.

The excellent vascularity of this flap makes distal flap necrosis unusual and markedly reduces the risk of infection. This characteristic of the paramedian forehead flap also accounts for its most common complication, namely, hematoma formation. Often, the distal aspect of the flap is stripped of its muscle and subcutaneous tissue and has a propensity to bleed postoperatively.[14] The potential dead space between the thinned flap and the underlying nasal defect is an area where hematoma formation can occur. To avoid this complication, much attention is given to achieving hemostasis over the entire area of the raw surface of the flap. Compression dressings applied with several bolster sutures passing full thickness through the flap to the nasal passage and back again may be helpful if bleeding is significant.[14] However, bolster dressings are not used routinely as they may impair circulation to the distal part of the flap.

COMPLICATIONS IN MICROVASCULAR FREE FLAPS

Microvascular free tissue transfer (MFTT) after tumor extirpation or trauma is extremely reliable in achieving successful reconstruction of the head and neck. Foremost of the advantages of MFTT is the ability to tailor the donor flap to the specific needs of the ablative site. For example, a thin and pliable radial forearm flap would be ideal for a defect of the floor of the mouth or tongue, whereas the muscular bulk and large skin paddle of a rectus abdominus flap may be better suited for total glossectomy or maxillectomy defects. The pedicled flaps described earlier in this chapter are less suitable for defects that require either extreme bulk of tissue or very thin, pliable, and mobile tissue.

Due to the increased operating time and need for technical expertise, MFTT is often perceived as being a less reliable and more costly procedure than rotational flap reconstruction. However, several studies that compared MFTT to rotational flaps for reconstruction of the head and neck have suggested that this may not be true. Brown et al. showed that the risk of postoperative complications in patients who underwent free flap reconstruction was not significantly greater than those matched patients who received pedicled flap reconstruction.[15] Their data suggested a trend toward shorter intensive care unit (ICU) and overall hospital stays with MFTT, although the differences were not statistically significant. In addition, several reviews identified the pectoralis major myocutaneous flap as having a higher risk of major postoperative complications such as fistula formation, flap loss, infection, and hematoma compared with radial forearm or rectus abdominus flaps.[16,17]

The disadvantages of MFTT include the technical demands on the surgical team, operating room staff, anesthesiology, and the ICU. The initial anesthetic time for MFTT is longer than for nonmicrovascular reconstructions, but studies have shown that the overall cost, length of hospital and ICU stay, and incidence of complications is not significantly increased with MFTT.[15,18] The potential for total flap loss is also a distinct disadvantage of MFTT. Even the most experienced microsurgeons will have failures, usually due to thrombosis. However, as mentioned previously, the radial forearm and the rectus abdominus flaps have shown lower incidence of flap loss than the pectoralis major myocutaneous flap.[16,17] Several large studies have shown a 0.8% to 2.9% incidence of free flap failure and a 3% incidence of partial flap necrosis.[19,20] The current state of MFTT has evolved from a radical, last-resort procedure with a high failure rate to the first and most reliable choice in many types of soft tissue reconstruction of the head and neck.

Hypercoagulable states are the only true contraindications to MFTT (Table 14.1).[21] This includes diseases such as polycythemia, thrombocytosis, and possibly sickle cell anemia. The risk of thrombosis in these conditions is too high to justify MFTT. Patients taking the antiestrogen medication tamoxifen for prevention or treatment of breast cancer should be taken off this medication prior to surgery due to its known thrombogenic activity.[22] Also, smokers should be encouraged to stop at least 1 week prior to surgery for similar reasons, in addition to risk for decreased flap perfusion and overall impaired wound healing.

Age has not been shown to be a significant risk factor for postoperative complications with MFTT. Although studies have implied that advanced age has a greater risk for prolonged hospital stay, medical complication, and in-hospital death,[23,24] others have shown no significant difference in complications following major head and neck reconstructive surgery.[25] However, advanced age is associated with atherosclerotic disease and increased vessel fragility, which may pose a specific potential, though not absolute,

Table 14.1. Hypercoagulable States

INHERITED	ACQUIRED
Antithrombin III deficiency	Prolonged immobilization
Protein C deficiency	Pregnancy
Protein S deficiency	Surgery/trauma
Activated protein C resistance	Oral contraceptives/antiestrogens
Factor V Leiden	Homocystinuria
Dysfibrinogenemia	Vitamin K deficiency
Plasminogen activator deficiency	Disseminated intravascular coagulation
Plasminogen deficiency	Smoking
Factor XII deficiency	Nephrotic syndrome
Polycythemia	L-asparaginase
Thrombocytosis	Diabetes mellitus
Sickle cell anemia	Hyperlipidemia
Heparin cofactor II deficiency	Malignancy
	Lupus anticoagulant
	Anticardiolipin antibody

problem in MFTT. Atherosclerosis is most problematic when evaluating the patient for harvest of the fibula flap due to concerns of distal lower extremity vessel perfusion. However, the actual effect of atherosclerosis on a microvascular anastomosis is not known. Diabetes mellitus can predispose patients to microvascular disease and atherosclerosis, which may result in delayed wound healing, infection, and possible flap loss.

Finally, pediatric patients may have very small caliber vessels that will make anastomosis difficult and less reliable, especially when the vessels are less than 1 mm in diameter.

The postoperative management of patients receiving MFTT is as important as the intraoperative MFTT technique. Protocols vary by institution and are not based on scientific evidence of efficacy but rather surgeon preference and experience. However, in order to minimize postoperative complications, certain standards should be applied to all free flap reconstructions regardless of site.

Pressure on the microvascular pedicle should be avoided at all times. In head and neck reconstruction, circumferential ties or straps such as those for tracheostomies or oxygen tents can easily compress the vessels in the neck. Similarly, kinking or undue tension on the vessels must be avoided, especially during the immediate postoperative period. The position of the neck that optimizes vessel geometry should be strictly maintained. This position can be sustained by using postoperative sedation with ventilator support. A paralytic agent can also be added to this pharmacologic management. It is the authors' preference not to sedate most patients in the postoperative period as long as the patient is able understand and follow instructions to maintain a neutral head position.

Hemodynamics should be maintained as close to normal limits as possible. Avoiding extreme hyper- or hypotension is crucial to preventing hematoma formation while maintaining perfusion of the flap. A balance in the oxygen-carrying capacity of blood and blood viscosity must also be achieved. Although little scientific evidence exists, a hematocrit of 28% to 30% is generally accepted as the desired goal for the immediate postoperative period.

Flap monitoring protocols vary drastically between institutions. Although many modalities of monitoring flaps are currently available, with most oral and maxillofacial reconstructions, the skin paddle is readily examinable and its clinical appearance is the current standard for flap monitoring (Fig. 14.4). The parameters evaluated include color, capillary refill, flap turgor, and warmth. The frequency of serial postoperative evaluations of flaps also varies by institution, from every 1 hour to every 4 hours. The frequency is based on the fact that the time between the onset of a thrombotic event and its recognition may be critical to

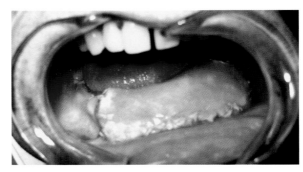

Fig. 14.4. Early postoperative appearance of healthy skin paddle of mandibular reconstruction. Notice natural skin color and texture, minimal swelling. This flap would be soft, warm, and have good capillary refill. (From Kim D, and Ghali GE. "Postablative reconstruction techniques for oral cancer." *Oral and Maxillofacial Surgery Clinics of North America*, Vol. 18 No. 4, Elsevier, Nov. 2006, 573–604.)

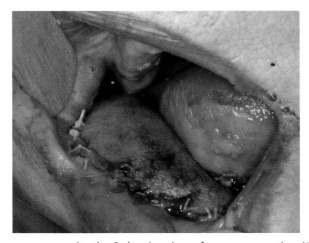

Fig. 14.5. Radial forearm flap on postoperative day 3 showing signs of venous congestion. Note the presence of significant flap edema and ecchymotic appearance of the skin. A pin-prick test on this flap would result in rapid return of dark colored blood.

the flap's salvage.[26] In pig skin flaps, this critical time is reported as 7 hours.[27] After 8–12 hours it may not be possible to reestablish the flap's circulation.[28]

Possibly the most commonly used adjunct to the clinical exam is the pin-prick test. A 25-gauge needle is used at the center of the skin paddle, and the rapidity, color, and amount of blood return is evaluated. A healthy flap will bleed bright red blood after a slight delay (within 1–3 seconds). Rapid return of dark-colored blood, combined with an ecchymotic skin paddle, suggests venous insufficiency (Fig. 14.5). The blood consistency of a venous congested flap has been compared with crankcase fluid. Finally, no blood return, with a flap that is cool to the touch with a pale color, suggests arterial thrombosis. Although this widely used exam is subject to much interobserver error, it can be a valuable aid to the clinical assessment.

The next most commonly used modality in postoperative flap monitoring is the handheld surface Doppler probe. The practical utilization of the Doppler probe is mainly for confirmation of arterial flow, but its ability to confirm venous outflow has been proposed.[29] Observance of a change in the character of the "phases" of the Doppler signal may help the clinician identify the impending failure of a flap. However, because thrombotic complications are usually venous in nature, the utility of this modality is severely limited. In addition, one must be aware that Doppler signals obtained at the anastomotic site may be unreliable due to the proximity of the carotid arteries.

Avoiding Complications at the Vascular Anastomosis Stage

Prior to vascular anastomosis, the flap should be inset to the defect, and any tunneling necessary for the passage of the pedicle should be performed. For oral cavity reconstruction, a watertight closure of the flap to the oral mucosa must be obtained to prevent catastrophic complication of a salivary leak and fistula formation. Salivary contamination of the vascular anastomosis will result in thrombosis. Nonresorbing or slowly resorbing (Vicryl®) sutures passed in a simple interrupted or horizontal mattress fashion, so as to provide wound edge eversion and a water tight seal, are preferred. Once the inset is complete or nearly complete, attention can then be turned to preparing both the recipient and donor vessels.

Regardless of the vessel type or the anastomosis technique being performed, the initial preparation of all the recipient vessels is essentially the same. Extreme care should be employed when dissecting the vessels to be utilized. At no time should the vessel wall be grasped directly with any instrument. The only part of the vessel that should be handled is the adventitia. Careless dissection can result in apparently intact vessels having intimal damage that will promote thrombus formation.

Particular care must be utilized during venous anastomosis as the vessel walls are much thinner and more susceptible to damage from aggressive traction, dissection, or other manipulations. Smaller, more controlled movements are necessary to avoid damaging veins.

Another potential pitfall of venous anastomosis is a higher likelihood of "back-wall" suturing. The placing of jeweler's forceps into the lumen of the vessel to facilitate needle passage helps to avoid this error. Alternatively, a skilled assistant can help prevent back-wall suturing by applying a gentle stream of heparinized saline irrigation to the vessel lumen allowing it to balloon while placing the sutures. However, this technique creates a change in the optics of the procedure because the surgeon must visualize the vessel through a pool of fluid that decreases depth perception and may affect the accuracy of needle placement.

Flap Salvage

The threatened flap must be identified as early as possible in order to maximize the possibility of salvaging the reconstruction. Depending on the timing of the thrombotic event, return to the operating room may be necessary to surgically revise one or more of the microvascular anastomoses. Alternatively, nonsurgical methods of salvage may be indicated if the event occurs in the late postoperative period. Techniques for flap salvage are not well documented. The specific procedures will depend on the clinical situation and the appearance of the anastomosed vessels.

For example, an expanding hematoma in the neck may compress the venous outflow of a flap, causing it to appear ecchymotic and edematous. In this circumstance, the neck should be explored and the only necessary salvage procedure may be evacuation of the hematoma along with bipolar coagulation or clipping of any bleeding vessels so that venous outflow can be restored. However, in other instances it may be necessary to open and revise both venous and arterial anastomoses. In rat femoral veins, most venous thromboses occurred within 24 hours of anastomosis.[30] In a clinical situation, this would equate to an early thrombosis of the venous anastomosis that warrants immediate surgical exploration.

Once a thrombosed artery or vein is identified, the length of the vessels should be palpated to determine the extent of the clot. At the site of the clot the thrombosis will be firm whereas the vessels will be compressible proximal and distal to the clot. If the thrombosis cannot be identified by palpation, then a strip test can be performed by occluding the lumen of the vessel downstream, applying a stripping motion upstream, and then releasing (Fig. 14.6). Rapid refill of the vessel usually indicates adequate flow.

If a thrombosis is present, the anastomosis can be opened by removing some or all of the sutures or by excising the existing anastomosis. The area of the thrombosis can either be resected and a new anastomosis attempted at the new site, or the thrombus can be removed using vascular balloon catheters. The choice of technique will depend on the clinical circumstance, length and caliber of vessel, and quality of the existing vessel opening. For example, if the thrombosis occurred due to endothelial damage at the original site of anastomosis, that section of artery or vein should be removed and a new anastomosis created at an undamaged site.

Other situations that may require revision of microvascular anastomoses are kinking or compression of the vascular pedicle. Such compression can occur due to a hematoma, from external sources such as tracheal

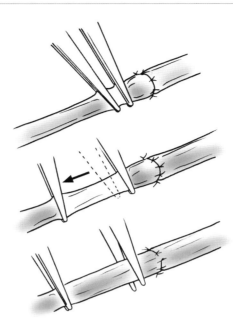

Fig. 14.6. The strip test. (From: Kim D. "Microvascular free tissue reconstruction of the oral cavity." *Selected Readings in Oral and Maxillofacial Surgery*, Vol. 12 No. 4. Elsevier, August 2004.)

ties or from poor orientation of the vascular pedicle in the neck. These situations are best avoided entirely, but when they do occur the remedy would be to reorient the pedicle and suspend it with carefully placed sutures. Alternatively, the anastomosis can be resected, the vessel trimmed and the anastomosis revised, or an alternative recipient vessel may be chosen to improve the pedicle geometry.

Exsanguination therapies must be discussed as an option for those flaps whose venous anastomoses cannot be revised or whose revision has failed. These modalities maintain perfusion, allowing continued viability of tissue while neovascularization occurs. These therapies are known to be useful in finger replantations, but head and neck reconstruction requires the exsanguination of a much larger surface area of tissue, possibly leading to considerable blood loss and the need for a transfusion. Indeed, one paper reported that an average of 13 units of packed red blood cells per patient was necessary to maintain adequate hemoglobin concentrations.[31] Medicinal leech therapy in head and neck MFTT should proceed with much care so the leeches do not migrate down the esophagus or larynx. Furthermore, antibiotic prophylaxis with antipseudomonal penicillin or a fluoroquinolone should be instituted prior to leech treatment to prevent infection by *Aeromonas hydrophila*.[32]

MICROVASCULAR FREE FLAP DONOR SITE COMPLICATIONS FROM MICROVASCULAR DONOR SITE

Donor site morbidity is of great concern to reconstructive surgeons. Different free flap donor sites have very different morbidity profiles. However, many of the most commonly used flaps, such as the radial forearm, rectus abdominus, and the anterolateral thigh flaps have very acceptable levels of postoperative morbidity with few long-term deficits.

Radial Forearm Free Flap

The radial forearm free flap (RFFF) has become a work horse flap for oral cavity soft tissue reconstruction. Studies report success rates for the RFFF in head and neck reconstruction to be as high as 98%.[19] Even with the high success rate of the RFFF itself, donor site morbidity remains a problem.

Attempts at primary closure can result in compartment syndrome, a possibly catastrophic complication. Commonly, the radial forearm donor defect is closed with a split- or full-thickness skin graft. This often

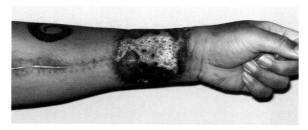

Fig. 14.7. Partial skin graft loss due to inadequate "pin cushion" suturing and compression dressing of the graft.

results in the primary problem with RFFF, namely, poor cosmetic outcome of the donor site. Various authors report partial skin graft loss and delayed wound healing in 22% to 40% of patients, with exposure of tendons in as many as 13% of patients(Fig. 14.7).

Creating an ideal bed for donor site skin grafting begins with careful flap dissection. Attention must be given to leave a thin film of paratenon on the tendons of the wrist flexors or wound complications due to skin graft failure will be a problem. Vascular clips will be necessary to control the numerous branches to the surrounding musculature and prevent formation of a hematoma under the skin graft. Additionally, the graft should be perforated to allow for seepage of fluid during healing. The graft should be compressed to the recipient bed by Vaseline® gauze and by gauze that is supported by a plaster splint fabricated to the volar aspect of the lower arm and hand. This splint should be left in place for 7 days to prevent sheer forces on the skin graft. Prior to placing the final dressing, perfusion to the index finger and thumb should be verified by checking capillary refill.

Critical ischemia of the hand has been described and is a catastrophic complication of the RFFF. The blood supply to the lower arm and hand is by the radial and ulnar branches of the brachial artery. The radial artery terminates in the deep palmar arch and the ulnar leads to the superficial palmar arch. Once the radial forearm flap is harvested, the blood supply to the hand and digits will be completely reliant on the ulnar artery. The blood supply to the third, fourth, and fifth digits are normally supplied by the ulnar artery, so the perfusion to the thumb and index finger is at greatest risk when harvesting this flap.

In order for ischemia of the thumb or index finger to occur, two anatomic variations must be present. First, the superficial palmar arch must lack branches to the thumb and index finger. Second, the superficial and deep palmar arches must completely lack communicating branches. A cadaveric study showed this combination of anomalies to be present in approximately 12% of specimens.[33] An accurate Allen's test is essential for avoiding potential ischemic complications after flap harvest. If the Allen's test is equivocal or difficult to interpret, radial artery mapping can objectively determine the pattern of flow and reversal of flow following occlusion of the radial artery.

Donor site infection is a rare but potentially serious complication. Management involves early recognition for signs and symptoms of infection (wound erythema, drainage, fever, etc.), administration of intravenous antibiotics, debridement of necrotic material, and serial irrigation of the wound [Figs. 14.8(a), (b)].

Rectus Abdominus Myocutaneous Flap

The foremost concern for donor site complications of the rectus abdominus myocutaneous flap (RAMF) is postoperative hernias. When considering the RAMF, the anatomy of the anterior abdominal wall should be reviewed because preservation of the fascial sheaths is critical to preventing the formation of postoperative abdominal hernias. The rectus sheath extends from the pubis to the xiphoid and is formed by the fibrous aponeuroses of the abdominal muscles. However, it is important to realize that the composition of the posterior wall of the sheath changes at the level of the anterior superior iliac spine, demarcated by the arcuate line (Fig. 14.9). Above the arcuate line, the posterior rectus sheath is formed by extensions of the transversalis fascia and part of the internal oblique aponeurosis, and this double-layered sheath is adequate to prevent hernias. Below the arcuate line, the posterior rectus sheath is formed by the transversalis fascia alone. Therefore, below the arcuate line bulging or hernia complications may occur if the fascia is not reinforced by preserving the anterior sheath and closing it as a separate layer.

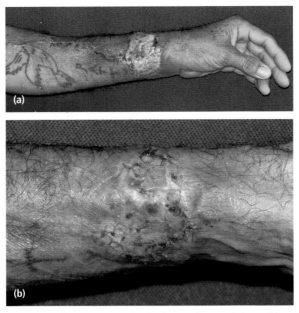

Fig. 14.8. (a) Radial forearm donor site infection and split thickness skin graft loss. (b) Donor site after administration of IV antibiotics, debridement of necrotic skin graft, serial saline irrigation of the wound bed, and repeat split-thickness skin graft.

1. External obligue aponeurosis
2. Internal oblige aponeurosis
3. Transversus abdominis

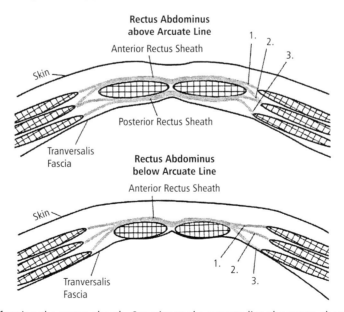

Fig. 14.9. Aponeuroses forming the rectus sheath. Superior to the arcuate line the rectus sheath is complete posteriorly. Below the arcuate line the muscle contacts transversalis fascia. (From: Kim D. "Microvascular free tissue reconstruction of the oral cavity." *Selected Readings in Oral and Maxillofacial Surgery*, Vol. 12 No. 4. Elsevier, August 2004.)

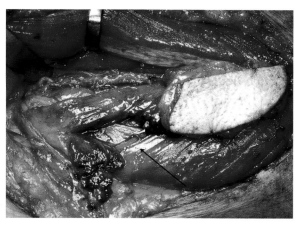

Fig. 14.10. The dissection through the vastus lateralis muscle for the anterolateral thigh flap. Dark arrow—vastus lateralis. (From Miloro M, et al. 2011. *Peterson's Principles of Oral and Maxillofacial Surgery*, 3rd ed. PmPH-USA, Shelton, CT.)

Thus, closure of the RAMF should begin with the reapproximation of the inferior portion of the cut anterior wall of the rectus sheath. The superior portion, which is harvested with the flap, may also be closed with relatively large, slowly resorbable sutures. Care should be taken not to puncture the posterior rectus sheath with suture needles or other sharp instruments that could produce visceral injury.

Anterolateral Thigh Flap

Although many of the aforementioned free flaps have very reasonable morbidity profiles, a new standard may be developing for acceptable donor site morbidity in free flap reconstruction. With perforator flaps, the skin territory to be harvested is dissected directly with the skin perforator through intervening tissue to the source vessel. For example, the deep inferior epigastric perforator flap avoids the morbidity of harvesting the rectus muscle with skin, along with its attendant sequelae.

The anterolateral thigh flap (ALTF) is a perforator flap based on the cutaneous perforators of the descending branch of the lateral circumflex femoral artery, a branch of the profunda femoris. Care must be taken when dissecting the source artery and vein to avoid injury to the nerve to the vastus lateralis. If intramuscular dissection is necessary the muscle should be reapproximated after adequate hemostasis is achieved (Fig. 14.10).

This flap has the benefit of primary closure of the donor site if the skin paddle dimensions are less than 6 to 9 cm (Fig. 14.11). Larger skin paddles may require skin grafting. Very few donor site complications are associated with this flap aside from temporary weakness of the vastus lateralis if an intramuscular dissection is necessary or if nerve injury is sustained to the nerve that innervates this muscle.

MANAGEMENT OF SELECTED COMPLICATIONS

Total/Partial Flap Loss

Total flap necrosis occurs in less than 8% of most major studies of myocutaneous flaps (e.g., the pectoralis major flap) and even less in most series of free flap transfers.[1,3,7,19,20] (Figs. 14.12(a), (b). Physical factors causing impaired arterial inflow or obstructed venous outflow are usually the cause. This may be caused by pressure on the pedicle resulting from dressings, tracheostomy ties, hematoma, or overlying skin flaps as mentioned earlier. Careful attention to these factors will prevent flap loss or, if recognized and corrected early, save a compromised flap. Also, several technical details can affect the flow of blood from the muscle to skin. Inwardly beveled skin incisions can alter the number of perforating vessels to the skin paddle, failure to suture the paddle to the underlying muscle and fascia can lead to shearing of perforating vessels during manipulation and insetting of the flap into the defect site, failure to suspend the muscle bulk of myocutaneous flaps to periosteum or reconstruction plates can place tension between the muscle and skin,

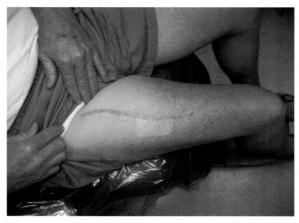

Fig. 14.11. Result after primary closure of anterolateral thigh flap.

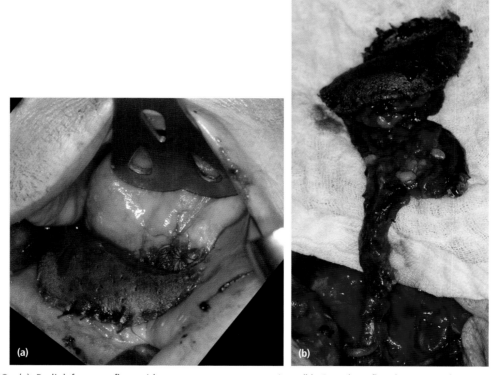

Fig. 14.12. (a) Radial forearm flap with severe venous congestion. (b) Complete flap loss secondary to venous clot formation.

and the final position of the skin paddle can lead to skin necrosis if the skin is being pulled away from the muscle or excessively compressed or folded.[34] Total flap necrosis should be managed by removing the necrotic tissue, debriding and irrigating the wound bed, and salvaging reconstruction by a secondary flap or primary closure.

Partial flap loss in rotational flaps occurs more frequently than total flap necrosis and usually involves loss of all or part of the skin paddle and its subcutaneous fat with retained viability of the underlying muscle [Fig. 14.1(b)].[1,3] When significant skin necrosis does occur, prompt debridement is necessary to prevent infection and progression to loss of any underlying muscle.[34] Attempts at primary closure of the resulting wound should be made with gentle undermining of surrounding tissues. In instances where primary closure cannot be obtained, the wound may be left to heal by secondary intention if fistula formation is not a concern or a secondary soft tissue flap may be indicated to close the defect.

Infection

The reported incidence of infection in head and neck oncologic surgery approaches 90% in clean-contaminated wounds without perioperative antibiotics. This rate has been reduced to 10–20% with antibiotic prophylaxis. Wound infections are a constant concern to the surgeon who is involved in head and neck soft tissue reconstruction because of their impact on patient prognosis, morbidity, length of stay, and overall cost. Prevention, identification, and appropriate treatment remain priorities for every surgeon.

Preoperative identification of patients at higher risk for wound infection can be difficult. Factors believed to increase the incidence of infection include the patient's physical status according to the guidelines of the American Society of Anesthesiologists (ASA), duration of surgery, preoperative tracheostomy, previous radiation or chemotherapy, nutritional status, and comorbid medical conditions. The literature is replete with conflicting data on the significance of each of these variables and its association with wound infection.[35–38]

Research has indicated that a bacterial inoculums of 1×10^5 bacteria per gram of tissue is necessary for a wound infection to occur.[39] Salivary contamination in surgical wounds allows for the introduction of $1 \times 10^{8-9}$ bacteria per milliliter of saliva,[40] and these organisms are most commonly cultured in wound sepsis after head and neck surgery. The role of perioperative antibiotic prophylaxis is to decrease this bacterial inoculum at the time of surgery. Many studies on prophylactic intravenous antibiotic administration have concluded unanimously that perioperative antibiotics have a profound effect on decreasing the incidence of wound infections. Antibiotic selection is targeted at the organisms that inhabit the oral cavity. *Eikenella corrodens, Bacteroides* spp., coagulase-negative *Staphylococcus, Streptococcus* spp., *Enterobacter* spp., *Fusobacterium,* and *Escherichia coli* have been the commonly isolated bacteria in head and neck infections. Ampicillin/sulbactam (3 g intravenously every 6 hours) and clindamycin (900 mg intravenously every 8 hours) have emerged from numerous trials evaluating different antibiotics for use in this context.[41] The duration of these perioperative antibiotics has been shown to have no additional benefit of intravenous antibiotics beyond 24 hours after surgery. Indeed, much of the data is derived from studies of general head and neck patients undergoing clean-contaminated procedures so their applicability to flap reconstruction has been in question. However, Carroll, et al. studied this question in a randomized prospective single-blind trial that encompassed 74 patients. The study groups were divided into short-course and long-course antibiotic groups (900 mg clindamycin every 8 hours); no significant difference in infection rates was noted between them.

Finally, the use of topical antibiotics in clean-contaminated head and neck surgery has also been studied but to a lesser extent. Pilot studies of the use of various antibiotics (clindamycin, piperacillin/tazobactam, Peridex™ [3M, St. Paul, MN]) in the form of oral rinses and added to the irrigation solution have been reported.[42–45] All of these pilot studies have shown a significant decrease in the aerobic and anaerobic bacteria cultured from intraoperative wounds. In one study, 99% of some species were reduced in the cultured neck sites after a single preoperative oral rinse with clindamycin.[43] Though these pilot studies are encouraging, no large prospective trials have been published to verify these findings.

For the flap reconstruction patient suspected of having an infection, clinical signs and symptoms will be analogous to any postoperative infection. Namely, fever, redness around the incision site, increased swelling, fluctuance, drainage, and foul odor may be present. Initial management may simply require a bedside procedure to release a few neck staples/sutures, open the abscess cavity and obtain specimens for culture and sensitivity. If this is inadequate, formal drainage in the operating room may be required particularly in free flap reconstructions due to the possibility of the infection promoting thrombosis in the microvascular anastomoses. It may be advantageous to formally explore the suspected infection site to identify any inciting areas such as chronic salivary contamination through an intraoral wound dehiscence.

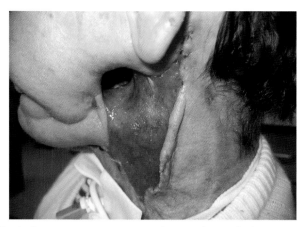

Fig. 14.13. Oral-cutaneous fistula in a recurrent tongue carcinoma after radiation treatment and surgical salvage with pectoralis major flap reconstruction.

Fistula Formation

A particularly troublesome complication after head and neck surgery is formation of oral and pharyngo-cutaneous fistulas (OCFs) (Fig. 14.13). The occurrence has been reported to be as high as 30% after composite resections. Many of the same variables implicated in wound infection are also applicable to OCF formation, including nutritional status, previous radiation therapy, operative technique, comorbidity, and flap reconstruction. Regardless of cause, once an OCF is present, it must be identified quickly and treated appropriately to prevent catastrophic complications.

Early identification of OCFs can be difficult. Fever, wound erythema, and drainage approximately 1 week after surgery are suggestive of the presence of an OCF. With the probable mechanism of inadequate closure or breakdown of the mucosal defect, this symptom chronologically seems plausible. An earlier sign of OCF may be the presence of clear, bubbly fluid in the closed suction drains.[46] Identification of OCFs and wound infections in the early postoperative period may decrease the morbidity, overall length of hospital stay, and cost incurred by these complications.[42,47]

The treatment of an OCF is aimed at preventing life-threatening complications while minimizing functional and cosmetic sequelae. As with all wound infections, drainage of any collections, culture and sensitivity testing, surgical debridement, and the appropriate use of antibiotics are the initial steps in management. Many small fistulas in nonirradiated patients heal with conservative measures.[48] It is imperative, however, that the tracheobronchial tree be protected from salivary or purulent fluids with cuffed tracheostomy tubes and fistula divergence to prevent aspiration.[46]

Of concern is contamination of the carotid artery system with saliva or infectious material. Any fistula that threatens the carotid artery should be treated as a surgical emergency because the threat of arterial rupture may be imminent. This rare but catastrophic complication is most commonly seen at the carotid bifurcation. Prevention includes use of nontrifurcate incisions, thick subplatysmal skin flaps, gentle tissue handling, and prevention of wound infection. Treatment includes adequate debridement of infected material and necrotic tissue around the arteries as necessary and coverage by muscle flaps (usually the pectoralis major) for protection. Microvascular free tissue transfer is also an option for carotid coverage when regional tissue is unavailable.[46]

Hematoma Formation

The risk of hematoma formation is a possibility whenever a surgical procedure is undertaken [Figs. 14.14(a)–(d)]. This is especially true in the highly vascularized area of the head and neck. The best means of dealing with this complication is by prevention. This starts with a detailed patient history, including medication history and the use of over-the-counter drugs. Aspirin is present in many over-the-counter medications, and it has an irreversible effect on platelets.[34]

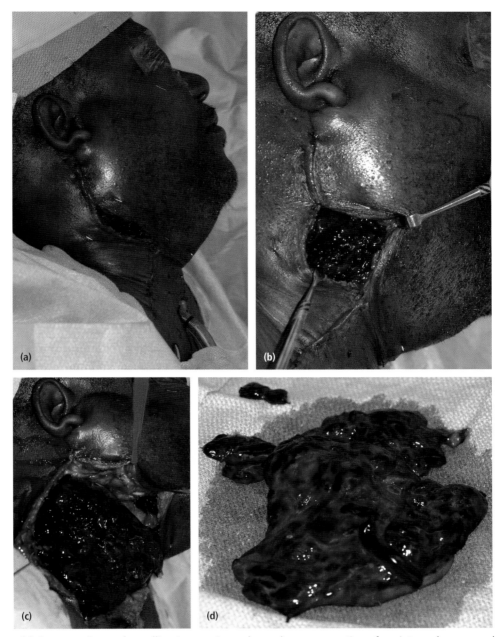

Fig. 14.14. (a) Postoperative neck swelling in a patient who underwent resection of an intraoral mass, neck dissection and microvascular free flap reconstruction. (b), (c), Wound exploration reveals a large neck hematoma. (d) Evacuation of neck hematoma.

Intraoperatively, the surgeon must achieve good hemostasis during the procedure by means of hemoclip/ tie ligature and electrocautery. In addition, a drain should be placed in certain wounds. The use of a closed system as opposed to an open Penrose drain acts to lower the likelihood of infection.[34] However, a drain should not be used as a substitute for achieving proper intraoperative hemostasis.

Once a hematoma does occur, it should be evacuated to lessen the likelihood of wound infections and skin flap necrosis. The iron present in hematomas is a nutrient for bacteria, making the wound more prone to infection.[34,49] Additionally, some feel that incidence of skin flap necrosis in the setting of a hematoma is increased by way of a free radical mechanisms.[34,50]

CONCLUSIONS

The goals of surgical reconstruction of the oral and maxillofacial patient are restoration of function and preservation of normal appearance. This involves negotiation of a complex anatomic region with the added obstacle of oral and pharyngeal contamination. Total or partial flap failure, suture line dehiscence, donor site morbidity, wound infection, hematoma and seroma formation, and fistulas are only a few of the possible complications that can be encountered. These complications can occur either at the donor site, recipient site, or both. The use of preventive measures to forestall complications and the prompt recognition and appropriate treatment when they do occur helps to minimize the associated morbidity of treatment.

SUGGESTED READINGS

1. Kroll SS, Goepfert H, et al. 1990. "Analysis of complications in 168 pectoralis major myocutaneous flaps used for head and neck reconstruction." *Ann Plast Surg* 25(2): 93–97.
2. Liu R, Gullane P, et al. 2001. "Pectoralis major myocutaneous pedicled flap in head and neck reconstruction: Retrospective review of indications and results in 244 consecutive cases at the Toronto General Hospital." *J Otolaryngol* 30(1): 34–40.
3. El-Marakby HH. 2006. "The reliability of pectoralis major myocutaneous flap in head and neck reconstruction." *J Egypt Natl Canc Inst* 18(1): 41–50.
4. Zou H, Zhang WF, et al. 2007. "Salvage reconstruction of extensive recurrent oral cancer defects with the pectoralis major myocutaneous flap." *J Oral Maxillofac Surg* 65(10): 1935–1939.
5. Ethier JL, Trites J, et al. 2009. "Pectoralis major myofascial flap in head and neck reconstruction: Indications and outcomes." *J Otolaryngol Head Neck Surg* 38(6): 632–641.
6. Vartanian JG, Carvalho AL, et al. 2004. "Pectoralis major and other myofascial/myocutaneous flaps in head and neck cancer reconstruction: Experience with 437 cases at a single institution." *Head Neck* 26(12): 1018–1023.
7. Ramakrishnan VR, Yao W, et al. 2009. "Improved skin paddle survival in pectoralis major myocutaneous flap reconstruction of head and neck defects." *Arch Facial Plast Surg* 11(5): 306–310.
8. Myers EN, ed. 2008. *Operative Otolaryngology: Head and Neck Surgery*. Philadelphia: Saunders Elsevier.
9. Abouchadi A, Capon-Degardin N, et al. 2007. "The submental flap in facial reconstruction: Advantages and limitations." *J Oral Maxillofac Surg* 65(5): 863–869.
10. Parmar PS, and Goldstein DP. 2009. "The submental island flap in head and neck reconstruction." *Curr Opin Otolaryngol Head Neck Surg* 17(4): 263–266.
11. Kim JT, Kim SK, et al. 2002. "An anatomic study and clinical applications of the reversed submental perforator-based island flap." *Plast Reconstr Surg* 109(7): 2204–2210.
12. Sterne GD, Januszkiewicz JS, et al. 1996. "The submental island flap." *Br J Plast Surg* 49(2): 85–89.
13. Pistre V, Pelissier P, et al. 2001. "Ten years of experience with the submental flap." *Plast Reconstr Surg* 108(6): 1576–1581.
14. Baker SR. 2007. *Local Flaps in Facial Reconstruction*. St. Louis: Mosby Elsevier.
15. Brown MR, McCulloch TM, et al. 1997. "Resource utilization and patient morbidity in head and neck reconstruction." *Laryngoscope* 107(8): 1028–1031.
16. Schusterman MA, Kroll SS, et al. 1991. "Intraoral soft tissue reconstruction after cancer ablation: A comparison of the pectoralis major flap and the free radial forearm flap." *Am J Surg* 162(4): 397–399.
17. Kroll SS, Reece GP, et al. 1992. "Comparison of the rectus abdominis free flap with the pectoralis major myocutaneous flap for reconstructions in the head and neck." *Am J Surg* 164(6): 615–618.
18. Huang RD, Silver SM, et al. 1992. "Pectoralis major myocutaneous flap: Analysis of complications in a VA population." *Head Neck* 14(2): 102–106.
19. Suh JD, Sercarz JA., et al. 2004. "Analysis of outcome and complications in 400 cases of microvascular head and neck reconstruction." *Arch Otolaryngol Head Neck Surg* 130(8): 962–966.
20. Pohlenz P, Blessmann M, et al. 2007. "Postoperative complications in 202 cases of microvascular head and neck reconstruction." *J Craniomaxillofac Surg* 35(6–7): 311–315.
21. Ayala C, and Blackwell KE. 1999. "Protein C deficiency in microvascular head and neck reconstruction." *Laryngoscope* 109(2 Pt 1): 259–265.
22. Peverill RE. 2003. "Hormone therapy and venous thromboembolism." *Best Pract Res Clin Endocrinol Metab* 17(1): 149–164.
23. Bhattacharyya N, and Fried MP. 2001. "Benchmarks for mortality, morbidity, and length of stay for head and neck surgical procedures." *Arch Otolaryngol Head Neck Surg* 127(2): 127–132.
24. Polanczyk CA, Marcantonio E, et al. 2001. "Impact of age on perioperative complications and length of stay in patients undergoing noncardiac surgery." *Ann Intern Med* 134(8): 637–643.
25. Shaari CM, and Urken ML. 1999. "Complications of head and neck surgery in the elderly." *Ear Nose Throat J* 78(7): 510–512.
26. Hidalgo DA, and Jones CS. 1990. "The role of emergent exploration in free-tissue transfer: A review of 150 consecutive cases." *Plast Reconstr Surg* 86(3): 492–498; discussion 499–501.

27. Kerrigan CL, Zelt RG, et al. 1984. "Secondary critical ischemia time of experimental skin flaps." *Plast Reconstr Surg* 74(4): 522–526.

28. May JW, Jr., Chait LA, et al. 1978. "The no-reflow phenomenon in experimental free flaps." *Plast Reconstr Surg* 61(2): 256–267.

29. Jones NF. 1992. "Intraoperative and postoperative monitoring of microsurgical free tissue transfers." *Clin Plast Surg* 19(4): 783–797.

30. Hui KC, Zhang F, et al. 2002. "Assessment of the patency of microvascular venous anastomosis." *J Reconstr Microsurg* 18(2): 111–114.

31. Chepeha DB, Nussenbaum B., et al. 2002. "Leech therapy for patients with surgically unsalvageable venous obstruction after revascularized free tissue transfer." *Arch Otolaryngol Head Neck Surg* 128(8): 960–965.

32. Kubo T, Yano K, et al. 2002. "Management of flaps with compromised venous outflow in head and neck microsurgical reconstruction." *Microsurgery* 22(8): 391–395.

33. Urken ML. 1995. "Free flaps. Fascial and fasciocutaneous flaps. Radial forearm." In: *Atlas of Regional and Free Flaps for Head and Neck Reconstruction*, Urken ML, Sullivan MJ, and Biller HF, eds., 149–168. New York: Raven Press.

34. Eisele DW. 1993. *Complications in Head and Neck Surgery*. St. Louis: Mosby.

35. Becker GD. 1986. "Identification and management of the patient at high risk for wound infection." *Head Neck Surg* 8(3): 205–210.

36. Brown BM, Johnson JT, et al. 1987. "Etiologic factors in head and neck wound infections." *Laryngoscope* 97(5): 587–590.

37. Coskun H, Erisen L, et al. 2000. "Factors affecting wound infection rates in head and neck surgery." *Otolaryngol Head Neck Surg* 123(3): 328–333.

38. Penel N, Lefebvre D, et al. 2001. "Risk factors for wound infection in head and neck cancer surgery: A prospective study." *Head Neck* 23(6): 447–455.

39. Cruse P. 1977. "Infection surveillance: Identifying the problems and the high-risk patient." *South Med J* 70(Suppl 1): 4–8.

40. Bartlett JG, and Gorbach SL. 1976. "Anaerobic infections of the head and neck." *Otolaryngol Clin North Am* 9(3): 655–678.

41. Blanchaert RH, Jr. 2002. "Oral and oral pharyngeal cancer: An update on incidence and epidemiology, identification, advances in treatment, and outcomes." *Compend Contin Educ Dent* 23(12 Suppl): 25–29.

42. Simons JP, Johnson JT, et al. 2001. "The role of topical antibiotic prophylaxis in patients undergoing contaminated head and neck surgery with flap reconstruction." *Laryngoscope* 111(2): 329–335.

43. Balbuena L, and Stambaugh KI, et al. 1998. "Effects of topical oral antiseptic rinses on bacterial counts of saliva in healthy human subjects." *Otolaryngol Head Neck Surg* 118: 625–629.

44. Grandis JR, Vickers RM, et al. 1994. "The efficacy of topical antibiotic prophylaxis for contaminated head and neck surgery." *Laryngoscope* 104: 719–724.

45. Kirchner JC, Edberg SC, et al. 1988. "The use of topical oral antibiotics in head and neck prophylaxis: Is it justified?" *Laryngoscope* 98: 26–29.

46. Bumpous JM, and Johnson JT. 1995. "The infected wound and its management." *Otolaryngol Clin North Am* 28(5): 987–1001.

47. Mandell-Brown M, Johnson JT, et al. 1984. "Cost-effectiveness of prophylactic antibiotics in head and neck surgery." *Otolaryngol Head Neck Surg* 92(5): 520–523.

48. Coleman JJ, 3rd, 1986. "Complications in head and neck surgery." *Surg Clin North Am* 66(1): 149–167.

49. Krizek TJ, and Davis JH. 1965. "The role of the red cell in subcutaneous infection." *J Trauma* 5: 85–95.

50. Angel, MF, Narayanan K, et al. 1986. "The etiologic role of free radicals in hematoma-induced flap necrosis." *Plast Reconstr Surg* 77(5): 795–803.

15

Microvascular Composite Bone Flaps

Rui Fernandes, MD, DMD, FACS
Phil Pirgousis, MD, DMD, FRCS, FRACDS(OMS)

INTRODUCTION

The use of microvascular free tissue transfer has become an established and routine reconstructive option in head and neck surgery. Furthermore, it has been embraced by oral and maxillofacial units worldwide wherein free flap reconstruction of such defects is now considered gold standard of care.[1] Microvascular reconstructive surgery remains both technically challenging and operator sensitive, yet reported success rates of free flap surgery have consistently been between 96% and 99%.[2–5]

Despite continual refinement in microsurgical techniques, technological advances, and accumulation of experience, a small percentage of free flaps fail in most major centers. Unlike other less technically demanding reconstructive options, failure in microsurgery represents a potentially devastating situation for both patients and surgeons.[6] For patients, psychological and physical suffering escalates, in addition to prolonged hospitalization, further surgery, and increasing treatment costs. Patient comorbidities and additional general anesthesia may adversely impact patient recovery and outcome. For surgeons, free flap failure represents a unique and stressful situation where a persistent defect requires coverage with fewer donor sites available, especially if composite tissue is needed to achieve optimal functional and aesthetic results. Furthermore, recipient vessel availability for reanastomosis in the vicinity of the previous failed anastomoses is frequently compromised. The original defect size is often larger following necessary debridement, and critically exposed vascular structures that need prompt coverage may complicate the situation. This chapter will aim to outline the various complications associated with composite bone flaps for head and neck reconstruction with reference to the literature, and provide strategies to avoid and mange these where appropriate.

OSTEOCUTANEOUS RADIAL FOREARM FLAP

The radial forearm flap has enjoyed much popularity especially for soft tissue reconstruction; however, its osteocutaneous counterpart has been superseded by other bone flaps due to the poor volume bone stock and significant donor site morbidity.

Hand Ischemia

Vascular insufficiency of the hand following harvest of the radial forearm flap remains the most devastating complication. Numerous reports exist supporting this phenomenon despite normal preoperative Allen's testing.[7,8] Such ischemic events frequently arise from an incomplete superficial palmar arch with absent branches to the thumb and index finger combined and no communication with the deep palmar arch.[9]

Management of Complications in Oral and Maxillofacial Surgery, First Edition. Edited by Michael Miloro, Antonia Kolokythas.
© 2012 John Wiley & Sons, Inc. Published 2012 by John Wiley & Sons, Inc.

Management requires immediate surgical exploration and reestablishment of radial flow with vein graft reconstruction. Other causes include too tight a skin closure and compression from the forearm dressing, which produces a compartment syndrome. Limiting the splint to only volar coverage and maintaining exposure of the hand for postoperative monitoring can avoid this.

Radius Fracture

The radial osteocutaneous flap initially became established as the first reliable free flap for reconstruction of mandibular continuity defects.[10] This flap has rapidly lost popularity and has been superseded by superior bone flaps due to its limited bone stock and significant incidence of postoperative radius fracture. Early reports showed an incidence of fracture as high as 28% to 43%,[10–13] while larger series reported incidences of 23% (Ref. 14) and 31%.[15] Refinements in osteotomy technique and prophylactic internal fixation have reduced this functionally disabling complication to 15%.[16] Serious frequent sequelae of pathologic radius fracture include wrist deformity, and reduced wrist and grip strength from impaired flexor pollicis longus function. Biomechanical studies have confirmed loss of 75% or more of the strength of the human radius in bending,[17] and the sheep tibia in torsion,[18] when 50% of the circumference is removed. Beveling the proximal and distal osteotomy cuts has a minimal strengthening effect on the remaining radius of up to 5%.[18] Postoperative radius fracture can be minimized by strictly adhering to bony dimensions not exceeding 30% of its cross-sectional area, and 40% of its circumference.[19] Additional radius protection can be afforded by external support with an above-elbow cast or preformed splint to ensure 6 to 8 weeks of immobilization; however, fracture rates remain as high as 19%.[20] Prophylactic internal fixation with dynamic compression plate (DCP) is the most effective method of increasing both the torsional and bending strength of the osteotomized radius, supported by several large clinical series.[21–24] Both anterior and posterior positions of the plate are equally effective in reducing overall fracture rates to 2.6% with the posterior position providing greater reinforcement and significantly fewer healing problems.[22] Secondary revision surgery in the above instances is very uncommon necessary in only 0.4% of cases.

Sensory/Motor Deficit

Neurologic injury resulting from radial forearm flap harvest varies in the literature but is generally significantly worse in the osteocutaneous flap.[25] Direct median and ulnar nerve injury are uncommon; however, when present, they result in significant patient disability. Richardson et al.,[25] in their prospective study, noted a 36% incidence of reduction in grip strength, pinch strength, and range of wrist movement compared with the nonoperated control arm and the fasciocutaneous group (16%). More importantly, functional impairment was worse in patients suffering radius fracture following composite flaps. Other authors have found similar results with respect to functional morbidity.[13,14,26] Sensory deficit from radial forearm flap harvest remains common with similar incidences in both composite and fasciocutaneous flap variants, and in subfascial and suprafascial dissection methods.[27] Objective and subjective sensory deficits are greatest in the radial nerve distribution compared to median and ulnar nerve dermatomes.[25,28] Kerawala et al.[28] identified a 76% incidence of subjective sensory loss in the radial nerve distribution with 84% of patients exhibiting objective evidence of sensory deficit associated with pinprick, light touch, temperature, and two-point discrimination modalities. Painful neuromas and dysaesthesia are relatively infrequent with a 2–10% incidence. Sensory recovery appears to improve with time, with most long-term studies reporting resolution at about 12 months postoperatively.[25,28] Thorough familiarity of the regional anatomy and cognizance of the location of the superficial branch of the radial nerve can avoid this complication.

Donor Site Skin Graft Failure

This remains the most problematic complication in both the composite and fasciocutaneous radial forearm free flap donor site defect and has been one of the most intensely studied areas.[29,30] Numerous authors have demonstrated statistically significant objective functional and aesthetic deficits in the form of tendon exposure, contracture, and pain resulting from skin graft loss and delayed wound healing. Split thickness skin graft failure ranges from 19% to 53% in the literature. Tendon exposure has been reported in 13% to 33% of patients and tendon adhesion in 18.7% to 33%.[27] Full thickness skin graft take has a reported success rate of 93%, and produces superior aesthetic results.[30] Other published methods of skin donor site

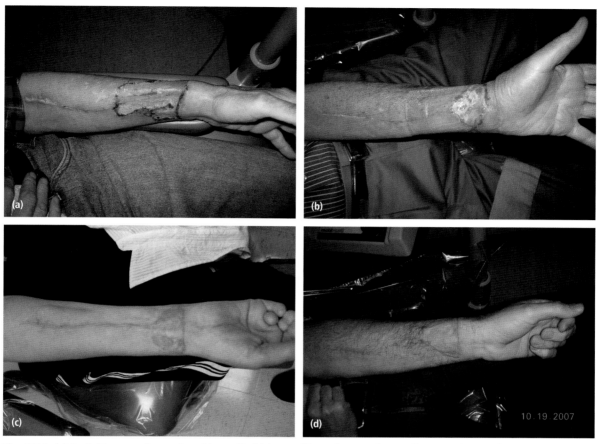

Fig. 15.1 (a) Radial forearm donor site with a split thickness skin graft; note the excellent initial take of the graft. (b) Donor site after partial skin graft failure with exposure of the underlying structures. These patients are initially treated with wet-to-dry dressing to stimulate healing by secondary intention or they may be taken back to the operating room and have a reapplication of the skin graft. (c) Donor site after complete take of a full thickness skin graft. (d) Donor site after complete take of a split thickness skin graft.

repair include preoperative tissue expansion, purse string wound closure,[31] prefabricated fascial split thickness skin grafts,[32] allogenic dermis,[33] and negative pressure vacuum wound dressings.[34] However, reported numbers in these series are small, and superior outcomes to conventional skin grafting are not demonstrable.

Maximizing skin graft take is facilitated through meticulous surgical technique, good homeostasis, paratenon preservation during flap harvest and wrist immobilization with a volar splint for 10 days postoperatively [Figs. 15.1(a)–(d)].

OSTEOCUTANEOUS FIBULA FLAP

The first successful microvascular transfer of a fibula free flap for mandibular reconstruction in the canine model was in 1974.[35] In 1975, Ian Taylor first reported on free fibula transfer for reconstruction of lower extremity defects.[36] Later, Hidalgo adapted this flap for mandibular reconstruction.[37] Since that time, the fibula flap has achieved universal popularity as the bone flap of first choice for most maxillofacial defects. Its thick cortical bone, tubular shape, long length (up to 25 cm), associated skin paddle, tolerability to multiple bony osteotomies, long vascular pedicle, and large vessel caliber make it well suited to facial bone reconstruction.[38]

Foot Ischemia/Vascular Compromise

Vascular compromise of the foot is the most devastating complication arising from fibula free flap harvest. The anatomic basis for this resides in congenital or acquired vascular anomalies of the lower extremity vasculature. Normally, the peroneal artery contributes minimally to the vascular supply of the foot with the dominant supply provided by the anterior and posterior tibial vessels. In 7–10% of cases, these two normally dominant vessels may be significantly attenuated or individually absent, and the primary vascular supply is derived from the peroneal artery (peroneal arteria magna). Congenital absence of the peroneal vessels is rare with a population incidence of 0.1%.[39] Acquired vascular insufficiency of the lower extremities is frequently associated with atherosclerosis, particularly in elderly patients. Preoperative imaging with computed tomography (CT) angiography, magnetic resonance (MR) angiography, or routine angiography can avoid limb-threatening ischemia. Compartment syndrome from wound closure under excessive tension can produce disastrous ischemic complications.

Gait Disturbance

Significant early and late morbidity relating to gait disturbance is reported by numerous authors, although objectively measurable parameters frequently exceed subjectively perceived morbidity.[40] Despite reports of alterations in gait, paresis of the flexors of the toes and hallux, and sensitivity changes, the majority of patients are able to ambulate normally. The loss of the fibula and interosseous membrane, which form the origin of the deep muscles, produces muscle disturbance with consequent loss of function.[41] Antalgic gait is a common phenomenon following fibula flap harvest with gait analysis studies demonstrating a characteristically short stance phase of the affected lower extremity.[42] Foot drop is an uncommon but disabling complication that impacts markedly on ambulation and arises from surgical trauma to the extensor hallucis longus musculature.[43] Ankle instability and stiffness have also been reported and arise when less than 6 cm of distal fibula is preserved, leading to external rotation of the talus beneath the tibial plateau and resultant valgus deformity.[44] Isokinetic studies reveal significant decreases in ankle mobility and strength during all four ankle motions. Knee mobility remains unaffected; however, diminished strength during knee flexion and extension on objective assessment is apparent.[41,42]

Limited Great Toe Flexion

Almost all patients develop limited flexion capability of the hallux consistent with inclusion of the flexor hallucis longus muscle with the flap. This phenomenon does not interfere with ambulation.[45] Damage to branches of the peroneal nerve and posterior compartment muscle scarring are additional causes.

Neurologic Injuries

The common peroneal nerve is the nerve at risk during fibula flap harvest. It has both sensory and motor functions, with sensory disturbance reported in up to 24% of cases in either the superficial or deep peroneal nerve distribution.[46] Motor disturbances lead to weakness in dorsiflexion in about 7% of cases resulting from damage to peroneal nerve branches and associated equinovarus deformity.[47] Common peroneal nerve damage is avoided by limiting proximal dissection to greater than 6 cm from the fibula head and avoidance of overzealous traction during proximal dissection.

Delayed Wound Healing

Primary closure of the skin paddle donor site is often possible when skin paddle widths are less than 5 cm. Larger skin paddles typically require the use of split thickness skin grafts from a second donor site for defect coverage. Partial or total split thickness skin graft loss is estimated to range from 17% to 28% of cases, with partial necrosis of the peroneal tendons and/or muscles in up to 5%. Donor wound infections occur in about 7% of patients.[48] Optimizing graft take is facilitated by careful application of pressure dressings and lower leg immobilization with splint for 10 days postoperatively. Intravenous broad-spectrum antibiotics postoperatively will reduce infections rates [Figs. 15.2(a), (b)].

Skin Paddle Loss

The reliability of the skin paddle associated with the composite fibula flap was initially questioned by some,[37] after ischemic necrosis due to the tenuous vascular supply to the fibula skin. More recently, however,

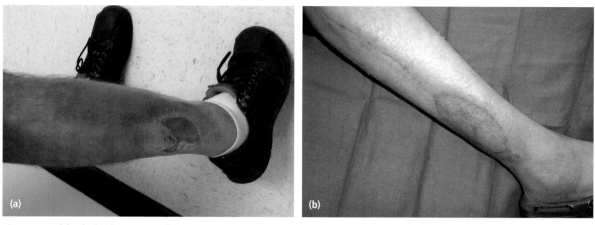

Fig. 15.2. (a) Fibula donor site after partial loss of the split thickness skin graft. Note the healing by secondary intention and contraction of the defect. (b) Fibula donor site after complete healing of the split thickness skin graft.

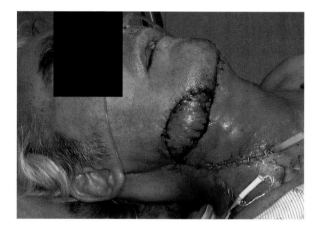

Fig. 15.3. Osteocutaneous fibula flap showing venous congestion of the skin paddle component.

Wei et al.[49] described two types of perforators supplying the fibula skin. Septocutaneous perforators traverse the posterior crural septum only, whereas septomyocutaneous perforators first travel through flexor hallucis longus, tibialis posterior, or soleus prior to entering the septum and then the skin. The latter perforators are important to identify during dissection in order to include a protective cuff of muscle around these. Yoshimura et al.[50] noted that 71% of cutaneous perforators are septomyocutaneous and only 29% are septocutaneous. Further angiographic cadaveric studies identified that 20% of 80 cadaver leg dissections lacked septocutaneous perforators while an additional 6.25% lacked septomyocutaneous perforators but did not mention cases of total absence of both. Absolute skin paddle reliability thus ranged from 93% to 94%.[51] It is recommended that a cuff of flexor hallucis longus and soleus be included in the dissection to protect these delicate perforators and avoid ischemic compromise to the skin island (Fig. 15.3).

SCAPULA FREE FLAP

The scapula free flap has proven to be an extremely valuable reconstructive option in head and neck surgery. Its ability to carry multiple skin flaps, latissimus dorsi muscle, serratus anterior muscle, and scapula bone, all based on a single pedicle, makes this system of flaps uniquely suited for the complex three-dimensional (3D) sculpting necessary in the head and neck. A distinct advantage in the elderly population is the unimpeded early postoperative ambulation not shared by the fibula and iliac crest flaps.[52]

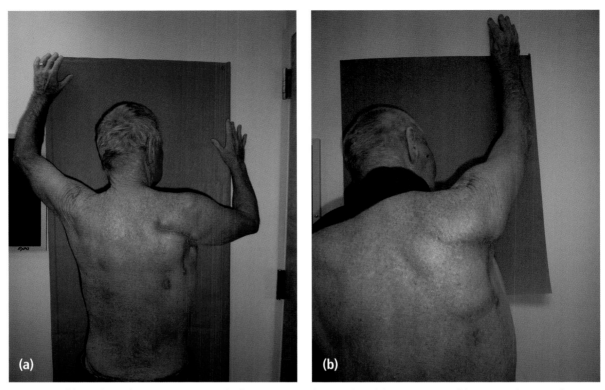

Fig. 15.4. (a) Healing of a composite scapula flap site; note the initial mobility restriction. (b) Increased range of motion with resolution of initial mobility restriction as well as softening of the scar at the donor site.

Shoulder Dysfunction

Shoulder weakness results from division of the rotator cuff muscles—teres major and minor—from the lateral border of the scapula during flap harvest. Significant disability may result particularly when coupled with shoulder dysfunction associated with accessory nerve paresis following neck dissection. Restricted arm elevation, extension, and adduction are the commonest impaired shoulder movements.[53]

Scapula Winging

This complication typically results from detachment of the teres major and minor muscles from the lateral border of the scapula, and failure to reattach these following completion of the flap harvest.[54] Scarred, denervated fibrotic teres muscles may also produce this complication. Specific attention to anchoring these muscles to holes drilled in the remaining scapula bone often avoids this problem. Intense postoperative physical therapy has also been shown to maximize shoulder mobility with return to premorbid function by 6 months post surgery [Figs. 15.4(a), (b)].[55,56]

ILIAC CREST FREE FLAP

The iliac crest free flap arguably provides the greatest quantity of bone stock for head and neck reconstruction. Its site distant from the ablative head and neck team permits synchronous harvest, while its inherent shape is well suited for reconstruction of the facial bones.[57] This flap is often avoided due to an apparent technically demanding flap harvest, relatively short vascular pedicle, and small caliber vessels. Others, however, have shown excellent outcomes with this flap.[58]

Taylor et al.[59] and Sanders and Mayou[60] in 1979 separately identified and reported the deep circumflex iliac artery and vein as the most reliable and favorable pedicle for free transfer of the ilium. Taylor et al.[59] further elucidated the endosteal and periosteal blood supply of the ilium through dye injection studies.

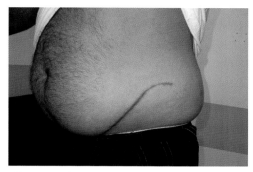

Fig. 15.5. Donor site of a DCIA free flap; note the absence of any hernia or weakness of the abdominal wall.

Experimental work by Ramasastry et al.[61] in 1984 identified the ascending branch of the deep circumflex iliac artery (DCIA) as the primary blood supply to the internal oblique muscle allowing for composite flap transfer.

Ventral Hernias

This complication results from weakening of the abdominal wall through harvest of the internal oblique muscle and denervation of the rectus muscle whose motor nerves run in the neurovascular plane between the internal oblique and tranversus abdominus.[62] Incisional hernias, although infrequent and asymptomatic, occur in 3% (Ref. 63) to 9% (Ref. 64) of patients. Mesh repair to reinforce the abdominal wall can eliminate this phenomenon.

Contour Deformity

Despite this being clinically obvious, patients subjectively deny any significant aesthetic dissatisfaction (Fig. 15.5).[65]

Neurologic Sequelae

Transection or traction injury to the lateral femoral cutaneous nerve results in impaired sensation to the lateral thigh.[66] Severe trauma to the lateral femoral and ilioinguinal nerves may potentially produce thigh pain and dysesthesia.

Ambulation/Gait Disturbance

Immediate postoperative and short-term effects on ambulation are common following iliac crest free flaps, with antalgic gait and weakness of the operated hip being usual sequelae. Reports in the literature have demonstrated through controlled orthopedic objective testing that ambulation resolves by 6 months postoperatively.[63,65] Gait disturbance has also been reported to arise secondary to femoral paresis resulting from traction injury or tight surgical wound closure.[58,63]

FLAP FAILURE

A wide spectrum of causes are involved in flap failure apart from inadequate perfusion and necrosis. Management of flap failure varies for the *failing flap* and the *failed flap*. A *failing flap* is one that is potentially salvageable provided prompt action is taken to reverse the cause or causes of failure. A *failed flap* is one where irreversible ischemia has led to partial or total tissue necrosis requiring urgent wound care, local debridement, or additional reconstruction.

Management of the Failing Flap

Timing of the presentation of vascular compromise is critical to successful flap salvage and is critically dependent on the accuracy of postoperative flap monitoring. Chen et al.[67] in a large series of 1,142 free flaps reexplored 113 patients (9.9%) due to vascular compromise where 51.3% of these displayed signs of compromise within the first 4 postoperative hours, 82.3% within the first 24 hours, and 95.6% within the first 72 hours. It was also apparent that flaps with early signs of circulatory compromise had significantly lower salvage rates, lending further support and emphasis on diligent postoperative flap monitoring for rapid intervention. Early reexploration of the failing flap is paramount if successful salvage is expected prior to the stage of the no-reflow phenomenon.[68] Success rates following salvage of compromised flaps vary from 28% to 87.5% in published reports [Figs. 15.6(a), (b)].[69,70]

Nonsurgical Management

Medicinal leech therapy, *Hirudo medicinalis*, dates back to the fourteenth century BC ancient Egypt. It has proved effective in relieving venous congestion in compromised free flaps. The mechanism relates to the secretion of hirudin, a potent anticoagulant, and hyaluronidase, which allows the dissipation of hirudin in the local wound environment combined with antihistamine for prolonged bleeding through vasodilation. Smoot et al.[71] and Soucacos et al.[72] successfully salvaged 17 of 20 patients with flaps suffering venous insufficiency for upper and lower extremity coverage (Fig. 15.7).

Radiologic Evaluation

Bone scintigraphy using Technetium-99m-methylene diphosphonate (Tc-99m MDP) has been frequently utilized to check the anastomotic patency of microvascular flaps as well as the viability of the composite bone. It represents a safe, sensitive, and noninvasive technique for sequential evaluation of bone viability,

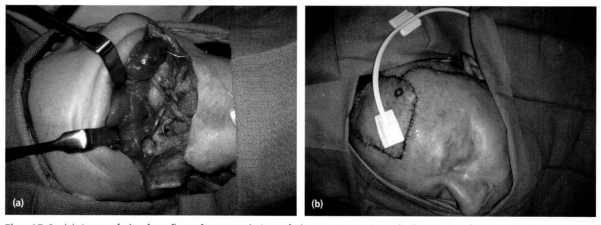

Fig. 15.6. (a) Inset of the free flap after completion of the anastomosis and placement of an implantable doppler. (b) Monitoring of the flap with an oxygen saturation probe.

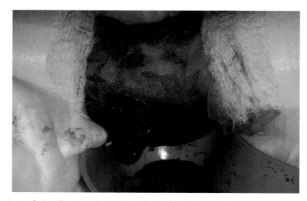

Fig. 15.7. Significant congestion of the flap with application of leeches to improve venous outflow.

and it maintains an important role in the assessment of composite bone flap viability with accuracy out to 6 weeks postoperatively.[73] Similarly, single photon emission computed tomography (SPECT) scintigraphy has been successfully used to evaluate bone viability in free flaps providing improved imaging characteristics and structural detail in the transplanted bone.[74] Furthermore, ^{18}F- positron emission tomography has also been shown to be highly accurate in determining early postoperative graft viability based on the quantity of fluoride influx.[75] All the above imaging modalities have proven sensitive and accurate in determining the early and late postoperative viability of composite bone flaps including situations of vascular insufficiency.

SUGGESTED READINGS

1. Brown JS, Magennis P, Rogers SN, et al. 2006. "Trends in head and neck microvascular reconstructive surgery in Liverpool (1992–2001)." *British Journal of Oral and Maxillofacial Surgery* 44(5): 364–370.
2. Khouri RK, and Shaw WW. 2009. "Reconstruction of the lower extremity with microvascular free flaps: A 10-year experience with 304 consecutive cases." *Head & Neck* 31: 45–51.
3. Bianci B, Copelli C, Ferrari S, et al. 2009. "Free flaps: Outcomes and complications in head and neck reconstructions." *Journal of Cranio-Maxillofacial Surgery* 37(8): 438–442.
4. Urken ML, Buchbinder D, Costantino PD, et al. 1998. "Oromandibular reconstruction using microvascular composite flaps: Report of 210 cases." *Archives of Otolaryngology Head and Neck Surgery* 124(1): 46–55.
5. Nakatsuka T, Harii K, Asato H, et al. 2003. "Analytical review of 2372 free flap transfers for head and neck reconstruction following cancer resection." *Journal of Reconstructive Microsurgery* 19: 363–368.
6. Yu P, Chang DW, Miller MJ, et al. 2009. "Analysis of 49 cases of flap compromise in 1310 free flaps for head and neck reconstruction." *Head & Neck* 31: 45–51.
7. Jones BM, and O'Brien CJ. 1985. "Acute ischaemia of the hand resulting from elevation of a radial forearm flap." *British Journal of Plastic Surgery* 38(3): 396–397.
8. Varley I, Carter LM, Wales CJ, et al. 2008. "Ischaemia of the hand after harvest of a radial forearm flap." *British Journal of Oral and Maxillofacial Surgery* 46(5): 403–405.
9. Coleman T, and Anson B. 1961. "Arterial patterns in the hand based upon a study of 650 specimens." *Surgical Gynaecology & Obstetrics* 113: 409–424.
10. Soutar DS, and McGregor IA. 1986. "The radial forearm flap in intraoral reconstruction: The experience of 60 consecutive cases." *Plastic & Reconstructive Surgery* 78: 1–8.
11. McGregor IA. 1985. "Fasciocutaneous flaps in intraoral reconstruction." *Clinics in Plastic Surgery* 12: 453–461.
12. Timmons MJ, Missotten FE, Poole MD, et al. 1986. "Complications of radial forearm flap donor sites." *British Journal of Plastic Surgery* 39: 176–178.
13. Boorman JG, Brown JA, and Sykes PJ. 1987. "Morbidity in the forearm flap donor arm." *British Journal of Plastic Surgery* 40: 207–212.
14. Bardsley AF, Soutar DS, Elliot D, et al. 1990. "Reducing morbidity in the radial forearm flap donor site." *Plastic & Reconstructive Surgery* 86: 287–294.
15. Vaughan ED. 1990. "The radial forearm free flap in orofacial reconstruction. Personal experience in 120 consecutive cases." *Journal of Craniomaxillofacial Surgery* 18: 2–7.
16. Thoma A, Khadaroo R, Grigenas O, et al. 1999. "Oromandibular reconstruction with the radial-forearm osteocutaneous flap: Experience with 60 consecutive cases." *Plastic & Reconstructive Surgery* 104: 368–380.
17. Swanson E, Boyd JB, and Mulholland RS. 1990. "The radial forearm flap: A biomechanical study of the osteotomized radius." *Plastic & Reconstructive Surgery* 85: 267–272.
18. Meland NB, Maki S, Chao EY, et al. 1992. "The radial forearm flap: A biomechanical study of donor-site morbidity utilizing sheep tibia." *Plastic & Reconstructive Surgery* 90: 763–773.
19. Collyer J, and Goodger NM. 2005. "The composite radial forearm free flap: An anatomical guide to harvesting the radius." *British Journal of Oral & Maxillofacial Surgery* 43: 205–209.
20. Clark S, Greenwood M, Banks RJ, et al. 2004. "Fracture of the radial donor site after composite free flap harvest: A ten-year review." *Surgical Journal of the Royal College of Surgeons of Edinburgh & Ireland* 2: 281–286.
21. Avery CM, Danford M, and Johnson PA. 2007. "Prophylactic internal fixation of the radial osteocutaneous donor site." *British Journal of Oral & Maxillofacial Surgery* 45: 576–578.
22. Werle AH, Tsue TT, Toby EB, et al. 2000. "Osteocutaneous radial forearm free flap: Its use without significant donor site morbidity." *Otolaryngology Head & Neck Surgery* 123: 711–717.
23. Villaret DB, and Futran NA. 2003. "The indications and outcomes in the use of osteocutaneous radial forearm free flap." *Head Neck* 25: 475–481.
24. Kim JH, Rosenthal EL, Ellis T, et al. 2005. "Radial forearm osteocutaneous free flap in maxillofacial and oromandibular reconstructions." *Laryngoscope* 155: 1697–1701.
25. Richardson D, Fisher SE, Vaughan ED, et al. 1997. "Radial forearm flap donor-site complications and morbidity: Prospective study." *Plastic & Reconstructive Surgery* 99: 109–115.

26. Brown MT, Cheney ML, Glicklich RL, et al. 1996. "Assessment of functional morbidity in the radial forearm free flap donor site." *Archives of Otolaryngology Head and Neck Surgery* 122: 991–994.

27. Lutz BS, Wei FC, Chang SC, et al. 1999. "Donor site morbidity after suprafascial elevation of the radial forearm flap: A prospective study in 95 consecutive cases." *Plastic & Reconstructive Surgery* 103: 132–137.

28. Kerawala CJ, and Martin IC. 2006. "Sensory deficit in the donor hand after harvest of radial forearm free flaps." *British Journal of Oral & Maxillofacial Surgery* 44: 100–102.

29. Emerick KS, and Deschler DG. 2007. "Incidence of donor site skin graft loss requiring surgical intervention with the radial forearm free flap." *Head & Neck* 29: 573–576.

30. Sidebottom AJ, Stevens L, Moore M, et al. 2000. "Repair of the radial free flap donor site with full or partial thickness skin grafts: A prospective randomized controlled trial." *International Journal of Oral & Maxillofacial Surgery* 29: 194–197.

31. Winslow CP, Hansen J, Mackenzie D, et al. 2000. "Pursestring closure of radial forearm fasciocutaneous donor sites." *Laryngoscope* 110: 1815–1818.

32. Wolff KD, Ervens J, and Hoffmeister B. 1996. "Improvement of the radial forearm donor site by prefabrication of fascial-split thickness skin grafts." *Plastic & Reconstructive Surgery* 98: 358–362.

33. Lee J-W, Jang Y-C, and Oh S-J. 2005. "Use of the artificial dermis for free radial forearm flap donor site." *Annals of Plastic Surgery* 55: 500–502.

34. Avery C, Pereira A, Moody M, et al. 2000. "Negative pressure wound dressing of the radial forearm donor site." *International Journal of Oral & Maxillofacial Surgery* 29: 198–200.

35. Ostrup LT, and Fredrickson JM. 1974. "Distant transfer of a free, living bone graft by microvascular anastomoses. An experimental study." *Plastic & Reconstructive Surgery* 54: 274–284.

36. Taylor GI, Miller GD, and Ham FJ. 1975. "The free vascularized bone graft. A clinical extension of microvascular techniques." *Plastic & Reconstructive Surgery* 55: 533–544.

37. Hidalgo DA. 1989. "Fibula free flap: A new method of mandible reconstruction." *Plastic & Reconstructive Surgery* 84: 71–79.

38. Kim D, Orron DE, and Skillman JJ. 1989. "Surgical significance of popliteal artery variants: A unified angiographic classification." *Annals of Surgery* 210: 776.

39. Lippert H, and Pabst R. 1985. *Arterial Variations in Man: Classification,*" 60–63. New York: JF Bergman Verlag.

40. Zimmermann CE, Borner B-I, Hasse A, et al. 2001. "Donor site morbidity after microvascular fibula transfer." *Clinical Oral Investigation* 5: 214–219.

41. Youdas JW, Wood MB, Cahalan TD, et al. 1988. "A quantitative analysis of donor site morbidity after vascularized fibula transfer." *Journal of Orthopaedic Research* 6: 621–629.

42. Lee J-H, Chung C-Y, Myoung H, et al. 2008. "Gait analysis of donor leg after free fibular flap transfer." *International Journal of Oral & Maxillofacial Surgery* 37: 625–629.

43. Coghlan BA, and Townsend PL. 1993. "The morbidity of the free vascularised fibula flap." *British Journal of Plastic Surgery* 46: 466–469.

44. Pacelli LL, Gillard J, McLoughlin SW, et al. 2003. "A biomechanical analysis of donor-site ankle instability following free fibula graft harvest." *Journal of Bone & Joint Surgery of America* 85: 597–603.

45. Hidalgo DA, and Rekow A. 1995. "A review of 60 consecutive fibula free flap mandible reconstructions." *Plastic & Reconstructive Surgery* 96: 585–596; discussion 597–602.

46. Anthony JP, Rawnsley JD, Benhaim P, et al. 1995. "Donor leg morbidity and function after fibula free flap mandible reconstruction." *Plastic & Reconstructive Surgery* 96: 146–152.

47. Goodacre TE, Walker CJ, Jawad AS, et al. 1990. "Donor site morbidity following osteocutaneous free fibula transfer." *British Journal of Plastic Surgery* 43: 410–412.

48. Papadopoulos NA, Schaff J, Bucher H, et al. 2002. "Donor site morbidity after harvest of free osteofasciocutaneous fibular flaps with an extended skin island." *Annals of Plastic Surgery* 49: 138–144.

49. Wei FC, Chen HC, Chuang CC, et al. 1986. "Fibula osteoseptocutaneous flap: Anatomic study and clinical application." *Plastic & Reconstructive Surgery* 78: 191–199.

50. Yoshimura M, Shimada T, Hosokawa M. 1990. "The vasculature of the peroneal tissue transfer." *Plastic & Reconstructive Surgery* 85: 917–921.

51. Shusterman MA, Reece GP, Miller MJ, et al. 1992. "The osteocutaneous free fibula flap: Is the skin paddle reliable?" *Plastic & Reconstructive Surgery* 90: 787–793.

52. Hallock GG. 1997. "Permutations of combined free flaps using the subscapular system." *Journal of Reconstructive Microsurgery* 13: 47–54.

53. Swartz WM, Banis JC, Newton ED, et al. 1986. "The osteocutaneous scapular flap for mandibular and maxillary reconstruction." *Plastic & Reconstructive Surgery* 77: 530.

54. Coleman SC, Burkey BB, Day TA, et al. 2000. "Increasing use of the scapula osteocutaneous free flap." *Laryngoscope* 110: 1419–1424.

55. Clark JR, Vesely M, and Gilbert R. 2008. "Scapular angle osteomyogenous flap in postmaxillectomy reconstruction: Defect, reconstruction, shoulder function, and harvest technique. *Head & Neck* 30: 10–20.

56. Nkenke E, Vairaktaris E, Stelzle F, et al. 2009. "Osteocutaneous free flap including medial and lateral scapular crests: Technical aspects, viability and donor site morbidity." *Journal of Reconstructive Microsurgery* 25: 545–554.

57. Brown JS. 1996. "Deep circumflex iliac artery free flap with internal oblique muscle as a new method of immediate reconstruction of maxillectomy defect." *Head & Neck* 412–421.

58. Urken ML, Vickery C, Weinberg H, et al. 1989. "The internal oblique-iliac crest osseomyocutaneous free flap in oromandibular reconstruction: Report of 20 cases." *Archives of Otolaryngology Head and Neck Surgery* 115: 339–349.

59. Taylor GI, Townsend P, and Corlett R. 1979. "Superiority of the deep circumflex iliac vessels as the supply for free groin flaps: Experimental work." *Plastic & Reconstructive Surgery* 64: 595–604.

60. Sanders R, and Mayou B. 1979. "A new vascularized bone graft transferred by microvascular anastomosis as a free flap." *British Journal of Surgery* 66: 787–788.

61. Ramasastry SS, Tucker JB, Swartz WM, et al. 1984. "The internal oblique muscle flap: An anatomic and clinical study." *Plastic & Reconstructive Surgery* 73: 721–733.

62. Urken ML, Weinberg H, Vickery C, et al. 1991. "The internal oblique-iliac crest free flap in composite defects of the oral cavity involving bone, skin and mucosa." *Laryngoscope* 101: 257–270.

63. Boyd JB, Rosen I, Rotstein L, et al. 1990. "The iliac crest and the radial forearm flap in vascularized oromandibular reconstruction." *American Journal of Surgery* 159: 301–308.

64. Duncan MJ, Manktelow RT, Zuker RM, et al. 1985. "Mandibular reconstruction in the radiated patient: The role of osteocutaneous free tissue transfers." *Plastic & Reconstructive Surgery* 76: 829–840.

65. Rogers SN, Lakshmiah SR, Narayan B, et al. 2003. "A comparison of the long-term morbidity following deep circumflex iliac and fibula free flaps for reconstruction following head and neck cancer." *Plastic & Reconstructive Surgery* 112: 1517–1525.

66. Boyd JB. 1989. "Deep circumflex iliac groin flaps." In: *Microsurgical Reconstruction of the Head and Neck*, Baker SR, ed., 55–81. New York: Churchill Livingstone.

67. Chen K-T, Mardini S, Chuang DC-C, et al. 2007. "Timing of presentation of the first signs of vascular compromise dictates the salvage outcome of free flap transfers." *Plastic & Reconstructive Surgery* 120: 187–195.

68. Ames A, Wright RL, Kowada M, et al. 1968. "Cerebral ischaemia II. The no-reflow phenomenon." *American Journal of Pathology* 52: 437–453.

69. Nakatsuka T, Harii K, Asato H, et al. 2003. "Analytical review of 2372 free flap transfers for head and neck reconstruction following cancer resection." *Journal of Reconstructive Microsurgery* 19: 363–368.

70. Bui DT, Cordeiro PG, Hu QY, et al. 2007. "Free flap reexploration: Indications, treatment, and outcomes in 1193 free flaps." *Plastic & Reconstructive Surgery* 119: 2092–2100.

71. Smoot EC, Ruiz-Inchaustegui JA, and Roth AC. 1995. "Mechanical leech therapy to relieve venous congestion." *Journal of Reconstructive Microsurgery* 11: 51–55.

72. Soucacos PN, Beris AE, Malizos KN, et al. 1994. "Successful treatment of venous congestion in free skin flaps using medicinal leeches." *Microsurgery* 496–501.

73. Takato T, Harii K, and Nakatsuka T. 1988. "The sequential evaluation of bone scintigraphy: An analysis of revascularised bone grafts." *British Journal of Plastic Surgery* 41: 262–269.

74. Moskowitz GW, and Lukash F. 1988. "Evaluation of bone graft viability." *Seminars in Nuclear Medicine* 3: 246–254.

75. Schliephake H, Berding G, Knapp WH, et al. 1999. "Monitoring of graft perfusion and osteoblast activity in revascularised fibula segments using ^{18}F- positron emission tomography." *International Journal of Oral & Maxillofacial Surgery* 28: 349–355.

Index

Page numbers followed by f indicate figures. Page numbers followed by t indicate tables.

Management of Complications in Oral and Maxillofacial Surgery, First Edition. Edited by Michael Miloro, Antonia Kolokythas.
© 2012 John Wiley & Sons, Inc. Published 2012 by John Wiley & Sons, Inc.

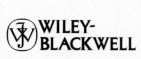
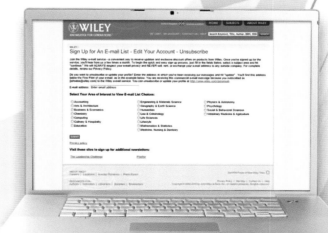